Aging: Anatomical, Physiological and Biochemical Changes in the Nervous System

Aging: Anatomical, Physiological and Biochemical Changes in the Nervous System

Edited by Isla Pearson

STATES
ACADEMIC PRESS
www.statesacademicpress.com

States Academic Press,
109 South 5th Street,
Brooklyn, NY 11249, USA

Visit us on the World Wide Web at:
www.statesacademicpress.com

ISBN: 978-1-63989-030-9

Cataloging-in-Publication Data

Aging : anatomical, physiological and biochemical changes in the nervous system / edited by Isla Pearson.
p. cm.
Includes bibliographical references and index.
ISBN 978-1-63989-030-9
1. Aging--Molecular aspects. 2. Aging--Physiological aspects. 3. Nervous system--Aging. I. Pearson, Isla.
QP86 .A35 2022
612.67--dc23

Table of Contents

Preface ... VII

Chapter 1 **Site-specific differences in the association between plantar tactile perception and mobility function in older adults** ... 1
Yenisel Cruz-Almeida, Mieniecia L. Black, Evangelos A. Christou and David J. Clark

Chapter 2 **Age-related changes in motor cortical representation and interhemispheric interactions: a transcranial magnetic stimulation study** ... 7
Elisabetta Coppi, Elise Houdayer, Raffaella Chieffo, Francesca Spagnolo, Alberto Inuggi, Laura Straffi, Giancarlo Comi and Letizia Leocani

Chapter 3 **Motor variability during sustained contractions increases with cognitive demand in older adults** ... 16
Marnie L. Vanden Noven, Hugo M. Pereira, Tejin Yoon, Alyssa A. Stevens, Kristy A. Nielson and Sandra K. Hunter

Chapter 4 **Utilization of central nervous system resources for preparation and performance of complex walking tasks in older adults** ... 30
David J. Clark, Dorian K. Rose, Sarah A. Ring and Eric C. Porges

Chapter 5 **Development and decline of upright gait stability** ... 39
Marco Iosa, Augusto Fusco, Giovanni Morone and Stefano Paolucci

Chapter 6 **Aging induced loss of complexity and dedifferentiation: consequences for coordination dynamics within and between brain, muscular and behavioral levels** ... 51
Rita Sleimen-Malkoun, Jean-Jacques Temprado and S. Lee Hong

Chapter 7 **Benefits of physical exercise on basic visuo-motor functions across age** ... 68
Marika Berchicci, Giuliana Lucci, Rinaldo Livio Perri, Donatella Spinelli and Francesco Di Russo

Chapter 8 **The neuromuscular junction: aging at the crossroad between nerves and muscle** ... 76
Marta Gonzalez-Freire, Rafael de Cabo, Stephanie A. Studenski and Luigi Ferrucci

Chapter 9 **Increased bilateral interactions in middle-aged subjects** ... 87
Jolien Heetkamp, Tibor Hortobágyi and Inge Zijdewind

Chapter 10 **Aging interferes central control mechanism for eccentric muscle contraction** ... 101
Wan X. Yao, Jinqi Li, Zhiguo Jiang, Jia-Hong Gao, Crystal G. Franklin, Yufei Huang, Jack L. Lancaster and Guang H. Yue

Chapter 11 **Safety margins in older adults increase with improved control of a dynamic object** ... 110
Christopher J. Hasson and Dagmar Sternad

Chapter 12 **Using the zebrafish model for Alzheimer's disease research** 119
Morgan Newman, Esmaeil Ebrahimie and Michael Lardelli

Chapter 13 **Worming forward: amyotrophic lateral sclerosis toxicity mechanisms and genetic interactions in *Caenorhabditis elegans*** 129
Martine Therrien and J. Alex Parker

Chapter 14 **A semi-automated motion-tracking analysis of locomotion speed in the *C. elegans* transgenics overexpressing beta-amyloid in neurons** 142
Kevin Machino, Christopher D. Link, Susan Wang, Hana Murakami and Shin Murakami

Chapter 15 **Using mice to model Alzheimer's dementia: an overview of the clinical disease and the preclinical behavioral changes in 10 mouse models** 148
Scott J. Webster, Adam D. Bachstetter, Peter T. Nelson, Frederick A. Schmitt and Linda J. Van Eldik

Chapter 16 **Longevity pathways and memory aging** 171
Ilias Gkikas, Dionysia Petratou and Nektarios Tavernarakis

Chapter 17 **Emerging functional similarities and divergences between *Drosophila* Spargel/dPGC-1 and mammalian PGC-1 protein** 181
Subhas Mukherjee1, Mohammed A. Basar, Claudette Davis and Atanu Duttaroy

Chapter 18 **Insulin signaling in the aging of healthy and proteotoxically stressed mechanosensory neurons** 186
Courtney Scerbak, Elena M. Vayndorf, J. Alex Parker, Christian Neri, Monica Driscoll and Barbara E. Taylor

Chapter 19 **Use of *Caenorhabditis elegans* as a model to study Alzheimer's disease and other neurodegenerative diseases** 200
Adanna G. Alexander, Vanessa Marfil and Chris Li

Chapter 20 **Phospholipase A_2 – nexus of aging, oxidative stress, neuronal excitability, and functional decline of the aging nervous system? Insights from a snail model system of neuronal aging and age-associated memory impairment** 221
Petra M. Hermann, Shawn N. Watson and Willem C. Wildering

Permissions

List of Contributors

Index

Preface

I am honored to present to you this unique book which encompasses the most up-to-date data in the field. I was extremely pleased to get this opportunity of editing the work of experts from across the globe. I have also written papers in this field and researched the various aspects revolving around the progress of the discipline. I have tried to unify my knowledge along with that of stalwarts from every corner of the world, to produce a text which not only benefits the readers but also facilitates the growth of the field.

Aging is a gradual and continuous process that leads to a decline in bodily functions over time. With an increase in age, the brain and nervous system go through some natural changes such as losing nerve cells and weight. The process of passing messages also slows down with age. As a result of the breakdown of nerve cells, waste products and other chemicals get accumulated in the brain tissues. This may lead to abnormal changes in the brain and buildup of fatty brown pigment in nerve tissue. Breakdown of nerves can lead to reduced or lost reflexes, resulting in problems with movement. Different approaches, evaluations, methodologies and advanced studies on the changes in nervous system with age have been included in this book. It explores all the important aspects of this field. This book will provide comprehensive knowledge to the readers.

Finally, I would like to thank all the contributing authors for their valuable time and contributions. This book would not have been possible without their efforts. I would also like to thank my friends and family for their constant support.

Editor

1

Site-specific differences in the association between plantar tactile perception and mobility function in older adults

Yenisel Cruz-Almeida*[1], *Mieniecia L. Black*[2], *Evangelos A. Christou*[3] and *David J. Clark*[2,4] *

[1] Pain Research and Intervention Center of Excellence, University of Florida, Gainesville, FL, USA
[2] Department of Aging and Geriatric Research, University of Florida, Gainesville, FL, USA
[3] Department of Applied Physiology and Kinesiology, University of Florida, Gainesville, FL, USA
[4] Brain Rehabilitation Research Center, Malcom Randall VA Medical Center, Gainesville, FL, USA

Edited by:
Brian C. Clark, Ohio University, USA

Reviewed by:
Matthieu Pascal Boisgontier, KU Leuven, Belgium
Guang H. Yue, Kessler Foundation Research Center, USA

****Correspondence:***
David J. Clark, Brain Rehabilitation Research Center (151A), Malcom Randall VA Medical Center, 1601 SW Archer Road, Gainesville, FL 32608, USA
e-mail: davidclark@ufl.edu

Introduction: Impaired somatosensation is common in older adults and contributes to age-related loss of mobility function. However, little is known about whether somatosensation at different sites on the plantar surface of the foot are differentially related to mobility function. Such a finding may have important implications for clinical care of older adults and other at-risk populations, such as for optimizing interventions (e.g., footwear for augmenting somatosensory feedback) and for improving the efficiency of clinical assessment.

Materials and Methods: Tactile perception was evaluated with a 10 g monofilament at four sites on the plantar surface of each foot: great toe (GT), first metatarsal head (MT1), heel (H) and fifth metatarsal head (MT5). Mobility function was assessed with the Berg Balance Scale and walking speed.

Results: Sixty-one older adults participated. Tactile perception was significantly positively associated with Berg Balance Score (adjusted $r = 0.30 - 0.75$; $p = 0.03 - < 0.001$), with the strongest association found at the site of the MT1. Only at this site was tactile perception found to be significantly associated with usual walking speed (adjusted $r = 0.51$; $p < 0.001$) and maximal walking speed (adjusted $r = 0.38$, $p = 0.004$). Clinically mild somatosensory impairment at MT1, but not at other sites, was found to yield substantial deficits in both Berg Balance Score and walking speed.

Discussion: The present findings indicate that tactile perception at MT1 is more closely linked to mobility function than is tactile perception at GT, MT5 or H. These findings warrant further research to examine whether interventions (e.g., textured insoles) and assessments that preferentially or exclusively focus on the site of MT1 may be more effective for optimizing clinical care.

Keywords: somatosensation, aging, mobility, walking, balance

INTRODUCTION

Impaired somatosensation is common in older adults (Mold et al., 2004; Shaffer and Harrison, 2007). A large study of peripheral nerve function in older adults found bilateral somatosensory deficits in approximately 26% of individuals 65–74 years of age, 36% of individuals 75–84 and 54% of individuals ≥85 (Mold et al., 2004). This age-related impairment of somatosensation has important functional implications for older adults, as it has been linked to deficits in balance and walking ability (Resnick et al., 2000; Mold et al., 2004; Deshpande et al., 2008; Buchman et al., 2009). A particular concern with somatosensory impairment is increased risk of injurious falls (Sorock and Labiner, 1992; Richardson and Hurvitz, 1995), which are a major contributor to disability and death in older adults (Soriano et al., 2007). The issue is compounded by the fact that many older adults are unaware that they have peripheral neurological impairment (Mold et al., 2004), and are therefore unlikely to seek preemptive intervention.

Given the importance of somatosensory function to mobility in older adults, there is a clear need for research that can contribute to enhanced clinical assessment and intervention of somatosensory deficits. A potentially important question is whether mobility outcomes are differentially affected by the site of somatosensory deficits. For example, the presence of site-specific differences in the relationship with balance or walking function could have important implications for intervening with sensory augmentation footwear. Sensory augmentation footwear involves placing specialized insoles in the shoes (i.e., textured or vibrating insoles), and has shown promise for enhancing mobility function in older adults (Priplata et al., 2003; Palluel et al., 2008, 2009; Qiu et al., 2012; Stephen et al., 2012; Hatton et al., 2013). However, there are also studies which report no benefit or possibly even deleterious effects of somatosensory augmentation (Hatton et al., 2009, 2012; Hartmann et al., 2010). Knowledge of site-specific associations with mobility function may be helpful for explaining such discrepancies and for guiding future development of footwear. This knowledge may also be valuable for refining clinical assessment protocols so that somatosensory screening can be conducted in a time and cost-effective manner. Accordingly, the objective of the present study is to investigate the extent to which tactile perception at four different sites on the plantar surface of the foot may be differentially associated with mobility function, including tests of balance and walking speed.

MATERIALS AND METHODS

PARTICIPANTS

Older adult volunteers were recruited by newspaper advertisement and mass mailing to a research recruitment database. The database consisted of a heterogeneous mix of older adults who had previously indicated willingness to volunteer for research studies. Screening of inclusion/exclusion criteria was conducted by telephone. Inclusion criteria for this study were: (1) age between 65 and 85 years and (2) agreement with the statement "You find it physically tiring to walk a quarter mile, or climb two flights of stairs, or perform household chores (at least one of these should be true)". Exclusion criteria included use of an assistive device for walking (cane, crutch, walker, brace, etc.); lower extremity pain while walking; involuntary weight gain or loss exceeding 10 pounds within the past 6 months; myocardial infarction or symptomatic cardiovascular disease in the past year; bone fracture in the past year; injury or illness to the central nervous system; uncontrolled hypertension exceeding 160 systolic and/or 95 diastolic; or terminal illness. Volunteers who met these criteria were invited to our research center to participate in the assessments described below. During this visit, we also acquired demographic and health-related information (e.g., medication use, weight and height) and administered the Mini Mental State Examination to assess cognitive status. In order to determine if volunteers were aware of the presence of a clinically significant neuropathy, they were asked to reply "Yes" or "No" to the question: "Do you regularly experience either numbness or tingling in your feet (when sitting or walking)?" All study procedures were approved by the University of Florida Institutional Review Board. All individuals participating in on-site assessments provided their written informed consent.

ASSESSMENT OF CUTANEOUS TACTILE PERCEPTION

Cutaneous tactile perception was assessed at four sites on the plantar surface of each foot using a Semmes–Weinstein 5.07 (10 g) monofilament. The sites tested were the great toe (GT), first metatarsal head (MT1), fifth metatarsal head (MT5) and heel (H). Participants laid flat on their back on an examination table. They were provided with an illustration of a set of "footprints" (**Figure 1**), with each testing site labeled with a code that specified side and testing site. When prompted by the examiner, the participants were instructed to indicate whether they felt a touch and, if so, at what site. The examiner performed 24 trials (three trials at each of the four sites for both feet) in random order. At each site, one of the three trials was a "sham" in which the examiner did not actually touch the participant but still asked for a response. One point was awarded for each correct response (including a "no" response for a sham trial) for a total cutaneous tactile score of up to 24 points (12 points per foot). For ease of interpretation, the number of correct responses was converted to a percent value.

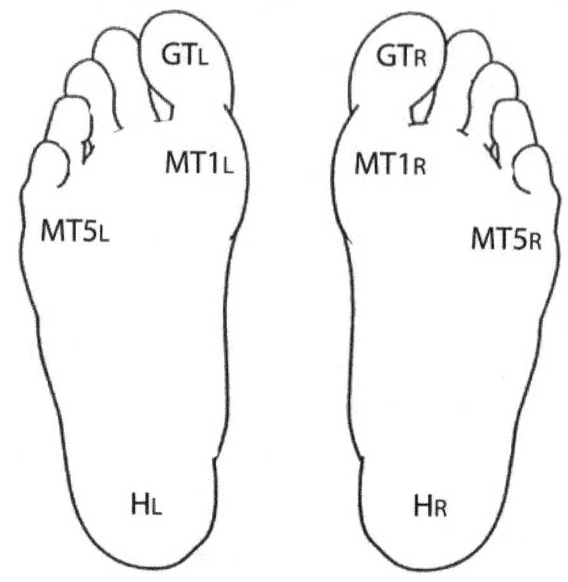

FIGURE 1 | Testing sites for tactile perception. Using the figure shown, participants were instructed to report which site was touched by the monofilament. A total of 24 trials were conducted, including 16 with a tactile stimulus and 8 sham trials with no stimulus.

FUNCTIONAL MEASURES

Balance was assessed with the Berg Balance Scale (Berg et al., 1989), which is a 14-item performance assessment of balance related tasks. Each task is scored on an ordinal scale from 0 (unable) to 4 (independent). The sum of all scores is used as the final outcome. Both walking tests (usual and maximal speed) were timed with a stopwatch. In order to ensure that we recorded steady state walking speed during the 10 m fast walk, the beginning and end of the course included 5 m acceleration/deceleration zones such that the total distance walked was 20 m. The watch was started and stopped when the individual's torso passed over the lines marking the start and end, respectively, of the 10 m course. Three fast walking trials were conducted, and the average was used for subsequent analysis. Only one trial was conducted for 400 m usual walking speed.

STATISTICS

Values are reported as mean ± standard deviation unless otherwise stated. The data were checked for normality and homoscedasticity. Consistency of results for left and right sides (i.e., inter-item reliability) was assessed by examining Cronbach's α coefficients. For the primary analysis, associations between continuous variables were quantified by Pearson's moment correlations, and partial correlations accounted for age, sex, body mass index, MMSE score and number of medications. Regression models were used to compare the strength of associations between different somatosensory sites and mobility tests, after adjusting for confounding variables. Statistical analysis was conducted using SPSS 21, and significance level was set to $\alpha < 0.05$. For the secondary analysis, two tailed t-tests were used to compare subgroups of participants. The False Discovery Rate Procedure was used to correct for multiple comparisons (Curran-Everett, 2000).

RESULTS

PARTICIPANT CHARACTERISTICS

A total of 198 individuals underwent screening by telephone. Of these, 72 passed the phone screen and were invited to our research center for on-site screening and assessment. Ultimately, 61 (38 females and 23 males) were found to meet all criteria and were able to complete all necessary assessments. The mean age was 74.5 ± 6.6 years. The mean body mass index was 28.0 ± 3.6 (range 16.2–34.5) and the mean score on the Mini-Mental State Exam was 27.5 ± 1.7 (range 24–30). Participants used on average 3 prescription medications (range 0–13 medications).

SOMATOSENSORY FUNCTION

Tactile perception data were examined for the statistical assumptions of normality, independence and homoscedasticity. The data were found to be significantly non-normally distributed (skewness statistic = −1.961 ± 0.31, $p < 0.01$), and were transformed with a square root transformation prior to conducting regression analysis. Tactile perception for the left and right sides (including data from all four testing sites) were significantly correlated (r = 0.73, $p < 0.001$), with high inter-item reliability (Cronbach's $\alpha = 0.85$). Therefore, the left and right sides were averaged by testing site to yield four tactile perception scores, which were used for subsequent analysis. The group mean scores for each testing site were: GT: 86.1 ± 22.2%, MT1: 89.0 ± 21.1%, H: 87.1 ± 21.0% and MT5: 90.6 ± 19.9%. Scores from the four sites were significantly positively associated with one another, with correlations ranging from 0.48 to 0.62 ($p < 0.001$). Seventeen participants (out of 61) had at least one false positive response to the sham trials, with the overall proportion of false positive responses being about 6%.

Approximately 37% of participants self-reported regularly experiencing tingling and/or numbness in their feet (i.e., abnormal somatosensation). Tactile perception at MT1 was significantly worse in those reporting abnormal somatosensation compared to those who did not report this deficit (81.8% vs. 95.2%, $p = 0.005$). Similar non-significant trends were also observed at MT5 (p = 0.05) and GT ($p = 0.11$).

RELATIONSHIP BETWEEN SOMATOSENSATION AND MOBILITY FUNCTION

Tactile perception at each site was significantly associated with performance on the Berg Balance Scale. These findings were maintained after adjusting for age, sex, body mass index, MMSE score and medication use (**Table 1**). Tactile perception at MT1 was the only site found to be significantly associated with usual and maximal walking speed. The strength of the association between Berg Balance score and tactile perception at MT1 was significantly stronger than the associations between Berg Balance score and tactile perception at each other site (adjusted $p < 0.05$). The results also show that the strength of the association between MT1 and Berg Balance score was stronger than the association between MT1 and maximal speed (adjusted $p < 0.05$). The same trend was evident for the relationship between MT1 and Berg Balance score relative to that of MT1 and usual walking speed (adjusted p = 0.07).

A secondary analysis was conducted to examine the extent to which the occurrence of clinically mild somatosensory impairment at each plantar testing site may affect mobility function. For each testing site, we compared subgroups of older adults with no clinically detectable impairment (i.e., no incorrect responses at the plantar site) to those with clinically mild impairment (i.e., only one incorrect response at the plantar site). Results of this analysis are shown in **Table 2**. Compared to participants with no impairment at MT1, those with mild impairment at MT1 had lower scores for the Berg Balance Scale (53.0 ± 3.1 vs. 50.3 ± 3.0, $p = 0.006$), usual walking speed (1.12 ± 0.12 vs. 0.97 ± 0.12 m/s, $p = 0.007$), and a trend for lower maximal walking speed (1.61 ± 0.23 vs. 1.45 ± 0.37 m/s, $p = 0.073$). For each other site (GT, H, MT5) there were no statistically significant differences for any mobility test between the subgroup with no impairment vs. the subgroup with mild impairment (all $p > 0.17$).

DISCUSSION

The primary objective of this study was to investigate the extent to which tactile perception at four different sites on the plantar surface of the foot may be differentially related to mobility function in older adults. The results indicate that tactile perception at MT1 is more closely linked to mobility function than is tactile perception at GT, H or MT5. The strength of the association

Table 1 | Associations between somatosensory scores and mobility function.

	GT	MT1	H	MT5
Adjusted r*				
Berg Balance Score	0.41, $p < 0.002$	0.75, $p < 0.001$	0.39, $p = 0.003$	0.30, $p = 0.03$
400m Usual (m/s)	0.17, $p = 0.22$	0.51, $p < 0.001$	0.17, $p = 0.21$	0.07, $p = 0.59$
10m Maximal (m/s)	0.11, $p = 0.44$	0.38, $p = 0.004$	0.00, $p = 0.98$	−0.15, $p = 0.25$

** adjusted for age, sex, body mass index, MMSE score and number of medications.*

Abbreviations: GT (great toe); MTI (first metatarsal head); H (heel); MT5 (fifth metatarsal head).

Table 2 | Mobility function for subgroups without somatosensory impairment vs. with mild somatosensory impairment.

	GT		MT1		H		MT5	
	Not Impaired (n = 40)	**Mildly Impaired (n = 10)**	**Not Impaired (n = 41)**	**Mildly Impaired (n = 11)**	**Not Impaired (n = 37)**	**Mildly Impaired (n = 14)**	**Not Impaired (n = 44)**	**Mildly mpaired (n = 10)**
Berg Balance Score	52.0 ± 3.6	52.3 ± 3.5	***53.0 ± 3.1***	***50.3 ± 3.0****	52.8 ± 3.4	50.1 ± 5.5	52.1 ± 3.5	50.9 ± 6.0
Usual Speed (m/s)	1.09 ± 0.13	1.04 ± 0.14	***1.12 ± 0.12***	***0.97 ± 0.12****	1.07 ± 0.13	1.05 ± 0.19	1.07 ± 0.12	1.09 ± 0.20
Maximal Speed (m/s)	1.59 ± 0.29	1.5 ± 0.16	1.61 ± 0.23	1.45 ± 0.37	1.55 ± 0.26	1.58 ± 0.37	1.53 ± 0.22	1.62 ± 0.44

** indicates adjusted p < 0.05.*

Abbreviations: GT (great toe); MTI (first metatarsal head); H (heel); MT5 (fifth metatarsal head).

between Berg Balance score and tactile perception at MT1 was significantly stronger than the associations between Berg Balance score and tactile perception at each other site. Furthermore, MT1 was the only site that was significantly associated with usual and maximal walking speed. What accounts for the finding that tactile perception at MT1 is especially highly linked to mobility function? It might be explained in part by the prior finding that somatosensory thresholds are lower (i.e., more sensitive) in the ball of the foot, which includes MT1, compared to the heel and toe regions (Inglis et al., 2002). This could be due to the relatively high density of slow and fast adapting cutaneous receptors at MT1 (Kennedy and Inglis, 2002; Fallon et al., 2005). These anatomical characteristics may be an evolutionary adaptation in response to the important role of the forefoot in control of walking. The forefoot, including MT1, is highly involved in the crucial biomechanical task of forward propulsion during gait (Melai et al., 2013). In this role, the forefoot bears high levels of pressure that likely provides important neural input that is relevant to controlling speed and directional steering during walking.

Even clinically mild somatosensory impairment at MT1 appears to have a marked influence on mobility function. This was evidenced by our subgroup analyses of individuals with clinically mild somatosensory impairment vs. those with no clinically detectable somatosensory impairment. For tactile perception at MT1, Berg Balance Scale score was 2.7 points lower for the subgroup with mild impairment vs. the subgroup with no impairment (50.3 vs. 53.0 points). This difference approaches the value of 3.3 points that has been reported as a meaningful change for independently ambulating older adults (Donoghue and Stokes, 2009). Furthermore, the score of 53 in the subgroup with no impairment remains above the threshold of 51 that is indicative of a higher fall risk in elders who have a prior history of falling (Shumway-Cook et al., 1997). Equally alarming is the group difference of 0.15 m/s for usual walking speed, which well exceeds the threshold of 0.10 m/s that is considered a clinically meaningful change in older adults (Perera et al., 2006). The importance of MT1 relative to other plantar sites is further confirmed by the absence of significant differences in mobility function between subgroups at the other plantar sites.

Another interesting finding from this study is the distinct difference in the extent to which tactile perception is linked to Berg Balance score vs. walking speed. At sites GT, MT5 and H, there was a significant association between tactile perception and Berg Balance score, but not between tactile perception and walking speed. At site MT1, the strength of the association between tactile perception and Berg Balance score was significantly stronger than the association with maximal walking speed ($p < 0.05$) and there was a trend for a stronger association compared to usual walking speed ($p = 0.07$). The finding that somatosensation is more closely linked to balance is consistent with prior reports (Mold et al., 2004; Deshpande et al., 2008; Zhang and Li, 2013), although the reason remains unclear. It may be that processing of movement control for balance is less "automatic" than processing for walking, and relies more heavily on utilization of peripheral inputs to provide real-time information (Brandt et al., 1999; Jahn et al., 2004; Zwergal et al., 2012; Lau et al., 2014), such as for integration with the visual and vestibular systems. Another possible explanation is that there is an age-related increase in controlled processing of balance (Boisgontier et al., 2013) that is less pronounced for gait. It may also be that somatosensory information is more likely to be deficient during balance tasks. This is because activation thresholds of peripheral receptors are more likely to be reached during walking due to higher pressure and impact forces compared to balance tasks (Jonely et al., 2011).

Overall, the results of this study strongly agree with prior work demonstrating that impaired somatosensation is detrimental to mobility function (Resnick et al., 2000; Mold et al., 2004; Deshpande et al., 2008; Buchman et al., 2009). We have expanded on this knowledge by demonstrating site-specific differences in the association between tactile perception and mobility function. There are some methodological considerations that should be noted when interpreting the results of this study. We assessed somatosensation of the plantar surface of the feet because they are the primary interface between ground and body, and because peripheral age-related neural impairments are most profound distally (Shaffer and Harrison, 2007). However, the relationship between somatosensation and mobility may also be affected by other types of somatosensory information (e.g., muscle spindles and joint receptors) from other lower extremity regions. We used a clinical assessment of somatosensation (monofilament) as opposed to more rigorous assessments (e.g., sensory thresholds). Accordingly, our data should be interpreted in the context of clinically detectable levels of impairment.

The findings from this research may have important implications for clinical care of older adults, such as in the design of footwear that is used to augment somatosensation. Our finding that mobility function is most closely associated with somatosensory function at MT1 warrants further research to examine whether insoles that preferentially or exclusively augment somatosensation at MT1 provide an advantage for enhancing functional outcomes. The potential importance of this topic is supported by evidence showing that the site of somatosensory stimulation on the plantar surface of the foot can yield different postural responses (Kavounoudias et al., 1998, 2001). Our findings also have implications for clinical assessment. An ideal assessment of somatosensory function would involve testing at multiple sites with multiple modalities (tactile, vibratory, proprioception, etc.). However, this rigorous level of assessment may be excessively time consuming and costly for use in regular screenings. Single-site assessment is more feasible and may encourage more widespread use of somatosensory screening in older adults. Although more research is warranted, our data suggest that assessment at MT1 may prove to be the most relevant site in the context of gauging risk for adverse mobility outcomes.

AUTHOR CONTRIBUTIONS

This study was designed by David J. Clark and Evangelos A. Christou. Data collection was conducted by Mieniecia L. Black and David J. Clark. Data analysis was conducted by Yenisel Cruz-Almeida and David J. Clark. The content of the manuscript was prepared by Yenisel Cruz-Almeida, Mieniecia L. Black, Evangelos A. Christou and David J. Clark.

ACKNOWLEDGMENTS

This work was supported by the National Institute on Aging (2P30-AG028740-06 to David J. Clark and Evangelos A. Christou; AG039659-02S1 to Yenisel Cruz-Almeida). Support was also provided by the U.S. Department of Veterans Affairs Rehabilitation Research and Development Service (B7176-W to David J. Clark).

REFERENCES

Berg, K., Wood-Dauphinee, S., Williams, J. I., and Gayton, D. (1989). Measuring balance in the elderly: preliminary development of an instrument. *Physiother Can* 41, 304–311. doi: 10.3138/ptc.41.6.304

Boisgontier, M. P., Beets, I. A., Duysens, J., Nieuwboer, A., Krampe, R. T., and Swinnen, S. P. (2013). Age-related differences in attentional cost associated with postural dual tasks: increased recruitment of generic cognitive resources in older adults. *Neurosci. Biobehav. Rev.* 37, 1824–1837. doi: 10.1016/j.neubiorev.2013.07.014

Brandt, T., Strupp, M., and Benson, J. (1999). You are better off running than walking with acute vestibulopathy. *Lancet* 354, 746. doi: 10.1016/s0140-6736(99)03179-7

Buchman, A. S., Wilson, R. S., Leurgans, S., and Bennett, D. A. (2009). Vibratory thresholds and mobility in older persons. *Muscle Nerve* 39, 754–760. doi: 10.1002/mus.21263

Curran-Everett, D. (2000). Multiple comparisons: philosophies and illustrations. *Am. J. Physiol. Regul. Integr. Comp. Physiol.* 279, R1–R8.

Deshpande, N., Ferrucci, L., Metter, J., Faulkner, K. A., Strotmeyer, E., Satterfield, S., et al. (2008). Association of lower limb cutaneous sensitivity with gait speed in the elderly: the health ABC study. *Am. J. Phys. Med. Rehabil.* 87, 921–928. doi: 10.1097/phm.0b013e31818a5556

Donoghue, D., Physiotherapy Research and Older People (PROP) Group, Stokes, E. K. (2009). How much change is true change? The minimum detectable change of the Berg Balance Scale in elderly people. *J. Rehabil. Med.* 41, 343–346. doi: 10.2340/16501977-0337

Fallon, J. B., Bent, L. R., McNulty, P. A., and Macefield, V. G. (2005). Evidence for strong synaptic coupling between single tactile afferents from the sole of the foot and motoneurons supplying leg muscles. *J. Neurophysiol.* 94, 3795–3804. doi: 10.1152/jn.00359.2005

Hartmann, A., Murer, K., de Bie, R. A., and de Bruin, E. D. (2010). The effect of a training program combined with augmented afferent feedback from the feet using shoe insoles on gait performance and muscle power in older adults: a randomised controlled trial. *Disabil. Rehabil.* 32, 755–764. doi: 10.3109/09638280903295441

Hatton, A. L., Dixon, J., Martin, D., and Rome, K. (2009). The effect of textured surfaces on postural stability and lower limb muscle activity. *J. Electromyogr. Kinesiol.* 19, 957–964. doi: 10.1016/j.jelekin.2008.04.012

Hatton, A. L., Dixon, J., Rome, K., Newton, J. L., and Martin, D. J. (2012). Altering gait by way of stimulation of the plantar surface of the foot: the immediate effect of wearing textured insoles in older fallers. *J. Foot Ankle Res.* 5:11. doi: 10.1186/1757-1146-5-s1-o21

Hatton, A. L., Rome, K., Dixon, J., Martin, D. J., and McKeon, P. O. (2013). Footwear interventions: a review of their sensorimotor and mechanical effects on balance performance and gait in older adults. *J. Am. Podiatr. Med. Assoc.* 103, 516–533.

Inglis, J. T., Kennedy, P. M., Wells, C., and Chua, R. (2002). The role of cutaneous receptors in the foot. *Adv. Exp. Med. Biol.* 508, 111–117. doi: 10.1007/978-1-4615-0713-0_14

Jahn, K., Deutschlander, A., Stephan, T., Strupp, M., Wiesmann, M., and Brandt, T. (2004). Brain activation patterns during imagined stance and locomotion in functional magnetic resonance imaging. *Neuroimage* 22, 1722–1731. doi: 10.1016/j.neuroimage.2004.05.017

Jonely, H., Brismee, J. M., Sizer, P. S. Jr., and James, C. R. (2011). Relationships between clinical measures of static foot posture and plantar pressure during static standing and walking. *Clin. Biomech. (Bristol, Avon)* 26, 873–879. doi: 10.1016/j.clinbiomech.2011.04.008

Kavounoudias, A., Roll, R., and Roll, J. P. (1998). The plantar sole is a 'dynamometric map' for human balance control. *Neuroreport* 9, 3247–3252. doi: 10.1097/00001756-199810050-00021

Kavounoudias, A., Roll, R., and Roll, J. P. (2001). Foot sole and ankle muscle inputs contribute jointly to human erect posture regulation. *J. Physiol.* 532(Pt. 3), 869–878. doi: 10.1111/j.1469-7793.2001.0869e.x

Kennedy, P. M., and Inglis, J. T. (2002). Distribution and behaviour of glabrous cutaneous receptors in the human foot sole. *J. Physiol.* 538(Pt. 3), 995–1002. doi: 10.1113/jphysiol.2001.013087

Lau, T. M., Gwin, J. T., and Ferris, D. P. (2014). Walking reduces sensorimotor network connectivity compared to standing. *J. Neuroeng. Rehabil.* 11:14. doi: 10.1186/1743-0003-11-14

Melai, T., Schaper, N. C., Ijzerman, T. H., de Lange, T. L., Willems, P. J., Meijer, K., et al. (2013). Increased forefoot loading is associated with an increased plantar flexion moment. *Hum. Mov. Sci.* 32, 785–793. doi: 10.1016/j.humov.2013.05.001

Mold, J. W., Vesely, S. K., Keyl, B. A., Schenk, J. B., and Roberts, M. (2004). The prevalence, predictors, and consequences of peripheral sensory neuropathy in older patients. *J. Am. Board Fam. Pract.* 17, 309–318. doi: 10.3122/jabfm.17.5.309

Palluel, E., Nougier, V., and Olivier, I. (2008). Do spike insoles enhance postural stability and plantar-surface cutaneous sensitivity in the elderly? *Age (Dordr.)* 30, 53–61. doi: 10.1007/s11357-008-9047-2

Palluel, E., Olivier, I., and Nougier, V. (2009). The lasting effects of spike insoles on postural control in the elderly. *Behav. Neurosci.* 123, 1141–1147. doi: 10.1037/a0017115

Perera, S., Mody, S. H., Woodman, R. C., and Studenski, S. A. (2006). Meaningful change and responsiveness in common physical performance measures in older adults. *J. Am. Geriatr. Soc.* 54, 743–749. doi: 10.1111/j.1532-5415.2006.00701.x

Priplata, A. A., Niemi, J. B., Harry, J. D., Lipsitz, L. A., and Collins, J. J. (2003). Vibrating insoles and balance control in elderly people. *Lancet* 362, 1123–1124. doi: 10.1016/s0140-6736(03)14470-4

Qiu, F., Cole, M. H., Davids, K. W., Hennig, E. M., Silburn, P. A., Netscher, H., et al. (2012). Enhanced somatosensory information decreases postural sway in older people. *Gait Posture* 35, 630–635. doi: 10.1016/j.gaitpost.2011.12.013

Resnick, H. E., Vinik, A. I., Schwartz, A. V., Leveille, S. G., Brancati, F. L., Balfour, J., et al. (2000). Independent effects of peripheral nerve dysfunction on lower-extremity physical function in old age: the Women's Health and Aging Study. *Diabetes Care* 23, 1642–1647. doi: 10.2337/diacare.23.11.1642

Richardson, J. K., and Hurvitz, E. A. (1995). Peripheral neuropathy: a true risk factor for falls. *J. Gerontol. A Biol. Sci. Med. Sci.* 50, M211–M215. doi: 10.1093/gerona/50a.4.m211

Shaffer, S. W., and Harrison, A. L. (2007). Aging of the somatosensory system: a translational perspective. *Phys. Ther.* 87, 193–207. doi: 10.2522/ptj.20060083

Shumway-Cook, A., Baldwin, M., Polissar, N. L., and Gruber, W. (1997). Predicting the probability for falls in community-dwelling older adults. *Phys. Ther.* 77, 812–819.

Soriano, T. A., DeCherrie, L. V., and Thomas, D. C. (2007). Falls in the community-dwelling older adult: a review for primary-care providers. *Clin. Interv. Aging* 2, 545–554.

Sorock, G. S., and Labiner, D. M. (1992). Peripheral neuromuscular dysfunction and falls in an elderly cohort. *Am. J. Epidemiol.* 136, 584–591.

Stephen, D. G., Wilcox, B. J., Niemi, J. B., Franz, J. R., Kerrigan, D., and D'Andrea, S. E. (2012). Baseline-dependent effect of noise-enhanced insoles on gait variability in healthy elderly walkers. *Gait Posture* 36, 537–540. doi: 10.1016/j.gaitpost.2012.05.014.

Zhang, S., and Li, L. (2013). The differential effects of foot sole sensory on plantar pressure distribution between balance and gait. *Gait Posture* 37, 532–535. doi: 10.1016/j.gaitpost.2012.09.012

Zwergal, A., Linn, J., Xiong, G., Brandt, T., Strupp, M., and Jahn, K. (2012). Aging of human supraspinal locomotor and postural control in fMRI. *Neurobiol. Aging* 33, 1073–1084. doi: 10.1016/j.neurobiolaging.2010.09.022

2

Age-related changes in motor cortical representation and interhemispheric interactions: a transcranial magnetic stimulation study

Elisabetta Coppi, Elise Houdayer, Raffaella Chieffo, Francesca Spagnolo, Alberto Inuggi, Laura Straffi, Giancarlo Comi and Letizia Leocani*

Neurological Department and Experimental Neurophysiology Unit, Institute of Experimental Neurology (INSPE), University Hospital-IRCCS San Raffaele, Milan, Italy

Edited by:
Brian C. Clark, Ohio University, USA

Reviewed by:
Martin Lotze, University of Greifswald, Germany
Ashleigh Elizabeth Smith, University of South Australia, Australia

***Correspondence:**
Letizia Leocani, Experimental Neurophysiology Unit, INSPE-Institute of Experimental Neurology, Hospital San Raffaele, Via Olgettina 60, 20132, Milan, Italy
e-mail: letizia.leocani@hsr.it

To better understand the physiological mechanisms responsible for the differential motor cortex functioning in aging, we used transcranial magnetic stimulation to investigate interhemispheric interactions and cortical representation of hand muscles in the early phase of physiological aging, correlating these data with participants' motor abilities. Right-handed healthy subjects were divided into a younger group ($n = 15$, mean age 25.4 ± 1.9 years old) and an older group ($n = 16$, mean age 61.1 ± 5.1 years old). Activity of the bilateral abductor pollicis brevis (APB) and abductor digiti minimi (ADM) was recorded. Ipsilateral silent period (ISP) was measured in both APBs. Cortical maps of APB and ADM were measured bilaterally. Mirror movements (MM) were recorded during thumb abductions. Motor abilities were tested using Nine Hole Peg Test, finger tapping, and grip strength. ISP was reduced in the older group on both sides, in terms of duration ($p = 0.025$), onset ($p = 0.029$), and area ($p = 0.008$). Resting motor threshold did not differ between groups. APB and ADM maps were symmetrical in the younger group, but were reduced on the right compared to the left hemisphere in the older group ($p = 0.008$). The APB map of the right hemisphere was reduced in the older group compared to the younger ($p = 0.021$). Older subjects showed higher frequency of MM and worse motor abilities ($p < 0.001$). The reduction of right ISP area correlated significantly with the worsening of motor performances. Our results showed decreased interhemispheric interactions in the early processes of physiological aging and decreased cortical muscles representation over the non-dominant hemisphere. The decreased ISP and increased frequency of MM suggest a reduction of transcallosal inhibition. These data demonstrate that early processes of normal aging are marked by a dissociation of motor cortices, characterized, at least, by a decline of the non-dominant hemisphere, reinforcing the hypothesis of the right hemi-aging model.

Keywords: physiological aging, transcranial magnetic stimulation, ipsilateral silent period, muscle cortical maps, motor performances

INTRODUCTION

During physiological aging, the human brain undergoes a series of morphological and functional changes. In healthy aging, cognitive and simple motor tasks produce more symmetrical and widespread cortical activation compared to young adults, due to a higher recruitment of cortical areas of both hemispheres, as supported by functional neuroimaging (Hutchinson et al., 2002; Mattay et al., 2002; Riecker et al., 2006; Ward et al., 2007) and electroencephalographic (EEG) studies (Sailer et al., 2000; Labyt et al., 2006; Vallesi et al., 2010).

In cognitive processes, this greater bilateral cortical activation seems to reflect compensatory mechanisms, in order to support cognitive abilities in healthy older people (Cabeza et al., 2002; Dolcos et al., 2002). Conversely, evidence for a positive effect of this cortical hyperactivation on motor functions is less clear. Functional neuroimaging (Riecker et al., 2006) and EEG (Inuggi et al., 2011) studies demonstrated that this bilateral cortical activation was still characterized by reduced motor abilities in aging. These results suggest that the more symmetrical motor cortex activity observed in physiological aging would not be due to a compensatory mechanism (Inuggi et al., 2011). Therefore, the functional modulations revealed in motor cortices during physiological aging are likely to be related to a loss of balance between excitatory and inhibitory circuits.

A major hypothesis is that this could be related to changes in interhemispheric connections between motor cortices (Talelli et al., 2008), due to either a loss of transcallosal fibers or to a decreased excitability of interhemispheric connections. Transcranial magnetic stimulation (TMS) has been used to investigate the effects of aging on interhemispheric inhibition (IHI). A paired-pulse TMS study, with conditioning stimulus on the hemisphere ipsilateral to the moving hand and a contralateral test stimulus, showed no age-related differences in IHI at rest, but demonstrated an enhanced IHI in young subjects during unilateral movements (from the activated hemisphere to the resting one) (Talelli et al., 2008). This IHI modulation during movement was absent in the older group, showing functional alteration of the IHI in physiological aging.

More recently, single-pulse TMS was used to study IHI in aging using the ipsilateral silent period (ISP) (Davidson and Tremblay, 2013; Petitjean and Ko, 2013). These studies demonstrated a reduction in ISP in terms of duration (Petitjean and Ko, 2013) and area (Davidson and Tremblay, 2013) in older subjects compared to younger participants. The ISP consists in stimulating one motor cortex during maximal voluntary contraction of the ipsilateral hand (Ferbert et al., 1992). The stimulated motor cortex would induce a transcallosal IHI of the opposite motor cortex (Meyer et al., 1995). This inhibition is detectable as a pause in the ipsilateral electromyographic (EMG) trace (ISP). Although both IHI and ISP represent a phenomenon of IHI, they are due to different neuronal mechanisms (Chen et al., 2003). The advantage of studying ISP is that, unlike IHI, representing a reduction of motor evoked potential (MEP) amplitude, ISP represents a direct measure of the interhemispheric control of voluntary cortical motor output (Giovannelli et al., 2009).

In line with decreased interhemispheric interactions, physiological aging can be accompanied by an increased in mirror movements (MM), or more generally motor overflow (MO), reflecting all kinds of involuntary movements that appear in other muscular districts during the execution of a voluntary muscle contraction (Hoy et al., 2004). MM are due to an impaired transcallosal inhibition (Bodwell et al., 2003) and are generally observed in neurological disorders involving the corpus callosum, such as complex congenital syndromes (Galléa et al., 2011) or also post-stroke (Chieffo et al., 2013).

The increased symmetrical motor cortex activation observed in aging could also be due to an increased cortical representation of the different muscles involved in the movement, or to an increased excitability of these motor representations. Regarding the excitability of the motor cortex in physiological aging, no consensus has been found since some authors found no significant differences in resting motor threshold (RMT) between young and older people (Pitcher et al., 2003; Oliviero et al., 2006; Fujiyama et al., 2012), while others revealed a significant increase in RMT (indicating a lower excitability) in older subjects (Rossini et al., 1992; Petitjean and Ko, 2013). Peinemann et al. (2001) found only a trend toward a slightly lower RMT in younger compared with older subjects.

Thus, in order to better understand the physiological mechanisms responsible for this differential motor cortex functioning in aging, it is necessary to provide complementary data on the different aspects of motor control. To this aim, we investigated interhemispheric interactions (using ISP) in physiological aging and correlated this functional data with cortical representation of various hand muscles (using TMS mapping) and with participants' motor performance (using hand motor function tests). Moreover, in order to better understand the mechanisms of physiological aging, we decided to focus on the early phase of aging and included healthy people in the age-range 50–70 years old.

MATERIALS AND METHODS

POPULATION

Thirty-one healthy volunteers were included in this study and divided into two groups: younger (15 subjects, 6 females, mean age ± SD: 25.4 ± 1.9 years, range 21–28 years old) and older (16 subjects, 7 females, mean age ± SD: 61.1 ± 5.1 years, range 51–72 years old). All subjects were fully right-handed, having obtained the maximal score at a translated modified version of the Edinburgh Handedness Inventory (Oldfield, 1971). Participants had no history of neurologic or psychiatric disorders, drug abuse, current use of psychoactive medications, neurosurgery, and metal/electronic implants or other contraindications for the use of TMS (Rossi et al., 2009). Subjects gave their written informed consent before participating in the study, which was approved by the Institutional Ethics Committee.

TRANSCRANIAL MAGNETIC STIMULATION

Transcranial magnetic stimulation was delivered by a Magstim 200 simulator (Magstim Company, Ltd., Whitland, Dyfed, UK) connected to a figure-of-eight coil (Magstim second generation, 70 mm of external diameter). EMG activity of the bilateral abductor pollicis brevis (APB) and abductor digiti minimi (ADM) muscles were recorded using surface Ag/AgCl electrodes in a belly tendon montage. The coil was positioned over the best scalp location (hotspot, marked on a fitting polyester cap that subjects were wearing) for optimal MEPs over the contralateral target muscle (APB or ADM). RMT was defined as the lowest intensity that could induce a 50 μV peak-to-peak amplitude MEP in at least 5 out of 10 trials (Rossi et al., 2009). RMTs were measured on each side. For ISPs measurements, 15 stimuli were applied at an intensity of 90% of the stimulator output (Chen et al., 2003; Trompetto et al., 2004; Spagnolo et al., 2013) while subjects were performing a voluntary maximal contraction of the ipsilateral APB muscle. In between the TMS pulses, subjects were instructed to relax for 4–8 s. Both hemispheres were tested.

For the cortical maps registration, a grid centered on the vertex was placed on the polyester cap. Intersection points of the grid lines were spaced 1 cm apart and served as visual references for coil positioning. Over each hemisphere, a total of 144 intersection points were drawn. TMS pulses were delivered at 115% RMT, starting from point 1, placed 6 cm laterally to the vertex. Then, the coil was moved following growing clockwise (for the right hemisphere) or anticlockwise (left hemisphere) spirals, from one point to another until no MEP could be evoked. Four TMS pulses were applied over each stimulating point. At the end of the session, each stimulating point as well as anatomical references (nasion, vertex, left, and right tragus) were digitized (Polhemus©, FastTrak, Colchester, VT, USA).

Electromyographic signals were sampled at 2 kHz, amplified and bandpass filtered (30–1000 Hz). Impedances were kept below 5 kΩ. Data were acquired using the SynAmp/SCAN 4.3 system (Compumedics Germany GmbH, Singen, Germany) and stored on a computer for off-line analyses.

HAND MOTOR PERFORMANCE

Mirror movements

Participants were comfortably seated on an armchair, their forearms and pronated hands resting on a table in front of them. They performed voluntary phasic ("brief and brisk") thumb abductions in response to a verbal "go" command (10 trials at inter-trial interval of 4 s). EMG was recorded bilaterally. The occurrence of MM in the opposite muscles was inspected off-line. For each trial, the single rectified EMG traces were averaged. If EMG average showed an involuntary activity in the contralateral homologous muscle, MM was considered positive (MM score = 1), otherwise MM score was considered as 0 (Spagnolo et al., 2013).

Nine Hole Peg Test

Nine Hole Peg Test (NHPT) score (Oxford Grice et al., 2003) consisted of the time taken by the subject to insert every peg in the empty holes and then remove them and place them back in the shallow container, as quickly as possible. The test was performed twice. The fastest speed among the two trials was kept for further analyses.

Finger tapping

Subjects were comfortably seated on a chair, their forearm and hands resting on a table placed in front of them. Participants were instructed to press on a left-button mouse as fast as possible during 10 s with their index finger. The test was performed three times, with both hands, in random sequence. Tapping frequency was calculated using STIM software (Compumedics Germany GmbH, Singen, Germany). The mean frequency of the three trials, for each hand, was kept for analyses.

Martin's vigorimeter

Grip strength was measured using the Martin's dynamometer (Martin's Vigorimeter; BCB Ltd., Cardiff, Wales, UK). Subjects were comfortably seated on a chair, their back leaning against the back of the chair and their feet fully resting on the floor. They were asked to grab the dynamometer with their elbow flexed at 90° and their wrist extended between 0° and 30° and squeeze as hard as they could for a few seconds. Three trials per side were recorded for each subject, and the averages of the three scores were kept for further analyses.

Hand motor function scores asymmetry was calculated by subtracting left hand (L) from the right (R) values, and normalizing by their sum:

$$\text{Asym} = \frac{R - L}{R + L}$$

TMS DATA ANALYSES

Ipsilateral silent period durations were determined by rectifying the EMG traces before average. ISP onset was defined as the latency at which the averaged EMG activity became constantly (for at least 10 ms) smaller than the averaged baseline contraction level (between −60 and −10 ms before stimulus; Spagnolo et al., 2013). ISP offset was set at the first point after ISP onset at which the EMG activity regained the baseline activity for at least 10 ms. ISP duration was defined as:

$$\text{ISP}_{\text{duration}} = \text{ISP}_{\text{offset}} - \text{ISP}_{\text{onset}}$$

We also measured the ISP_{area}, which was normalized according to the degree of muscle contraction pre-trigger, in order to correct for intersubject variability. The ISP_{area} (in mV × s), was calculated as $[\text{ISP}_{\text{amplitude}} \times \text{ISP}_{\text{duration}}]$, and then normalized according to the pre-trigger EMG amplitude as follows: [(ISP area − baseline area)/(baseline area × 100)]. $\text{ISP}_{\text{duration}}$ and normalized ISP_{area} asymmetry were calculated by subtracting L from R-hand values, and normalizing by their sum:

$$\text{Asym} = \frac{R - L}{R + L}$$

To analyze the cortical maps, the four MEPs obtained at each stimulating point were averaged, and the mean peak-to-peak amplitude was measured. Then, the following parameters were calculated for each considered muscle (APB and ADM):

(1) maximal MEP amplitude;
(2) map area (total number of stimulating sites in which the mean MEP was at least 50 μV of amplitude).

STATISTICAL ANALYSES

All statistical analyses were performed with SPSS/PC+ 13.0 (SPSS, Inc., Chicago, IL, USA). Normality of the data was assessed using the Kolmogorov–Smirnov test. For each variable, outliers were identified according to Tukey's method, implemented in SPSS, and excluded from the corresponding statistical analyses. Hand motor performance scores, RMTs, ISPs, and map parameters were analyzed either with an ANOVA for repeated measures, or the Conover's free distribution method, a non-parametric ANOVA based on ranks, depending on the data normality (Conover and Iman, 1982). For the ISP and motor performance analyses the two main factors were SIDE (two levels: right and left) and GROUP (two levels: younger and older). For the cortical maps analyses, the main factors were MUSCLE (two levels: APB and ADM) and HEMISPHERE (two levels: right and left). If a main effect or an interaction between the main factors was found, *t*-tests, Mann–Whitney, or Wilcoxon tests (for unpaired or paired data) were used for *post hoc* analyses. Asymmetry values were compared between groups using Mann–Whitney or *t*-tests, depending on the normality of the data. MM frequency was compared between groups using Chi-square analyses. After having subdivided subjects according to the occurrence of MM (including both younger and older subjects), we used non-parametric Mann–Whitney tests to confront ISP parameters between these latter subgroups (group 1: presence of MM, group 2: no MM). Cross-sectional and longitudinal correlations between TMS and behavioral data were assessed using Pearson or Spearman tests, according to the data distribution. Data were considered significant when $p \leq 0.05$.

RESULTS

Eight participants (four older subjects) did not tolerate the high intensity used during ISP measurements and were thus excluded from the ISP analyses, leading thus to $n = 12$ in the older group, and $n = 11$ in the younger group for ISP and correlation analyses. However, these subjects were kept for hand motor performance and cortical map analyses.

TMS DATA

Conover analysis showed no group differences in terms of RMT, but showed a significant SIDE effect ($F_{1,29} = 13.931$; $p = 0.001$), left hemisphere RMTs being lower than right hemisphere [mean

RMT ± SD (% stimulator output); older group: left hemisphere = 50.9 ± 8.4, right hemisphere = 58.1 ± 12.1; younger group: left hemisphere = 48 ± 4.9, right hemisphere = 53.4 ± 11.1].

The ANOVA for repeated measures showed a significant SIDE effect ($F_{1,18} = 9.841$; $p = 0.006$) and a significant GROUP effect ($F_{1,18} = 5.614$; $p = 0.029$) for the ISP_{onset} (one upper outlier for right ISP_{onset} in the older group and two lower outliers for right ISP_{onset} in the older group). $ISP_{duration}$ showed a significant SIDE effect ($F_{1,21} = 5.047$; $p = 0.036$) as well as a significant GROUP effect ($F_{1,21} = 5.798$; $p = 0.025$). In ISP_{area} analyses, the ANOVA demonstrated also a significant GROUP effect ($F_{1,19} = 8.82$; $p = 0.008$), and a trend for a SIDE effect ($F_{1,19} = 3.567$; $p = 0.074$) (one upper outlier for right ISP_{area} in the older group and one lower outlier for right ISP_{area} in the younger group). Thus, in the older group ISP_{onset} was delayed, $ISP_{duration}$ and ISP_{area} were reduced on both sides (see **Figure 1**). Moreover, in both groups, left hand ISP was significantly greater than right hand ISP (except for ISP_{area} where only a trend was observed). It is noteworthy that pre-trigger EMG levels were similar in both groups ($p > 0.05$). ISP data are presented in **Table 1**.

Regarding the map areas (**Figure 2**), in the younger group the repeated measures ANOVA showed a significant main effect of MUSCLE ($F_{1,28} = 4.460$; $p = 0.04$) and no significant main effect of HEMISPHERE ($F_{1,28} = 1.219$; $p = 0.279$), demonstrating that APB had a greater cortical representation than ADM on both hemispheres.

The older group showed no significant effect of MUSCLE ($F_{1,30} = 0.327$; $p = 0.572$), but a significant main effect of HEMISPHERE ($F_{1,30} = 8.085$; $p = 0.008$), showing that APB and ADM maps had similar areas and were reduced on the right hemisphere compared with the left hemisphere. *Post hoc* between-group t-test comparisons within the right hemisphere confirmed a significant

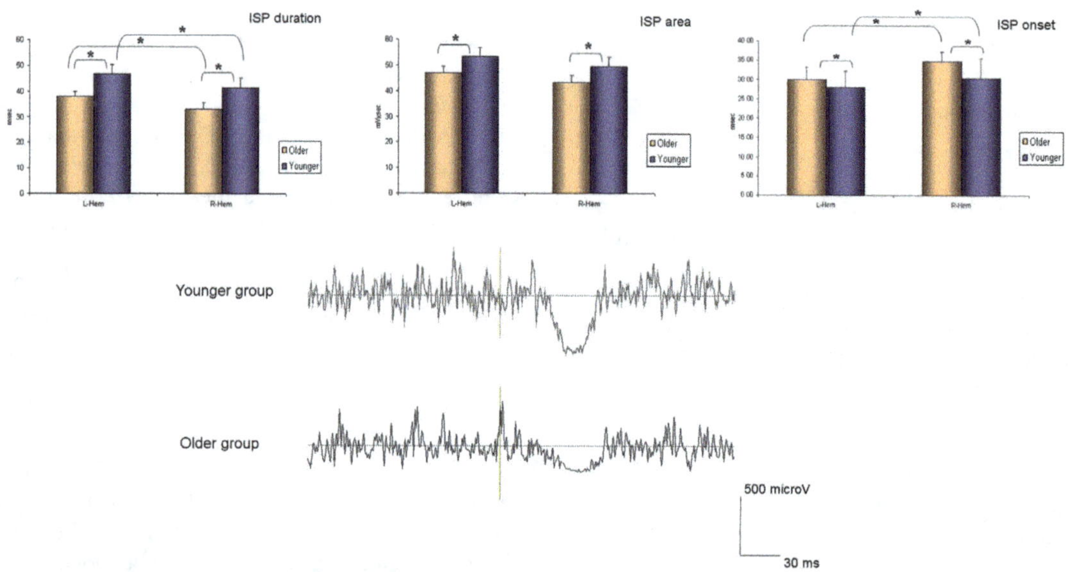

FIGURE 1 | Ipsilateral silent period parameters (duration, area, and onset) according to group and side (average ± SD). L-Hem, left hemisphere; R-Hem, right hemisphere. *$p < 0.05$. Examples of ISP traces in one older and one younger subject are exposed on the lower part of the figure.

Table 1 | ISP parameters (onset, area, duration, and offset) are shown in both groups of participants (younger and older).

ISP parameters	Younger Average ± SD	*p*-Value R vs. L	Older group Average ± SD	*p*-Value R vs. L	*p*-Value Younger vs. older
Onset (ms)	**L** 27.95 ± 4.34 **R** 30.38 ± 5.01	$p = 0.006$*	**L** 30.99 ± 3.01 **R** 35.41 ± 11.69	$p = 0.006$*	$p = 0.029$* $p = 0.029$*
Area (mV x s)	**L** 53.28 ± 13.28 **R** 49.62 ± 11.88	ns	**L** 46.93 ± 13.03 **R** 43.42 ± 9.43	ns	$p = 0.008$* $p = 0.008$*
Duration (ms)	**L** 46.48 ± 11.39 **R** 41.5 ± 12.3	$p = 0.036$*	**L** 38.05 ± 6.59 **R** 32.89 ± 9.88	$p = 0.036$*	$p = 0.025$* $p = 0.025$*
Offset (ms)	**L** 74.63 ± 11.34 **R** 71.88 ± 11.34	ns	**L** 69.04 ± 5.68 **R** 68.3 ± 11.89	ns	ns ns

L, left; R, right; SD, standard deviation; ns, non-significant.
**Statistically significant differences.*

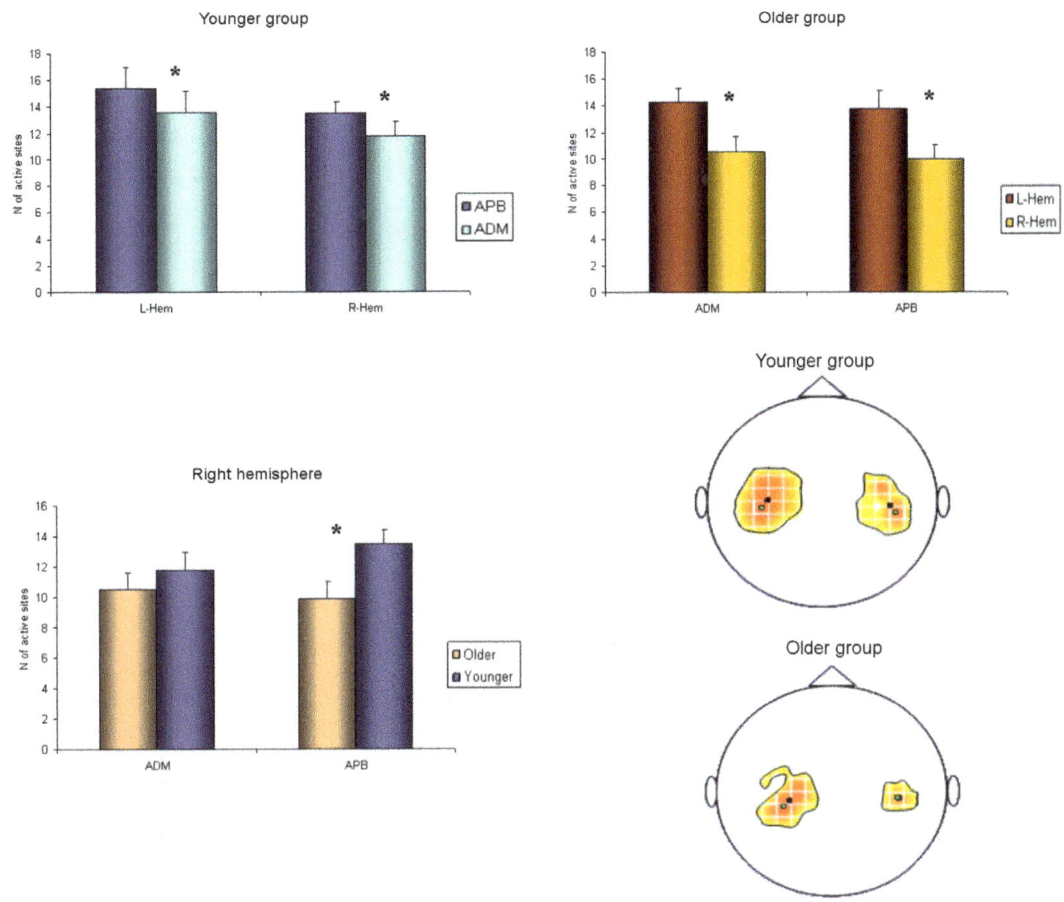

FIGURE 2 | Cortical maps of APB and ADM muscles in the younger and older groups. Upper left graph shows representations of APB and ADM muscles in the younger group, demonstrating a significantly reduced ADM map compared to the APB, on both hemispheres. Upper right graph illustrates the significant reduction of the right hemisphere maps of both APB and ADM muscles, respected to the left hemisphere, in the older group. The lower part of Figure 2 represents the significant reduction of the APB map over the right hemisphere in the older group, compared to the younger group. *$p < 0.05$.

reduction of APB map in the older compared to the younger group ($p = 0.021$). No such differences were observed on the left hemisphere ($p = 0.269$). For ADM maps no significant differences were found between older and younger subjects, on both hemispheres.

Conversely, the analyses of the maximal MEP amplitude (concerning both APB and ADM) did not demonstrate any significant differences, either between groups or between hemispheres ($p > 0.05$). The analyses of the asymmetry confirmed this latter result ($p = 0.774$). Cortical maps data are presented in **Tables 2** and **3**.

HAND MOTOR PERFORMANCE

Brisk thumb movements induced significantly more MM in the older than in the younger group (in 9 older subjects and 1 younger subject for right finger movements, $p < 0.001$; and in 13 older subjects and 5 younger subjects for left thumb extension, $p = 0.001$) (see **Figure 3**). Subjects showing MM did not have significantly different ISP parameters compared to subjects without MM ($p > 0.05$).

Regarding the NHPT analyses, the repeated measures ANOVA showed a significant main effect of SIDE ($F_{1,26} = 17.219$; $p < 0.001$) and GROUP ($F_{1,26} = 29.742$; $p < 0.001$), as the younger had faster scores than the older group, and the right hand scores were better than the left hand, in both groups (one upper outlier for right NHPT in the younger group, one upper outlier for left NHPT in the younger group, and one upper outlier for left NHPT in the older group). The same results were obtained for the finger tapping (FT) frequency (one upper outlier for left FT in the younger group): the younger group was faster than the older group ($F_{1,28} = 30.337$; $p < 0.001$), and performances were faster on the right compared with the left hand ($F_{1,28} = 60.681$; $p < 0.001$). The ANOVA for repeated measures showed greater grip strength in the younger group ($F_{1,29} = 6.545$; $p = 0.016$), and a strong trend for better scores with the right hand in both groups (although non-significant, $F_{1,29} = 4.189$; $p = 0.051$). The paired t-tests demonstrated that the asymmetrical hand motor performances (right better than left) did not differ between groups. Motor performances data are presented in **Table 4**.

CORRELATIONS

We found that hand motor performances (NHPT, FT, and grip strength) of both hands correlated significantly with the

Table 2 | Maps parameters for APB muscles are shown in both group of participants (younger and older).

APB MAPS parameters	Younger group Average ± SD	*p*-Value R vs. L	Older group Average ± SD	*p*-Value R vs. L	*p*-Value Younger vs. older
Map area (*N* of active sites)	**L** 15.4 ± 6.17	ns	**L** 13.87 ± 5.27	$p = 0.008$*	ns
	R 13.53 ± 3.37		**R** 9.93 ± 4.69		$p = 0.021$*
MEP amplitude (μV)	**L** 798.77 ± 546.29	ns	**L** 819.19 ± 948.7	ns	ns
	R 589.18 ± 345.83		**R** 583.06 ± 652.87		ns

APB, abductor pollicis brevis; L-Hem, left hemisphere (dominant); R-Hem, right hemisphere (non-dominant); MEP, motor evoked potential; SD, standard deviation; ns, non-significant; L, Left; R, Right.

**Statistically significant differences.*

Table 3 | Maps parameters for ADM muscles are shown in both group of participants (younger and older).

ADM MAPS parameters	Younger group Average ± SD	*p*-Value R vs. L	Older group Average ± SD	*p*-Value R vs. L	*p*-Value Younger vs. older
Map area (*N* of active sites)	**L** 13.66 ± 6.18	ns	**L** 14.37 ± 4.16	$p = 0.008$*	ns
	R 11.8 ± 4.26		**R** 10.56 ± 4.81		ns
MEP amplitude (μV)	**L** 705.38 ± 527.19	ns	**L** 1299.85 ± 1256.05	Ns	ns
	R 554.63 ± 330.29		**R** 631.55 ± 623.91		ns

ADM, abductor digiti minimi; L-Hem, left hemisphere (dominant); R-Hem, right hemisphere (non-dominant); MEP, motor evoked potential; SD, standard deviation; ns, non-significant; L, Left; R, Right.

**Statistically significant differences.*

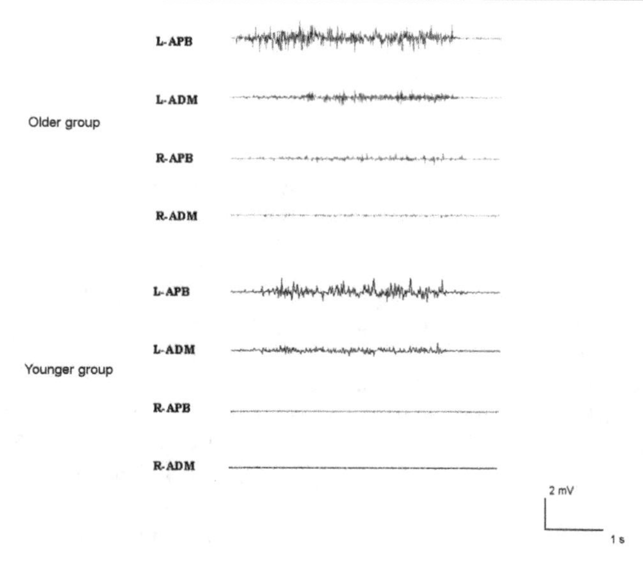

FIGURE 3 | Examples of mirror movements in an older subject (upper traces), compared to a young subject (lower traces).

right ISP_{area}: a smaller right ISP_{area} is associated with worse motor performances with both upper limbs in NHPT (for right NHPT $p = 0.021$, $\rho = 0.499$; for left NHPT $p = 0.006$, $\rho = 0.576$), FT (for right FT $p = 0.009$, $\rho = -0.555$; for left FT $p = 0.027$, $\rho = -0.483$), and grip strength (R: $p = 0.024$, $\rho = -0.492$; L: $p = 0.049$, $\rho = -0.435$). There were no further significant correlations with the other variables analyzed.

DISCUSSION

Our data are consistent with the fact that physiological aging is characterized by a deterioration of interhemispheric inhibition, as previously reported in recent TMS studies (Davidson and Tremblay, 2013; Petitjean and Ko, 2013). The present results bring further details on these abnormal interactions by reporting all components of ISP (duration, onset, and area) and correlating them with other measurements of motor control.

The reduction of all ISP parameters, bilaterally, reflects a declined efficiency of interhemispheric interactions, most probably due to a decreased transcallosal inhibition (Bodwell et al., 2003). Indeed, physiological aging is accompanied by a progressive degeneration of the cerebral tissue as demonstrated by the reduction in fractional anisotropy in the cerebral white matter (Pfefferbaum et al., 2000; Pfefferbaum and Sullivan, 2003; Rovaris et al., 2003; Head et al., 2004). This progressive degeneration involves also the corpus callosum, especially in its anterior portions (Abe et al., 2002; Head et al., 2004; Ota et al., 2006) that connects bilateral motor cortices (Zarei et al., 2006). The defective interhemispheric communication might thus be responsible for the more symmetrical cerebral activity observed in EEG or fMRI studies (Sailer et al., 2000; Hutchinson et al., 2002; Mattay et al., 2002; Labyt et al., 2006; Riecker et al., 2006; Ward et al., 2007; Vallesi et al., 2010) and might also be responsible for the increased frequency of MM, as previously shown in patients with agenesis of the corpus callosum (Mayston et al., 1999; Galléa et al., 2011). Indeed, our older group showed an increase in MM frequency, as the expression of a reduced ability to inhibit the tendency to activate bilateral motor cortices during a simple unimanual motor task (Cincotta and Ziemann, 2008). Thus, our results support the

Table 4 | Hand motor performances are shown in both groups of participants (younger and older).

Hand motor perfomances	Younger group Average ± SD	p-Value R vs. L	Older group Average ± SD	p-Value R vs. L	p-Value Younger vs. older
FT (Hz)	**L** 4.9 ± 0.79 **R** 6.44 ± 1.13	$p < 0.001$*	**L** 3.65 ± 0.55 **R** 4.51 ± 0.68	$p < 0.001$*	$p < 0.001$* $p < 0.001$*
Grip strength (kg)	**L** 0.92 ± 0.24 **R** 0.96 ± 0.26	$p = 0.051$	**L** 0.71 ± 0.18 **R** 0.73 ± 0.22	$p = 0.051$	$p = 0.016$* $p = 0.016$*
NHPT (s)	**L** 17.05 ± 1.62 **R** 15.82 ± 1.6	$p < 0.001$*	**L** 20.69 ± 3.06 **R** 18.87 ± 2.14	$p < 0.001$*	$p < 0.001$* $p < 0.001$*

FT, finger tapping; NHPT, Nine Hole Peg Test; R-Hand, right hand; L-Hand, left hand; SD, standard deviation; L, Left; R, Right.
**Statistically significant differences.*

hypothesis of an abnormal bilateral cortical activation in the early processes of physiological aging, as described in the literature during the execution of unilateral simple motor tasks, probably due to a disruption of inter-cortical inhibitory circuits.

In our older group, the declined IHI was associated with a reduction of the cortical representation of hand muscle on the right (non-dominant) hemisphere. More specifically, while in the younger group APB and ADM muscles were symmetrically represented on the two motor cortices, in our older subjects the cortical maps resulted smaller on the right hemisphere compared with the left (dominant) one. Moreover, in older subjects, APB cortical representation on the right hemisphere was significantly reduced compared with the younger ones. No significant differences were found between groups for ADM map on the right hemisphere, probably because ADM muscle is physiologically poorly represented on motor cortices even in young people (Menon et al., 2014). As a consequence, physiological changes in hand muscles representations would be more apparent on the APB map.

This finding of a reduced cortical hand muscles representation on the right hemisphere in older subjects recalls the "right hemi-aging model" (Dolcos et al., 2002). This model is based on some evidence, especially in cognitive functions, of a progressive involution of the right cerebral hemisphere during physiological aging, but has never been demonstrated through neurophysiological studies, so far. Moreover, the hypothesis of a right hemisphere involution could explain previous findings of strong hand-dominance with a reduction of the prevalence of left-handedness in older subjects (Gilbert and Wysocki, 1992). Indeed, the progressive decline in left hand muscle representation at the cortical level could lead aging subjects to use preferentially their right hand.

We did not find significant differences in RMTs between the two groups, confirming the results of previous studies (Peinemann et al., 2001; Pitcher et al., 2003; Oliviero et al., 2006; Fujiyama et al., 2012). Thus, it seems that normal aging would not be accompanied by a change in the excitability of the pyramidal cells membrane, suggesting that Na+ and Ca2+ channels of the pyramidal cells' axons are not modified by physiological aging (Ziemann et al., 1996). A previous study showed increased RMTs in older subjects (Rossini et al., 1992). This divergence could be explained by the higher age of the subjects (age-range 51–86 years) and the use of a different (circular) coil. Interestingly, Petitjean and Ko (2013) also found an increased RMT in the older group, but only on the right hemisphere (Petitjean and Ko, 2013). This latter result could be compatible with the "right hemi-aging model."

As expected, the older group had slower hand motor performances. One could attribute such decline to the loss of muscle mass and strength primarily due to the loss of alpha motoneurons and the subsequent denervation of muscle fibers in aging (Doherty et al., 1993). However, these motoneuron losses are seen only after the seventh or eighth decade of age (Tomlinson and Irving, 1997). Thus, earlier changes may be attributable to supraspinal mechanisms. Indeed, Pitcher et al. (2003) demonstrated a greater trial-to-trial variability in MEP amplitudes in older subjects, attributed to a reduced synchronization of I waves in the descending volleys. Moreover, aging is associated with changes in NMDA-receptors function, in particular at the striatal level (Landfield and Pitler, 1984; Disterhoft et al., 1996; Thibault et al., 2001), leading to less efficient striatal processing of cortical information. Akopian and Walsh (2006) demonstrated age-related differences in long-term potentiation, associated with reduced sensitivity to block NMDA receptors. These modulations of corticostriatal functioning in normal aging might thus contribute to age-related deficits in striatum control of movement. These data suggest that normal aging is accompanied by impaired glutamatergic (excitatory) transmission. Moreover, inhibitory circuits would also be involved in the mechanisms of physiological aging since TMS studies demonstrated a reduced efficacy of intra-cortical inhibitory interneurons in older people. Indeed, apart from IHI deficits, age-related decreased short-interval intra-cortical inhibition (SICI) and cortical silent period durations have been shown, illustrating deficits in GABAergic (a and b) transmission (Peinemann et al., 2001; Oliviero et al., 2006; Fujiyama et al., 2012). Thus, all these previous data combined with ours suggest that early processes of physiological aging are accompanied by an imbalance in the regulation of inhibitory and excitatory circuits that might participate to the age-related worsening of motor abilities.

Degradation of motor performance in normal aging would also be related to several other factors, such as corpus callosum functions. Even unilateral movements require the functional integrity of the corpus callosum. Indeed, lesions of the corpus callosum increase the incidence of MM (Cox et al., 2012), which are also often observed in young children who have an immature corpus callosum (Mayston et al., 1999). It is thus not surprising that motor performances and ISP were significantly correlated in our study. This result might be an indirect correlation reflecting deficient corpus callosum connections and/or intrahemispheric inhibition. Indeed, ISP measurements reflect bilateral mechanisms involving activation of transcallosal fibers from one hemisphere to the other and local intra-cortical inhibitory interneurons. Thus, an ISP reduction could be due to dysfunction of one or both of these components. This could explain why right ISP area reduction correlated significantly with motor performance of both hands. If the functional decline within the right hemisphere tends to appear earlier than the left hemisphere, we may hypothesize that the right ISP measurements might be more sensitive to highlight correlations between motor performances and interhemispheric interactions. It would now be of great interest to study older aging populations in order to determine how these intra- and interhemispheric interactions evolve with time.

To conclude, our present findings suggest that early processes of physiological aging are marked by interhemispheric dissociation of motor cortices, characterized, at least in right-handed subjects, by a decline of the non-dominant hemisphere and of transcallosal interactions. In order to better qualify these early age-related changes in motor control, it would be of great interest to explore the dynamics of such changes during skilled motor behavior.

ACKNOWLEDGMENTS

This study was partly supported by the Joint Italian-Israeli laboratory San Raffaele-Weizmann (Italian Ministry of Foreign Affairs).

REFERENCES

Abe, O., Aoki, S., Hayashi, N., Yamada, H., Kunimatsu, A., Mori, H., et al. (2002). Normal aging in the central nervous system: quantitative MR diffusion-tensor analysis. *Neurobiol. Aging* 23, 433–441. doi:10.1016/S0197-4580(01)00318-9

Akopian, G., and Walsh, J. P. (2006). Pre- and postsynaptic contributions to age-related alterations in corticostriatal synaptic plasticity. *Synapse* 60, 223–238. doi:10.1002/syn.20289

Bodwell, J. A., Mahurin, R. K., Waddle, S., Price, R., and Cramer, S. C. (2003). Age and features of movement influence motor overflow. *J. Am. Geriatr. Soc.* 51, 1735–1739. doi:10.1046/j.1532-5415.2003.51557.x

Cabeza, R., Anderson, N. D., Locantore, J. K., and McIntosh, A. R. (2002). Aging gracefully: compensatory brain activity in high-performing older adults. *Neuroimage* 17, 1394–1402. doi:10.1006/nimg.2002.1280

Chen, R., Yung, D., and Li, J. Y. (2003). Organization of ipsilateral excitatory and inhibitory pathways in the human motor cortex. *J. Neurophysiol.* 89, 1256–1264. doi:10.1152/jn.00950.2002

Chieffo, R., Inuggi, A., Straffi, L., Coppi, E., Gonzalez-Rosa, J., Spagnolo, F., et al. (2013). Mapping early changes of cortical motor output after subcortical stroke: a transcranial magnetic stimulation study. *Brain Stimul.* 6, 322–329. doi:10.1016/j.brs.2012.06.003

Cincotta, M., and Ziemann, U. (2008). Neurophysiology of unimanual motor control and mirror movements. *Clin. Neurophysiol.* 119, 744–762. doi:10.1016/j.clinph.2007.11.047

Conover, W. J., and Iman, L. (1982). Analysis of covariance using the rank transformation. *Biometrics* 38, 715–724. doi:10.2307/2530051

Cox, B. C., Cincotta, M., and Espay, A. J. (2012). Mirror movements in movement disorders: a review. *Tremor Other Hyperkinet. Mov. (N. Y.)* 2, tre-02-59-398-1.

Davidson, T., and Tremblay, F. (2013). Age and hemispheric differences in transcallosal inhibition between motor cortices: an ispsilateral silent period study. *BMC Neurosci.* 14:62. doi:10.1186/1471-2202-14-62

Disterhoft, J. F., Thompson, L. T., Moyer, J. R. Jr., and Mogul, D. J. (1996). Calcium-dependent afterhyperpolarization and learning in young and aging hippocampus. *Life Sci.* 59, 413–420. doi:10.1016/0024-3205(96)00320-7

Doherty, T. J., Vandervoort, A. A., and Brown, W. F. (1993). Effects of ageing on the motor unit: a brief review. *Can. J. Appl. Physiol.* 18, 331–358. doi:10.1139/h93-029

Dolcos, F., Rice, H. J., and Cabeza, R. (2002). Hemispheric asymmetry and aging: right hemisphere decline or asymmetry reduction. *Neurosci. Biobehav. Rev.* 26, 819–825. doi:10.1016/S0149-7634(02)00068-4

Ferbert, A., Priori, A., Rothwell, J. C., Day, B. L., Colebatch, J. G., and Marsden, C. D. (1992). Interhemispheric inhibition of the human motor cortex. *J. Physiol.* 453, 525–546.

Fujiyama, H., Hinder, M. R., Schmidt, M. W., Tandonnet, C., Garry, M. I., and Summers, J. J. (2012). Age-related differences in corticomotor excitability and inhibitory processes during a visuomotor RT task. *J. Cogn. Neurosci.* 24, 1253–1263. doi:10.1162/jocn_a_00201

Galléa, C., Popa, T., Billot, S., Méneret, A., Depienne, C., and Roze, E. (2011). Congenital mirror movements: a clue to understanding bimanual motor control. *J. Neurol.* 258, 1911–1919. doi:10.1007/s00415-011-6107-9

Gilbert, A. N., and Wysocki, C. J. (1992). Hand preference and age in the United States. *Neuropsychologia* 30, 601–608. doi:10.1016/0028-3932(92)90065-T

Giovannelli, F., Borgheresi, A., Balestrieri, F., Zaccara, G., Viggiano, M. P., Cincotta, M., et al. (2009). Modulation of interhemispheric inhibition by volitional motor activity: an ipsilateral silent period study. *J. Physiol.* 587, 5393–5410. doi:10.1113/jphysiol.2009.175885

Head, D., Buckner, R. L., Shimony, J. S., Williams, L. E., Akbudak, E., Conturo, T. E., et al. (2004). Differential vulnerability of anterior white matter in nondemented aging with minimal acceleration in dementia of the Alzheimer type: evidence from diffusion tensor imaging. *Cereb. Cortex* 14, 410–423. doi:10.1093/cercor/bhh003

Hoy, K. E., Fitzgerald, P. B., Bradshaw, J. L., Armatas, C. A., and Georgiou-Karistianis, N. (2004). Investigating the cortical origins of motor overflow. *Brain Res. Rev.* 46, 315–327. doi:10.1016/j.brainresrev.2004.07.013

Hutchinson, S., Kobayashi, M., Horkan, C. M., Pascual-Leone, A., Alexander, M. P., and Schlaug, G. (2002). Age-related differences in movement representation. *Neuroimage* 17, 1720–1728. doi:10.1006/nimg.2002.1309

Inuggi, A., Amato, N., Magnani, G., González-Rosa, J. J., Chieffo, R., Comi, G., et al. (2011). Cortical control of unilateral simple movement in healthy aging. *Neurobiol. Aging* 32, 524–538. doi:10.1016/j.neurobiolaging.2009.02.020

Labyt, E., Cassim, F., Szurhaj, W., Bourriez, J. L., and Derambure, P. (2006). Oscillatory cortical activity related to voluntary muscle relaxation: influence of normal aging. *Clin. Neurophysiol.* 117, 1922–1930. doi:10.1016/j.clinph.2006.05.017

Landfield, P. W., and Pitler, T. A. (1984). Prolonged Ca2+-dependent afterhyperpolarizations in hippocampal neurons of aged rats. *Science* 226, 1089–1092. doi:10.1126/science.6494926

Mattay, V. S., Fera, F., Tessitore, A., Hariri, A. R., Das, S., Callicott, J. H., et al. (2002). Neurophysiological correlates of age-related changes in human motor function. *Neurology* 58, 630–635. doi:10.1212/WNL.58.4.630

Mayston, M. J., Harrison, L. M., and Stephens, J. A. (1999). A neurophysiological study of mirror movements in adults and children. *Ann. Neurol.* 45, 583–594. doi:10.1002/1531-8249(199905)45:5<583::AID-ANA6>3.0.CO;2-W

Menon, P., Kiernan, M. C., and Vucic, S. (2014). Cortical excitability differences in hand muscles follow a split-hand pattern in healthy controls. *Muscle Nerve* 49, 836–844. doi:10.1002/mus.24072

Meyer, B. U., Röricht, S., Gräfin von Einsiedel, H., Kruggel, F., and Weindl, A. (1995). Inhibitory and excitatory interhemispheric transfers between motor cortical areas in normal humans and patients with abnormalities of the corpus callosum. *Brain* 118(Pt 2), 429–440. doi:10.1093/brain/118.2.429

Oldfield, R. C. (1971). The assessment and analysis of handedness: the Edinburgh inventory. *Neuropsychologia* 9, 97–113. doi:10.1016/0028-3932(71)90067-4

Oliviero, A., Profice, P., Tonali, P. A., Pilato, F., Saturno, E., Dileone, M., et al. (2006). Effects of aging on motor cortex excitability. *Neurosci. Res.* 55, 74–77. doi:10.1016/j.neures.2006.02.002

Ota, M., Obata, T., Akine, Y., Ito, H., Ikehira, H., Asada, T., et al. (2006). Age-related degeneration of corpus callosum measured with diffusion tensor imaging. *Neuroimage* 31, 1445–1452. doi:10.1016/j.neuroimage.2006.02.008

Oxford Grice, K., Vogel, K. A., Le, V., Mitchell, A., Muniz, S., and Vollmer, M. A. (2003). Adult norms for a commercially available Nine Hole Peg Test for finger dexterity. *Am. J. Occup. Ther.* 57, 570–573. doi:10.5014/ajot.57.5.570

Peinemann, A., Lehner, C., Conrad, B., and Siebner, H. R. (2001). Age-related decrease in paired-pulse intracortical inhibition in the human primary motor cortex. *Neurosci. Lett.* 313, 33–36. doi:10.1016/S0304-3940(01)02239-X

Petitjean, M., and Ko, J. Y. (2013). An age-related change in the ipsilateral silent period of a small hand muscle. *Clin. Neurophysiol.* 124, 346–353. doi:10.1016/j.clinph.2012.07.006

Pfefferbaum, A., and Sullivan, E. V. (2003). Increased brain white matter diffusivity in normal adult aging: relationship to anisotropy and partial voluming. *Magn. Reson. Med.* 49, 953–961. doi:10.1002/mrm.10452

Pfefferbaum, A., Sullivan, E. V., Hedehus, M., Lim, K. O., Adalsteinsson, E., and Moseley, M. (2000). Age-related decline in brain white matter anisotropy measured with spatially corrected echo-planar diffusion tensor imaging. *Magn. Reson. Med.* 44, 259–268. doi:10.1002/1522-2594(200008)44:2<259::AID-MRM13>3.0.CO;2-6

Pitcher, J. B., Ogston, K. M., and Miles, T. S. (2003). Age and sex differences in human motor cortex input-output characteristics. *J. Physiol.* 546, 605–613. doi:10.1113/jphysiol.2002.029454

Riecker, A., Groschel, K., Ackermann, H., Steinbrink, C., Witte, O., and Kastrup, A. (2006). Functional significance of age-related differences in motor activation patterns. *Neuroimage* 32, 1345–1354. doi:10.1016/j.neuroimage.2006.05.021

Rossi, S., Hallett, M., Rossini, P. M., Pascual-Leone, A., and Safety of TMS Consensus Group. (2009). Safety, ethical considerations, and application guidelines for the use of transcranial magnetic stimulation in clinical practice and research. *Clin. Neurophysiol.* 120, 2008–2039. doi:10.1016/j.clinph.2009.08.016

Rossini, P. M., Desiato, M. T., and Caramia, M. D. (1992). Age-related changes of motor evoked potentials in healthy humans: non-invasive evaluation of central and peripheral motor tracts excitability and conductivity. *Brain Res.* 593, 14–19. doi:10.1016/0006-8993(92)91256-E

Rovaris, M., Iannucci, G., Cercignani, M., Sormani, M. P., De Stefano, N., Gerevini, S., et al. (2003). Age-related changes in conventional, magnetization transfer, and diffusion-tensor MR imaging findings: study with whole-brain tissue histogram analysis. *Radiology* 227, 731–738. doi:10.1148/radiol.2273020721

Sailer, A., Dichgans, J., and Gerloff, C. (2000). The influence of normal aging on the cortical processing of a simple motor task. *Neurology* 55, 979–985. doi:10.1212/WNL.55.7.979

Spagnolo, F., Coppi, E., Chieffo, R., Straffi, L., Fichera, M., Nuara, A., et al. (2013). Interhemispheric balance in Parkinson's disease: a transcranial magnetic stimulation study. *Brain Stimul.* 6, 892–897. doi:10.1016/j.brs.2013.05.004

Talelli, P., Waddingham, W., Ewas, A., Rothwell, J. C., and Ward, N. S. (2008). The effect of age on task-related modulation of interhemispheric balance. *Exp. Brain Res.* 186, 59–66. doi:10.1007/s00221-007-1205-8

Thibault, O., Hadley, R., and Landfield, P. W. (2001). Elevated postsynaptic [Ca2+]i and L-type calcium channel activity in aged hippocampal neurons: relationship to impaired synaptic plasticity. *J. Neurosci.* 15, 9744–9756.

Tomlinson, B. E., and Irving, D. (1997). The numbers of limb motor neurons in the human lumbosacral cord throughout life. *J. Neurol. Sci.* 34, 213–219. doi:10.1016/0022-510X(77)90069-7

Trompetto, C., Bove, M., Marinelli, L., Avanzino, L., Buccolieri, A., and Abbruzzese, G. (2004). Suppression of the transcallosal motor output: a transcranial magnetic stimulation study in healthy subjects. *Exp. Brain Res.* 158, 133–140. doi:10.1007/s00221-004-1881-6

Vallesi, A., McIntosh, A. R., Kovacevic, N., Chan, S. C., and Stuss, D. T. (2010). Age effects on the asymmetry of the motor system: evidence from cortical oscillatory activity. *Biol. Psychol.* 85, 213–218. doi:10.1016/j.biopsycho.2010.07.003

Ward, N. S., Swayne, O. B., and Newton, J. M. (2007). Age-dependent changes in the neural correlates of force modulation: an fMRI study. *Neurobiol. Aging* 29, 1434–1446. doi:10.1016/j.neurobiolaging.2007.04.017

Zarei, M., Johansen-Berg, H., Smith, S., Ciccarelli, O., Thompson, A. J., and Matthews, P. M. (2006). Functional anatomy of interhemispheric cortical connections in the human brain. *J. Anat.* 209, 311–320. doi:10.1111/j.1469-7580.2006.00615.x

Ziemann, U., Lonnecker, S., Steinhoff, B. J., and Paulus, W. (1996). Effects of antiepileptic drugs on motor cortex excitability in humans: a transcranial magnetic stimulation study. *Ann. Neurol.* 40, 367–378. doi:10.1002/ana.410400306

3

Motor variability during sustained contractions increases with cognitive demand in older adults

Marnie L. Vanden Noven[1], Hugo M. Pereira[1], Tejin Yoon[1], Alyssa A. Stevens[1], Kristy A. Nielson[2] and Sandra K. Hunter[1]*

[1] *Exercise Science Program, Department of Physical Therapy, Marquette University, Milwaukee, WI, USA*
[2] *Department of Psychology, Marquette University, Milwaukee, WI, USA*

Edited by:
Brian C. Clark, Ohio University, USA

Reviewed by:
S. Lee Hong, Ohio University, USA
Shinichi Amano, Ohio University, USA

***Correspondence:**
Sandra K. Hunter, Exercise Science Program, Department of Physical Therapy, Marquette University, PO Box 1881, Milwaukee, WI, USA
e-mail: Sandra.Hunter@marquette.edu

To expose cortical involvement in age-related changes in motor performance, we compared steadiness (force fluctuations) and fatigability of submaximal isometric contractions with the ankle dorsiflexor muscles in older and young adults and with varying levels of cognitive demand imposed. Sixteen young (20.4 ± 2.1 year: 8 men, 9 women) and 17 older adults (68.8 ± 4.4 years: 9 men, 8 women) attended three sessions and performed a 40 s isometric contraction at 5% maximal voluntary contraction (MVC) force followed by an isometric contraction at 30% MVC until task failure. The cognitive demand required during the submaximal contractions in each session differed as follows: (1) *high-cognitive demand* session where difficult mental math was imposed (counting backward by 13 from a 4-digit number); (2) *low-cognitive demand* session which involved simple mental math (counting backward by 1); and (3) *control session* with no mental math. Anxiety was elevated during the high-cognitive demand session compared with other sessions for both age groups but more so for the older adults than young adults ($p < 0.05$). Older adults had larger force fluctuations than young adults during: (1) the 5% MVC task as cognitive demand increased ($p = 0.007$), and (2) the fatiguing contraction for all sessions ($p = 0.002$). Time to task failure did not differ between sessions or age groups ($p > 0.05$), but the variability between sessions (standard deviation of three sessions) was greater for older adults than young (2.02 ± 1.05 vs. 1.25 ± 0.51 min, $p < 0.05$). Thus, variability in lower limb motor performance for low- and moderate-force isometric tasks increased with age and was exacerbated when cognitive demand was imposed, and may be related to modulation of synergist and antagonist muscles and an altered neural strategy with age originating from central sources. These data have significant implications for cognitively demanding low-force motor tasks that are relevant to functional and ergonomic in an aging workforce.

Keywords: arousal, ankle dorsiflexor muscles, muscle fatigue, age, motor variability, steadiness, aging, stress

INTRODUCTION

Aging results in marked declines in both motor performance and cognitive function. For example, older adults are weaker and less steady (i.e., they exhibit greater fluctuations in force around a target force) than young adults (Enoka et al., 2003; Hunter et al., 2008). Decreased steadiness with age is greatest during low-intensity isometric contractions in lower and upper extremity muscles (Enoka et al., 2003; Tracy, 2007; Marmon et al., 2011) probably due to age-related changes in inputs to the motoneurone pool (Barry et al., 2007). Cognitive impairment can also be marked but subtle and often subclinical in early stages of cognitive dysfunction (Chen et al., 2001; Morris et al., 2001; Aine et al., 2011); it is often observed as degradation in short-term memory and executive function resulting in a decreased ability to perform daily tasks that are dependent upon memory-related abilities (Artero et al., 2001; Morris et al., 2001; Farias et al., 2012), including planning and decision-making in lower limb activities such as gait (Yogev-Seligmann et al., 2008). Age-related declines in motor and cognitive function are usually studied separately but are often performed simultaneously in daily tasks. The current study assessed motor function with a focus on steadiness and muscle fatigability in young and older adults while they were presented with low and high levels of cognitive demand.

In young adults, cognitive performance declines and force fluctuations increase when a cognitive task is imposed (reaction time) during sustained isometric tasks with hand muscles (Lorist et al., 2002; Zijdewind et al., 2006); however, force fluctuations were affected more during the isometric fatiguing contractions than during a 5% maximal voluntary contraction (MVC) non-fatiguing contraction (Lorist et al., 2002). We also previously found that steadiness of the elbow flexor muscles declined (increased force fluctuations) and time to failure of a sustained 20% MVC submaximal task was reduced (increased fatigability) in young adults when simultaneously performing a demanding cognitive task ('high-cognitive demand') that increased anxiety (counting backwards by 13). Accordingly, heart rate and blood pressure, which are indices of increased sympathetic activity with arousal (Kajantie and Phillips, 2006), were elevated during the "high-cognitive demand" session compared with control (Yoon et al., 2009; Keller-Ross et al., 2014a). Individuals who were weaker (primarily the women) showed the largest decrement in time to task failure when the stressful cognitive task was imposed during the fatiguing contraction (Yoon et al., 2009; Keller-Ross et al., 2014a). Older adults are typically weaker than young adults, and older women weaker than older men for upper and lower limb muscles (Galganski et al., 1993; Laidlaw et al., 2000; Tracy and Enoka, 2002), possibly increasing susceptibility to increased fatigability when a cognitive task is imposed. However, it is not known whether fatigability with increased cognitive demand is exacerbated with advanced age. Furthermore, the effects of increased cognitive demand on lower limb fatigability and steadiness in young or older adults are not known.

Initial evidence would suggest that age-related decrements in motor function of the upper limb (e.g., reduced steadiness) become larger with greater cortical involvement of non-motor centers (Voelcker-Rehage et al., 2006; Voelcker-Rehage and Alberts, 2007; Fraser et al., 2010) and may increase between- and within-participant variability particularly in older adults (Enoka et al., 2003; Sosnoff and Newell, 2006). Older adults display greater between- and within-participant variability than young in activation of supraspinal centers during maximal contractions with the upper limb (Hunter et al., 2008) indicating that variability within cortical motor areas is larger with advanced age. Increased cognitive involvement, particularly with tasks that tax attentional resources and that require the use of short-term memory or executive function, may contribute further to age-related variability in motor performance for older adults during functional tasks (Voelcker-Rehage et al., 2006; Yogev-Seligmann et al., 2008; Sommervoll et al., 2011).

Increased cognitive involvement however, can increase anxiety and stress levels (e.g., Noteboom et al., 2001), which may further decrease steadiness of upper limb muscles in older adults compared with young. Force fluctuations, for example, increased for older adults more than young when exposed to a noxious stressor (unpredictable electrical stimulation to the hand) prior to performing the pinch grip task (Christou et al., 2004). The increased force fluctuations therefore, could be due to age-related changes in monoaminergic drive modulating inputs to the motoneurone pool (Barry et al., 2007). A novel aspect of this current study is that we varied the level of cognitive demand administered simultaneously during motor task of the lower limbs to determine its influence on lower limb fatigability and steadiness and any accompanying changes in anxiety and stress.

The purpose of this study was to compare both the amplitude of force fluctuations (steadiness) and time to task failure (fatigability) for low-to-moderate-force isometric contractions in the presence and absence of varying levels of cognitive demand in young and older adults. Participants were exposed to two different levels of cognitive load, low- and high-cognitive demand while performing a motor task with the ankle dorsiflexor muscles, which are muscles that play a functional role controlling the position of the foot during walking and while maintaining balance. We *hypothesized* that older adults would show greater reductions in time to task failure and greater force fluctuations than young as cognitive demand increased. We also compared variability of fatigability between and within young and older adults with increased cognitive demand. We *hypothesized* that as cognitive demand increased, older adults would exhibit both greater between- and within-participant variability in fatigability. To understand the perceived and physiological arousal responses with the varying levels of cognitive demand in young and older adults, during each session we quantified perceived levels of exertion, stress and anxiety as well as heart rate and blood pressure.

MATERIALS AND METHODS

Sixteen young adults (8 men, 8 women; 18–24 years) and 17 older adults (9 men, 8 women; 62–79 years) participated in the study (see **Table 1** for physical characteristics). All participants were healthy with no known neurological or cardiovascular diseases, had controlled blood pressure and were naïve to the protocol. Six of the older adults were on medication to control blood pressure. Both young and older adults had low-to-moderate levels of anxiety (trait) according to the State-Trait Anxiety Inventory (STAI) (Spielberger et al., 1970) and reported no history of current mental or psychological pathology, including anxiety or depressive disorders. Participants were right-leg dominant (0.81 ± 0.40 vs. 0.80 ± 0.54 for young and older adults, respectively, with a ratio of 1 indicating complete dominance of the right leg) (Oldfield, 1971). The physical activity level for each participant was assessed with a questionnaire that estimated the relative kilocalorie expenditure of energy per week (Kriska and Bennett, 1992). Prior to participation, each participant provided informed consent, and the protocol was approved by the Institutional Review Board at Marquette University.

Each participant reported to the laboratory on four occasions to perform a protocol that involved a fatiguing contraction with the left ankle dorsiflexor muscles: once for a familiarization session and three experimental sessions (*control, low-cognitive demand,* and *high-cognitive demand*), with each experimental session being at least 5 days apart. During the low-cognitive demand and high-cognitive demand sessions, each participant performed either a simple mental math task (low-cognitive demand session) or difficult mental math task (high-cognitive demand session) at rest, and also while performing isometric contractions at 5% maximum voluntary contraction (MVC) force (40 s duration) and a 30% MVC for as long as possible until task failure (**Figure 1**). During the control session, each participant performed the motor tasks without performing any mental math. Session order was counterbalanced among participants within each age group.

MECHANICAL RECORDING OF FORCE

Each participant was seated upright in an adjustable chair (Biodex Medical Systems, NY, USA) with the hips and knees at 90° of flexion. The setup is similar to that described elsewhere (Griffith et al., 2010). In brief, the left foot rested on a footplate in a custom made dynamometer to measure forces of the lower leg, with the ankle in a neutral position (0° dorsiflexion). The foot was secured to the footplate via a strap placed over the anterior aspect of the ankle and another strap placed 1–2 cm proximal to the metatarsophalangeal joint. Isometric force of the dorsiflexor muscles was recorded using a force transducer (Transducer Techniques, Temecula, CA, USA) and recorded online at 500 Hz using a Power 1401 analog-to-digital (A/D) converter and Spike2 software

Table 1 | Demographic and physical characteristics and age group means (±SD) for control, low-cognitive demand (low-CD), and high-cognitive demand (high-CD) sessions.

Variable	Session	Young	Older
Number of participants		16	17
Age (years)		20.4 ± 2.1	68.8 ± 4.4[a]
Height (cm)		168.9 ± 23.6	167.5 ± 11.3
Women age (years)		19.3 ± 1.5	68.4 ± 3.6[a]
Men age (years)		21.5 ± 2.0	69.2 ± 4.9[a]
Weight (kg)		74.4 ± 27.9	77.8 ± 15.2
Physical activity (METS hours per week)		59.5 ± 38.3	22.0 ± 21.8[a]
Baseline trait STAI scores		36.4 ± 7	34.8 ± 7.3
Baseline state STAI scores		26.0 ± 6.7	26.2 ± 5.3
MVC torque (Nm)	Control	22.4 ± 6.9	19.1 ± 6.6
	Low-CD	22.2 ± 6.6	18.3 ± 5.8
	High-CD	22.8 ± 7.7	18.7 ± 6.3
	Total	22.5 ± 7.0	18.7 ± 6.1[a]
MVC torque recovery (% of initial)	Control	96.3 ± 7.4	97.9 ± 6.8
	Low-CD	95.4 ± 3.7	93.2 ± 8.5
	High-CD	94.8 ± 3.9	94.7 ± 5.5
	Total	96.2 ± 7.4	97.6 ± 6.5
Time to task failure (min)	Control	6.1 ± 2.2	8.0 ± 3.2
	Low-CD	6.1 ± 2.0	7.6 ± 3.1
	High-CD	7.1 ± 2.5	8.7 ± 3.8
	Total	6.4 ± 2.2	8.1 ± 3.4
30% MVC CV of torque (%)	Control	4.5 ± 1.2	6.0 ± 3.0
	Low-CD	4.5 ± 0.8	7.2 ± 4.1
	High-CD	4.6 ± 2.7	6.8 ± 2.3
	Total	4.5 ± 1.0	6.7 ± 3.2[a]
TA EMG[a] (% MVC)	Control	23.5 ± 5.6	29.1 ± 6.0
	Low-CD	23.5 ± 6.2	27.2 ± 4.7
	High-CD	24.1 ± 4.8	28.7 ± 8.4
	Total	23.7 ± 4.3	28.3 ± 5.9[a]
TA EMG bursting activity (bursts per min)	Control	10.3 ± 9.7	5.7 ± 5.7
	Low-CD	11.5 ± 10.6	9.0 ± 9.2
	High-CD	9.4 ± 9.6	7.7 ± 7.6
	Total	10.4 ± 9.8	7.4 ± 7.6
Soleus EMG (% MVC)	Control	20.3 ± 9.6	28.4 ± 14.2
	Low-CD	19.2 ± 5.3	28.8 ± 12.2
	High-CD	17.4 ± 6.1	30.0 ± 13.9
	Total	18.9 ± 7.2	29.1 ± 13.2[a]
Gastrocnemius EMG (% MVC)	Control	26.7 ± 15.8	32.9 ± 13.8
	Low-CD	26.3 ± 9.9	30.6 ± 11.8
	High-CD	21.1 ± 6.1	29.9 ± 13.8
	Total	24.2 ± 11.3	31.1 ± 12.9[a]
Rectus femoris EMG (% MVC)	Control	5.4 ± 3.8	17.3 ± 22.0
	Low-CD	5.3 ± 4.2	18.5 ± 22.9
	High-CD	5.0 ± 3.0	15.8 ± 20.8
	Total	5.8 ± 3.8	17.2 ± 21.5[a]

(Continued)

[a]*Variables reaching statistical significance for main effect of age ($p < 0.05$). STAI, State-Trait Anxiety Index; MVC, maximal voluntary contraction; TA, tibialis anterior; EMG, electromyography; METS hours per week = metabolic equivalents hours per week.*

[Cambridge Electronics Design (CED), Cambridge, UK]. Force displayed on a 19-inch monitor was located at eye level 1.5 m in front of the participant. Each participant was asked to trace a horizontal cursor placed in the middle of the screen with the force signal as it appeared on the screen from the right side of the monitor.

ELECTRICAL RECORDINGS

Whole muscle electromyographic (EMG) signals of the tibialis anterior, medial head of the gastrocnemius, soleus, and rectus femoris were recorded using bipolar surface electrodes (sintered pellet Ag-AgCl, 8 mm diameter, 20 mm between electrodes) taped to the skin over the belly of each muscle. Reference electrodes were placed on the patella. The recording electrodes on each muscle were placed in line with the muscle fibers and in accordance with locations recommended by the European Recommendations for Surface Electromyography (Hermens et al., 2000). The EMG signals were amplified (1,000 ×) and band-pass filtered (13–1,000 Hz) with Coulbourn bioamplifiers (Coulbourn Instruments, Allentown, PA, USA) prior to being recorded directly to a computer using the Power 1401 and Spike2 software (CED). The EMG signals were digitized at 2,000 samples/s and analyzed offline using Spike2 software (CED).

CARDIOVASCULAR MEASUREMENTS

Heart rate and blood pressure were monitored during submaximal and fatiguing contractions and periods of rest or mental math with an automated beat-by-beat blood pressure monitor (Finapress 2300, Datex-Ohmeda, Louisville, CO, USA). The blood pressure cuff was placed around the middle finger of the left hand, and the arm was placed on a platform to maintain the hand at heart level. Blood pressure was sampled at 500 samples/s and collected online to PC using Spike2 software (CED).

COGNITIVE ASSESSMENT OF ANXIETY AND STRESS

Cognitive levels of anxiety and stress were assessed throughout the protocol using a visual analog scale (VAS) (Yoon et al., 2009) and the *state* portion of the STAI questionnaire (Spielberger et al., 1970). Each VAS (one for anxiety and another for stress) had a 10-cm line anchored at the far left by "none" and at the far right by "as bad as it could be." The right anchor corresponded to the most stressful or most anxious moment in the life of the

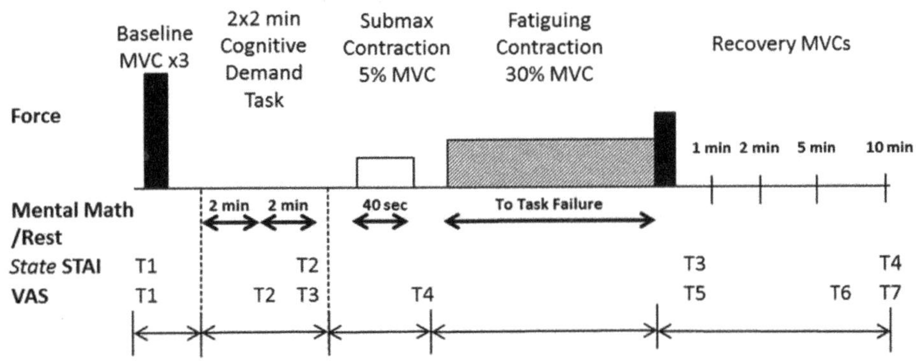

FIGURE 1 | Experimental protocol. The top panel illustrates in order the tasks performed by each participant with the ankle dorsiflexor muscles. Maximal voluntary contractions (MVC) (solid bars) were performed at the beginning of the experimental session and during recovery (immediately after the fatiguing contraction and at 1, 2, 5, and 10 min of recovery). The fatiguing contraction (30% MVC), symbolized by the hatched rectangle, was performed until task failure by each participant. The bottom panels indicate when the State-Trait Anxiety Inventory (STAI; four times) was performed and the Visual Analog Scale (VAS) for anxiety and stress were recorded (at seven time points, T1–T7). The schematic is not to scale for time or force.

participant. Anxiety was defined as the participant's negative feelings regarding the immediate future, whereas stress represented the physical changes (e.g., increase in heart rate and perspiration) occurring during the test perceived by the participant that were above and beyond the expectation for their level of exertion (Christou et al., 2004). VAS for anxiety and stress were recorded at seven time points (T1–T7) during the protocol: one baseline assessment before intended arousal (T1); during the rest period after each 2 × 2-min bout of mental math (low-cognitive demand or high-cognitive demand session) or quiet rest (control session) (T2, T3); immediately after the 5% MVC submaximal contraction (T4); immediately after the fatiguing contraction/MVC (T5); and 5 and 10 min after the fatiguing contraction (T6, T7) (**Figure 1**).

The *state* portion of the STAI-questionnaire consisted of 20 statements that required a response on a four-point Likert-type scale. Baseline *trait* and *state* assessments were conducted during the familiarization session. There was no significant difference between young and older adults in baseline *trait* STAI scores ($p = 0.54$) or baseline *state* STAI scores taken during the familiarization session ($p = 0.66$) (**Table 1**). *State* STAI assessments were also conducted at four different time points during the experimental protocol: baseline assessment before arousal; after 2 × 2-min bouts of quiet sitting (control session) or mental math (low-cognitive demand and high-cognitive demand sessions); immediately after the fatiguing contraction/MVC; and 10 min after completion of the fatiguing contraction (**Figure 1**).

COGNITIVE DEMAND CONDITIONS

Difficult mental math is an established psychosocial technique used to induce cognitive demand and increase levels of anxiety (Kajantie and Phillips, 2006) and was used for the *high-cognitive demand task* (Noteboom et al., 2001). Each participant performed serial subtraction from a four-digit number by 13 with one response required every 3 s (Noteboom et al., 2001). If the participant made an error in serial subtraction or was unable to provide the correct answer within 3 s, they were asked to restart the mental math from the first number in the series. After three errors, the investigator asked the participant to begin with a new four-digit number. The *simple mental math task*, performed during the *low-cognitive demand session*, was designed to increase cognitive demand above control without elevating arousal. Participants serially counted backward by 1's from 50 to 0 at a slow, even pace. If the participant made an error in counting, they were asked to restart counting from 50. During the *control session*, participants were instructed to rest quietly during the 2 × 2-min bouts, 5% MVC submaximal contraction (40 s) and 30% MVC fatiguing contraction. During the low-cognitive demand and high-cognitive demand sessions, participants performed the mental math task while at rest (2 × 2-min bouts), and then continuously during the 5% MVC submaximal contraction and 30% MVC fatiguing contraction until task failure.

EXPERIMENTAL PROTOCOL

The protocol for each experimental session (control, low-cognitive demand, and high-cognitive demand sessions) involved procedures in the following order: (1) MVCs of the ankle dorsiflexor, ankle plantarflexor, and knee extensor muscles; (2) assessment of cognitive and physiological arousal before and after 2 × 2-min bout of either quiet sitting (control session), simple mental math (low-cognitive demand session), or difficult mental math (high-cognitive demand session); (3) performance of one submaximal isometric contraction at 5% MVC force sustained for 40 s with assessment of cognitive and physiological arousal immediately following the contraction; (4) a submaximal fatiguing isometric contraction at 30% MVC force sustained until task failure; and (5) recovery MVCs immediately following the fatiguing contraction, and at 1, 2, 5, and 10 min recovery with assessment of anxiety and stress levels (**Figure 1**).

Participants performed two MVCs of the knee extensor and plantar flexor muscles each at the beginning of each experimental session in order to obtain peak EMG for the gastrocnemius, soleus, and rectus femoris muscles. Participants rested for 60 s between each trial. For both muscle groups, MVCs were performed with the participant seated in the same position as used for testing the ankle dorsiflexors muscles (described above). The aim was to obtain peak EMG values for each muscle group; forces were not recorded during knee extension and plantar flexion. Each participant was asked to push as hard as possible against an immovable restraint for 3–4 s to activate either the knee extensor or ankle plantar flexor muscles. For the knee extensor muscles, manual resistance was applied to the distal leg (just above the lateral malleolus) so that the lower leg was restrained at 90° of flexion while the participant performed maximal knee extension. For the ankle plantar flexor muscles, the foot of each participant was placed on the footplate, and vertical movement was minimized during each MVC by a block that eliminated movement of the footplate. The MVC trial with the greatest amount of EMG activity was used to normalize the EMG recordings of the rectus femoris, medial head of the gastrocnemius, and soleus muscles during the submaximal contractions.

Participants performed three to four MVC trials with the ankle dorsiflexors while their foot was attached to the footplate. Each participant was asked to dorsiflex as hard as possible for 3–4 s. Participants were given visual feedback on a display monitor and strong verbal encouragement to achieve and maintain maximal force. Participants rested for 60 s between each trial. If the peak force achieved for two of the first three trials was not within 5% of each other, additional trials were performed until this criterion was met. The greatest MVC force achieved with the ankle dorsiflexor muscles was used as the reference to calculate the target level for both the submaximal contractions at 5% MVC and the fatiguing contraction at 30% MVC. The MVC with the greatest amount of EMG activity was used to normalize the EMG recordings during the fatiguing contractions of the tibialis anterior muscle. MVCs of the ankle dorsiflexor muscles were also performed during recovery (**Figure 1**).

A fatiguing contraction was performed with the ankle dorsiflexor muscles at 30% MVC during each experimental session. Each participant was asked to trace a horizontal cursor with the force signal as it appeared from the right side of the monitor in order to match the vertical target force as displayed on the screen. Participants were encouraged to sustain the force for as long as possible. The fatiguing contraction was terminated when the force declined by 10% of the target force. To minimize the influence of transient fluctuations in motor output on the criteria for task failure, the task was terminated only after force fell below the predetermined threshold for 2.5 s of a 5 s interval. Participants were not informed of their time to task failure.

Rating of perceived exertion (RPE) was assessed using the modified Borg 10-point scale (Borg, 1982). Each participant was instructed to focus their assessment of exertion on the ankle muscles performing the fatiguing task. The scale was anchored so that 0 represented the resting state and 10 corresponded to the strongest contraction that the ankle muscles could perform. The RPE was recorded at the beginning of the fatiguing contraction and every minute thereafter until task failure. In order to obtain RPE while the participant was performing mental math during the low-cognitive demand and high-cognitive demand sessions, the participant was interrupted and asked to report their RPE. After reporting their RPE, participants resumed the mental math task of serial counting from 50 to 0 during the low-cognitive demand session or serial subtraction using a new four-digit number during the high-cognitive demand session.

DATA ANALYSIS

All data collected during the experiments were recorded online using a Power 1401 A/D converter and analyzed using Spike2 (CED). The MVC torque was quantified as the average value over a 0.5-s interval that was centered about the peak. The torque for the MVCs, submaximal and fatiguing contractions was calculated as the product of force and the distance between the ankle joint and the point at which the ankle was attached to the force transducer. The maximal EMG for each muscle was determined as the root mean square (RMS) value over a 0.5-s interval about the same peak interval of the MVC torque measurement. The maximal EMG value of the involved muscles was then used to normalize the RMS EMG values recorded during the 5% MVC task and the fatiguing contraction at 30% MVC. The RMS value of the 5% MVC task was averaged for each muscle over the middle 30 s of the 40 s contraction for the tibialis anterior, medial gastrocnemius, soleus, and rectus femoris. During the fatiguing contraction, the RMS EMG signal for each muscle was quantified at the following time intervals: the first 30 s; 15 s on both sides of 25, 50, and 75% of time to task failure; and the last 30 s of the task duration. The EMG activity of each muscle was normalized to the RMS EMG value obtained during the MVC for each respective muscle.

To quantify the bursts of EMG activity of the tibialis anterior during the fatiguing contraction at 30% MVC, the EMG signal was first rectified, smoothed (averages of 1 s duration, 500 data points), and then differentiated over 0.25 s averages. The differentiated signal represents the rate of change and was used to identify rapid changes in the rectified and smoothed EMG signal. The threshold for establishing if a burst of EMG had occurred was determined by first finding the minimum standard deviation (SD) of the differentiated EMG during the fatiguing contraction using a 30 s moving window; the threshold was then defined as the mean + 3 SD of the minimum differentiated signal. The minimal burst duration was 0.1 s. The EMG bursting activity (bursts/min) was quantified for five continuous intervals of 20% of the time to task failure.

The amplitude of the force fluctuations was quantified as the coefficient of variation (CV) ($CV = SD/mean \times 100$) for the 5% MVC task and 30% MVC fatiguing contraction. The fluctuations in torque during the 5% MVC task were quantified over the middle 30 s of the 40 s contraction. For the fatiguing contraction at 30% MVC, the fluctuations in torque were quantified for five continuous intervals of 20% of the time to task failure (between 0 and 100%).

Mean arterial pressure (MAP) and heart rate were evaluated only on participants not currently taking blood pressure medications with normal blood pressure. MAP and heart rate recorded during the fatiguing contraction at 30% MVC were analyzed by comparing ~15 s averages at 25% intervals throughout the fatiguing contraction; during the 5% MVC submaximal contraction they were quantified over the middle 30 s of the 40 s contraction. For each interval, the blood pressure signal was analyzed for the mean peaks [systolic blood pressure (SBP)], mean troughs [diastolic blood pressure (DBP)], and number of pulses per second (multiplied by 60 to determine heart rate). MAP was calculated for each epoch with the following equation: $MAP = DBP + 1/3 (SBP - DBP)$. Rate-pressure product (RPP) was calculated as the product of heart rate and MAP for the equivalent time periods as stated above.

STATISTICAL ANALYSIS

Data were reported as means ± SD within the text, and displayed as means ± SE in the figures. Analyses of variances (ANOVA) models were used to compare the various dependent variables. Specifically, separate ANOVAs with repeated measures on session (control, low-cognitive demand, and high-cognitive demand), and with age (young and old) and sex (men and women) as fixed factors, were used to compare MVC torque and STAI (state) and VAS for anxiety and stress at baseline, MAP, heart rate, CV of torque, and EMG activity during the 5% MVC task, error rates (only low- and high-cognitive demand sessions included for error rate analysis) during the fatiguing contraction and the time to task failure of the fatiguing contraction. This ANOVA model was also used to compare the SD of the time to failure from the three sessions, and the SD of the mean CV of torque during the fatiguing contraction obtained from the three sessions. ANOVAs with repeated measures on session and time, and with age and sex as fixed factors, were used to compare VAS for stress and anxiety, STAI (state) and MVC torques throughout the sessions, i.e., before and after the fatiguing contraction (see **Figure 1** for time points). ANOVAs with repeated measures on session and time (five time points for each: see Data Analysis), and with age and sex as fixed factors, were used to compare the following variables during the fatiguing contraction: CV of torque, RMS EMG, EMG bursting activity, heart rate, MAP, RPP, and RPE. *Post hoc* analyses (Tukey) were used to test for differences among pairs when appropriate. Univariate ANOVAs were used to compare young and old men and women for the following variables: physical characteristics (age, height, and weight), physical activity level, handedness, and STAI (trait). The strength of an association is reported as the Pearson product–moment correlation coefficient (r). The statistical significance adopted was 5% ($p < 0.05$) and all analysis were performed in IBM Statistical Package for Social Sciences (SPSS) version 19.

RESULTS

Young and older adults were of similar height and weight ($p > 0.05$) but the older adults were less active than the young ($p < 0.05$). See **Table 1** for subject characteristics.

MVC TORQUE

At baseline, young adults were stronger than the older adults (22.5 ± 7 vs. 18.7 ± 6.1 Nm, respectively: age effect, $p = 0.005$) and men were stronger than women (sex effect, $p = 0.0001$) on all 3 days of testing, with no interaction between sex and age (age × sex, $p = 0.69$) (**Table 1**). The relative reduction (%) in MVC torque after the fatiguing contraction was similar across sessions (session effect, $p = 0.98$), and similar for young and older adults (session × age, $p = 0.26$). During recovery, MVC torque increased to near baseline levels within 10 min of completing the fatiguing contraction similarly for young and older adults across all sessions (session × age, $p = 0.57$) (**Table 1**). Furthermore, at the end of the recovery period, the MVC (% of baseline) was similar for young and older men and women ($p > 0.05$).

ANXIETY AND STRESS LEVELS

State STAI scores

Baseline *state* STAI scores taken at the beginning of each experimental session were similar for young and older men and women (age effect, $p = 0.88$; sex effect, $p = 0.57$) (**Table 1**). *State* STAI scores taken after exposure to the 2 × 2 min of difficult mental math were higher during the high-cognitive demand session compared with the control and low-cognitive demand sessions (control, 25.1 ± 6.6; low-cognitive demand, 30.4 ± 10.0; high-cognitive demand, 42.8 ± 13.1; and session effect, $p = 0.0001$) and immediately after the fatiguing contraction (control, 36.2 ± 9.2; low-cognitive demand, 38 ± 9; high-cognitive demand, 50.4 ± 13.8; and session effect, $p = 0.0001$). There was no difference between young and older adults across all three session after completing the fatiguing contraction (age effect, $p = 0.72$). Older adults however, demonstrated higher *state* STAI scores than young adults after the fatiguing contraction when exposed to the high-cognitive demand (session × time × age, $p = 0.02$).

VAS for stress and anxiety

Visual analog scale scores for stress and anxiety were similar at baseline for young and older adults, and men and women ($p > 0.05$, **Figure 2**). *Anxiety VAS* was significantly higher during the high-cognitive demand session compared to the control and low-cognitive demand sessions (session × time, $p = 0.0001$), and increased more for older adults than young over time (time × age, $p = 0.01$) (**Figure 2A**). There were no other interactions. *Stress VAS* scores were significantly higher for older adults than young during the high-cognitive demand session compared with the control and low-cognitive demand sessions (session × age, $p = 0.02$, **Figure 2B**) and for older adults than young over time (time × age, $p = 0.001$). There were no main effects of sex and no other interactions.

LOW-INTENSITY SUSTAINED CONTRACTION (5% MVC)

Fluctuations in torque

Older adults had greater fluctuations in torque (CV of torque) compared with young across all three sessions (age effect, $p = 0.007$) (**Figure 3**) and women had higher fluctuations in torque than men (sex effect, $p = 0.001$). On average, the older adults had a linear increase in fluctuations in torque as cognitive demand increased while young adults showed no change (linear interaction for session × age, $p = 0.04$, **Figure 3A**). Women demonstrated higher force fluctuations than men ($p = 0.001$), but there were no other interactions ($p > 0.05$).

MAP and heart rate

Cardiovascular measures were analyzed for only those older participants who were *not* currently taking blood pressure medications at the time of the experiment (young, $n = 16$; older, $n = 11$). During the 5% MVC task, MAP was higher during the high-cognitive demand session (105.1 ± 18.8 mmHg) than the low-cognitive demand session (87.2 ± 28.3 mmHg) and the control session (88.8 ± 23 mmHg; session effect, $p = 0.001$). There was no influence of age or sex on MAP ($p > 0.05$). Similarly, heart rate was greater during the high-cognitive demand session

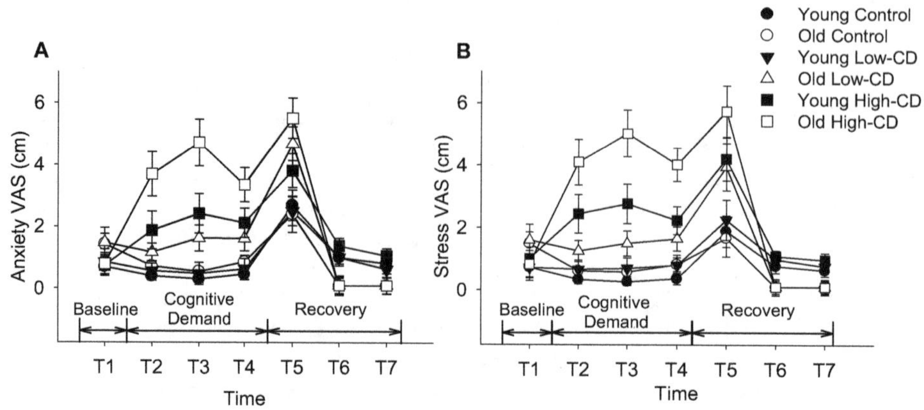

FIGURE 2 | Visual Analog Scale (VAS) scores for anxiety (A) and stress (B). Mean (±SE) VAS scores for young adults (closed symbols) and older adults (open symbols) are shown for anxiety **(A)** and stress **(B)** throughout the experimental protocol during the control session (circles), low-cognitive demand session (Low-CD, triangles), and high-cognitive demand session (High-CD, squares). Time intervals were as follows: baseline (T1), after the first bout of 2 min of quiet rest/mental math (T2), after the second bout of 2 min of quiet rest/mental math (T3), after the 5% submaximal contraction (T4), during recovery immediately after task failure (T5), and then at 5 min (T6) and 10 min of recovery (T7).

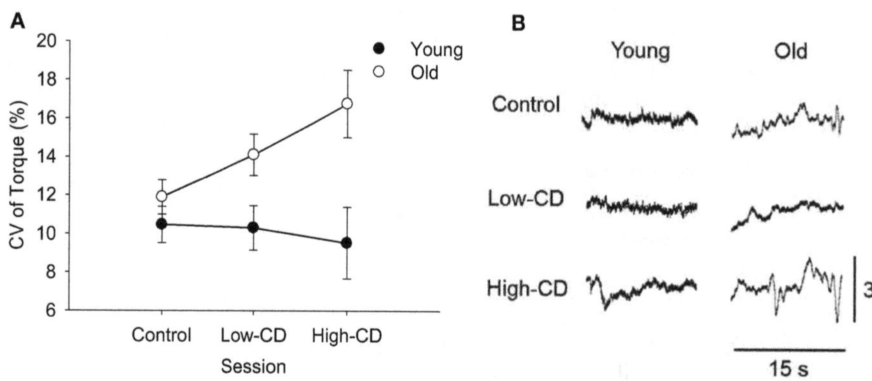

FIGURE 3 | Coefficient of Variation (CV) of torque during the 5% MVC task for young (closed symbols) and older (open symbols) adults during the control, low-cognitive demand (Low-CD), and high-cognitive demand (High-CD) sessions (A), and representative force tracings of a young and older adult (B). Shown are the mean (±SE) in **(A)**. Older adults had significantly higher CV of torque than young adults (age effect, $p = 0.007$).

(79.6 ± 15 beats/min) compared with the low-cognitive demand (71.6 ± 28 beats/min) and control sessions (68.2 ± 19.4 beats/min, session effect, $p = 0.04$) regardless of age of sex ($p > 0.05$, i.e., no interactions). Consequently, the *RPP* was higher during the high-cognitive demand session than the control and low-cognitive demand sessions (session effect, $p = 0.0001$), but there was no difference between young and older adults (age effect, $p = 0.52$) or men and women (sex effect, $p = 0.70$).

EMG activity

During the 5% MVC task, older adults had higher soleus RMS EMG (% MVC) (antagonist muscle) than young adults during the high-cognitive demand session (session × age, $p = 0.04$), but there were no other interactions, or main effects of age, sex or session for soleus or any other muscles (tibialis anterior, gastrocnemius, and rectus femoris).

FATIGUING CONTRACTION (30% MVC)

Time to task failure

There was no difference in time to task failure across sessions or with age ($p > 0.05$) (**Table 1**; **Figure 4**). There was no difference in time to task failure between men and women (sex effect, $p = 0.96$) and no interactions for age, sex, and session ($p > 0.05$). Variability between the three sessions in the time to task failure (comparison of SD generated from the three sessions for each participant) however, was greater for older adults than young adults (2.02 ± 1.05 vs. 1.25 ± 0.51 min, respectively, $p = 0.02$), but similar for men and women (sex effect, $p = 0.53$; sex × age, $p = 0.57$) (**Figure 4**). Furthermore, we compared the SD for time to task failure between sessions (SD for control and low-cognitive demand session vs. SD for control and high-cognitive demand session) to determine if variability increased with difficulty of the mental math. While the age effect remained (age effect, $p = 0.03$), there were no effects

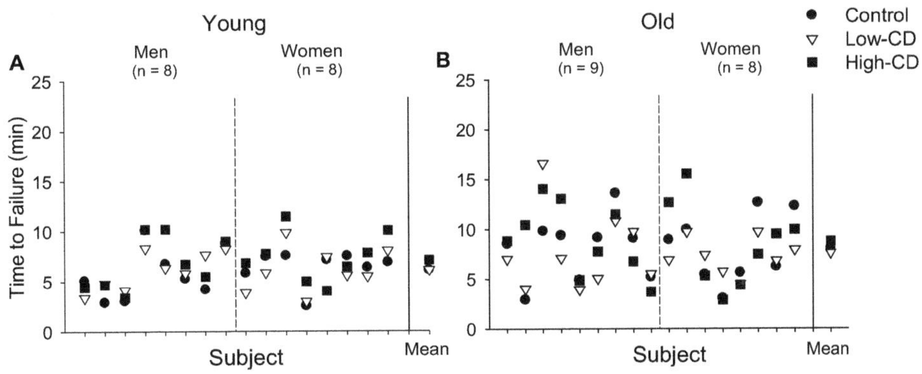

FIGURE 4 | Time to task failure during the fatiguing contraction for individual young (A) and older adults (B) during the control (circle), low-cognitive demand (Low-CD, triangle), and high-cognitive demand (High-CD, square) sessions. Time to task failure is shown for each young **(A)** and older **(B)** man and woman for each session (separated by dashed line). The aggregate mean (±SE) is shown for each session after the solid vertical line. The range and variability of time to task failure among the older adults was greater than for the young adults for each session. Older adults were more variable than young between the three sessions due to addition of a cognitive task (age effect, $p = 0.03$), but variability did not increase with task difficulty (session effect, $p = 0.38$).

of session (session effect, $p = 0.38$) or sex (sex effect, $p = 0.69$), and no interactions. Thus, although the older adults were more variable than young between the three sessions due to addition of a cognitive task, the variability between the older adults did not increase with to the difficulty of the cognitive task.

Fluctuations in torque

Fluctuations in torque (CV) increased over time during the sustained contraction (time, $p < 0.001$) similarly across sessions for both age groups (session × time, $p = 0.56$, **Figure 5C**). Older adults however, had larger fluctuations in torque than young adults (age effect, $p = 0.002$) and this difference was similar across sessions (session × age, $p = 0.11$). Women also had larger fluctuations in torque than men (sex effect, $p = 0.005$) and this sex difference was similar across sessions (session × sex, $p = 0.69$). There were no other interactions ($p > 0.05$). Because older and young adults can demonstrate more variability in motor performance than young adults, we evaluated variability of the fluctuations in torque (CV of torque) during the 30% MVC task (comparison of SD generated from the three sessions for each participant) between young and older adults. Variability was greater for older adults than young adults ($p = 0.01$), and greater for women than men (sex effect, $p = 0.02$), but there were no interactions (sex × age, $p = 0.94$) (**Figures 5A,B**).

EMG ACTIVITY OF AGONIST MUSCLES

The amplitude of the RMS EMG (% MVC) for the tibialis anterior (ankle dorsiflexors), increased during the fatiguing contraction (time effect, $p < 0.001$) and similarly across sessions (session × time, $p = 0.38$). Furthermore, tibialis anterior EMG activity was greater for the older adults than young during all three sessions (age effect, $p = 0.002$) (**Table 1**), but there was no difference between men and women (sex effect, $p = 0.80$), and no interactions.

Electromyographic bursting activity (bursts per minute) increased over time during the fatiguing contraction (30% MVC) for all three sessions (time effect, $p = 0.002$); however, there was no difference across the sessions (session effect, $p = 0.50$). Neither age nor sex influenced the bursting activity during the fatiguing contraction ($p > 0.05$, **Table 1**).

EMG ACTIVITY OF ANTAGONIST AND ACCESSORY MUSCLES

The RMS EMG amplitude (% MVC) for the soleus, gastrocnemius, and rectus femoris increased over time during the fatiguing contractions (time effect, $p < 0.001$ for all muscles) but was similar across sessions (session effect, $p > 0.05$ for all muscles). Older adults however, had higher RMS EMG for the soleus (age effect, $p = 0.04$), gastrocnemius ($p = 0.01$), and rectus femoris ($p = 0.03$) than young adults (see **Table 1**). There was no effect of sex for gastrocnemius and soleus (sex effect, $p > 0.05$) and there were no interactions ($p > 0.05$). For the rectus femoris, however, women had higher RMS EMG amplitudes than men (sex effect, $p = 0.04$), but there were no interactions ($p > 0.05$). There was a correlation between rectus femoris RMS EMG and CV of torque for the high-cognitive demand session only, indicating that participants who had greater torque fluctuations during the high-cognitive demand session also had greater rectus femoris EMG ($r_{33} = 0.31$, $p = 0.04$).

MAP AND HEART RATE

Cardiovascular measures were included only for older participants who were not currently taking blood pressure medications at the time of the experiment (young, $n = 16$; older, $n = 11$). MAP, heart rate, and RPP increased over time (time, $p < 0.05$) (**Figure 6**). MAP, heart rate, and RPP were higher during the high-cognitive demand session than the control or low-cognitive demand sessions (session effect, $p < 0.05$). MAP was higher for older adults during the fatiguing contraction in the high-cognitive demand session over time than other sessions (session × time × age, $p = 0.02$). Heart rate and RPP, however, were similar for older adults over time across sessions (session × time × age, $p > 0.05$), with no main effects of age or sex ($p > 0.05$).

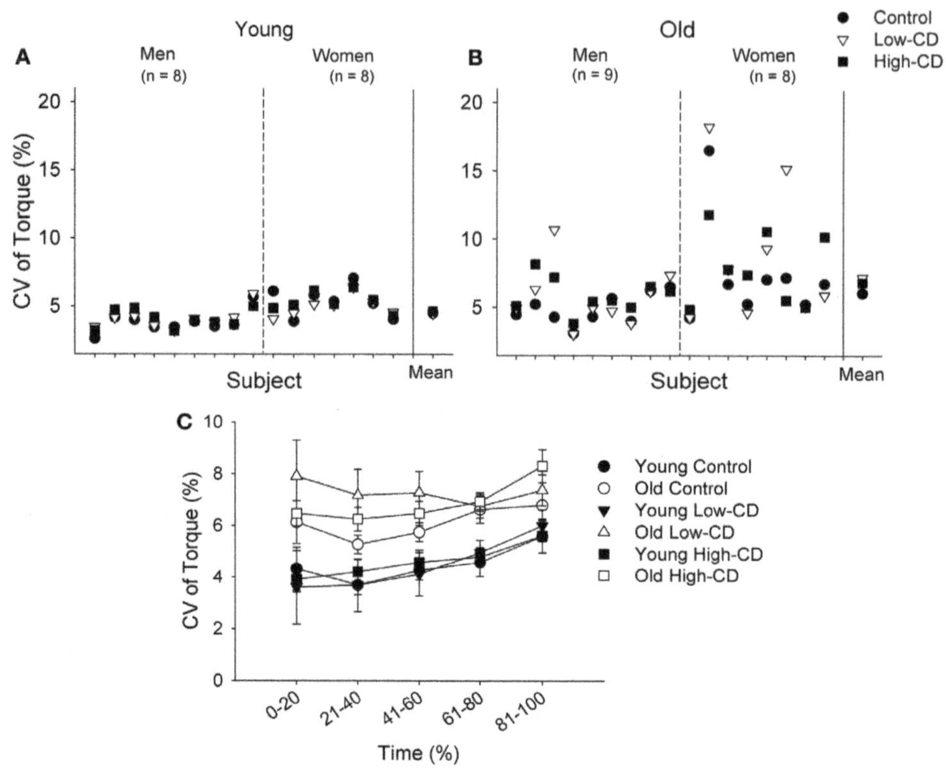

FIGURE 5 | Coefficient of variation of torque during the fatiguing contraction (30% MVC) for individual young (A) and older adults (B), and across time for young and older adults (C) during the control session (circle), low-cognitive demand session (Low-CD, triangle), and high-cognitive demand session (High-CD, square). CV of torque is shown for each young **(A)** and older **(B)** man and woman for each session. The aggregate mean (± SE) is shown for each session after the solid vertical line. The older adults and women exhibited greater variability in steadiness across sessions than the young and men respectively ($p < 0.05$). In **(C)**, the CV of torque (mean ± SE) is shown for the control (circle), low-CD demand (triangle), and high-CD (square) sessions for young (closed symbols) and older (open symbols) adults during five continuous intervals of 20% during the fatiguing contraction between 0 and 100% of the time to failure. Thus, the x axis intervals for **(C)** indicate the interval of data points averaged in each 20% interval. Older adults had significantly higher CV of torque than young adults (age effect, $p = 0.002$).

Rating of perceived exertion (RPE)

Perceived exertion increased during the fatiguing contraction (time effect, $p = 0.0001$) similarly across sessions (session effect, $p = 0.59$). RPE was similar for young and older adults (age effect, $p = 0.82$) and men and women (sex effect, $p = 0.62$), with no interactions ($p > 0.05$). Mean RPE across all three sessions was 4.2 ± 1.5 and 4.2 ± 1.8 at the beginning of the fatiguing contraction for young and older adults respectively and increased to 8.7 ± 2.3 vs. 9.1 ± 1.4 by the end of the fatiguing contraction.

Error rate

The mental math error rate during the fatiguing contraction (errors/min) was significantly higher during the high-cognitive demand session (2.9 ± 1.3 errors/min) compared with the low-cognitive demand session (0.4 ± 0.4 errors/min, session effect, $p < 0.001$). There was no main effect of age or sex ($p > 0.05$). There was also no correlation between error rate and CV of torque during the fatiguing contraction for the low-cognitive demand ($r_{33} = -0.17$, $p = 0.35$) or high-cognitive demand ($r_{33} = -0.26$, $p = 0.14$) sessions; nor were there significant associations between error rate during the fatiguing contraction and the time to task failure for the low-cognitive demand ($r_{33} = -0.12$, $p = 0.52$) or high-cognitive demand ($r_{33} = -0.06$, $p = 0.74$) sessions.

DISCUSSION

This study imposed several levels of cognitive demand during sustained low- and moderate-force isometric contractions with the ankle dorsiflexor muscles to determine the influence of increased cortical involvement on motor function and fatigability in young and older adults. The novel findings of this study were that as cognitive demand increased, steadiness decreased (i.e., CV of torque increased) during the very low-force contraction (5% MVC) for older adults but did not change for the young adults. While fatigability (time to failure) of a moderate intensity contraction (30% MVC) was not essentially different with imposed cognitive demand for young or older adults, variability in the time to failure and in the torque fluctuations across sessions was greater for the older adults than the young adults. These results provide evidence that increased cortical involvement of motor and non-motor cortical areas can disrupt motor performance of low-to-moderate intensity isometric contractions of the lower limb more so in older adults than young adults.

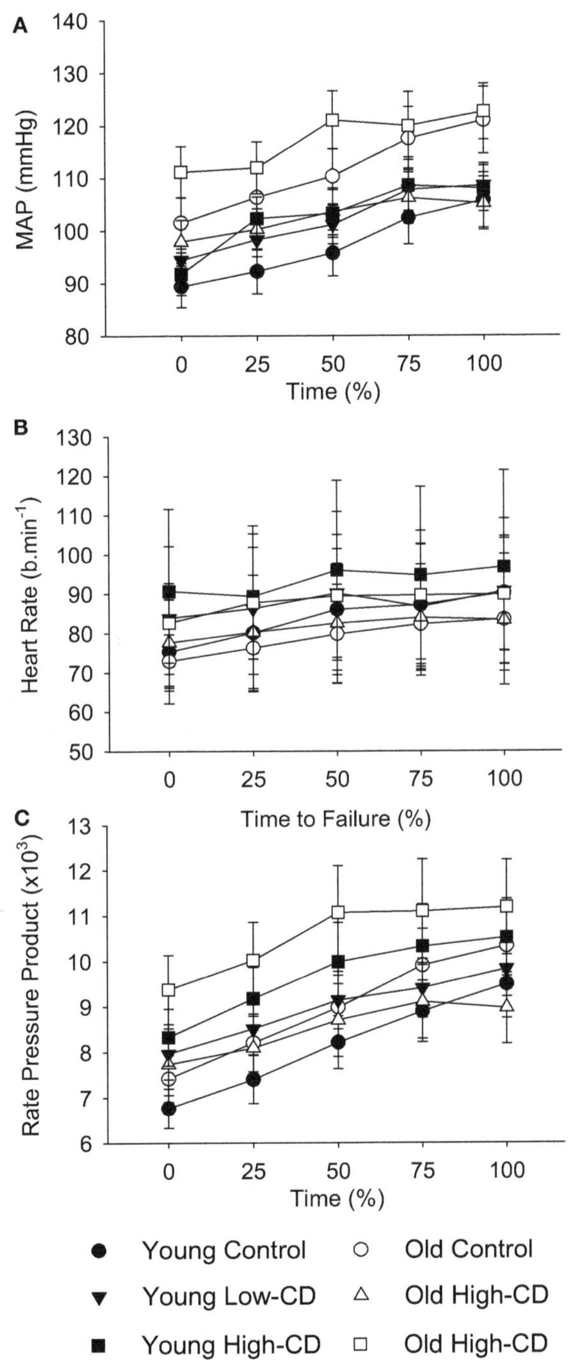

FIGURE 6 | Mean arterial pressure, heart rate, and rate-pressure product during the fatiguing contraction for young and older adults across sessions. The values are mean ± SE at 25% increments of time to task failure for young (closed symbols) and older (open symbols) adults during the control (circles), low-cognitive demand (Low-CD, triangles), and high-cognitive demand (High-CD, squares) sessions for mean arterial pressure **(A)**, heart rate **(B)**, and rate-pressure product **(C)** during the fatiguing contraction. Averages of 15-s intervals were used for the MAP and heart rate. Rate-pressure product was the product of heart rate and MAP for the equivalent time periods in **(A,B)**.

STEADINESS WAS REDUCED WITH AGE IN THE LOWER LIMB

Torque fluctuations (CV) were greater (steadiness reduced) during the low-intensity contraction (5% MVC) than at the start of the 30% MVC task (prior to fatigue), and also greater for older adults than young across all sessions. Larger torque fluctuations with advanced age have also been observed under control conditions across various muscle groups and particularly at the lower intensity contractions for both young and older men and women (Enoka et al., 2003; Tracy et al., 2005, 2007). Typically, the CV (%) will decrease as contraction intensity increases (Enoka et al., 2003; Taylor et al., 2003; Moritz et al., 2005; Tracy, 2007) and as we observed. Because we showed increased torque fluctuations during ankle dorsiflexion for the older adults during both 5% MVC and 30% MVC tasks compared with young, the age-related mechanism for reduced steadiness under control conditions influences both the low- and moderate-force tasks in the ankle dorsiflexor muscles. CV of torque across a range of low-to-high forces appear to be primarily modulated by low-frequency oscillations (<2–3 Hz) in neural drive found in motor unit action potentials trains (Negro et al., 2009; Dideriksen et al., 2012) with some contribution from increased motor unit variability at very low forces (Dideriksen et al., 2012; Jesunathadas et al., 2012). This low-frequency oscillating neural drive likely reflects an integration of both descending and afferent inputs onto the motoneurone pool (Negro et al., 2009; Dideriksen et al., 2012; Farina et al., 2012). With advanced age, the motoneurone pool undergoes remodeling that results in decreased motor units numbers and altered relations between discharge rates and recruitment thresholds (Barry et al., 2007); the age difference in torque fluctuations, therefore, appears to be due to age-related changes in the inputs to the motoneurone pool (Barry et al., 2007) with possibly some influence of greater motor unit discharge rate variability in older adults (Laidlaw et al., 2000; Kornatz et al., 2005; Tracy et al., 2005; Barry et al., 2007). Age-related changes in visual-motor processing may also contribute to altered motoneuronal inputs causing increased torque fluctuations during static contractions with age (Henningsen et al., 1997; Seidler-Dobrin and Stelmach, 1998; Tracy et al., 2007; Fox et al., 2013).

CARDIOVASCULAR RESPONSES AND ANXIETY WERE ELEVATED WITH HIGH-COGNITIVE DEMAND

While mental math was used to manipulate different levels of cognitive demand in this study, it can also increase anxiety and stress (Kajantie and Phillips, 2006) as it did for the young but more so in the older adults during the high-cognitive demand task (see **Figure 2**). Accordingly, MAP and heart rate were elevated when the difficult mental math was performed during both the 5% MVC and 30% MVC tasks, although similarly for the young and older adults. Older adults have reduced maximal heart rates compared with young, explaining the similar age-related increase in heart rate despite older adults reporting they felt more anxious and stressed. Because both MAP and heart rate were elevated, rate-pressure product was elevated for both young and older adults indicating increased cardiac work and myocardial oxygen consumption (Gobel et al., 1978; Wasmund et al., 2002) during the 5% MVC task and 30% MVC fatiguing contraction when cognitive demand was high. Chronicity of high blood pressure has been associated with an increased risk of stroke, cognitive decline, and dementia, especially in older adults with untreated high blood pressure (Tzourio et al., 1999; Tzourio, 2007). In the short term, increased stress and anxiety can increase monoaminergic drive; neuromodulatory inputs alter excitability of the motoneurone pool (Heckman et al., 2009) and potentially alter motor neuron output especially at low forces.

STEADINESS DECREASED WITH COGNITIVE DEMAND IN OLDER ADULTS

A novel finding was that the age difference in CV of torque grew linearly (i.e., steadiness decreased) with the increased levels of cognitive demand during a low-intensity contraction (5% MVC) of the lower limb. Although steadiness during the 30% MVC task was similar across sessions, older adults had greater variability in the CV of torque between sessions than the young. Increased torque fluctuations during the 5% MVC task between the low- and high-cognitive demand sessions indicate that the decline in steadiness was not solely due to the added distraction or challenge of talking because the low-cognitive demand task controlled for those factors. Because motor unit discharge rate variability can contribute to the force fluctuations at very low forces (Tracy et al., 2005; Jesunathadas et al., 2012), increased variability of the motor unit pool in the older adults may have been altered when high-cognitive demand was imposed.

Our findings indicate that increased antagonist muscle activation may also have contributed to the larger force fluctuations in the older adults when cognitive demand was high during the 5% MVC task. The older adults had greater soleus muscle activation during the high-cognitive demand session relative to the other sessions and compared with the young adults: this suggests less inhibition of the antagonist muscle from descending cortical sources. Increased antagonist muscle activity is a strategy adopted by older adults to stiffen joints and reduce movement variability with age (Hortobagyi and DeVita, 2006). For the higher force task (30% MVC) the torque fluctuations were larger with age, but there was no increase in the CV of torque with cognitive demand for young or older adults. Agonist (tibialis anterior), antagonist (gastrocnemius and soleus), and synergist (rectus femoris) activations were greater in the older adults than the young across all sessions, possibly contributing to the larger torque fluctuations with age. Because both the agonist (tibialis anterior) and antagonist activation were greater in the older adults compared with the young, activation differences had minimal effect on the greater CV of torque in the older adults.

There are numerous age-related changes along the neuroaxis that can alter inputs to the motoneurone pool and perhaps make it more susceptible to altering motor output when cognitive demand is imposed. Cortical size (Raz et al., 2007) and processing are diminished with age, along with reduced corticospinal fibers numbers (Eisen et al., 1996), and changes in spinal reflex pathways (Kido et al., 2004), which result in decreased cortical inhibition of both cognitive and motor processes with age (Peinemann et al., 2001; Sale and Semmler, 2005; Hunter et al., 2008). Age-related changes along the neuroaxis can also result in increased activation of antagonist muscles (Macaluso et al., 2002; Hortobagyi and DeVita, 2006) and as discussed may have been responsible for the greater activation of antagonist muscles with age in the current study.

Several theories of motor control assert that the division of attentional resources during a dual-task paradigm has limits and these limitations increase with advanced aging due to diminished cortical processing (Woollacott and Shumway-Cook, 2002). Consequently, some studies show older adults have less ability to simultaneously perform a cognitive task and motor task as well as they can be performed individually (Voelcker-Rehage and Alberts, 2007; Fraser et al., 2010; Johnson and Shinohara, 2012). Changes in performance for older adults in dual-tasks appear to be especially sensitive to cognitive tasks that require executive function (Yogev-Seligmann et al., 2008). Executive function (which included working memory, which was varied in this study), anxiety, and stress are modulated in prefrontal cortical regions and the anterior cingulate cortex (Miller, 2000; Owen et al., 2005; Banich et al., 2009; Schweizer et al., 2013). Prefrontal connections to motor areas (Takahara et al., 2012) along with input to neural connections between these and other cortical centers associated with cognition, anxiety, and motor function could directly alter motor output, as was observed in this study.

Capacity theories of attention that assume attentional resource limitations on the ability to perform multiple tasks simultaneously (Kahneman, 1973; McDowd, 2007; Hiraga et al., 2009) would predict even greater decrements in steadiness for older adults when descending drive from the motor cortex increased during the 30% MVC task and as the fatiguing contraction progressed. Interestingly, error rates in mental math (executive function task) during the fatiguing contraction did not differ across the age groups for the low-cognitive demand sessions and high-cognitive demand, indicating that mental math performance was not diminished in the older adults compared with the young. Although the variability in the CV of torque across the sessions was greater for the older adults than the young, the mean values in CV of torque were similar across the three sessions during the 30% MVC task and increased at similar rates to the young adults during the fatiguing contraction. Time to failure was also similar across sessions for each age group, and the increase in EMG activity, EMG bursting activity, and perceived effort during the fatiguing contraction progressed at similar rates across sessions. Increases in EMG and RPE during a fatiguing contraction are the result of increased descending drive to recruit more motor units in an effort to maintain the required force as the working muscle becomes progressively fatigued (Riley et al., 2008). Thus, while some older adults are clearly more affected than others by the increased cognitive demand during the sustained contractions (**Figure 5B**), capacity limitations in cortical regions of older adults cannot alone explain the loss of steadiness, especially at the very low forces when descending drive was not large.

Another explanation for the reduced steadiness in older adults as cognitive demand increased is that descending and afferent inputs to the motoneurone pool differed for the older and young adults. One input that likely differed between the young and older adults was monoaminergic drive (Christou et al., 2004). Increased monoaminergic drive to the spinal cord from the brainstem enables motoneurone activation and is essential for exercise

(Heckman, 2003), but monoaminergic drive is attenuated in older adults (Meltzer et al., 1998; Reynolds and Meltzer, 1999; Seals and Esler, 2000), potentially leading to decreased motor output and altered responses to increased anxiety and stress compared with young.

SEX DIFFERENCES IN STEADINESS

Both young and old women demonstrated heightened levels of stress and anxiety, and greater torque fluctuations during the very low-intensity and fatiguing contractions for all three sessions compared with men, regardless of the magnitude of cognitive demand. Similar sex differences in stress and anxiety (Christou et al., 2004) and in torque fluctuations have been shown previously in the upper limb (Yoon et al., 2009; Brown et al., 2010; Keller-Ross et al., 2014a); however, this is the first study to demonstrate increased torque fluctuations in women when performing submaximal contractions of the lower limb with varying levels of cognitive demand. Greater torque fluctuations in women when performing upper extremity tasks have been attributed to strength difference between men and women (Brown et al., 2010), although the mechanism is not known. When exposed to a stressful noxious stimulus prior to task performance, increased torque fluctuations have been attributed to greater activation of central neural mechanisms in response to increased stress and anxiety (Christou et al., 2004); however, in the current study, women demonstrated greater torque fluctuations and reported higher stress and anxiety than men regardless of the magnitude of cognitive demand (i.e., in both low- and high-cognitive demand tasks compared with control). Because both aging and decreased levels of estrogen in postmenopausal women possibly contribute to changes in monoaminergic drive (Meltzer et al., 1998), women may be even more vulnerable than men to diminished motor output with aging (see **Figure 5B**); however, it remains unclear if greater torque fluctuations in women are related to activation of alternate neural pathways, or a strength-related mechanism.

INCREASED VARIABILITY IN FATIGABILITY WITH COGNITIVE DEMAND AND AGING

Fatigability (time to task failure) of the ankle dorsiflexor muscles was similar across age groups and sessions. Hence, there was no systematic decrease in fatigability when cognitive demand was imposed during the sustained contraction with the ankle dorsiflexor muscles. In contrast, the elbow flexor muscles were more fatigable when high-cognitive demand was imposed in young men and women (Yoon et al., 2009; Keller-Ross et al., 2014a). Similarly, handgrip muscles were more fatigable in both young men and women when high-cognitive demand was imposed for high intensity contractions (Bray et al., 2008, 2012) but not for relatively strong men during a low-intensity sustained contraction (Keller-Ross et al., 2014b). The largest increases in fatigability were related to the initial muscle strength such that weaker participants experienced the greatest increases in fatigability (Yoon et al., 2009; Keller-Ross et al., 2014a). Perfusion associated changes within the muscle in response to a mental-math task (which was used to induce high-cognitive demand) was implicated but only partially explains these findings (Yoon et al., 2009; Keller-Ross et al., 2014a). In contrast to the elbow flexor muscles (Hunter et al., 2004), the ankle dorsiflexor muscles exhibit lesser differences between sub-populations including men and women (Avin et al., 2010), and young and older adults (Kent-Braun et al., 2002; Griffith et al., 2010) and we show here the fatigability of this muscle group is also less responsive to cognitive demand. Christie and Kamen (2009) attribute the lack of difference in fatigability of the dorsiflexor muscles between young and older adults to a lack of difference in motor unit discharge rates, suggesting young and older adults adopted similar neural adaptations during the fatiguing contractions. We found that the increase in EMG activity of the tibialis anterior muscle during the fatiguing contraction was similar across sessions for young and older adults, although older adults had greater EMG relative to the young. Another possible explanation for the different responses in fatigability with and without cognitive demand is a decreased number of corticospinal connections and larger motor unit ratio (motoneurone to fibers) in large lower limb muscles compared with the upper limb (Feinstein et al., 1955). A reduced number of corticomotor inputs to the dorsiflexor muscles relative to the upper limb muscles may minimize the modulating inputs from higher centers imposed with high-cognitive demand and lessen the responsiveness during the sustained fatiguing contractions at the moderate intensity.

While there was no systematic reduction in time to failure of the ankle dorsiflexor muscles as we have observed with the upper limb, older adults, particularly older women, demonstrated significantly more variability in their time to task failure between sessions than young adults (**Figure 4**). Variability between trials of a motor task can be exacerbated with increased cognitive demand in young people (Lorist et al., 2002) but is often greater with age as shown here. The greater variability in performance with advanced age can be due greater variability in cortical and motor nerve activation during motor tasks (Hunter et al., 2008; Yoon et al., 2008). This greater age-related variability in a motor task when a cognitive task was imposed further demonstrates the important role of cognitive control in determining reliability of performance of motor tasks especially during work-related tasks performed by an aging workforce.

CONCLUSION

This study demonstrated that older adults exhibit more variability than young adults in fatigability and less steadiness while performing low-force and moderate isometric with the ankle dorsiflexor muscles. For very low-force contractions, steadiness decreased further as greater cognitive demand increased. The reduced steadiness in older adults compared with the young, may be related to modulation of synergist and antagonist muscles and an altered neural strategy with age. Older adults also exhibited greater variability in steadiness between sessions and in fatigability as cognitive demand was imposed. Increased variability in lower extremity tasks may negatively impact activities of daily living and work tasks that require high-cognitive demand in an aging population. These data also expose differences within an older adult but also between older adults. Our results provide evidence that increased involvement of non-motor cortical areas can disrupt motor performance of low-to-moderate intensity isometric contractions of the lower limb more so in older adults than young adults. These findings have significant implications related to successful aging and performance of activities of daily living with advanced age especially those activities that require simultaneous execution of a cognitive task that involves working memory and maintenance of a static motor task.

REFERENCES

Aine, C. J., Sanfratello, L., Adair, J. C., Knoefel, J. E., Caprihan, A., and Stephen, J. M. (2011). Development and decline of memory functions in normal, pathological and healthy successful aging. *Brain Topogr.* 24, 323–339. doi:10.1007/s10548-011-0178-x

Artero, S., Touchon, J., and Ritchie, K. (2001). Disability and mild cognitive impairment: a longitudinal population-based study. *Int. J. Geriatr. Psychiatry* 16, 1092–1097. doi:10.1002/gps.477

Avin, K. G., Naughton, M. R., Ford, B. W., Moore, H. E., Monitto-Webber, M. N., Stark, A. M., et al. (2010). Sex differences in fatigue resistance are muscle group dependent. *Med. Sci. Sports Exerc.* 42, 1943–1950. doi:10.1249/MSS.0b013e3181d8f8fa

Banich, M. T., Mackiewicz, K. L., Depue, B. E., Whitmer, A. J., Miller, G. A., and Heller, W. (2009). Cognitive control mechanisms, emotion and memory: a neural perspective with implications for psychopathology. *Neurosci. Biobehav. Rev* 33, 613–630. doi:10.1016/j.neubiorev.2008.09.010

Barry, B. K., Pascoe, M. A., Jesunathadas, M., and Enoka, R. M. (2007). Rate coding is compressed but variability is unaltered for motor units in a hand muscle of old adults. *J. Neurophysiol.* 97, 3206–3218. doi:10.1152/jn.01280.2006

Borg, G. A. (1982). Psychophysical bases of perceived exertion. *Med. Sci. Sports Exerc.* 14, 377–381. doi:10.1249/00005768-198205000-00012

Bray, S. R., Graham, J. D., Martin Ginis, K. A., and Hicks, A. L. (2012). Cognitive task performance causes impaired maximum force production in human hand flexor muscles. *Biol. Psychol.* 89, 195–200. doi:10.1016/j.biopsycho.2011.10.008

Bray, S. R., Martin Ginis, K. A., Hicks, A. L., and Woodgate, J. (2008). Effects of self-regulatory strength depletion on muscular performance and EMG activation. *Psychophysiology* 45, 337–343. doi:10.1111/j.1469-8986.2007.00625.x

Brown, R. E., Edwards, D. L., and Jakobi, J. M. (2010). Sex differences in force steadiness in three positions of the forearm. *Eur. J. Appl. Physiol.* 110, 1251–1257. doi:10.1007/s00421-010-1600-x

Chen, P., Ratcliff, G., Belle, S. H., Cauley, J. A., Dekosky, S. T., and Ganguli, M. (2001). Patterns of cognitive decline in presymptomatic Alzheimer disease: a prospective community study. *Arch. Gen. Psychiatry* 58, 853–858. doi:10.1001/archpsyc.58.9.853

Christie, A., and Kamen, G. (2009). Motor unit firing behavior during prolonged 50% MVC dorsiflexion contractions in young and older adults. *J. Electromyogr. Kinesiol.* 19, 543–552. doi:10.1016/j.jelekin.2008.03.005

Christou, E. A., Jakobi, J. M., Critchlow, A., Fleshner, M., and Enoka, R. M. (2004). The 1- to 2-Hz oscillations in muscle force are exacerbated by stress, especially in older adults. *J. Appl. Physiol.* 97, 225–235. doi:10.1152/japplphysiol.00066.2004

Dideriksen, J. L., Negro, F., Enoka, R. M., and Farina, D. (2012). Motor unit recruitment strategies and muscle properties determine the influence of synaptic noise on force steadiness. *J. Neurophysiol.* 107, 3357–3369. doi:10.1152/jn.00938.2011

Eisen, A., Entezari-Taher, M., and Stewart, H. (1996). Cortical projections to spinal motoneurons: changes with aging and amyotrophic lateral sclerosis. *Neurology* 46, 1396–1404. doi:10.1212/WNL.46.5.1396

Enoka, R. M., Christou, E. A., Hunter, S. K., Kornatz, K. W., Semmler, J. G., Taylor, A. M., et al. (2003). Mechanisms that contribute to differences in motor performance between young and old adults. *J. Electromyogr. Kinesiol.* 13, 1–12. doi:10.1016/s1050-3411(02)00084-6

Farias, S. T., Mungas, D., Reed, B. R., Harvey, D., Cahn-Weiner, D., and Decarli, C. (2012). MCI is associated with deficits in everyday functioning: Alzheimer disease & associated disorders. *Alzheimer Dis. Assoc. Disord.* 20, 217–223. doi:10.1097/01.wad.0000213849.51495.d9

Farina, D., Negro, F., Gizzi, L., and Falla, D. (2012). Low-frequency oscillations of the neural drive to the muscle are increased with experimental muscle pain. *J. Neurophysiol.* 107, 958–965. doi:10.1152/jn.00304.2011

Feinstein, B., Lindegard, B., Nyman, E., and Wohlfart, G. (1955). Morphologic studies of motor units in normal human muscles. *Acta Anat. (Basel)* 23, 127–142. doi:10.1159/000140989

Fox, E. J., Baweja, H. S., Kim, C., Kennedy, D. M., Vaillancourt, D. E., and Christou, E. A. (2013). Modulation of force below 1 Hz: age-associated differences and the effect of magnified visual feedback. *PLoS ONE* 8:e55970. doi:10.1371/journal.pone.0055970

Fraser, S. A., Li, K. Z., and Penhune, V. B. (2010). Dual-task performance reveals increased involvement of executive control in fine motor sequencing in healthy aging. *J. Gerontol. B Psychol. Sci. Soc. Sci.* 65, 526–535. doi:10.1093/geronb/gbq036

Galganski, M. E., Fuglevand, A. J., and Enoka, R. M. (1993). Reduced control of motor output in a human hand muscle of elderly subjects during submaximal contractions. *J. Neurophysiol.* 69, 2108–2115.

Gobel, F. L., Norstrom, L. A., Nelson, R. R., Jorgensen, C. R., and Wang, Y. (1978). The rate-pressure product as an index of myocardial oxygen consumption during exercise in patients with angina pectoris. *Circulation* 57, 549–556. doi:10.1161/01.CIR.57.3.549

Griffith, E. E., Yoon, T., and Hunter, S. K. (2010). Age and load compliance alter time to task failure for a submaximal fatiguing contraction with the lower leg. *J. Appl. Physiol.* 108, 1510–1519. doi:10.1152/japplphysiol.01396.2009

Heckman, C. J. (2003). Active conductances in motoneuron dendrites enhance movement capabilities [article]. *Exerc. Sport Sci. Rev.* 31, 96–101. doi:10.1097/00003677-200304000-00008

Heckman, C. J., Mottram, C. J., Quinlan, K., Theiss, R., and Schuster, J. (2009). Motoneuron excitability: the importance of neuromodulatory inputs. *Clin. Neurophysiol.* 120, 2040–2054. doi:10.1016/j.clinph.2009.08.009

Henningsen, H., Knecht, S., and Ende-Henningsen, B. (1997). Influence of afferent feedback on isometric fine force resolution in humans. *Exp. Brain Res.* 113, 207–213. doi:10.1007/BF02450319

Hermens, H. J., Freriks, B., Disselhorst-Klug, C., and Rau, G. (2000). Development of recommendations for SEMG sensors and sensor placement procedures. *J. Electromyogr. Kinesiol.* 10, 361–374. doi:10.1016/S1050-6411(00)00027-4

Hiraga, C. Y., Garry, M. I., Carson, R. G., and Summers, J. J. (2009). Dual-task interference: attentional and neurophysiological influences. *Behav. Brain Res.* 205, 10–18. doi:10.1016/j.bbr.2009.07.019

Hortobagyi, T., and DeVita, P. (2006). Mechanisms responsible for the age-associated increase in coactivation of antagonist muscles. [article]. *Exerc. Sport Sci. Rev.* 34, 29–35. doi:10.1097/00003677-200601000-00007

Hunter, S. K., Critchlow, A., and Enoka, R. M. (2004). Influence of aging on sex differences in muscle fatigability. *J. Appl. Physiol.* 97, 1723–1732. doi:10.1152/japplphysiol.00460.2004

Hunter, S. K., Todd, G., Butler, J. E., Gandevia, S. C., and Taylor, J. L. (2008). Recovery from supraspinal fatigue is slowed in old adults after fatiguing maximal isometric contractions. *J. Appl. Physiol.* 105, 1199–1209. doi:10.1152/japplphysiol.01246.2007

Jesunathadas, M., Klass, M., Duchateau, J., and Enoka, R. M. (2012). Discharge properties of motor units during steady isometric contractions performed with the dorsiflexor muscles. *J. Appl. Physiol.* 112, 1897–1905. doi:10.1152/japplphysiol.01372.2011

Johnson, A. N., and Shinohara, M. (2012). Corticomuscular coherence with and without additional task in the elderly. *J. Appl. Physiol.* 112, 970–981. doi:10.1152/japplphysiol.01079.2011

Kahneman, D. (1973). *Attention and Effort.* Englewood Cliffs, NJ: Prentice Hall.

Kajantie, E., and Phillips, D. I. (2006). The effects of sex and hormonal status on the physiological response to acute psychosocial stress. *Psychoneuroendocrinology* 31, 151–178. doi:10.1016/j.psyneuen.2005.07.002

Keller-Ross, M., Pruse, J., Yoon, T., Harkins, A., and Hunter, S. (2014a). Stressor-induced increase muscle fatigability of young men and women is predicted by strength, but not voluntary activation. *J. Appl. Physiol.* 116, 767–778. doi:10.1152/japplphysiol.01129.2013

Keller-Ross, M. L., De-Lap, B. S., Doyel, R., Larson, G., and Hunter, S. K. (2014b). Muscle fatigability and control of force in men with posttraumatic stress disorder. *Med. Sci. Sports Exerc* doi:10.1249/MSS.0000000000000244

Kent-Braun, J. A., Ng, A. V., Doyle, J. W., and Towse, T. F. (2002). Human skeletal muscle responses vary with age and gender during fatigue due to incremental isometric exercise. *J. Appl. Physiol.* 93, 1813–1823. doi:10.1152/japplphysiol.00091.2002

Kido, A., Tanaka, N., and Stein, R. B. (2004). Spinal excitation and inhibition decrease as humans age. *Can. J. Physiol. Pharmacol.* 82, 238–248. doi:10.1139/y04-017

Kornatz, K. W., Christou, E. A., and Enoka, R. M. (2005). Practice reduces motor unit discharge variability in a hand muscle and improves manual dexterity in old adults. *J. Appl. Physiol.* 98, 2072–2080. doi:10.1152/japplphysiol.01149.2004

Kriska, A., and Bennett, P. (1992). An epidemiological perspective of the relationship between physical activity and NIDDM: from activity assessment to intervention. *Diabetes Metab. Rev.* 8, 355–372. doi:10.1002/dmr.5610080404

Laidlaw, D. H., Bilodeau, M., and Enoka, R. M. (2000). Steadiness is reduced and motor unit discharge is more variable in old adults. *Muscle Nerve* 23, 600–612. doi:10.1002/(SICI)1097-4598(200004)23:43.3.CO;2-4

Lorist, M. M., Kernell, D., Meijman, T. F., and Zijdewind, I. (2002). Motor fatigue and cognitive task performance in humans. *J. Physiol.* 545, 313–319. doi:10.1113/jphysiol.2002.027938

Macaluso, A., Nimmo, M. A., Foster, J. E., Cockburn, M., Mcmillan, N. C., and De Vito, G. (2002). Contractile muscle volume and agonist-antagonist coactivation account for differences in torque between young and older women. *Muscle Nerve* 25, 858–863. doi:10.1002/mus.10113

Marmon, A. R., Pascoe, M. A., Schwartz, R. S., and Enoka, R. M. (2011). Associations among strength, steadiness, and hand function across the adult life span. *Med. Sci. Sports Exerc.* 43, 560–567. doi:10.1249/MSS.0b013e3181f3f3ab

McDowd, J. M. (2007). An overview of attention: behavior and brain. *J. Neurol. Phys. Ther.* 31, 98–103. doi:10.1097/NPT.0b013e31814d7874

Meltzer, C. C., Smith, G., Dekosky, S. T., Pollock, B. G., Mathis, C. A., Moore, R. Y., et al. (1998). Serotonin in aging, late-life depression, and Alzheimer's disease: the emerging role of functional imaging. *Neuropsychopharmacology* 18, 407–430. doi:10.1016/S0893-133X(97)00194-2

Miller, E. K. (2000). The prefrontal cortex and cognitive control. *Nat. Rev. Neurosci.* 1, 59–65. doi:10.1038/35044578

Moritz, C. T., Barry, B. K., Pascoe, M. A., and Enoka, R. M. (2005). Discharge rate variability influences the variation in force fluctuations across the working range of a hand muscle. *J. Neurophysiol.* 93, 2449–2459. doi:10.1152/jn.01122.2004

Morris, J. C., Storandt, M., Miller, J. P., Mckeel, D. W., Price, J. L., Rubin, E. H., et al. (2001). Mild cognitive impairment represents early-stage Alzheimer disease. *Arch. Neurol* 58, 397–405. doi:10.1001/archneur.58.3.397

Negro, F., Holobar, A., and Farina, D. (2009). Fluctuations in isometric muscle force can be described by one linear projection of low-frequency components of motor unit discharge rates. *J. Physiol.* 587, 5925–5938. doi:10.1113/jphysiol.2009.178509

Noteboom, J. T., Fleshner, M., and Enoka, R. M. (2001). Activation of the arousal response can impair performance on a simple motor task. *J. Appl. Physiol.* 91, 821–831.

Oldfield, R. C. (1971). The assessment and analysis of handedness: the Edinburgh inventory. *Neuropsychologia* 9, 97–113. doi:10.1016/0028-3932(71)90067-4

Owen, A. M., Mcmillan, K. M., Laird, A. R., and Bullmore, E. (2005). N-back working memory paradigm: a meta-analysis of normative functional neuroimaging studies. *Hum. Brain Mapp.* 25, 46–59. doi:10.1002/hbm.20131

Peinemann, A., Lehner, C., Conrad, B., and Siebner, H. R. (2001). Age-related decrease in paired-pulse intracortical inhibition in the human primary motor cortex. *Neurosci. Lett.* 313, 33–36. doi:10.1016/S0304-3940(01)02239-X

Raz, N., Rodrigue, K. M., and Haacke, E. M. (2007). Brain aging and its modifiers: insights from in vivo neuromorphometry and susceptibility weighted imaging. *Ann. N. Y. Acad. Sci.* 1097, 84–93. doi:10.1196/annals.1379.018

Reynolds, C. C., and Meltzer, C. F. (1999). In vivo assessment of aging changes in serotonin function. *Neuropsychopharmacology* 21, 323–324. doi:10.1016/S0893-133X(99)00058-5

Riley, Z. A., Maerz, A. H., Litsey, J. C., and Enoka, R. M. (2008). Motor unit recruitment in human biceps brachii during sustained voluntary contractions. *J. Physiol.* 586, 2183–2193. doi:10.1113/jphysiol.2008.150698

Sale, M. V., and Semmler, J. G. (2005). Age-related differences in corticospinal control during functional isometric contractions in left and right hands. *J. Appl. Physiol.* 99, 1483–1493. doi:10.1152/japplphysiol.00371.2005

Schweizer, S., Grahn, J., Hampshire, A., Mobbs, D., and Dalgleish, T. (2013). Training the emotional brain: improving affective control through emotional working memory training. *J. Neurosci.* 33, 5301–5311. doi:10.1523/JNEUROSCI.2593-12.2013

Seals, D. R., and Esler, M. D. (2000). Human ageing and the sympathoadrenal system. *J. Physiol.* 528, 407–417. doi:10.1111/j.1469-7793.2000.00407.x

Seidler-Dobrin, R. D., and Stelmach, G. E. (1998). Persistence in visual feedback control by the elderly. *Exp. Brain Res.* 119, 467–474. doi:10.1007/s002210050362

Sommervoll, Y., Ettema, G., and Vereijken, B. (2011). Effects of age, task, and frequency on variability of finger tapping. *Percept. Mot. Skills* 113, 647–661. doi:10.2466/10.25.PMS.113.5.647-661

Sosnoff, J. J., and Newell, K. M. (2006). The generalization of perceptual-motor intra-individual variability in young and old adults. *J. Gerontol. B Psychol. Sci. Soc. Sci.* 61, 304–310. doi:10.1093/geronb/61.5.P304

Spielberger, C. D., Gorsuch, R. L., and Lushene, R. D. (1970). *STAI: Manual for the State-Trait Anxiety Inventory.* Palo Alto, CA: Consulting Psychologists Press.

Takahara, D., Inoue, K., Hirata, Y., Miyachi, S., Nambu, A., Takada, M., et al. (2012). Multisynaptic projections from the ventrolateral prefrontal cortex to the dorsal premotor cortex in macaques – anatomical substrate for conditional visuomotor behavior. *Eur. J. Neurosci.* 36, 3365–3375. doi:10.1111/j.1460-9568.2012.08251.x

Taylor, A. M., Christou, E. A., and Enoka, R. M. (2003). Multiple features of motor-unit activity influence force fluctuations during isometric contractions. *J. Neurophysiol.* 90, 1350–1361. doi:10.1152/jn.00056.2003

Tracy, B. L. (2007). Force control is impaired in the ankle plantarflexors of elderly adults. *Eur. J. Appl. Physiol.* 101, 629–636. doi:10.1007/s00421-007-0538-0

Tracy, B. L., Dinenno, D. V., Jorgensen, B., and Welsh, S. J. (2007). Aging, visuomotor correction, and force fluctuations in large muscles. *Med. Sci. Sports Exerc* 39, 469–479. doi:10.1249/mss.0b013e31802d3ad300005768-200703000-00010

Tracy, B. L., and Enoka, R. M. (2002). Older adults are less steady during submaximal isometric contractions with the knee extensor muscles. *J. Appl. Physiol.* 92, 1004–1012. doi:10.1152/japplphysiol.00954.2001

Tracy, B. L., Maluf, K. S., Stephenson, J. L., Hunter, S. K., and Enoka, R. M. (2005). Variability of motor unit discharge and force fluctuations across a range of muscle forces in older adults. *Muscle Nerve* 32, 533–540. doi:10.1002/mus.20392

Tzourio, C. (2007). Hypertension, cognitive decline, and dementia: an epidemiological perspective. *Dialogues Clin. Neurosci.* 9, 61–70.

Tzourio, C., Dufouil, C., Ducimetiere, P., and Alperovitch, A. (1999). Cognitive decline in individuals with high blood pressure: a longitudinal study in the elderly. *Neurology* 53, 1948–1952. doi:10.1212/WNL.53.9.1948

Voelcker-Rehage, C., and Alberts, J. L. (2007). Effect of motor practice on dual-task performance in older adults. *J. Gerontol. B Psychol. Sci. Soc. Sci.* 62, 141–148. doi:10.1093/geronb/62.3.P141

Voelcker-Rehage, C., Stronge, A. J., and Alberts, J. L. (2006). Age-related differences in working memory and force control under dual-task conditions. *Neuropsychol. Dev. Cogn. B Aging Neuropsychol. Cogn.* 13, 366–384. doi:10.1080/138255890969339

Wasmund, W. L., Westerholm, E. C., Watenpaugh, D. E., Wasmund, S. L., and Smith, M. L. (2002). Interactive effects of mental and physical stress on cardiovascular control. *J. Appl. Physiol.* 92, 1828–1834. doi:10.1152/japplphysiol.00019.2001

Woollacott, M., and Shumway-Cook, A. (2002). Attention and the control of posture and gait: a review of an emerging area of research. *Gait Posture* 16, 1–14. doi:10.1016/S0966-6362(01)00156-4

Yogev-Seligmann, G., Hausdorff, J. M., and Giladi, N. (2008). The role of executive function and attention in gait. *Mov. Disord.* 23, 329–342; quiz 472. doi:10.1002/mds.21720

Yoon, T., Keller, M. L., De-Lap, B. S., Harkins, A., Lepers, R., and Hunter, S. K. (2009). Sex differences in response to cognitive stress during a fatiguing contraction. *J. Appl. Physiol.* 107, 1486–1496. doi:10.1152/japplphysiol.00238.2009

Yoon, T., De-Lap, B. S., Griffith, E. E., and Hunter, S. K. (2008). Age-related muscle fatigue after a low-force fatiguing contraction is explained by central fatigue. *Muscle Nerve* 37, 457–466. doi:10.1002/mus.20969

Zijdewind, I., Van Duinen, H., Zielman, R., and Lorist, M. M. (2006). Interaction between force production and cognitive performance in humans. *Clin. Neurophysiol.* 117, 660–667. doi:10.1016/j.clinph.2005.11.016

4

Utilization of central nervous system resources for preparation and performance of complex walking tasks in older adults

David J. Clark[1,2]*, Dorian K. Rose[1,3], Sarah A. Ring[1,2] and Eric C. Porges[2]

[1] Brain Rehabilitation Research Center, Malcom Randall VA Medical Center, North Florida/South Georgia Veterans Health System, Gainesville, FL, USA
[2] Department of Aging and Geriatric Research, University of Florida, Gainesville, FL, USA
[3] Department of Physical Therapy, University of Florida, Gainesville, FL, USA

Edited by:
Brian C. Clark, Ohio University, USA

Reviewed by:
Sue Lord, Newcastle University, UK
Chia-Cheng Lin, University of Pittsburgh, USA

***Correspondence:**
David J. Clark, Brain Rehabilitation Research Center (151A), Malcom Randall VA Medical Center, North Florida/South Georgia Veterans Health System, 1601 SW Archer Road, Gainesville, FL 32608, USA
e-mail: davidclark@ufl.edu

Introduction: Walking in the home and community often involves performance of complex walking tasks. Understanding the control of such tasks is crucial to preserving independence and quality of life in older adults. However, very little research has been conducted in this area. Here, we assess the extent to which two measures of central nervous system (CNS) activity are responsive to the challenges posed by preparation and performance of complex walking tasks. Prefrontal cortical activity was measured by functional near-infrared spectroscopy (fNIRS) and sympathetic nervous system arousal was measured by skin conductance level (SCL).

Materials and methods: Sixteen older men and women (age: 77.2 ± 5.6 years) with mild mobility deficits participated in this study. Participants walked at their preferred speed without distractions along an unobstructed, well-lit course (*control* task) and also walked on the same course under five separate challenging conditions: performing a cognitive verbal fluency task (*verbal* task), dim lighting (*dim* task), carrying a tray (*carry* task), negotiating obstacles (*obstacles* task) and wearing a weighted vest (*vest* task). Mean prefrontal activation and SCL were calculated during the preparation and performance phases of each task. Gait spatiotemporal measurements were acquired by an instrumented gait mat.

Results: Prefrontal cortical activity and SCL were elevated during the preparation phase of complex walking tasks relative to the control task. During the performance phase, prefrontal activity remained elevated to a similar level as during task preparation. In contrast, SCL continued to increase beyond the level observed during task preparation. A larger increase in prefrontal activity was found to be linked to preserved quality of gait during complex walking tasks.

Discussion: These findings indicate that availability and utilization of CNS resources are important for optimizing performance of complex walking tasks in older adults.

Keywords: walking, aging, motor control, near infrared spectroscopy, skin conductance

INTRODUCTION

Walking in the home and community environment often involves performance of complex tasks (Patla and Shumway-Cook, 1999; Frank and Patla, 2003; Lord et al., 2010). Such tasks can encompass a variety of different conditions such as walking over obstacles, in low-lighting and while multi-tasking. Compared to typical steady-state walking, these tasks require heightened demand on motor and/or cognitive resources. A study of over 1200 older adults by Shumway-Cook et al. (2007) demonstrated that age-related performance decrements are more severe for complex walking tasks than for typical steady-state walking. Furthermore, age-related mobility disability has been shown to be characterized in part by avoidance of environments that require performance of complex walking tasks (Shumway-Cook et al., 2002, 2003). There is a crucial need for enhanced understanding of the control of complex walking tasks in older adults. This knowledge will contribute to the development of novel mobility assessments and to the design of new therapeutic interventions that seek to preserve independent ambulation in the home and community.

Very little research has been conducted to understand the central nervous system (CNS) determinants of complex walking task performance, especially in older adults. The present study sought to advance this area of research by examining prefrontal cortical activity and sympathetic nervous system (SNS) arousal during the preparation and performance phases of various complex walking tasks. Prefrontal cortical activity was quantified by functional near-infrared spectroscopy (fNIRS). fNIRS is a relatively new technology that non-invasively assesses tissue metabolic activity using near-infrared light, which is able to pass through bone and other biological tissues (Bunce et al., 2006). Metabolic activity is estimated based on the characteristic properties of infrared light absorption by oxygenated hemoglobin and deoxygenated hemoglobin (markers of oxygen delivery and utilization) (Bunce et al., 2006). Prefrontal activation has been shown to be broadly linked to the amount of attention/intention directed toward cognitive and motor tasks, including walking (Okamoto et al., 2004; Herrmann et al., 2006; Suzuki et al., 2008; Atsumori et al., 2010; Kaneko et al., 2011; Koenraadt et al., 2014). In some studies, higher levels of prefrontal activity have been linked to better performance under novel task conditions (Ohsugi et al., 2013; Ishikuro et al., 2014).

SNS arousal was quantified by skin conductance level (SCL), which measures the electrical conductance of the skin. SCL is affected by sweat gland activity, which is under the control of the SNS (Sato et al., 1989). One function of the SNS is to mobilize physiological resources (e.g., increase blood flow and glucose release) under physically or psychologically challenging conditions (Bear et al., 2007). It has been proposed to up-regulate the gain of the entire CNS to increase responsiveness (Sibley et al., 2010). Although increased arousal can be beneficial to task performance under certain conditions, excessive arousal is known to compromise performance (Yerkes and Dodson, 1908). The extent to which this may affect mobility performance in older adults remains unclear. It is possible that fear of falling due to the challenge of walking with an aged CNS and musculoskeletal system could lead to excessively heightened arousal. For instance, heightened arousal/anxiety due to fear of falling has previously been linked to abnormal responses for posture (Adkin et al., 2002; Carpenter et al., 2004) and gait (Brown et al., 2002; Hadjistavropoulos et al., 2012).

Our primary objective was to assess the extent to which prefrontal activity and SCL were responsive to the increased utilization of CNS resources that is expected to occur when preparing for and executing complex walking tasks. Our secondary objective was to assess the potential link between CNS responses and gait quality during performance of the complex walking tasks. We hypothesized that prefrontal activity (interpreted as utilization and availability of cognitive resources) would be increased during preparation and performance of complex walking tasks, and that higher responses would be linked to better gait performance. We also hypothesized that SCL (interpreted as cognitive load and arousal) would be increased during preparation and performance of complex walking tasks, but that higher responses would be linked to poorer gait performance.

MATERIALS AND METHODS

PARTICIPANTS

Men and women between the ages of 65–85 years with mild mobility deficits were recruited for this study. Mild mobility deficits were defined as 400 m walking speed less than 1.1 m/s and agreement with the statement "You find it physically tiring to walk a quarter mile, or climb two flights of stairs, or perform household chores." Preliminary screening of inclusion/exclusion criteria was conducted by telephone. Exclusion criteria included use of an assistive device for walking (cane, crutch, walker, brace, etc.); lower extremity pain while walking; involuntary weight gain or loss exceeding 10 pounds within the past six months; myocardial infarction or symptomatic cardiovascular disease in the past year; bone fracture in the past year; injury or illness to the CNS; uncontrolled hypertension exceeding 160 systolic and/or 95 diastolic; or terminal illness. Volunteers who met these criteria were invited to our research center for further screening. Additional inclusion criteria applied at the onsite visit were Berg Balance Scale (BBS, Berg et al., 1989) score $\geq$ 41, Mini-Mental State Exam (MMSE, Folstein et al., 1975) score $\geq$ 21, and body mass index (BMI) within the range of 19–35. All study procedures were approved by the University of Florida Institutional Review Board. All individuals provided their written informed consent at time of enrollment.

PROTOCOL AND EQUIPMENT

The assessments described here are a subset from a larger experimental protocol (PI: David J. Clark) that tested motor control of walking in older adults. The study was conducted over three separate visits to our research center. The first day consisted of functional assessments and questionnaires. This included the screening items mentioned in the prior section (BBS and MMSE) as well as the Activities-Specific Balance Confidence Scale (ABC Scale). The second and third day involved mechanistic assessments of walking including fNIRS of the prefrontal cortex, SCL and spatiotemporal gait measurement. The overground walking course consisted of five consecutive laps around an 18 m course in our laboratory, for a total walking distance of 90 m. The floor surface was smooth tile with the exception of the 5.2 m instrumented walkway, which has the texture of firm foam (GAITRite, CIR Systems, Sparta, NJ, USA). Participants walked at their preferred speed without distractions along an unobstructed, well-lit pathway (*control* task) and also walked on the same course while separately performing the following five additional challenging tasks on separate trials: cognitive verbal fluency task ("*verbal*"), dim lighting ("*dim*"), carrying a tray ("*carry*"), negotiating obstacles ("*obstacles*") and wearing a weighted vest ("*vest*"). The *control, verbal, dim,* and *carry* tasks were conducted on the second visit to our center, and the *control, obstacle,* and *vest* tasks were conducted on the third visit. For the *verbal* task, participants were asked to say as many words as possible that began with a randomly selected letter. In order to maintain a comparable level of cognitive effort over the duration of the trial, a new letter was provided to the participant for each lap. For the *dim* task the lights in the laboratory were turned off and the windows were blocked, but some light entered through the door of an adjoining room. The participant's eyes were allowed to adjust for approximately 2 min prior to starting the task. For the *carry* task, three rolls of athletic tape were stacked on the tray, and the participant was instructed to keep the tray stable to avoid having the stack fall over. For the *obstacle* task, the participant was instructed to step over six small obstacles (shoes) evenly spaced along the walking path. For the *vest* task, the participant wore an adjustable weighted vest with a load equal to 10% of body weight. The load was evenly distributed between the front and rear of the vest, and velcro straps were used to ensure that the vest remained snug against the body. Prior to performing each task, the participant stood quietly at the start of the course for about one minute to allow measurement of CNS activity during task preparation. The participants were given no specific instructions regarding how to perform or prioritize the objectives within each task, because our goal was to evaluate their natural/preferred walking behavior.

Metabolic activity of the left and right anterior prefrontal cortices (Brodmann Area 10) was evaluated with a commercially available fNIRS monitor (Niro 200NX, Hamamatsu Photonics, Japan). In accordance with prior studies, each set of probes (i.e., for left and right prefrontal cortices) were placed high on the forehead to avoid the temporalis muscle (but not over hair) and sufficiently lateral from the midline to avoid the superior sagittal sinus (Al-Rawi and Kirkpatrick, 2006; Tisdall et al., 2009). Optode spacing was 3 cm. fNIRS uses light of varying wavelengths to non-invasively record changes in blood flow and hemoglobin due to neuronal activation of cerebral cortex. SCL was measured using a commercially available data acquisition unit (Flexcomp Infiniti, Thought Technology Ltd., QC, Canada) and sensors (SA9309M, Thought Technology Ltd., QC, Canada). Sensors were secured to the proximal phalanges of the index and ring fingers using a velcro strap. SCL signals were acquired separately from both the left and right hands. fNIRS and SCL data were sampled at 2 and 32 Hz, respectively, and saved to a memory card in each data acquisition unit. Spatiotemporal gait data were acquired from the instrumented walkway.

DATA ANALYSIS

Raw data were converted into text files via each manufacturer's software, then analyzed with custom programs in Matlab version R2011b (The Mathworks, Natick, MA, USA). Prefrontal cortical activity was quantified as the tissue oxygenation index (TOI), which is the ratio (expressed as a percent) of oxygenated hemoglobin to total hemoglobin (sum of oxygenated and deoxygenated). TOI provides a real-time measure of the balance between cerebral oxygen delivery and utilization (Tisdall et al., 2009). For both TOI and SCL, the average magnitude was calculated for a 10-s epoch in which the participants were standing still immediately preceding task performance (preparation phase) and also for the full period of steady-state walking (performance phase). The transition periods for gait initiation and gait termination were excluded from the analysis. Gait variables extracted from the instrumented walkway included measures typically used to infer the use of a cautious gait pattern: decreased speed, increased stance width, increased double limb support time and increased variability (measured by standard deviation of step length and double support time).

STATISTICS

Statistical analysis was conducted with JMP Pro software (version 11.0.0). Two-way repeated-measures ANOVA models were used to assess task- and side-dependent differences in prefrontal TOI (task × hemisphere) and SCL (task × hand). Separate models were used for tasks that were assessed on the first day of evaluation (*control, verbal, dim* and *carry*) and the second day of evaluation (*control, obstacles,* and *vest*). Mauchly's sphericity test was used to test the assumption of sphericity in the ANOVA models. If sphericity was not achieved, the model was adjusted using the Huynh–Feldt correction (if $\epsilon > 0.75$) or the Greenhouse–Geisser correction (if $\epsilon < 0.75$). *Post hoc* testing of significant main effects was conducted using one-sided repeated-measures *t*-tests to test the hypothesis that complex walking tasks increased TOI and SCL relative to the preparation phase of each task and/or relative to performance of the *control* walking task. The false discovery rate procedure (Curran-Everett, 2000; Curran-Everett and Benos, 2004) was used to correct for multiple comparisons during *post hoc* testing. Secondary analyses were conducted to determine whether there was evidence to support a link between CNS responses and gait quality. For TOI, separate two-tailed *t*-tests were used to test the hypothesis that gait quality would be better in a high-response subgroup versus a low-response subgroup. For SCL, separate two-tailed *t*-tests were used to test the hypothesis that gait quality would be better in a low-response subgroup versus a high-response subgroup.

RESULTS

PARTICIPANTS

Sixteen older adults (8 male/8 female) participated in this study. The mean age of participants was 77.2 ± 5.6 years, with a range of 66–85 years. Additional information from clinical assessments is presented in **Table 1**.

fNIRS

Exemplar fNIRS data for one participant are shown in **Figure 1** and group average data are shown in **Figure 2**. For **Figure 2**, the TOI value shown for the performance phase of the control task is the average of the values from visit 1 and visit 2. These values did not differ significantly across visits (0.29 ± 1.13 versus 0.48 ± 1.24, respectively, $p = 0.38$).

Preparation for complex walking tasks

For TOI during the preparation phase preceding each walking task, there was a significant main effect of task ($p < 0.05$). The size of that effect across tasks is shown by the gray bars in **Figure 2**, which show the percent increase in TOI for the preparation phase of each complex walking task relative to the TOI for the preparation phase of the *control* task. *Post hoc* analysis revealed that, relative to $control_{\text{prepare}}$, TOI increased significantly for dim_{prepare} ($p = 0.003$), $carry_{\text{prepare}}$ ($p = 0.04$), $vest_{\text{prepare}}$ ($p = 0.006$) and $obstacles_{\text{prepare}}$ ($p = 0.001$). There was also a trend toward significance for $verbal_{\text{prepare}}$ ($p = 0.09$). The effects of hemisphere and task × hemisphere interaction were not significant.

Table 1 | Participant characteristics.

	Mean	Range
Body Mass Index (kg/m^2)	29.3 ± 2.7	24.3–33.8
Mini Mental State Exam	27.4 ± 1.7	24–30
Berg Balance Test	50.5 ± 3.9	42–56
400 m Walk speed (m/s)	0.92 ± 0.11	0.66–1.08
ABC Scale (% confidence)	83.0 ± 15.0	58–100

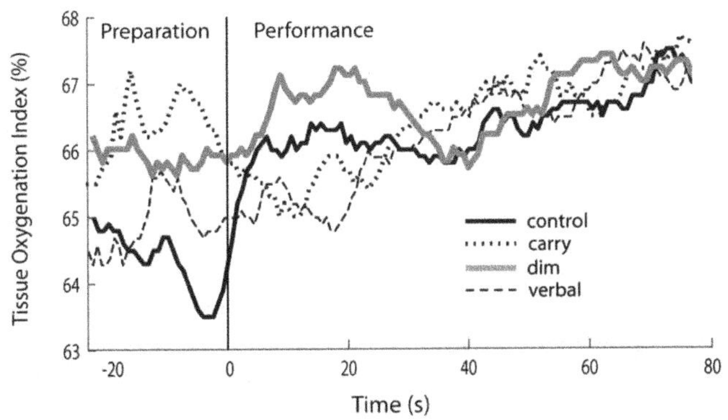

FIGURE 1 | Exemplar data demonstrating task-dependent differences in tissue oxygenation index (TOI). Prefrontal cortical activation, as indicated by TOI, for one study participant. Data are shown for walking along an unobstructed, well-lit pathway (*control* task; black solid line), walking while carrying a tray (*carry* task; dotted line), walking in dim lighting (*dim* task; gray solid line) and walking while performing a verbal fluency task (*verbal* task; dashed line). The participant is standing still for a short period of time at the start of the trial (preparation phase) and then walks at preferred speed (performance phase).

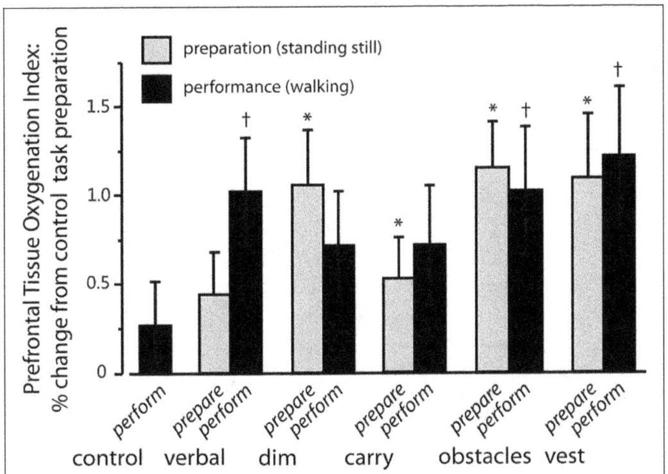

FIGURE 2 | Increase in prefrontal activation for complex tasks relative to preparation for control task. Gray bars indicate the average percentage increase in prefrontal activation during the preparation phase of each complex walking task relative to preparation for the *control* task. Significant changes are shown by an asterisk. Black bars indicate the percentage increase in prefrontal activation during the performance phase of each complex walking task relative to preparation for the *control* task. Significant changes are shown by a dagger. Error bars indicate group standard error.

Performance of complex walking tasks

For TOI during the performance phase of each task, a significant main effect of task was also found ($p < 0.05$). The size of that effect across tasks is indicated by the black bars of **Figure 2**, which show the percent increase in TOI for the performance phase of each complex walking task relative to the TOI for the preparation phase of the *control* task. *Post hoc* analysis revealed that, relative to $control_{prepare}$, TOI increased for $verbal_{perform}$ ($p = 0.006$), $vest_{perform}$ ($p = 0.005$), and $obstacles_{perform}$ ($p = 0.002$). There was a trend toward increased TOI during $dim_{perform}$ ($p = 0.06$) and $carry_{perform}$ ($p = 0.11$). The effects of hemisphere and task × hemisphere interaction were not significant.

Within-task comparison of preparation versus performance

Also examined was whether TOI increased from the preparation phase to the performance phase within each task (i.e., comparing gray bars to black bars for each task in **Figure 2**). TOI for preparation versus performance did not increase significantly between $dim_{prepare}$ and $dim_{perform}$ ($p = 0.95$), between $carry_{prepare}$ and $carry_{perform}$ ($p = 0.16$), between $obstacles_{prepare}$ and $obstacles_{perform}$ ($p = 0.84$), or between $vest_{prepare}$ and $vest_{perform}$ ($p = 0.30$). However, there was a trend for increased TOI between $verbal_{prepare}$ and $verbal_{perform}$ ($p = 0.05$).

SKIN CONDUCTANCE LEVEL

Exemplar SCL data for one participant are shown in **Figure 3** and group average data are shown in **Figure 4**. For **Figure 4**, the SCL value shown for the performance phase of the control task is the average of the values from visit 1 and visit 2. These values did not differ significantly across visits (8.02 ± 11.48 versus 9.85 ± 10.74, respectively, $p = 0.65$).

Preparation for complex walking tasks

For SCL during the preparation phase of each task, there was a significant main effect of task ($p < 0.05$). The size of that effect across tasks is shown by the gray bars in **Figure 4**, which show the change in SCL for the preparation phase of each complex walking task relative to the TOI for the preparation phase of the *control* task. *Post hoc* analysis revealed that, relative to $control_{prepare}$, SCL increased significantly for $verbal_{prepare}$ ($p = 0.03$), $dim_{prepare}$ ($p = 0.04$), $carry_{prepare}$ ($p = 0.02$), $obstacles_{prepare}$ ($p = 0.02$), and $vest_{prepare}$ ($p = 0.03$). The effects of side (right and left hands) and task × side interactions were not significant.

Performance of complex walking tasks

For SCL during the performance phase of each task, a significant main effect of task was also found ($p < 0.05$). The size of that effect across tasks is indicated by the black bars of **Figure 4**, which show the change in SCL for the performance phase of each complex walking task relative to the SCL for the preparation phase of the *control* task. *Post hoc* analysis revealed that, relative to $control_{prepare}$, SCL increased significantly for $verbal_{perform}$ ($p = 0.02$), $dim_{perform}$ ($p = 0.04$), $carry_{perform}$ ($p = 0.01$), $obstacles_{perform}$ ($p = 0.02$), and $vest_{perform}$ ($p = 0.03$). The effects of side (right and left hands) and task × side interaction were not significant.

Within-task comparison of preparation versus performance

Also examined was whether SCL increased from the preparation phase to the performance phase within each task (i.e., comparing gray bars to black bars for each task in **Figure 4**). Preparation and performance for TOI increased significantly between $dim_{prepare}$ to $dim_{perform}$ ($p = 0.001$), between $verbal_{prepare}$ and $verbal_{perform}$ ($p < 0.001$), between $carry_{prepare}$ and $carry_{perform}$ ($p < 0.001$), between $vest_{prepare}$ and $vest_{perform}$ ($p < 0.001$), and between $obstacles_{prepare}$ and $obstacles_{perform}$ ($p < 0.001$).

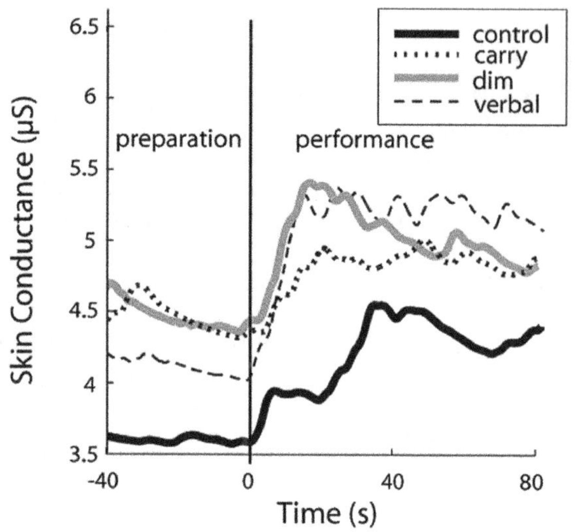

FIGURE 3 | Exemplar data demonstrating task-dependent differences in skin conductance level (SCL). Sympathetic nervous system (SNS) arousal, as indicated by SCL, for one study participant. Data are shown for walking along an unobstructed, well-lit pathway (*control* task; black solid line), walking while carrying a tray (*carry* task; dotted line), walking in dim lighting (*dim* task; gray solid line) and walking while performing a verbal fluency task (*verbal* task; dashed line). The participant is standing still for a short period of time at the start of the trial (preparation phase) and then walks at preferred speed (performance phase).

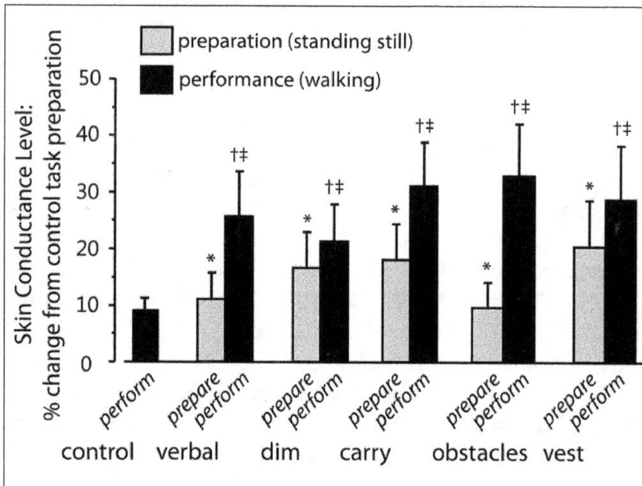

FIGURE 4 | Increase in skin conductance level (SCL) for complex tasks relative to preparation for control task. Gray bars indicate the average percentage increase in SCL during the preparation phase of each complex walking task relative to preparation for the *control* task. Significant changes are shown by an asterisk. Black bars indicate the percentage increase in SCL during the performance phase of each complex walking task relative to preparation for the *control* task. Significant changes are shown by a dagger. Significant within-task differences (preparation versus performance) are shows by a double dagger. Error bars indicate group standard error.

GAIT SPATIOTEMPORAL MEASUREMENTS

Gait spatiotemporal measurements were adversely affected by the complex walking tasks. Relative to *control*, walking speed was reduced for *carry* (−0.05 m/s, $p = 0.02$), *verbal* (−0.15 m/s, $p < 0.001$), *obstacles* (−0.15 m/s, $p < 0.001$) and tended to be reduced for *dim* (−0.02 m/s, $p = 0.09$). Base of support was increased for *carry* (0.89 cm, $p = 0.03$), *verbal* (0.82 cm, $p = 0.008$), and *dim* (0.94 cm, $p = 0.005$). Double support % was increased for *carry* (2.2%, $p = 0.002$), *verbal* (2.5%, $p < 0.001$), and *vest* (0.7%, $p = 0.02$). Variability of step length and double support time increased for *obstacles* (as expected due to the irregular terrain).

Secondary analyses were conducted to determine if the size of the response for prefrontal activation and/or SCL during the performance phase of complex walking tasks was related to the severity of the gait disturbance. For each CNS measure, the study sample was split in half to form two subgroups: low-response subgroup and high-response subgroup. For prefrontal activation, the "response" was calculated as the change in TOI that occurred between the preparation of the *control* task and the performance phase of each complex walking task. For each individual, the average response across all complex walking tasks was calculated. The low-response subgroup for TOI had an average change of −0.2 ± 1.1 percentage points (i.e., roughly unchanged prefrontal activity) and the high-response subgroup had a mean change in TOI of 2.1 ± 0.6 percentage points (i.e., increased prefrontal activity for complex tasks). For each TOI subgroup, average gait measurements during the *control* task are reported in **Table 2A**. The subgroups did not differ significantly for any *control* gait variable, with the exception of a trend for a wider base of support in the high-response subgroup. The subgroups also did not differ significantly for age, body mass index, or MMSE score (all p-values greater than 0.53). Significant differences between subgroups (or a trend) indicate that the high response subgroup had a smaller reduction of walking speed for *obstacles* ($p = 0.003$) and *vest* ($p = 0.001$); lower proportion of gait cycle spent in double limb support for *obstacles* ($p = 0.10$) and *vest* ($p = 0.04$); and less increase for step length variability for *carry* ($p = 0.02$), and *dim* ($p = 0.04$). Although the effect of complex walking tasks

Table 2 | Control task gait values for TOI and SCL response subgroups.

	High	Low	*p*
(A) TOI response subgroups			
Walking speed (m/s)	97.5 ± 9.5	102.5 ± 11.3	0.44
Base of support (cm)	12.5 ± 3.1	8.1 ± 2.7	0.04
Double support (% gait cycle)	34.1 ± 1.5	34.4 ± 2.8	0.85
Step length variability*	2.81 ± 2.10	1.66 ± 0.43	0.26
Double support time variability**	0.022 ± .009	0.021 ± .006	0.75
(B) SCL response subgroups			
Walking speed (m/s)	102.7 ± 14.0	95.9 ± 15.1	0.42
Base of support (cm)	9.9 ± 4.0	12.8 ± 3.0	0.18
Double support (% gait cycle)	34.5 ± 1.8	35.3 ± 3.5	0.59
Step length variability*	2.47 ± 2.04	2.4 ± 1.19	0.94
Double support time variability**	0.02 ± .009	0.026 ± .010	0.26

**Units are in cm SD. **Units are % gait cycle SD.*

Table 3 | Percentage change in gait variables for TOI response subgroups.

	High response	Low response	Effect size	p
Walking speed				
Carry	0.0 ± 7.3	−3.4 ± 5.5	0.51	0.40
Dim	0.6 ± 7.3	4.4 ± 5.3	0.61	0.35
Verbal	−13.6 ± 8.3	−12.5 ± 9.1	0.13	0.85
Obstacles	*−5.5 ± 6.2*	*−21.3 ± 5.8*	*1.72*	*0.003*
Vest	*7.0 ± 3.4*	*−5.3 ± 4.3*	*1.83*	*0.001*
Base of support				
Carry	6.9 ± 24.9	12.1 ± 15.8	0.28	0.69
Dim	11.1 ± 15.4	16.3 ± 18.3	0.34	0.63
Verbal	11.9 ± 9.8	0.7 ± 15.1	0.92	0.20
Obstacles	8.3 ± 24.0	6.8 ± 19.2	0.07	0.92
Vest	4.3 ± 20.0	−5.1 ± 18.3	0.54	0.46
Double support time				
Carry	1.0 ± 1.4	1.6 ± 2.7	0.27	0.67
Dim	0.9 ± 0.8	−0.1 ± 0.8	1.07	0.06
Verbal	2.1 ± 1.3	2.6 ± 2.5	0.26	0.69
Obstacles	−6.8 ± 1.9	−4.3 ± 2.2	1.16	0.10
Vest	*−0.2 ± 0.5*	*1.4 ± 1.2*	*1.36*	*0.04*
Step length variability				
Carry	*−4.3 ± 31.6*	*55.0 ± 37.7*	*1.39*	*0.02*
Dim	*−13.8 ± 35.8*	*16.2 ± 33.1*	*1.18*	*0.04*
Verbal	1.49 ± 50.6	63.6 ± 39.1	0.81	0.18
Obstacles	270.7 ± 184.1	376.9 ± 220.5	0.54	0.43
Vest	1.3 ± 42.6	20.0 ± 30.5	0.56	0.45
Double support time Variability				
Carry	−0.2 ± 30.1	44.8 ± 55.4	1.04	0.16
Dim	−0.5 ± 41.7	7.3 ± 37.9	0.22	0.75
Verbal	25.6 ± 47.2	65.9 ± 125.7	0.49	0.53
Obstacles	77.8 ± 77.3	91.6 ± 92.2	0.18	0.80
Vest	2.5 ± 33.8	13.7 ± 43.9	0.32	0.66

For each complex walking task, the percentage change for each gait variable is calculated relative to the control task. Results are shown for the subgroups determined by higher and lower response of prefrontal cortical activation. Italicized items indicate statistical significance as determined by two-tailed t-tests ($p < 0.05$). All values are mean ± SD.

was not statistically different between groups for most gait variables, it may be valuable to note that the direction of differences favored the high response subgroup as having less gait disturbance for 76% of the variables (19 out of 25; as indicated in **Table 3**). The mean effect size for this subset of gait variables was 0.76 ± 0.54.

The same type of exploratory subgroup analysis as just described was conducted for SCL. The low-response subgroup had an average change in SCL of −2.9 ± 4.2% (i.e., roughly unchanged SNS arousal) and the high-response subgroup had a mean change in SCL of 47.7 ± 29.7% (i.e., increased SNS arousal for complex tasks). For each SCL subgroup, average gait measurements during the *control* task are reported in **Table 2B**. The subgroups did not differ significantly for any *control* gait variable. The low and high SCL response subgroup differed significantly for age (73.6 versus 81.3 years, $p = 0.005$), but not for body mass index ($p = 0.24$) or MMSE score ($p = 0.74$). Accordingly, the gait variables were corrected for age prior to evaluating the effect of complex walking tasks. None of the age-corrected gait variables were found to differ significantly between the low and high SCL response subgroups (all p-values ≥ 0.23). Also examined was the potential association between the mean response size for prefrontal activity and the mean response size for SCL (means calculated across all tasks), in order to investigate the presence of a link between these physiological mechanisms. No association was found ($p = 0.90$).

DISCUSSION

Performance of complex walking tasks is adversely affected by aging (Shumway-Cook et al., 2007), which is concerning given the high relevance of such tasks to everyday ambulation in the home and community. Our choice of tasks was motivated by the "*person-environment interaction model*" of mobility proposed by Patla and Shumway-Cook (1999) and Shumway-Cook et al. (2002). This model describes multiple dimensions that must be mastered to attain successful community ambulatory function. Four dimensions are represented by the tasks in this study: terrain (*obstacles* task), physical load (*vest* task), ambient conditions (*dim* task), and attentional demands (*verbal* and *carry* tasks). The results of this study reveal that prefrontal cortical activity and SNS arousal are elevated during both the preparation and performance phases of complex walking tasks. Furthermore, the changes in prefrontal activity during performance of complex walking tasks were found to be linked to the quality of gait. These findings suggest that utilization of CNS resources is increased to optimize performance of complex walking tasks, and that a shortage of available resources contributes to performance decrements in some older adults.

Prefrontal cortical activation is important to complex walking tasks because of its role in preparing for and executing purposeful actions (Fuster, 2000; Jenkins et al., 2000; Tanji and Hoshi, 2001), including walking (Suzuki et al., 2008; Atsumori et al., 2010; Koenraadt et al., 2014). Our results show that prefrontal TOI increased bilaterally during preparation for all complex walking tasks with the exception of the *verbal* task. During the performance phase of the complex walking tasks, prefrontal TOI remained elevated but generally did not exceed the magnitude observed during the preparation phase. Again, the only notable exception was for *verbal*, where TOI was more strongly elevated during performance than during preparation. This is in agreement with the strongly increased demand for prefrontal resources that is associated with cognitive processing (Holtzer et al., 2011; Ohsugi et al., 2013). Our secondary analysis of subgroups with low versus high prefrontal response generally supported our hypothesis that a high response is linked to better gait performance. Most gait variables (19 out of the 25 when accounting for all tasks) seemed to favor the high-response subgroup, although only a small number were found to be statistically significantly because the analysis was underpowered. For these 19 variables, the average effect size was 0.76, which is considered to be a large effect (Cohen, 1988). Although these results are preliminary, the possible advantage for the high-response subgroup over the low-response subgroup provides encouraging rationale for pursuing this mechanistic finding in future research. We propose that a high response for prefrontal TOI indicates an available reserve supply of prefrontal resources that can contribute to control of complex walking tasks. This reserve supply helps to prevent against excessive competition for central neural resources, thereby preserving movement quality. This assertion is generally consistent with the "supply and demand framework" described by Seidler et al. (2010). These findings build upon prior work that has demonstrated an association between structural integrity of the cortex and gait performance under non-challenging walking conditions (Rosso et al., 2013; Holtzer et al., 2014). For instance, less cerebral gray matter volume of the prefrontal, medial temporal, frontoparietal and sensorimotor areas has been linked to walking decrements such as slow speed, shorter steps, and longer double support time (Rosano et al., 2007, 2008, 2012). The presence of cerebral white matter hyperintensities have also been shown to be linked to decrements in walking ability (Rosano et al., 2010; Wakefield et al., 2010; Viana-Baptista et al., 2011; Moscufo et al., 2012; Willey et al., 2013).

We quantified SNS arousal using the well-established measure of SCL. Our results show that SCL increases substantially when preparing for the complex walking tasks and increases even further when performing the complex walking tasks. However, our hypothesis of a link between SCL and gait performance during complex walking tasks was not supported. Future research is warranted to determine whether a link between SCL response and gait performance may be revealed by comparing cohorts with different characteristics (such as low versus high functioning elders). No association was found between the magnitude of SCL and prefrontal responses. The difference in SCL and prefrontal responses was also evident in the pattern of change that was observed across testing conditions. The elevation in SCL occurred in a stepwise manner, such that (1) SCL for complex task preparation increased over *control* task preparation, and (2) SCL for complex task performance increased over complex task preparation. In agreement with SCL, prefrontal TOI for complex task preparation increased over *control* task preparation. However, in contrast to SCL, no further increase was seen between complex task preparation and complex task performance. Cumulatively, our findings suggest that SCL and prefrontal TOI represent different functions of the CNS for control of walking.

An important finding from our data is that CNS assessments provide the advantage of being more broadly responsive to neurophysiological demand than any single spatiotemporal measure of gait performance. The spatiotemporal gait parameters that were affected by complex walking tasks differed depending on the task. Likewise, the gait parameters that were linked to prefrontal TOI response also differed depending on the task. This finding is not particularly surprising, because the gait modification that is adopted by an individual can be expected to depend on task objectives and also on what facet of performance is prioritized (Al-Yahya et al., 2009; Hobert et al., 2011; Oh-Park et al., 2013). For instance, if a person adopts a cautious gait pattern characterized by greater stance width, then it may be possible to preserve walking speed. In contrast, if a person adopts a slower walking speed, then it may be possible to preserve stance width. Therefore, caution should be used when attempting to interpret isolated gait parameters.

The relative supply and demand of CNS resources during complex walking tasks can be expected to differ among different people (Seidler et al., 2010). This is because the relative challenge of each task will be highly dependent on the specific motor, sensory, and/or cognitive capabilities of the individual. These capabilities were not thoroughly quantified for our participants, so explaining the precise reasons for heightened CNS activity and/or diminished gait quality during complex walking tasks is outside the scope of the present study. However, we did institute a number of exclusion criteria pertaining to medical history (as described in the section "Methods"). These criteria help to ensure that our findings are not overly influenced by the presence of overt health conditions. For instance, we excluded individuals with evidence of more than mild cognitive impairment, based on the MMSE. Cognitive impairment is well known to compromise performance on tasks requiring heightened attentional demand, and may therefore strongly affect task performance. We also screened out individuals who are considered to have a heightened fall risk due to balance impairment, as indicated by the Berg Balance Test. Based on the cumulative criteria employed by our study, it is reasonable to conclude that the observed demand for CNS resources is typical of what can be expected in pre-frail older adults who are free from major medical conditions. Another factor that is known to influence performance on complex tasks is the instructions given to the participants, and the resultant prioritization of different aspects of task performance. For the present study, we gave the participants no specific information regarding how performance would be evaluated, and no instructions regarding prioritization of dual tasks. The rationale for this approach was to observe each participants natural/preferred behavior in order to maximize the relevance of our findings to actual home and community ambulation.

In summary, preparation and performance of complex walking tasks requires heightened utilization of CNS resources in older adults. The findings from this study warrant additional investigation into the role of the CNS in loss of mobility function. The non-invasive measures presented here may be valuable for identifying individuals who are at risk of adverse mobility outcomes and falls, and for gauging the effectiveness of various rehabilitation approaches.

AUTHOR CONTRIBUTIONS

This study was designed by David J. Clark. Data collection was conducted by David J. Clark and Sarah A. Ring. Data analysis was conducted by David J. Clark and Eric C. Porges. Data interpretation was conducted by David J. Clark, Dorian K. Rose, and Eric C. Porges. The content of the manuscript was prepared by David J. Clark, Sarah A. Ring, Dorian K. Rose, and Eric C. Porges.

ACKNOWLEDGMENTS

This work was supported by the North Florida/South Georgia Veterans Health System Rehabilitation Research and Development Service (B7176W, B6862W, B6793C, and 0512BRRC-3), by the

National Institute on Aging via the University of Florida Claude Pepper Older Americans Independence Center (2P30AG028740-06) and by the University of Florida McKnight Brain Research Foundation endowment to the Cognitive Aging and Memory Clinical Translational Research Program.

REFERENCES

Adkin, A. L., Frank, J. S., Carpenter, M. G., and Peysar, G. W. (2002). Fear of falling modifies anticipatory postural control. *Exp. Brain Res.* 143, 160–170. doi: 10.1007/s00221-001-0974-8

Al-Rawi, P. G., and Kirkpatrick, P. J. (2006). Tissue oxygen index: thresholds for cerebral ischemia using near-infrared spectroscopy. *Stroke* 37, 2720–2725. doi: 10.1161/01.STR.0000244807.99073.ae

Al-Yahya, E., Dawes, H., Collett, J., Howells, K., Izadi, H., Wade, D. T., et al. (2009). Gait adaptations to simultaneous cognitive and mechanical constraints. *Exp. Brain Res.* 199, 39–48. doi: 10.1007/s00221-009-1968-1

Atsumori, H., Kiguchi, M., Katura, T., Funane, T., Obata, A., Sato, H., et al. (2010). Noninvasive imaging of prefrontal activation during attention-demanding tasks performed while walking using a wearable optical topography system. *J. Biomed. Opt.* 15, 046002. doi: 10.1117/1.3462996

Bear, M. F., Connors, B. W., and Paradiso, M. A. (2007). *Neuroscience: Exploring the Brain*, 3rd Edn. Philadelphia: Lippincott Williams & Wilkins.

Berg, K., Wood-Dauphinee, S., Williams, J. I., and Gayton, D. (1989). Measuring balance in the elderly: preliminary development of an instrument. *Physiother. Can.* 41, 304–311. doi: 10.3138/ptc.41.6.304

Brown, L. A., Gage, W. H., Polych, M. A., Sleik, R. J., and Winder, T. R. (2002). Central set influences on gait. Age-dependent effects of postural threat. *Exp. Brain Res.* 145, 286–296. doi: 10.1007/s00221-002-1082-0

Bunce, S. C., Izzetoglu, M., Izzetoglu, K., Onaral, B., and Pourrezaei, K. (2006). Functional near-infrared spectroscopy. *IEEE Eng. Med. Biol. Mag.* 25, 54–62. doi: 10.1109/MEMB.2006.1657788

Carpenter, M. G., Frank, J. S., Adkin, A. L., Paton, A., and Allum, J. H. (2004). Influence of postural anxiety on postural reactions to multi-directional surface rotations. *J. Neurophysiol.* 92, 3255–3265. doi: 10.1152/jn.01139.2003

Cohen, J. (1988). *Statistical Power Analysis for the Behavioral Sciences*, 2nd Edn. Hillsdale, NJ: Lawrence Erlbaum.

Curran-Everett, D. (2000). Multiple comparisons: philosophies and illustrations. *Am. J. Physiol. Regul. Integr. Comp. Physiol.* 279, R1–R8.

Curran-Everett, D., and Benos, D. J. (2004). Guidelines for reporting statistics in journals published by the American Physiological Society. *Am. J. Physiol. Regul. Integr. Comp. Physiol.* 287, R247–R249. doi: 10.1152/ajpregu.00346.2004

Folstein, M. F., Folstein, S. E., and McHugh, P. R. (1975). "Mini-mental state". A practical method for grading the cognitive state of patients for the clinician. *J. Psychiatr. Res.* 12, 189–198. doi: 10.1016/0022-3956(75)90026-6

Frank, J. S., and Patla. A. E. (2003). Balance and mobility challenges in older adults: implications for preserving community mobility. *Am. J. Prev. Med.* 25(3 Suppl. 2), 157–163. doi: 10.1016/S0749-3797(03)00179-X

Fuster, J. M. (2000). Executive frontal functions. *Exp. Brain Res.* 133, 66–70. doi: 10.1007/s002210000401

Hadjistavropoulos, T., Carleton, R. N., Delbaere, K., Barden, J., Zwakhalen, S., Fitzgerald, B., et al. (2012). The relationship of fear of falling and balance confidence with balance and dual tasking performance. *Psychol. Aging* 27, 1–13. doi: 10.1037/a0024054

Herrmann, M. J., Walter, A., Ehlis, A. C., and Fallgatter, A. J. (2006). Cerebral oxygenation changes in the prefrontal cortex: effects of age and gender. *Neurobiol. Aging* 27, 888–894. doi: 10.1016/j.neurobiolaging.2005.04.013

Hobert, M. A., Niebler, R., Meyer, S. I., Brockmann, K., Becker, C., Huber, H., et al. (2011). Poor trail making test performance is directly associated with altered dual task prioritization in the elderly–baseline results from the TREND study. *PLoS ONE* 6:e27831. doi: 10.1371/journal.pone.0027831

Holtzer, R., Epstein, N., Mahoney, J. R., Izzetoglu, M., and Blumen, H. M. (2014). Neuroimaging of mobility in aging: a targeted review. *J. Gerontol. A Biol. Sci. Med. Sci.* doi: 10.1093/gerona/glu052

Holtzer, R., Mahoney, J. R., Izzetoglu, M., Izzetoglu, K., Onaral, B., and Verghese, J. (2011). fNIRS study of walking and walking while talking in young and old individuals. *J. Gerontol. A Biol. Sci. Med. Sci.* 66, 879–887. doi: 10.1093/gerona/glr068

Ishikuro, K,. Urakawa, S., Takamoto, K., Ishikawa, A., Ono, T., and Nishijo, H. (2014). Cerebral functional imaging using near-infrared spectroscopy during repeated performances of motor rehabilitation tasks tested on healthy subjects. *Front. Hum. Neurosci.* 8:292. doi: 10.3389/fnhum.2014.00292

Jenkins, I. H., Jahanshahi, M., Jueptner, M., Passingham, R. E., and Brooks, D. J. (2000). Self-initiated versus externally triggered movements. II. The effect of movement predictability on regional cerebral blood flow. *Brain* 123(Pt 6), 1216–1228. doi: 10.1093/brain/123.6.1216

Kaneko, H., Yoshikawa, T., Nomura, K., Ito, H., Yamauchi, H., Ogura, M., et al. (2011). Hemodynamic changes in the prefrontal cortex during digit span task: a near-infrared spectroscopy study. *Neuropsychobiology* 63, 59–65. doi: 10.1159/000323446

Koenraadt, K. L., Roelofsen, E. G., Duysens, J., and Keijsers, N. L. (2014). Cortical control of normal gait and precision stepping: an fNIRS study. *Neuroimage* 85(Pt 1), 415–422. doi: 10.1016/j.neuroimage.2013.04.070

Lord, S. E., Weatherall, M., and Rochester, L. (2010). Community ambulation in older adults: which internal characteristics are important? *Arch. Phys. Med. Rehabil.* 91, 378–383. doi: 10.1016/j.apmr.2009.11.008

Moscufo, N., Wolfson, L., Meier, D., Liguori, M., Hildenbrand, P. G., Wakefield, D., et al. (2012). Mobility decline in the elderly relates to lesion accrual in the splenium of the corpus callosum. *Age* 34, 405–414. doi: 10.1007/s11357-011-9242-4

Oh-Park, M., Holtzer, R., Mahoney, J., Wang, C., Raghavan, P., and Verghese, J. (2013). Motor dual-task effect on gait and task of upper limbs in older adults under specific task prioritization: pilot study. *Aging Clin. Exp. Res.* 25, 99–106. doi: 10.1007/s40520-013-0014-0

Ohsugi, H., Ohgi, S., Shigemori, K., and Schneider, E. B. (2013). Differences in dual-task performance and prefrontal cortex activation between younger and older adults. *BMC Neurosci.* 14:10. doi: 10.1186/1471-2202-14-10

Okamoto, M., Dan, H., Shimizu, K., Takeo, K., Amita, T., Oda, I., et al. (2004). Multimodal assessment of cortical activation during apple peeling by NIRS and fMRI. *Neuroimage* 21, 1275–1288. doi: 10.1016/j.neuroimage.2003.12.003

Patla, A. E., and Shumway-Cook, A. (1999). Dimensions of mobility: defining the complexity and difficulty associated with community mobility. *J. Aging Phys. Act.* 7, 7–19.

Rosano, C., Aizenstein, H., Brach, J., Longenberger, A., Studenski, S., and Newman, A. B. (2008). Special article: gait measures indicate underlying focal gray matter atrophy in the brain of older adults. *J. Gerontol. A Biol. Sci. Med. Sci.* 63, 1380–1388. doi: 10.1093/gerona/63.12.1380

Rosano, C., Aizenstein, H. J., Studenski, S., and Newman, A. B. (2007). A regions-of-interest volumetric analysis of mobility limitations in community-dwelling older adults. *J. Gerontol. A Biol. Sci. Med. Sci.* 62, 1048–1055. doi: 10.1093/gerona/62.9.1048

Rosano, C., Bennett, D. A., Newman, A. B., Venkatraman, V., Yaffe, K., Harris, T., et al. (2012). Patterns of focal gray matter atrophy are associated with bradykinesia and gait disturbances in older adults. *J. Gerontol. A Biol. Sci. Med. Sci.* 67, 957–962. doi: 10.1093/gerona/glr262

Rosano, C., Sigurdsson, S., Siggeirsdottir, K., Phillips, C. L., Garcia, M., Jonsson, P. V., et al. (2010). Magnetization transfer imaging, white matter hyperintensities, brain atrophy and slower gait in older men and women. *Neurobiol. Aging* 31, 1197–1204. doi: 10.1016/j.neurobiolaging.2008.08.004

Rosso, A. L., Studenski, S. A., Chen, W. G., Aizenstein, H. J., Alexander, N. B., Bennett, D. A., et al. (2013). Aging, the central nervous system, and mobility. *J. Gerontol. A Biol. Sci. Med. Sci.* 68, 1379–1386. doi: 10.1093/gerona/glt089

Sato, K., Kang, W. H., Saga, K., and Sato, K. T. (1989). Biology of sweat glands and their disorders. I. Normal sweat gland function. *J. Am. Acad. Dermatol.* 20, 537–563. doi: 10.1016/S0190-9622(89)70063-3

Seidler, R. D., Bernard, J. A., Burutolu, T. B., Fling, B. W., Gordon, M. T., Gwin, J. T., et al. (2010). Motor control and aging: links to age-related brain structural, functional, and biochemical effects. *Neurosci. Biobehav. Rev.* 34, 721–733. doi: 10.1016/j.neubiorev.2009.10.005

Shumway-Cook, A., Guralnik, J. M., Phillips, C. L., Coppin, A. K., Ciol, M. A., Bandinelli, S., et al. (2007). Age-associated declines in complex walking task performance: the Walking InCHIANTI toolkit. *J. Am. Geriatr. Soc.* 55, 58–65. doi: 10.1111/j.1532-5415.2006.00962.x

Shumway-Cook, A., Patla, A., Stewart, A., Ferrucci, L., Ciol, M. A., and Guralnik, J. M. (2003). Environmental components of mobility disability in community-living older persons. *J. Am. Geriatr. Soc.* 51, 393–398. doi: 10.1046/j.1532-5415.2003.51114.x

Shumway-Cook, A., Patla, A. E., Stewart, A., Ferrucci, L., Ciol, M. A., and Guralnik, J. M. (2002). Environmental demands associated with community mobility in older adults with and without mobility disabilities. *Phys. Ther.* 82, 670–681.

Sibley, K. M., Mochizuki, G., Frank, J. S., and McIlroy, W. E. (2010). The relationship between physiological arousal and cortical and autonomic responses to postural instability. *Exp. Brain Res.* 203, 533–540. doi: 10.1007/s00221-010-2257-8

Suzuki, M., Miyai, I., Ono, T., and Kubota, K. (2008). Activities in the frontal cortex and gait performance are modulated by preparation. An fNIRS study. *Neuroimage* 39, 600–607. doi: 10.1016/j.neuroimage.2007.08.044

Tanji, J., and Hoshi, E. (2001). Behavioral planning in the prefrontal cortex. *Curr. Opin. Neurobiol.* 11, 164–170. doi: 10.1016/S0959-4388(00)00192-6

Tisdall, M. M., Taylor, C., Tachtsidis, I., Leung, T. S., Elwell, C. E., and Smith, M. (2009). The effect on cerebral tissue oxygenation index of changes in the concentrations of inspired oxygen and end-tidal carbon dioxide in healthy adult volunteers. *Anesth. Analg.* 109, 906–913. doi: 10.1213/ane.0b013e3181aedcdc

Viana-Baptista, M., Bugalho, P., Jordao, C., Ribeiro, O., Esperanca-Pina, J. A., and Ferro, J. (2011). Motor dysfunction correlates with frontal white matter ischemic changes in patients with leukoaraiosis. *J. Aging Res.* 2011, 950341. doi: 10.4061/2011/950341

Wakefield, D. B., Moscufo, N., Guttmann, C. R., Kuchel, G. A., Kaplan, R. F., Pearlson, G., et al. (2010). White matter hyperintensities predict functional decline in voiding, mobility, and cognition in older adults. *J. Am. Geriatr. Soc.* 58, 275–281. doi: 10.1111/j.1532-5415.2009.02699.x

Willey, J. Z., Scarmeas, N., Provenzano, F. A., Luchsinger, J. A., Mayeux, R., and Brickman, A. M. (2013). White matter hyperintensity volume and impaired mobility among older adults. *J. Neurol.* 260, 884–890. doi: 10.1007/s00415-012-6731-z

Yerkes, R. M., and Dodson, J. D. (1908). The relation of strength of stimulus to rapidity of habit formation. *J. Comp. Neurol. Psychol.* 18, 459–482. doi: 10.1002/cne.920180503

5

Development and decline of upright gait stability

Marco Iosa*, Augusto Fusco, Giovanni Morone and Stefano Paolucci

Clinical Laboratory of Experimental Neurorehabilitation, Fondazione Santa Lucia, Istituto di Ricovero e Cura a Carattere Scientifico (IRCCS), Rome, Italy

Edited by:
Brian C. Clark, Ohio University, USA

Reviewed by:
Shinichi Amano, Ohio University, USA
Jacob Sosnoff, University of Illinois at Urbana-Champaign, USA

***Correspondence:**
Marco Iosa, Clinical Laboratory of Experimental Neurorehabilitation, Fondazione Santa Lucia, IRCCS, Via Ardeatina 306, Rome 00179, Italy
e-mail: m.iosa@hsantalucia.it

Upright gait is a peculiar characteristic of humans that requires the ability to manage upper body dynamic balance while walking, despite the perturbations that are generated by movements of the lower limbs. Most of the studies on upright gait stability have compared young adults and the elderly to determine the effects of aging. In other studies, the comparison was between healthy subjects and patients to examine specific pathologies. Fewer researches have also investigated the development of upright gait stability in children. This review discusses these studies in order to provide an overview of this relevant aspect of human locomotion. A clear trend from development to decline of upright gait stability has been depicted across the entire lifespan, from toddlers at first steps to elderly. In old individuals, even if healthy, the deterioration of skeletal muscle, combined with sensorial and cognitive performance, reduces the ability to maintain an upright trunk during walking, increasing the instability and the risk of falls. Further, the pathological causes of altered development or of a sudden loss of gait stability, as well as the environmental influence are investigated. The last part of this review is focused on the control of upper body accelerations during walking, a particularly interesting topic for the recent development of low-cost wearable accelerometers.

Keywords: locomotion, walking, balance, falls, accelerometry, motor control, aging, neuromuscular diseases

INTRODUCTION

An experience of great pleasure for a person is surely when his/her child begins to walk independently. Those first few unstable steps are considered a fundamental stage of human development. Arguably, the child's clear pronunciation of his first word rivals this milestone.

Differently from other animals, human children need more time to develop independent gait (Garwicz et al., 2009). Fourteen months are in mean needed (Bosch et al., 2007) because baby's rudimentary lower limb flexion–extension movements evolve into sophisticated coordination that permits upright walking (Dominici et al., 2011). Upright walking was not only a fundamental stage in the ontogenesis of a child but also a basic step in phylogenetic human evolution that about 1.5 million years ago evolved to *Homo erectus*. Erectus should not be considered a synonym of bipedal walking but as a stable, upright upper body posture during walking.

The expression "stable gait" may refer to a step-to-step repeatable walking (Ingwell and Marin, 2006), to a gait resilient to external and internal perturbations (Terrier and Dériaz, 2011), or to the ability of maintaining upright balance during walking (Menz et al., 2003). A recent review identified 92 different linear and non-linear quantitative measures of "gait stability" obtained using five different categories of devices and mainly related to spatio-temporal gait parameters, lower limb joint kinematics, and upper body kinematics (Hamacher et al., 2011). About this latter aspect, "upright gait stability" refers to the capacity of humans to minimize oscillations during walking, in a progressive way from the lower to upper levels of the human body, with the head moved on a straight line at quite constant speed (Cappozzo, 1981; Inman et al., 1981). The stabilization of the head during human gait allows steadying the optic flow and increasing the control of equilibrium with more effective processing of vestibular system signals (Berthoz and Pozzo, 1994; Spoor et al., 1994). These and other advantages, such as keeping the hands free and seeing farther, might have spurred the development of upright walking in humans (Friedman, 2006). In general, both exploratory and performative activities can benefit from the upright posture maintained also during gait (Reed, 1996).

The purpose of this review was to investigate the development and the decline of upright gait stability during the lifespan, both in unimpaired and impaired subjects. In the second part of this review, particular attention was deserved to the upright gait stability, i.e., to the upper body dynamic balance evaluated in terms of the capacity of smoothing accelerations during walking.

DEVELOPMENT OF UPRIGHT GAIT STABILITY

PHYSIOLOGICAL DEVELOPMENT

In typical development, gait mechanism becomes predominantly functional and efficient by the age of 2 years [walking speed (WS) close to 0.8 stature/s (Sutherland et al., 1980) and 60% of energy recovery (Ivanenko et al., 2004)]. However, children may need more time to achieve a stable gait and to manage the emerging instability that accompanies the progressive increase in WS (Iosa et al., 2012f). The beginning of independent walking, averaging at 14 months (Bosch et al., 2007) is characterized by extensive trunk oscillations and a wide base of support, which help the control of instability in new walkers (Ivanenko et al., 2007). At this age, both motor and somatosensory systems need to be developed in order to improve balance and dynamic equilibrium control (Bosch and

Rosenbaum, 2010). Unlike the adults, the lateral component of kinetic energy of the center of mass is not negligible, compared to its sagittal components, in toddlers (Ivanenko et al., 2004).

Upper limbs play an important role in this scenario. Healthy adults move their upper and lower limbs in a contralaterally synchronized fashion, to reduce the moment of inertia and maintain upright gait stability (Sparrow and Newell, 1994). At the early stages of gait development, however, healthy toddlers keep their upper limbs high, similar to the spastic limbs observed in children with cerebral palsy. During development, children lower this "high guard" position of the upper limbs, increasing their WS (Kubo and Ulrich, 2006a). The interaction between arm posture and upper trunk position creates a variety of changes in forces and torque between individuals that can be explained by the need for healthy toddlers to explore their dynamics and gait stability in the early stages of gait development (Pozzo et al., 1990).

From age 7, upper body gait stability is related to the adoption of head stabilization (Pozzo et al., 1990), which appears to be more difficult in the latero-lateral (LL) compared to the antero-posterior (AP) direction (Assaiante and Amblard, 1993; Mazzà et al., 2010). At age 9, children show upper body stability, similar to that of adults (Mazzà et al., 2010). Unfortunately, few data are available about individuals between 10 and 20 years of age, preventing a detailed examination on what occurs in teenagers: in this age, cultural habits and psychological features may be also have an impact on functional development and anthropometric growth.

ALTERED DEVELOPMENT

In children with impaired development, such as those with cerebral palsy, the ability to walk at a proper speed is limited in the first phase of independent walking, even if they are not severely affected (Iosa et al., 2012f). Later, they develop a faster speed, implying high trunk instability (Iosa et al., 2012f). Higher vertical oscillations in these children are likely related to their equinus foot or crouch gait, two typical features of cerebral palsy (Perry, 1992; Gage, 1993). Along LL direction, an increased distance has been found between the body center of mass and the center of pressure under the foot of standing leg in children with diplegia due to cerebral palsy during single support phase of gait (Hsue et al., 2009a,b). This could be due to three possibly concomitant reasons: (1) hip muscle weakness (see Gait Instability and Risk of Fall for details); (2) facilitating contralateral foot lift; (3) facilitating the control of forward progression by transferring part of forward momentum to lateral momentum.

The high trunk accelerations and gait asymmetry that are observed in children with cerebral palsy are likely to be related to certain compensatory mechanisms that facilitate walking at a speed that is similar to that of unimpaired children (Meyns et al., 2012). Greater arm swing on the unaffected side is often required to compensate for the reduced movement on the affected side and to counteract the substantial increases in angular momentum that are generated by functional asymmetry in the legs (Bruijn et al., 2011). Thus, it is conceivable that this compensatory strategy destabilizes gait patterns (Bruijn et al., 2011), reducing upright gait stability (Iosa et al., 2012f).

In children with Down syndrome, the development of independent walking usually occurs approximately 1 year later than in children who undergo typical development (Henderson, 1986). At the early stages of walking, children with Down syndrome have similar gait spatio-temporal patterns as typically developed toddlers but appear to be less able to manage the coupling of AP–LL oscillations at the level of the center of mass, i.e., at the lower trunk level (Kubo and Ulrich, 2006b).

The altered development of upright gait stability is an interesting topic, and further studies are needed to examine the development of gait stability in toddlers with and without developmental disability. The possibility of easily assessing gait related features by wearable devices (rather than with more complex stereophotogrammetric systems) might be helpful for early clinical analysis and, in general, for a greater understanding of this processes (Masci et al., 2013).

DECLINE OF UPRIGHT GAIT STABILITY

PHYSIOLOGICAL DECLINE WITH AGING

Many studies reported a decline of gait stability in the elderly. Experimental evidence shows that this reduction in the ability to stabilize the upper body during walking is due to the loss of skeletal muscle strength (Doherty, 2003) and a reduction in the ability to detect and process proprioceptive and sensorial information (Scaglioni et al., 2003).

From a motor point of view, after the age of 50, approximately 1–2% of muscle mass is lost per year. This muscle mass and strength reduction, called sarcopenia, is also accompanied by intramuscular fat accumulation, muscle atrophy (especially the type IIa fibers), decreased satellite cell proliferation and differentiation capacity, and reduction in motor unit number (Muscaritoli et al., 2013). The loss in body mass density, which is related to muscle weakness, is greater in women compared to men aged 60 years and older (Daly et al., 2013). From a skeletal point of view, the age-related degradation of joints, including articular cartilage and bone epiphysis, especially at knee level, can cause gait impairments, especially when it suddenly degenerates in pathological osteoarthritis (van Baar et al., 1998).

A recent study had also suggested that vitamin D may be involved in gait stability. Vitamin D metabolism is in fact involved in muscular contraction speed and one of the consequence of its concentration reduction, typically occurring in the elderly, was found to be an increased stride-to-stride duration variability that is related to a reduction of gait stability and hence to an increased risk of fall (Beauchet et al., 2011).

Aging implies not only a loss in musculoskeletal functioning, but also a decline in vision, reaction time, peripheral and vestibular sensations: all of which can reduce upper body stability during walking (Menz et al., 2003). The vestibular system becomes impaired with age, altering the vestibulospinal reflex function (Allum et al., 1997). With regard to the chief function of the vestibular system in upright gait stability, it is noteworthy that the inner ear of *Homo erectus* was more developed than in earlier hominids, who possessed ape-like inner ears (Spoor et al., 1994).

Considering these reduction in sensorimotor ability, older persons have a more conservative gait pattern, characterized by reduced velocity that is a result of a shorter step length and accompanied by increased variability in step timing (Menz et al., 2003). These differences are particularly pronounced when they walk on irregular surfaces (Menz et al., 2003; Marigold and Patla, 2008). The conservative basic gait patterns, evident in older people, might be a compensatory strategy to ensure adequate stabilization of the upper body (Menz et al., 2003). It has been proposed that these gait patterns in older people are attributed in part to a decline in leg strength and a reluctance to walk quickly, so that their upper body accelerations do not increase (Menz et al., 2003). Notably, the elderly experience an abrupt increase in instability in the LL direction. These results are also supported by the excessive lateral momentum found in balance-impaired during gait (Kaya et al., 1998) and by the increased center of mass – center of pressure inclination angle measured in lateral direction (frontal plane) (Lee and Chou, 2006) that were both found as sensitive measures of loss of equilibrium in elderly during gait. Lateral trunk bending has been described as a typical compensation mechanism for hip abductor weakness: lateral trunk movements toward the stance limb align the body's center of mass over the hip joint center, supporting the body in the single stance when the hip abductor muscles are weak (Perry, 1992). This trunk bending strategy, helpful for compensation hip muscle weakness, is typical not only of old age, but also of many pathologies (as described below), including children with cerebral palsy with lateral excessive trunk bending, as reported above.

Not only motor and sensorial impairment have been shown to affect upright gait stability in the elderly. Indeed, physiological reduction of cognitive functions might also have a significant role, as suggested by studies that reported decreased gait stability in subjects with cognitive impairment (see Pathological Loss of Gait Stability) (Lamoth et al., 2011; Ijmker and Lamoth, 2012). This topic appears rather controversial, as the study entitled "walking without thinking" (Ruchinskas et al., 2000) questions the role of cognitive function on gait control, observing that, while it could affect the overall geriatric rehabilitation course, it may not predict walking or stair climbing ability. It must be remembered, however that cognitive status and thinking are two different things. Another study, in fact, observed that in elderly persons without cognitive impairment, gait patterns were altered when subjects were asked to walk and perform a cognitive naming task simultaneously (Lamoth et al., 2011). In response to dual tasking, subjects decreased their WS by increasing stride time. Despite the lower speed, trunk acceleration patterns were more irregular and variable, and local stability declined in the dual task condition. These results highlight the importance to take into account the control of functional resource allocation, with a reduction in upright gait stability when subjects are asked to walk and perform a cognitive task simultaneously, as occurs often in everyday life.

Finally, upright gait stability has been found adversely associated to subclinical cerebrovascular lesions. Silent infarcts (detectable in 7.2–28% of the general population, i.e., in the absence of a history of clinical stroke), cerebral microbleedings (occurring in 4.7–23.5% of the general population), and cerebral white matter microlesions (present in 90% of people aged >60 years) affect gait ability and stability in elderly (Choi et al., 2012).

GAIT INSTABILITY AND RISK OF FALL

All the difficulties described above in controlling dynamic balance during walking in the elderly have also been associated with the risk of falls (Marigold and Patla, 2008; Senden et al., 2012). There are currently over 400 known risk factors for falls, broadly classified into environmental, task-related, and personal factors (Masud and Morris, 2001). Age is one of the most important risk factor, and many other personal factors may be related to age: among others, muscular strength, reaction time, visual ability, use of drugs and medications, living alone, sedentary behavior, psychological status, and impaired cognition and foot problems (Hamacher et al., 2011). As above reported, most of them are also associated to higher upper body accelerations and higher step-by-step gait variability.

Environmental, task-related, and personal factors may also increase the risk of fall. For example, this risk increases when older individuals can not reduce their WS by controlling their trunk acceleration. This event may occur when they want to cross a street and must time their gait speed with the traffic lights, which usually requires a mean speed of at least 0.9 m/s (Hesse et al., 2009), higher than what many older subjects can attain (see **Table 1**; Mazzà et al., 2008; Lamoth et al., 2011; Senden et al., 2012). For example, in UK, such as in other Western countries, 1.2 m/s is the value of theoretical WS utilized to set the crossing timing of traffic lights (Asher et al., 2012). However, the comfortable speed of many elderly is lower than these values (Asher et al., 2012). A speed lower than 0.8 m/s has been defined as a pathological gait velocity and resulted associated with repeated falls, even when observed in healthy elderly (without any specific pathology) (Montero-Odasso et al., 2004). But a low steady speed is not the only factor affecting the safety in road crossing. The presence of obstacles (Hahn and Chou, 2004), the visual attention and the time-to-arrival estimation (Dommes and Cavallo, 2011), the fear of falling (Avineri et al., 2012), the time spent in selecting the proper motor strategy (Sueur et al., 2013), as well as the management of accelerations (for example in the start of walking, or for further increasing speed if traffic green light is going to expire or if a car is arriving) or deceleration for terminating road crossing (Bollard and Fleming, 2013) are all factors that can reduce gait stability and increase the risk of fall or of an accident.

Regarding acceleration, upper body cranio-caudal (CC) accelerations were found significantly increased in elderly with balance impairment compared to elderly without balance impairment (Senden et al., 2012). Furthermore, it has been reported that the harmonicity of trunk movements (assessed by analysis of trunk accelerations in the domain of frequency) is a reliable predictor of the risk of falls in elderly, independently of their physical performance, in 1 year after the assessment (Doi et al., 2013) (for details about these last two studies, see Assessment of Dynamic Equilibrium by Trunk Accelerations).

A recent review analyzed the available kinematic measures for assessing gait stability, taking into account old versus young subjects' comparisons and fallers versus no-fallers comparisons (Hamacher et al., 2011). The authors found that, regarding the 92 different outcome measures identified in literature, linear measures of gait stability showed a higher sensitivity concerning age-related differences than non-linear measures. In detail,

Table 1 | Healthy subject trunk accelerations during walking ordered by age.

Authors (year)	Age (years)	WS (m/s)	Gender	Trunk level	*n*	RMS_{AP} (m/s^2)	RMS_{LL} (m/s^2)	RMS_{CC} (m/s^2)
Iosa et al. (2012f)	4 ± 1	0.94 ± 0.22	M and F	L2–L3	8	2.23 ± 0.60	2.14 ± 0.47	2.95 ± 0.81
	7 ± 2	1.09 ± 0.13	M and F	L2–L3	9	1.72 ± 0.40	1.54 ± 0.48	2.44 ± 0.86
Mazzà et al. (2010)	9 ± 1	1.34 ± 0.14	M	Pelvis	15	1.93 ± 0.31	1.76 ± 0.23	2.90 ± 0.67
	9 ± 1	1.32 ± 0.16	F	Pelvis	15	1.97 ± 0.31	1.79 ± 0.31	2.93 ± 0.85
Mazzà et al. (2009)	23 ± 2	1.33 ± 0.13	M	Pelvis	20	1.91 ± 0.40	1.57 ± 0.36	2.70 ± 0.72
	23 ± 3	1.34 ± 0.09	F	Pelvis	20	2.06 ± 0.40	1.90 ± 0.22	2.88 ± 0.13
Moe-Nilssen (1998)	23 ± 2	1.2[a]	M and F	L3	19	1.57 ± 0.18	1.33 ± 0.17	2.06 ± 0.23
Kavanagh (2009)	23 ± 3	1.32 ± 0.18	M and F	L3	13	1.63 ± 0.17	1.23 ± 0.16	1.91 ± 0.23
Iosa et al. (2012b)	28 ± 5	1.12 ± 0.11	M and F	L2–L3	28	1.72 ± 0.28	1.51 ± 0.36	2.76 ± 0.56
Iosa et al. (2010)	31 ± 9	1.25 ± 0.08	M and F	Pelvis	13	1.53 ± 0.25	0.56 ± 0.07	1.79 ± 0.35
Henriksen et al. (2004)	35	1.35[a]	M and F	L3	20	1.75 ± 0.20	1.35 ± 0.25	2.47 ± 0.24
Iosa et al. (2012d)	63 ± 10	1.17 ± 0.18	M and F	L2–L3	10	1.49 ± 0.30	1.02 ± 0.22	2.21 ± 0.70
Iosa et al. (2012e)	29 ± 5	1.13 ± 0.11	M and F	L2–L3	15	1.75 ± 0.35	1.57 ± 0.39	2.87 ± 0.65
	65 ± 9	1.02 ± 0.16	M and F		15	1.37 ± 0.26	0.96 ± 0.22	1.94 ± 0.54
Mazzà et al. (2008)	24 ± 4	1.30 ± 0.28	F	Pelvis	16	1.41 ± 0.23	0.48 ± 0.18	1.66 ± 0.92
	72 ± 4	0.97 ± 0.18	F	Pelvis	20	1.06 ± 0.24	0.48 ± 0.14	0.99 ± 0.32
Kavanagh et al. (2004)	23 ± 4	1.28 ± 0.15	M and F	L2–L3	8	1.47 ± 0.98	1.10 ± 0.78	1.77 ± 1.17
	74 ± 3	1.23 ± 0.15		L2–L3	8	1.37 ± 0.98	1.10 ± 0.69	1.77 ± 1.10
Marigold and Patla (2008)	26 ± 5	1.0[a]	M and F	Iliac crests	10	0.95 ± 0.10	0.57 ± 0.09	1.65 ± 0.21
	74 ± 7				10	1.05 ± 0.16	0.74 ± 0.13	1.56 ± 0.17
Ijmker and Lamoth (2012)	64 ± 3	1.19 ± 0.08	M and F	L3	12	1.40 ± 0.16	1.28 ± 0.19	Not eval.
	77 ± 4	1.14 ± 0.11			14	0.84 ± 0.32	0.95 ± 0.31	
Lamoth et al. (2011)	79 ± 5	0.95 ± 0.21	M and F	L3	13	1.04 ± 0.23	0.96 ± 0.18	Not eval.
Menz et al. (2003)	29 ± 4	1.33 ± 0.19	M and F	Pelvis	30	1.86 ± 0.39	1.86 ± 0.39	2.55 ± 0.69
	79 ± 3	1.17 ± 0.16		Pelvis	30	1.67 ± 0.29	1.57 ± 0.49	1.96 ± 0.49
Senden et al. (2012)	74 ± 5	1.23 ± 0.22	M and F	Sacrum	50	Not eval.	Not eval.	2.45 ± 0.69
	79 ± 6	0.86 ± 0.26			50			1.57 ± 0.69

The columns report authors and year of publication, the reference number for each study, the mean age (±SD) of groups of subjects, walking speed ([a] in some studies a reference value of WS has been used to identify trunk acceleration from interpolant curves), gender, analyzed level of trunk (in many of these studies, other parts of the body are analyzed), number of subjects enrolled (n), and mean acceleration RMS along the antero-posterior (AP), latero-lateral (LL), and cranio-caudal (CC) axis. In some of the original studies, accelerations were reported in g, in which case they were transformed to m/s^2, or reported in terms of mean and standard error of the mean, in which case they were transformed to mean ± SD. For study Henderson (1986), the data are related to the first 6 min of walking. Finally, not all studies evaluated accelerations along all three body axes.

variability of step width and stride velocity were capable of distinguishing between old and young subjects, whereas variability of stride, stance, and swing between fallers and non-fallers. Step width variability had higher discriminative power in the comparison between elderly and young subjects than in the faller versus non-faller comparisons, suggesting that although it may increase with age, it is not necessarily a dominant factor in fall risk. This suggestion has also been supported by the fact that differences between fit and frail older adults were better highlighted by interstride trunk acceleration variability, than by step width variability (Moe-Nilssen and Helbostad, 2005). Another study reported increased trunk acceleration and trunk roll variability along LL direction in elderly walking, despite having similar step width of the control group formed by younger subjects (Marigold and Patla, 2008).

According to all these studies, the increased LL trunk acceleration observed in advanced age seems to be a particularly important risk of fall given its association with gait instability. Moreover, hip fractures occur most frequently in association with lateral falls.

PATHOLOGICAL LOSS OF GAIT STABILITY

The loss of stability can be abrupt when a pathological event occurs, wherein more severe pathologies affect a greater loss of upright gait stability.

Upright gait stability has been studied extensively in subjects after stroke. In these patients, upper body accelerations are significantly lower than in age-matched healthy controls in all axes due to the reducing WS. However, acceleration root mean square (RMS) values that have been normalized by speed are higher than in healthy subjects along all body axes in subjects with chronic (Mizuike et al., 2009) and subacute stroke (Iosa et al., 2012e). As shown in **Table 1**, the mean WS of young healthy adults was about 1.3 m/s. Although WS in stroke patients (reported in **Table 2**) declines by approximately 50% versus young healthy adults, their CC acceleration (in terms of its RMS), their AP and LL accelerations do not. Yet, in patients with stroke, trunk control is a prognostic factor for gait recovery (Masiero et al., 2007; Di Monaco et al., 2010): their trunk asymmetries are more marked than their

Table 2 | Gait stability data of subjects with a pathology or healthy subjects walking on uneven floor or without vision support, with respect to reference values obtained as the average of means (±SDMs) reported in studies on young healthy adults.

Condition	Reference	Age (years)	WS (m/s)	Trunk level	*n*	RMS_{AP} (m/s^2)	RMS_{LL} (m/s^2)	RMS_{CC} (m/s^2)
Cerebral palsy	Iosa et al. (2012f)	4 ± 1	0.76 ± 0.19	L2–L3	11	2.29 ± 0.78	2.26 ± 0.93	3.04 ± 1.43
		7 ± 2	1.15 ± 0.09	L2–L3	6	2.86 ± 0.91	2.50 ± 0.68	4.29 ± 1.31
Stroke	Iosa et al. (2012e)	61 ± 15	0.60 ± 0.29	L2–L3	15	0.98 ± 0.33	0.80 ± 0.24	1.16 ± 0.50
	Iosa et al. (2012d)	64 ± 13	0.55 ± 0.31	L2–L3	20	0.91 ± 0.37	0.87 ± 0.41	1.13 ± 0.61
Dystrophy	Iosa et al. (2010)	39 ± 11	1.04 ± 0.15	Pelvis	13	1.31 ± 0.36	0.59 ± 0.16	1.30 ± 0.40
Dementia	Lamoth et al. (2011)	83 ± 4	0.88 ± 0.27	L3	13	1.03 ± 0.26	0.82 ± 0.18	Not eval.
	Ijmker and Lamoth (2012)	82 ± 6	0.67 ± 0.21	L3	15	0.56 ± 0.22	0.59 ± 0.21	Not eval.
Uneven floor	Moe-Nilssen (1998)	23 ± 2	1.2[a]	L3	19	1.72 ± 0.22	1.57 ± 0.18	2.28 ± 0.23
No vision	Iosa et al. (2012b)	28 ± 5	0.83 ± 0.18	L2–L3	28	1.32 ± 0.36	1.23 ± 0.36	1.87 ± 0.68
Reference values	Mazzà et al. (2009), Iosa et al. (2012e), Menz et al. (2003), Kavanagh et al. (2004), Moe-Nilssen (1998), Henriksen et al. (2004), Marigold and Patla (2008)	26 ± 4	1.26 ± 0.10	Lower trunk	183	1.67 ± 0.30	1.40 ± 0.39	2.36 ± 0.47

[a]*A reference value of WS from interpolant curve.*

asymmetries with regard to step length and single support timing (Hodt-Billington et al., 2008).

Overexertion and fatigue can compromise the control of gait stability following stroke. Two alternative strategies have been highlighted in these patients for prolonged (6-min) walking. Some subjects maintain their speed during long-lasting walking, despite a slight but progressive reduction in upper body stability. Other subjects apply a compensatory strategy, based on a reduction in WS for maintaining low upper body accelerations (Iosa et al., 2012d).

Patients with Parkinson's disease show increased stride time variability, reduced trunk rotation, reduced arm swing as signs of gait impairments as well as increased time spent in the double support phase that is probably due to the need of improving dynamic equilibrium during gait (Horak and Mancini, 2013). L-DOPA reduces stride time variability, decreases double support time, and increases gait speed, all consistent with improvements in gait dynamic balance (Rebula et al., 2013). Interesting studies showed a reduced coordination between the rhythmic processes of the two legs in these patients (Plotnik et al., 2007). In particular, reduced inter-lower limb coordination and higher stride time variability can expose these subjects to a higher risk of falls. Furthermore, during the execution of a cognitive task while walking, gait symmetry was reduced in these patients (Plotnik et al., 2011).

Subjects who are affected by muscular impairment, such as dystrophy, have wider and less symmetrical upper body oscillations than healthy controls in the AP and LL directions. Further, the ability of these subjects to attenuate accelerations from the lower body to the head is weakened. It has been suggested that these features are related not only to upper body muscle impairments but also indirectly to the above described strategy that compensates for hip muscle weakness (Iosa et al., 2010).

As above mentioned, increased LL trunk bending, as described in the elderly, is a typical compensatory mechanism for hip abductor weakness also in other pathologies, such as dystrophy (Iosa et al., 2010), myelomeningocele (Gutierrez et al., 2005), and spinal muscular atrophy (Armand et al., 2005).

Upright gait stability in patients with vestibular deficits is a notable area of study. However, most researches on such patients have investigated their postural standing stability, instead of gait dynamic stability. Nevertheless, one of the few studies on upper body stability during walking in persons with vestibular hypofunction reported lower regularity of upper body movements compared with healthy subjects, consistent with the function of the vestibular system in controlling the dynamic stability of walking (Sylos-Labini et al., 2012). Also, in patients with small vestibular schwannomas and an apparently normal gait who are asked to walk without vision support, gait variability increases, reducing their gait steadiness (Yin et al., 2011). After unilateral vestibular neurotomy, used as curative surgery in patients with Menière syndrome, robust walking deviations develop toward the damaged side on walking with the eyes closed (Borel et al., 2004).

Another sensorial impairment that affects gait stability is altered vision (Perry et al., 2001). However, few studies have examined upright gait stability in a population with visual impairment. Yet, significant differences exist between subjects with and without visual impairments and between conditions of full vision and no vision. Further, these differences reflect a more cautious walking strategy and adaptive changes under challenging conditions. In particular, subjects with visual impairments undergo adaptations that are related to a shorter stride length and prolonged plantar foot contact. These patterns might reflect a strategy to overcome the problems that arise from sensory deprivation, compensated by the use of the feet to probe the ground for haptic exploration, to maintain adequate upper body stability (Hallemans et al., 2010).

In less disabling pathologies, such as low back pain, subjects exhibit altered coordination of the pelvis and trunk, resulting in a less harmonic and less stable gait (Lamoth et al., 2002).

Finally, reductions in cognitive functions, such as those that are related to dementia (Allali et al., 2008; Lamoth et al., 2011; Ijmker and Lamoth, 2012) and Alzheimer disease (Sheridan et al., 2003), contribute to changes in the variability and stability of the gait pattern when the task becomes more challenging, increasing the risk of falls.

OTHER FACTORS INFLUENCING UPRIGHT GAIT STABILITY

Upright gait stability also depends on the capacity of subjects to exploit information on the orientation of the swaying body during walking with respect to the environment. This information is provided primarily by the vestibular system, lower-extremity mechanoreceptors, and vision (Lee, 1980; Perry et al., 2001), but also environmental features can affect upright gait stability (Iosa et al., 2012b) and hence the risk of fall (Hamacher et al., 2011). For example, under impaired physical conditions, subjects usually adopt a strategy to reduce velocity in challenging environments, decreasing upper body accelerations.

A typical situation is when one walks on uneven ground, implying greater upper body acceleration, even in young healthy adults (Moe-Nilssen, 1998). Also, a sudden reduction in environmental light implies an increase in trunk accelerations and inter-step trunk acceleration variability (Moe-Nilssen et al., 2006). Conversely, optic flow can alter locomotion parameters (Pailhous et al., 1990) and mediates the maintenance of a steady gait (Pailhous and Bonnard, 1992).

When vision is blocked completely, the stability, in terms of normalized accelerations, decrease drastically and the harmony of movements in the AP direction falls significantly (Iosa et al., 2012b). These findings demonstrated the fundamental role of vision in upright gait stability, confirming that vestibular, proprioceptive, acoustic, and tactile information can not fully compensate for the loss of visual information to produce a normal gait pattern (Hallemans et al., 2009; Iosa et al., 2012b). There is also a slight difference between walking outdoors and indoors, with higher AP accelerations outdoors, a difference that increases in the absence of visual feedback (Iosa et al., 2012b). It has been suggested that when visual information is lacking, the memorized environment acts as a selective tuner between various walking strategies that is based more on sensory feedback versus on an internal representation of the own body and the external world (Iosa et al., 2012c).

Upper body stability during walking can be also affected by cultural habits, as already suggested (Mazzà et al., 2009), but this relationship has not been investigated in detail. Walking with books over the head was a common exercise for young aristocratic ladies. Certain gender differences in upright gait stability have recently been studied: females have better control strategy, allowing them to reach head accelerations that are equivalent to those of males, despite having higher LL pelvis accelerations (Mazzà et al., 2009). However, this difference was not found significant at the level of L2–L3 (Iosa et al., 2012b), of shoulders and head (Mazzà et al., 2008). Furthermore, the most of the studies did not separate data between males and females. Nevertheless, gender-related features of upright gait stability are reported and the absence of visual feedback exacerbates these gender-based differences in LL movements (Iosa et al., 2012b). The development of upright gait could have had sexual implications: it has even been suggested that permanent sexuality that replaced female estrus, was an effect of the phylogenetic development of upright gait (Graslund, 1995).

Finally, it is noteworthy that in some areas of the world that lack a transportation infrastructure, people routinely carry extraordinary loads supported by their heads, for example the sherpa of the Himalayas and the women of East Africa. It needs a very stable head during walking and it is a result of a greater conservation of mechanical energy resulting from an improved gait control (Heglund et al., 1995).

Thus, it is conceivable that differences in upright stable gait could be related not only to differences in motor abilities, but also to the dictates of social and cultural prescriptions specific for each phase of life and probably also to geographical differences. These hypotheses, however, are unconfirmed and should be further investigated.

THE CONTROL OF UPPER BODY ACCELERATIONS DURING GAIT

ASSESSMENT OF DYNAMIC EQUILIBRIUM BY TRUNK ACCELERATIONS

In the early 1990s, gait analysis was focused on hip, knee, and ankle angular kinematics, and the mainstream idea was that the upper body was a static passenger unit of a locomotor apparatus that was located primarily at the lower limb level (Perry, 1992). This idea was then challenged by empirical evidence. In fact, many following studies confirmed as the trunk plays a fundamental dynamic role during walking, attenuating acceleration, ensuring the upright posture, and stabilizing the optic flow and vestibular signals (Winter, 1995; Menz et al., 2003; Kavanagh et al., 2004). This stability is achieved through a combination of passive mechanical damping and active feed-forward control of paraspinal muscles (Prince et al., 1994).

According to these studies, interest in upper body movements during walking has even increased in the past decade. A large and growing body of literature has investigated movements of the pelvis, center of mass, trunk, shoulder, and head during walking, primarily for two reasons: the function of upper body during gait and the development of wearable wireless accelerometers for quantifying gait stability. Accelerometers are usually small, lightweight, wireless, and wearable, allowing subjects to walk relatively unrestricted and without the limitations of the test environment of a laboratory (Kavanagh and Menz, 2008; Iosa et al., 2012a).

The second part of this review is mainly focused on the stability of upper body during gait in terms of control of upper body accelerations during gait.

In a 2008 review, Kavanagh and Menz (2008) analyzed 33 reports on the use of accelerometry for gait analysis, noting that the most common location for these devices was the lower trunk (12 of 33 studies, 36%), followed by head (21%) and lower limbs (21%). The authors concluded that the available literature indicates accelerometry as an accurate and reliable measure of basic spatio-temporal gait parameters and segmental accelerations of the body when walking, and a suitable measure for highlighting age-related differences in dynamic balance control during gait in people with movement disorders.

Examples of accelerometric signals that are obtained during walking are reported in **Figure 1** for a child, an adult, and an elderly subject along the AP direction. It is possible to observe how upper body AP acceleration was higher and less repeatable in the child and elderly, whereas it was lower and less variable in the young adult.

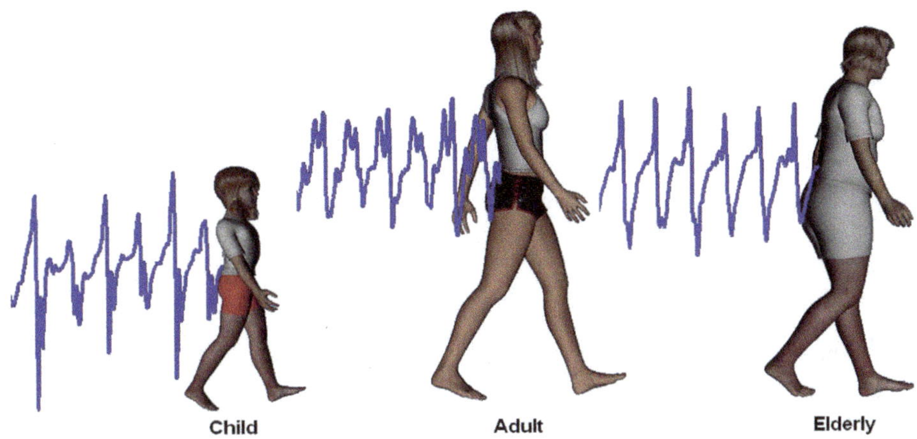

FIGURE 1 | Upper body accelerations. Upper body accelerations along the antero-posterior direction in a child (data obtained for a 2-year-old female), an adult (35 years, female), and an elderly subject (69 years, female).

The root mean square of an acceleration signal is the most commonly used parameter in assessing upper body stability using accelerometric-based gait analysis (Menz et al., 2003; Kavanagh et al., 2004; Marigold and Patla, 2008; Mazzà et al., 2008; Mizuike et al., 2009; Lamoth et al., 2011; Iosa et al., 2012e). It simply corresponds to the standard deviation of acceleration signals at which it has been removed its mean, indicating the dispersion of acceleration. Triaxial accelerometers allow one to measure accelerations along the three body axes: AP, LL, and CC, so the RMS can be evaluated along each one of the three body axes (RMS_{AP}, RMS_{LL}, RMS_{CC}, respectively).

Since the 90s, it has been suggested that RMS of accelerations could be a valid parameter for assessing balance during walking, differentiating between subjects with and without balance impairment or between walking on solid and soft terrains (Moe-Nilssen, 1998). These results were then confirmed by two studies of Menz et al. In the first one, the authors showed the age-related differences in walking stability measured using accelerometers fixed to head and trunk of subjects (Menz et al., 2003). In the second one, they showed as the RMS of pelvis accelerations increases when subjects were asked to walk on irregular surfaces (Menz et al., 2003). Subsequently, many other studies showed as acceleration RMS was a suitable parameter for discriminating between patients with unstable gait and healthy subjects (Mizuike et al., 2009; Lamoth et al., 2011; Iosa et al., 2012e). High reliability of three dimensional accelerometric approach at head, neck, trunk, and shank level was found in test–retest conditions (a mean coefficient of multiple determination across all conditions of 0.87) (Kavanagh et al., 2006).

Senden et al., enrolled 100 elderly subjects that were divided into two groups: with and without unspecific balance disorders clinically assessed by Tinetti scale. Many gait parameters were found correlated with the score of Tinetti scale, but only WS, step length, and acceleration RMS showed moderate to strong correlations and high discriminative power to classify elderly according to their clinical balance assessment. As reported in Section "Gait Instability and Risk of Fall," another study conducted using an accelerometric-based gait analysis found that the harmonic ratio of trunk acceleration (a parameter extracted by frequency analysis on accelerometric signals) may predict the risk of falls in elderly, independently of their physical performance, in 1 year after the accelerometric assessment (Doi et al., 2013). The harmonic ratio of trunk acceleration was taken into account also in the study of Senden et al. It showed moderate association with the Tinetti score, but did not enter into the final regression model for identifying subjects with unstable gait (Senden et al., 2012). All these studies showed as the analysis of trunk accelerations can be informative about the excessive and disperse trunk movements strictly interconnected with upright gait instabilities. The relationship between gait harmony and risk of falls needs further studies, however it has recently been suggested that the involuntary control of locomotion can be favored by the intrinsic gait temporal harmony, implying that its lost can increase the difficulties in controlling gait (Iosa et al., 2013).

Several studies have advocated normalizing upper body acceleration as a function of gait speed (Marigold and Patla, 2008; Kavanagh, 2009; Iosa et al., 2012e). In fact, increasing or decreasing gait speed effects a corresponding quadratic rise or decline in acceleration amplitude, thus, RMS values need to be normalized between subjects and populations at different walk speeds to assess only the upper body dynamic instabilities that are imputable to some balance impairment suitably (Mizuike et al., 2009; Iosa et al., 2012e). To take into account the relationship between acceleration RMS and WS, many different methods have been suggested (Moe-Nilssen and Helbostad, 2004; Marigold and Patla, 2008; Mizuike et al., 2009; Iosa et al., 2012e,f). Clinicians should hence keep clearly in mind that an increase in upper body accelerations could be attributed to an unsteady speed due to gait instabilities or a rise in WS, in absence of a suitable normalization of accelerometric values (Iosa et al., 2012e).

In this last part of the review, we summarize the results of the studies that compared upright gait stability between elderly and young adults or between subjects with a specific pathology or impairment and age-matched healthy controls, providing an overview of the development and the decline of upright gait stability in terms of upper body acceleration control.

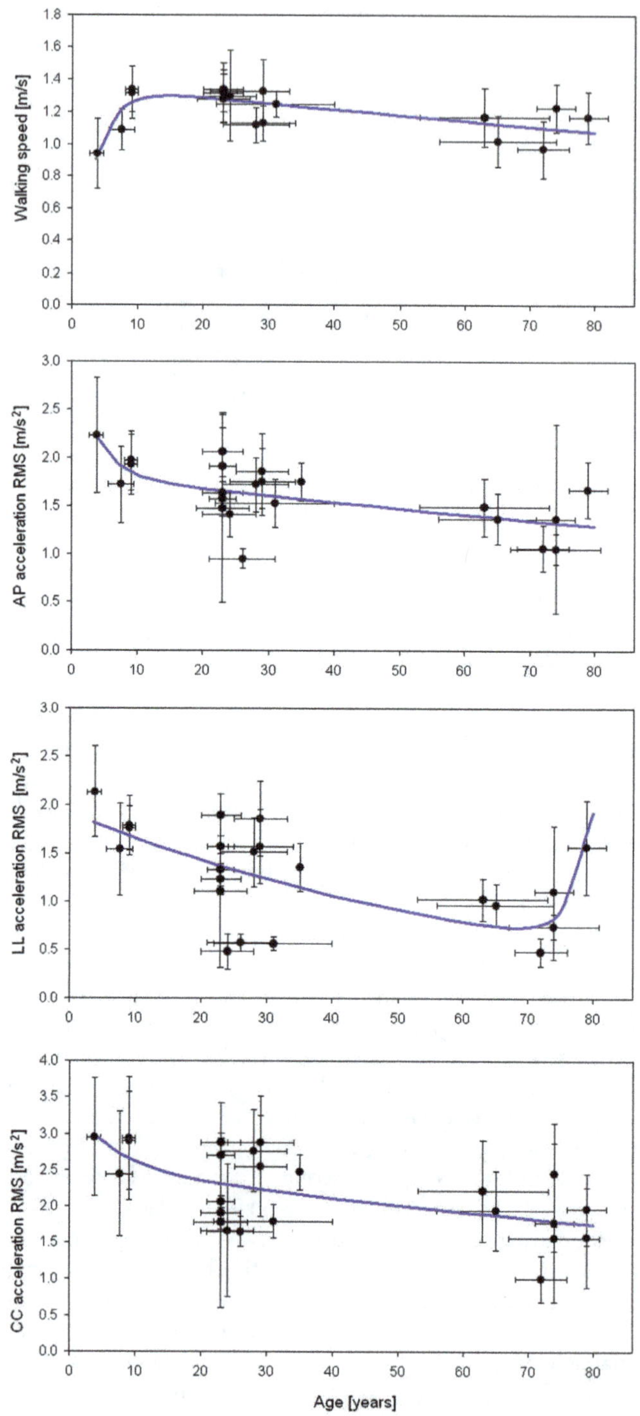

FIGURE 2 | Walking speed and acceleration RMSs. Mean (±SD) of walking speed, AP, LL, and CC acceleration RMSs with respect to mean (±SD) age for the studies in **Table 1**. Regression lines (in blue) were obtained with a bi-exponential fit.

DEVELOPMENT AND DECLINE OF UPPER BODY ACCELERATION CONTROL DURING GAIT

Table 1 reports the results of 15 studies regarding the measurements of upper body accelerations in 552 healthy subjects during walking. Only the data related to healthy subjects enrolled in these studies are reported in the table, and they were ordered by age. Most of these studies used accelerometers to assess upper body gait stability; two studies used stereophotogrammetry (Mazzà et al., 2008; Iosa et al., 2010) and one used an optoelectronic system (Marigold and Patla, 2008). The stereophotogrammetric analysis studies generated lower values of acceleration RMS along the LL direction compared with other studies, probably because analyzing a virtual point inside of the body, rendering them less sensitive to rotations around the CC axis.

Many of these studies compared upper body accelerations between healthy subjects (reported in **Table 1**) and patients. **Figure 2** graphs the results of the studies in **Table 1**. WS and RMSs were found significantly correlated with age (Pearson correlation: $p = 0.031$ for WS, $p < 0.001$ for RMS_{AP}, $p = 0.013$ for RMS_{LL}, $p = 0.003$ for RMS_{CC}). However, bi-exponential curves better fitted the data than linear regression fits (mean coefficient of determination 0.43 versus 0.30). The equation of the bi-exponential fit, applied using the least mean square method, was: $y = a \cdot e^{-\frac{x}{\tau_1}} + b \cdot e^{-\frac{x}{\tau_2}} + c$, with WS and accelerations as dependent variable y and age as independent variable x (**Figure 2**).

As expected, WS increased quickly in the first years of life, based on the rise in anthropometric dimensions, and slowly decreasing for the remainder of life after the teenage years. In details, RMS_{AP} declined rapidly in the first years of life, then being progressively reduced, despite an increase toward the end of life. RMS_{CC} decreased in childhood, becoming progressive and smooth for the remainder of life. The coefficient of determinations (R^2) of all four fits graphed in **Figure 2** was between 0.34 and 0.53, showing goodness of fits from moderate to good (Cohen, 1988). The lower value was for the RMS_{LL}. In this case, in fact, the bi-exponential trend lacks to fit the initial abrupt decrement occurred in childhood, well matching the data only after 7 years. It is noteworthy that lateral acceleration rose again in persons older than 70 toward values similar to those of children.

Because most studies have compared two groups of subjects, usually young versus elderly persons, little attention has been paid to the ages between 10–20 and 35–60 years. Nevertheless, we noted clear trends of rapid improvement in upright gait stability in the first period of life (reduction of RMS) despite the improvements in WS, and a loss of stability (increase of RMS) in older ages.

Because the quadratic relationship between WS and the three RMSs (Menz et al., 2003), a linear relationship exists between WS^2 and RMSs as shown by Mazzà et al. (2008). Hence, more regular quadrilateral shapes are expected for healthy subjects than for toddlers or patients for the plots reported in **Figure 3A** and formed by the mean values of WS^2 and of the three RMS values (obtained averaging the values over studies). On the left plot of this figure these quadrangles were reported for healthy subjects aged 1.5–5, 5–15, 20–30, 60–70, and over 70 years. Five of the studies in **Table 1** were not taken into account in generating this figure [two due to the instruments that were used (Mazzà et al., 2008; Iosa et al.,

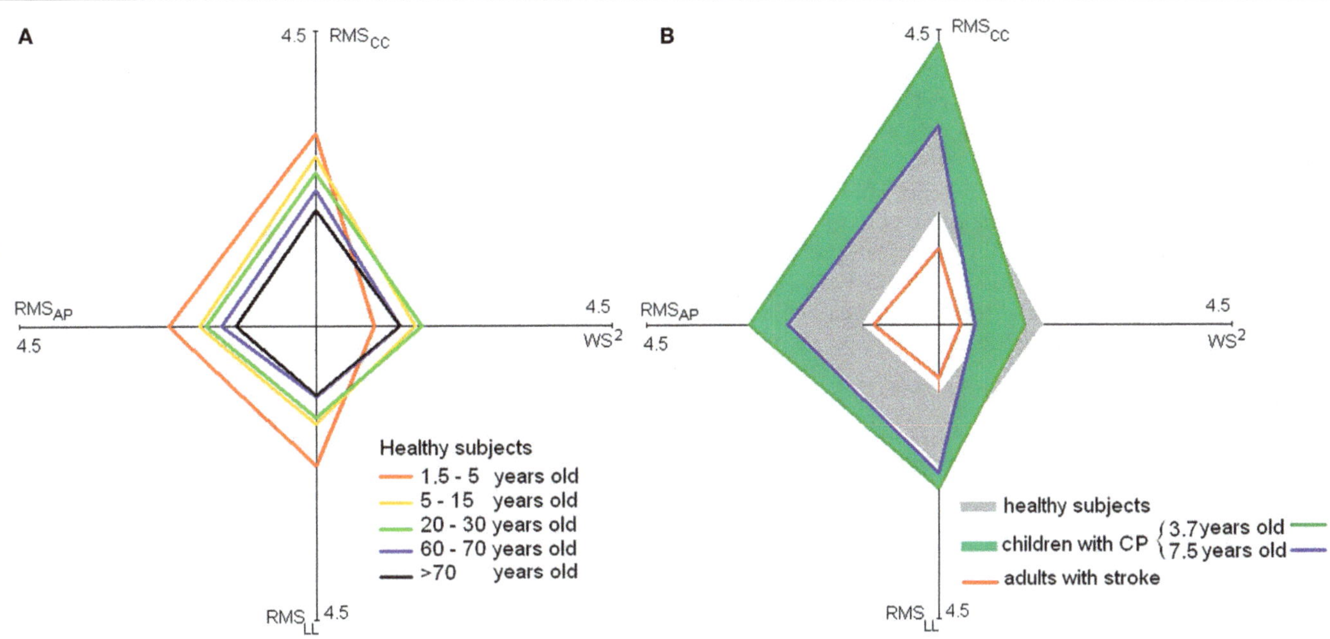

FIGURE 3 | Stability and velocity of walking. Values of mean RMSs [along the antero-posterior (AP), latero-lateral, (LL) and cranio-caudal (CC) axes] and WS^2 for healthy subjects at various ages [**(A)**, on the left] and for children with cerebral palsy and adults with stroke [**(B)**, on the right]. In the latter graph, the large gray rhomboidal area is formed by joining the extremes of values of healthy subjects [reported in **(A)**], and blue–green rhomboidal area by joining the extremes of values of children with cerebral palsy.

2010), two due to the absence of data along all the three body axes (Lamoth et al., 2011; Senden et al., 2012), and one due to subjects with a mean age of 35 years (Henriksen et al., 2004)].

The quadrilateral shape of younger children trended toward higher acceleration and lower speed. Older children and young adults generated a more rhomboidal shape, with lower acceleration and increased speed. Finally, elderly showed a reduction both in terms of speed and accelerations.

The reduction of gait instability was fast both along AP- and LL-axes during gait development, followed by a slight sloped trend, positive along AP and negative along LL-axis. Finally, after 65 years of age, an abrupt increase of instability occurred. Unfortunately, only sporadic data are available for age ranges between 10 and 20 years and between 40 and 60 years included; thus, upright gait stability in these ranges requires further investigation. On the right side of **Figure 3**, on the quadrilateral shape of healthy subjects were superimposed those of children with cerebral palsy (a range was shown to take into account the different ages) and subjects with stroke extracting the data by the relevant studies reported in **Table 2**.

CONCLUSION

Upright gait is a peculiar characteristic of human beings. This feature usually needs approximately 1 year to evolve but continues to improve during development. Body growth implies the possibility of increasing WS and the need to manage higher instabilities. In challenging environments or with existing physical impairments, the easiest solution to maintain upright gait stability is to reduce WS. This approach is also used by elderly subjects to compensate for the effects of aging on sensorimotor and cognitive functions.

The decline of upright gait stability with age is a slow but progressive process that increased drastically after 70 years. Pathologies can abruptly increase this loss proportionally to the severity of the impairment. The increase in upper body accelerations may be a direct effect of the impairment or a mixed result of impairment and compensatory strategies, as in children with atypical development (such as those with cerebral palsy) and persons with a progressively impairing pathology (such as muscular dystrophy).

A decrease in upright gait stability also exposes subjects to the risk of falls, which is particularly dangerous in the elderly. The development of low-cost and easy-to-use wearable sensors can facilitate the introduction of instrumented movement analysis in clinical settings (Iosa et al., 2012e). The clinical monitoring of upper body accelerations may provide a quantitative and hence objective outcome measure of the benefit of a rehabilitative pathway, evaluating the same parameters measured by vestibular system for maintaining balance.

Wireless and wearable technology have now provided us the possibility to quantify a feature, the importance of which was already noted in ancient time, when Aristotle wrote: "Man alone among all living beings walks erect, because his nature and his being are divine."

AUTHOR CONTRIBUTIONS

Marco Iosa conceived this review, analyzed the data, and wrote the first draft. Augusto Fusco and Giovanni Morone provided a critical revision of manuscript for important clinical intellectual content. Stefano Paolucci supervised the entire work and obtained funding.

ACKNOWLEDGMENTS

This material is the result of work supported by and use of facilities at the Italian Ministry of Health (projects: assessment of altered motor schemas in the pathologies of central nervous system; inability and instability of gait in patients with stroke) and the Fondazione Santa Lucia, IRCCS (Santa Lucia Foundation, Scientific Institute for Research Hospitalization and Health Care), Rome, Italy. The authors would thank Claudine J. C. Lamoth, Daniel S. Marigold, and Justin J. Kavanagh for having provided the data of their studies in order to allow the analyses performed in this review. The authors would thank Francesca Fusco Lynch for English Editing of this manuscript.

REFERENCES

Allali, G., Assal, F., Kressig, R. W., Dubost, V., Herrmann, F. R., and Beauchet, O. (2008). Impact of impaired executive function on gait stability. *Dement. Geriatr. Cogn. Disord.* 26, 364–369. doi:10.1159/000162358

Allum, J. H., Gresty, M., Keshner, E., and Shupert, C. (1997). The control of head movements during human balance corrections. *J. Vestib. Res.* 7, 189–218. doi:10.1016/S0957-4271(97)00029-3

Armand, S., Mercier, M., Watelain, E., Patte, K., Pelissier, J., and Rivier, F. (2005). A comparison of gait in spinal muscular atrophy, type II and duchenne muscular dystrophy. *Gait Posture* 21, 369–378. doi:10.1016/j.gaitpost.2004.04.006

Asher, L., Aresu, M., Falaschetti, E., and Mindell, J. (2012). Most older pedestrians are unable to cross the road in time: a cross-sectional study. *Age Ageing* 41, 690–694. doi:10.1093/ageing/afs076

Assaiante, C., and Amblard, B. (1993). Ontogenesis of head stabilization in space during locomotion in children: influence of visual cues. *Exp. Brain Res.* 93, 499–515. doi:10.1007/BF00229365

Avineri, E., Shinar, D., and Susilo, Y. O. (2012). Pedestrians' behaviour in cross walks: the effects of fear of falling and age. *Accid. Anal. Prev.* 44, 30–34. doi:10.1016/j.aap.2010.11.028

Beauchet, O., Annweiler, C., Verghese, J., Fantino, B., Herrmann, F. R., and Allali, G. (2011). Biology of gait control: vitamin D involvement. *Neurology* **76**, 1617–1622. doi:10.1212/WNL.0b013e318219fb08

Berthoz, A., and Pozzo, T. (1994). "Head and body coordination during locomotion and complex movements," in *Interlimb Coordination*, eds S. Swinnen, H. Heuer, J. Massion, and P. Casaer (San Diego: Academic Press), 147–165.

Bollard, E., and Fleming, H. (2013). A study to investigate the walking speed of elderly adults with relation to pedestrian crossings. *Physiother. Theory Pract.* 29, 142–149. doi:10.3109/09593985.2012.703760

Borel, L., Harlay, F., Lopez, C., Magnan, J., Chays, A., and Lacour, M. (2004). Walking performance of vestibular-defective patients before and after unilateral vestibular neurotomy. *Behav. Brain Res.* 150, 191–200. doi:10.1016/S0166-4328(03)00257-2

Bosch, K., Gerss, J., and Rosenbaum, D. (2007). Preliminary normative values for foot loading parameters of the developing child. *Gait Posture* 26, 238–247. doi:10.1016/j.gaitpost.2006.09.014

Bosch, K., and Rosenbaum, D. (2010). Gait symmetry improves in childhood – a 4-year follow-up of foot loading data. *Gait Posture* 32, 464–468. doi:10.1016/j.gaitpost.2010.07.002

Bruijn, S. M., Meyns, P., Jonkers, I., Kaat, D., and Duysens, J. (2011). Control of angular momentum during walking in children with cerebral palsy. *Res. Dev. Disabil.* 32, 2860–2866. doi:10.1016/j.ridd.2011.05.019

Cappozzo, A. (1981). Analysis of the linear displacement of the head and trunk during walking at different speeds. *J. Biomech.* 14, 411–425. doi:10.1016/0021-9290(81)90059-2

Choi, P., Ren, M., Phan, T. G., Callisaya, M., Ly, J. V., Beare, R., et al. (2012). Silent infarcts and cerebral microbleeds modify the associations of white matter lesions with gait and postural stability: population-based study. *Stroke* 43, 1505–1510. doi:10.1161/STROKEAHA.111.647271

Cohen, J. (1988). *Statistical Power Analysis for the Behavioral Sciences.* Hillsdale, NJ: Lawrence Erlbaum Associates, Inc.

Daly, R. M., Rosengren, B. E., Alwis, G., Ahlborg, H. G., Sernbo, I., and Karlsson, M. K. (2013). Gender specific age-related changes in bone density, muscle strength and functional performance in the elderly: a-10 year prospective population-based study. *BMC Geriatr.* 13:71. doi:10.1186/1471-2318-13-71

Di Monaco, M., Trucco, M., Di Monaco, R., Tappero, R., and Cavanna, A. (2010). The relationship between initial trunk control or postural balance and inpatient rehabilitation outcome after stroke: a prospective comparative study. *Clin. Rehabil.* 24, 543–554. doi:10.1177/0269215509353265

Doherty, T. J. (2003). Invited review: aging and sarcopenia. *J. Appl. Physiol.* 95, 1717–1727. doi:10.1152/japplphysiol.00347.2003

Doi, T., Hirata, S., Ono, R., Tsutsumimoto, K., Misu, S., and Ando, H. (2013). The harmonic ratio of trunk acceleration predicts falling among older people: results of a 1-year prospective study. *J. Neuroeng. Rehabil.* 10, 7. doi:10.1186/1743-0003-10-7

Dominici, N., Ivanenko, Y. P., Cappellini, G., d'Avella, A., Mondí, V., Cicchese, M., et al. (2011). Locomotor primitives in newborn babies and their development. *Science* 334, 997–999. doi:10.1126/science.1210617

Dommes, A., and Cavallo, V. (2011). The role of perceptual, cognitive, and motor abilities in street-crossing decisions of young and older pedestrians. *Ophthalmic Physiol. Opt.* 31, 292–301. doi:10.1111/j.1475-1313.2011.00835.x

Friedman, M. J. (2006). *The Evolution of Hominid Bipedalism.* Honors Projects, Wesleyan University, Bloomington.

Gage, J. R. (1993). Gait analysis. An essential tool in the treatment of cerebral palsy. *Clin. Orthop. Relat. Res.* 288, 126–134.

Garwicz, M., Christensson, M., and Psouni, E. (2009). A unifying model for timing of walking onset in humans and other mammals. *Proc. Natl. Acad. Sci. U.S.A.* 106, 21889–21893. doi:10.1073/pnas.0905777106

Graslund, B. (1995). *Early Humans and Their World.* Abingdon: Routledge.

Gutierrez, E. M., Bartonek, A., Haglund-Akerlind, Y., and Saraste, H. (2005). Kinetics of compensatory gait in persons with myelomeningocele. *Gait Posture* 21, 12–23. doi:10.1016/j.gaitpost.2003.11.002

Hahn, M. E., and Chou, L. S. (2004). Age-related reduction in sagittal plane center of mass motion during obstacle crossing. *J. Biomech.* 37, 837–844. doi:10.1016/j.jbiomech.2003.11.010

Hallemans, A., Beccu, S., Van Loock, K., Ortibus, E., Truijen, S., and Aerts, P. (2009). Visual deprivation leads to gait adaptations that are age- and context-specific: II. Kinematic parameters. *Gait Posture* 30, 307–311. doi:10.1016/j.gaitpost.2009.05.017

Hallemans, A., Ortibus, E., Meire, F., and Aerts, P. (2010). Low vision affects dynamic stability of gait. *Gait Posture* 32, 547–551. doi:10.1016/j.gaitpost.2010.07.018

Hamacher, D., Singh, N. B., Van Dieën, J. H., Heller, M. O., and Taylor, W. R. (2011). Kinematic measures for assessing gait stability in elderly individuals: a systematic review. *J. R. Soc. Interface* 8, 1682–1698. doi:10.1098/rsif.2011.0416

Heglund, N. C., Willems, P. A., Penta, M., and Lavagna, G. A. (1995). Energy-saving gait mechanics with head-supported loads. *Nature* 375, 52–54. doi:10.1038/375052a0

Henderson, S. E. (1986). "Some aspects of the development of motor control in Down's syndrome," in *Themes in Motor Development*, eds H. T. A. Whiting and M. G. Wade (Boston: Martinus Nijhoff), 147–186.

Henriksen, M., Lund, H., Moe-Nilssen, R., Bliddal, H., and Danneskiod-Samsøe, B. (2004). Test-retest reliability of trunk accelerometric gait analysis. *Gait Posture* 19, 288–297. doi:10.1016/S0966-6362(03)00069-9

Hesse, S., Welz, A., Assmann, E., Quentin, B., and Waldner, A. (2009). Pedestrians in Berlin after stroke. Recommendations for street and subway transit. *Nervenarzt* 80, 953–958. doi:10.1007/s00115-009-2700-x

Hodt-Billington, C., Helbostad, J. L., and Moe-Nilssen, R. (2008). Should trunk movement or footfall parameters quantify gait asymmetry in chronic stroke patients? *Gait Posture* 27, 552–558. doi:10.1016/j.gaitpost.2007.07.015

Horak, F. B., and Mancini, M. (2013). Objective biomarkers of balance and gait for Parkinson's disease using body-worn sensors. *Mov. Disord.* 28, 1544–1551. doi:10.1002/mds.25684

Hsue, B. J., Miller, F., and Su, F. C. (2009a). The dynamic balance of the children with cerebral palsy and typical developing during gait. Part I: spatial relationship between COM and COP trajectories. *Gait Posture* 29, 465–470. doi:10.1016/j.gaitpost.2008.11.007

Hsue, B. J., Miller, F., and Su, F. C. (2009b). The dynamic balance of the children with cerebral palsy and typical developing during gait. Part II: instantaneous velocity and acceleration of COM and COP and their relationship. *Gait Posture* 29, 471–476. doi:10.1016/j.gaitpost.2008.11.008

Ijmker, T., and Lamoth, C. J. (2012). Gait and cognition: the relationship between gait stability and variability with executive function in persons with and without dementia. *Gait Posture* 35, 126–130. doi:10.1016/j.gaitpost.2011.08.022

Ingwell, J. B., and Marin, L. C. (2006). Kinematic variability and local dynamic stability of upper body motions when walking at different speeds. *J. Biomech.* 39, 444–452. doi:10.1016/j.jbiomech.2004.12.014

Inman, V. T., Ralston, H. J., and Todd, F. (1981). *Human Walking*. Baltimore: Williams & Wilkins.

Iosa, M., Fusco, A., Marchetti, F., Morone, G., Caltagirone, C., Paolucci, S., et al. (2013). The golden ratio of gait harmony: repetitive proportions of repetitive gait phases. *Biomed Res. Int.* 2013, 918642. doi:10.1155/2013/918642

Iosa, M., Mazzà, C., Pecoraro, F., Aprile, I., Ricci, E., and Cappozzo, A. (2010). Control of the upper body movements during level walking in patients with facioscapulohumeral dystrophy. *Gait Posture* 31, 68–72. doi:10.1016/j.gaitpost.2009.08.247

Iosa, M., Morone, G., Fusco, A., Bragoni, M., Coiro, P., Multari, M., et al. (2012a). Seven capital devices for the future of stroke rehabilitation. *Stroke Res. Treat.* 2012, 187965. doi:10.1155/2012/187965

Iosa, M., Fusco, A., Morone, G., and Paolucci, S. (2012b). Effects of visual deprivation on gait dynamic stability. *ScientificWorldJournal* 2012, 974560. doi:10.1100/2012/974560

Iosa, M., Fusco, A., Morone, G., and Paolucci, S. (2012c). Walking there: environmental influence on walking-distance estimation. *Behav. Brain Res.* 226, 124–132. doi:10.1016/j.bbr.2011.09.007

Iosa, M., Morone, G., Fusco, A., Pratesi, L., Bragoni, M., Coiro, P., et al. (2012d). Effects of walking endurance reduction on gait stability in patients with stroke. *Stroke Res. Treat.* 2012, 810415. doi:10.1155/2012/810415

Iosa, M., Fusco, A., Morone, G., Pratesi, L., Coiro, P., Venturiero, V., et al. (2012e). Assessment of upper body dynamic stability during walking in patients with subacute stroke. *J. Rehabil. Res. Dev.* 49, 439–450. doi:10.1682/JRRD.2011.03.0057

Iosa, M., Marro, T., Paolucci, S., and Morelli, D. (2012f). Stability and harmony of gait in children with cerebral palsy. *Res. Dev. Disabil.* 33, 129–135. doi:10.1016/j.ridd.2011.08.031

Ivanenko, Y. P., Dominici, N., Cappellini, G., Dan, B., Cheron, G., and Lacquaniti, F. (2004). Development of pendulum mechanism and kinematic coordination from the first unsupported steps in toddlers. *J. Exp. Biol.* 207, 3797–3810. doi:10.1242/jeb.01214

Ivanenko, Y. P., Dominici, N., and Lacquaniti, F. (2007). Development of independent walking in toddlers. *Exerc. Sport Sci. Rev.* 35, 67–73. doi:10.1249/JES.0b013e31803eafa8

Kavanagh, J. J. (2009). Lower trunk motion and speed-dependence during walking. *J. Neuroeng. Rehabil.* 9, 6–9. doi:10.1186/1743-0003-6-9

Kavanagh, J. J., Barrett, R. S., and Morrison, S. (2004). Upper body accelerations during walking in healthy young and elderly men. *Gait Posture* 20, 291–298. doi:10.1016/j.gaitpost.2003.10.004

Kavanagh, J. J., and Menz, H. B. (2008). Accelerometry: a technique for quantifying movement patterns during walking. *Gait Posture* 28, 1–15. doi:10.1016/j.gaitpost.2007.10.010

Kavanagh, J. J., Morrison, S., James, D. A., and Barrett, R. (2006). Reliability of segmental accelerations measured using a new wireless gait analysis system. *J. Biomech.* 39, 2863–2872. doi:10.1016/j.jbiomech.2005.09.012

Kaya, B. K., Krebs, D. E., and Riley, P. O. (1998). Dynamic stability in elders: momentum control in locomotor ADL. *J. Gerontol. A Biol. Sci. Med. Sci.* 53, M126–M134. doi:10.1093/gerona/53A.2.M126

Kubo, M., and Ulrich, B. D. (2006a). A biomechanical analysis of the "high guard" position of arms during walking in toddlers. *Infant Behav. Dev.* 29, 509–517. doi:10.1016/j.infbeh.2006.05.001

Kubo, M., and Ulrich, B. D. (2006b). Early stage of walking: development of control in mediolateral and antoposterior directions. *J. Mot. Behav.* 38, 229–237. doi:10.3200/JMBR.38.3.229-237

Lamoth, C. J., Meijer, O. G., Wuisman, P. I., van Dieen, J. H., Levin, M. F., and Beek, P. J. (2002). Pelvis-thorax coordination in the transverse plane during walking in persons with nonspecific low back pain. *Spine* 27, E92–E99. doi:10.1097/00007632-200202150-00016

Lamoth, C. J., van Deudekom, F. J., van Campen, J. P., Appels, B. A., de Vries, O. J., and Pijnappels, M. (2011). Gait stability and variability measures show effects of impaired cognition and dual tasking in frail people. *J. Neuroeng. Rehabil.* 8, 2. doi:10.1186/1743-0003-8-2

Lee, D. N. (1980). The optic flow field: the foundation of vision. *Philos. Trans. R. Soc. Lond. B Biol. Sci.* 290, 169–179. doi:10.1098/rstb.1980.0089

Lee, H. J., and Chou, L. S. (2006). Detection of gait instability using the center of mass and center of pressure inclination angles. *Arch. Phys. Med. Rehabil.* 87, 569–575. doi:10.1016/j.apmr.2005.11.033

Marigold, D. S., and Patla, A. E. (2008). Age-related changes in gait for multi-surface terrain. *Gait Posture* 27, 696696. doi:10.1016/j.gaitpost.2007.09.005

Masci, I., Vannozzi, G., Bergamini, E., Pesce, C., Getchell, N., and Cappozzo, A. (2013). Assessing locomotor skills development in childhood using wearable inertial sensor devices: the running paradigm. *Gait Posture* 37, 570–574. doi:10.1016/j.gaitpost.2012.09.017

Masiero, S., Avesani, R., Armani, M., Verena, P., and Ermani, M. (2007). Predictive factors for ambulation in stroke patients in the rehabilitation setting: a multivariate analysis. *Clin. Neurol. Neurosurg.* 109, 763–769. doi:10.1016/j.clineuro.2007.07.009

Masud, T., and Morris, R. O. (2001). Epidemiology of falls. *Age Ageing* 30, 3–7. doi:10.1093/ageing/30.suppl_4.3

Mazzà, C., Iosa, M., Pecoraro, F., and Cappozzo, A. (2008). Control of the upper body accelerations in young and elderly women during level walking. *J. Neuroeng. Rehabil.* 5, 30. doi:10.1186/1743-0003-5-30

Mazzà, C., Iosa, M., Picerno, P., and Cappozzo, A. (2009). Gender differences in the control of the upper body accelerations during level walking. *Gait Posture* 29, 300–303. doi:10.1016/j.gaitpost.2008.09.013

Mazzà, C., Zok, M., and Cappozzo, A. (2010). Head stabilization in children of both genders during level walking. *Gait Posture* 31, 429–432. doi:10.1016/j.gaitpost.2010.01.012

Menz, H. B., Lord, S. R., and Fitzpatrick, R. C. (2003). Acceleration patterns of the head and pelvis when walking on level and irregular surfaces. *Gait Posture* 18, 35–46. doi:10.1016/S0966-6362(02)00159-5

Meyns, P., Van Gestel, L., Bruijn, S. M., Desloovere, K., Swinnen, S. P., and Duysens, J. (2012). Is interlimb coordination during walking preserved in children with cerebral palsy? *Res. Dev. Disabil.* 33, 1418–1428. doi:10.1016/j.ridd.2012.03.020

Mizuike, C., Ohgi, S., and Morita, S. (2009). Analysis of stroke patient walking dynamics using a tri-axial accelerometer. *Gait Posture* 30, 60–64. doi:10.1016/j.gaitpost.2009.02.017

Moe-Nilssen, R. (1998). Test-retest reliability of trunk accelerometry during standing and walking. *Arch. Phys. Med. Rehabil.* 79, 1377–1385. doi:10.1016/S0003-9993(98)90231-3

Moe-Nilssen, R., and Helbostad, J. L. (2004). Estimation of gait cycle characteristics by trunk accelerometry. *J. Biomech.* 37, 121–126. doi:10.1016/S0021-9290(03)00233-1

Moe-Nilssen, R., and Helbostad, J. L. (2005). Interstride trunk acceleration variability but not step width variability can differentiate between fit and frail older adults. *Gait Posture* 21, 164–170. doi:10.1016/j.gaitpost.2004.01.013

Moe-Nilssen, R., Helbostad, J. L., Akra, T., Birdedal, L., and Nygaard, H. A. (2006). Modulation of gait during visual adaptation to dark. *J. Mot. Behav.* 38, 118–125. doi:10.3200/JMBR.38.2.118-125

Montero-Odasso, M., Schapira, M., Varala, C., Pitteri, C., Soriano, E. R., Kaplan, R., et al. (2004). Gait velocity in senior people. An easy test for detecting mobility impairment in community elderly. *J. Nutr. Health Aging* 8, 340–343. doi:10.1093/brain/117.4.715

Muscaritoli, M., Lucia, S., Molfino, A., Cederholm, T., and Rossi Fanelli, F. (2013). Muscle atrophy in aging and chronic diseases: is it sarcopenia or cachexia? *Intern. Emerg. Med.* 8, 553–560. doi:10.1007/s11739-012-0807-8

Pailhous, J., and Bonnard, M. (1992). Steady-state fluctuations of human walking. *Behav. Brain Res.* 47, 181–189. doi:10.1016/S0166-4328(05)80124-X

Pailhous, J., Ferrandez, A. M., Flückiger, M., and Baumberger, B. (1990). Unintentional modulations of human gait by optical flow. *Behav. Brain Res.* 38, 275–281. doi:10.1016/0166-4328(90)90181-D

Perry, J. (1992). *Gait Analysis: Normal and Pathological Function*. Thorofare, NJ: Slack Incorporated.

Perry, S. D., Santos, L. C., and Patla, A. E. (2001). Contribution of vision and cutaneous sensation to the control of centre of mass (COM) during gait termination. *Brain Res.* 913, 27–34. doi:10.1016/S0006-8993(01)02748-2

Plotnik, M., Giladi, N., Dagan, Y., and Hausdorff, J. M. (2011). Postural instability and fall risk in Parkinson's disease: impaired dual tasking, pacing, and bilateral coordination of gait during the "ON" medication state. *Exp. Brain Res.* 210, 529–538. doi:10.1007/s00221-011-2551-0

Plotnik, M., Giladi, N., and Hausdorff, J. M. (2007). A new measure for quantifying the bilateral coordination of human gait: effects of aging and Parkinson's disease. *Exp. Brain Res.* 181, 561–570. doi:10.1007/s00221-007-0955-7

Pozzo, T., Berthoz, A., and Lefort, L. (1990). Head stabilization during various locomotor tasks in humans. I. Normal subjects. *Exp. Brain Res.* 82, 97–106. doi:10.1007/BF00230842

Prince, F., Winter, D. A., Stergiou, P., and Walt, S. E. (1994). Anticipatory control of upper body balance during human locomotion. *Gait Posture* 2, 19–25. doi:10.1371/journal.pone.0056313

Rebula, J. R., Ojeda, L. V., Adamczyk, P. G., and Kuo, A. D. (2013). Measurement of foot placement and its variability with inertial sensors. *Gait Posture* 38, 974–980. doi:10.1016/j.gaitpost.2013.05.012

Reed, E. S. (1996). *Encountering the World: Toward an Ecological Psychology*. New York: Oxford University Press.

Ruchinskas, R. A., Singer, H. K., and Repetz, N. K. (2000). Cognitive status and ambulation in geriatric rehabilitation: walking without thinking? *Arch. Phys. Med. Rehabil.* 81, 1224–1228. doi:10.1053/apmr.2000.6976

Scaglioni, G., Narici, M. V., Maffiuletti, N. A., Pensini, M., and Martin, A. (2003). Effect of ageing on the electrical and mechanical properties of human soleus motor units activated by the H reflex and M wave. *J. Physiol.* 548, 649–661. doi:10.1113/jphysiol.2002.032763

Senden, R., Savelberg, H. H., Grimm, B., Heyligers, I. C., and Meijer, K. (2012). Accelerometry-based gait analysis, an additional objective approach to screen subjects at risk for falling. *Gait Posture* 36, 296–300. doi:10.1016/j.gaitpost.2012.03.015

Sheridan, P. L., Solomont, J., Kowall, N., and Hausdorff, J. M. (2003). Influence of executive function on locomotor function: divided attention increases gait variability in Alzheimer's disease. *J. Am. Geriatr. Soc.* 51, 1633–1637. doi:10.1046/j.1532-5415.2003.51516.x

Sparrow, W. A., and Newell, K. M. (1994). The coordination and control of human creeping with increases in speed. *Behav. Brain Res.* 63, 151–158. doi:10.1016/0166-4328(94)90086-8

Spoor, F., Wood, B., and Zonneveld, F. (1994). Implications of early hominid labyrinthine morphology for evolution of human bipedal locomotion. *Nature* 369, 645–648. doi:10.1038/369645a0

Sueur, C., Class, B., Hamm, C., Meyer, X., and Pelé, M. (2013). Different risk thresholds in pedestrian road crossing behaviour: a comparison of French and Japanese approaches. *Accid. Anal. Prev.* 58, 59–63. doi:10.1016/j.aap.2013.04.027

Sutherland, D. H., Olshen, R., Cooper, L., and Woo, S. L. (1980). The development of mature gait. *J. Bone Joint Surg. Am.* 62, 336–353.

Sylos-Labini, F., Meli, A., Ivanenko, Y. P., and Tufarelli, D. (2012). Recurrence quantification analysis of gait in normal and hypovestibular subjects. *Gait Posture* 35, 48–55. doi:10.1016/j.gaitpost.2011.08.004

Terrier, P., and Dériaz, O. (2011). Kinematic variability, fractal dynamics and local dynamic stability of treadmill walking. *J. Neuroeng. Rehabil.* 8, 12. doi:10.1186/1743-0003-8-12

van Baar, M. E., Dekker, J., Lemmens, J. A., Oostendorp, R. A., and Bijlsma, J. W. (1998). Pain and disability in patients with osteoarthritis of hip or knee: the relationship with articular, kinesiological, and psychological characteristics. *J. Rheumatol.* 25, 125–133.

Winter, D. A. (1995). Human balance and posture control during standing and walking. *Gait Posture* 3, 193–214. doi:10.1016/0966-6362(95)99069-W

Yin, M., Ishikawa, K., Omi, E., Saito, T., Itasaka, Y., and Angunsuri, N. (2011). Small vestibular schwannomas can cause gait instability. *Gait Posture* 34, 25–28. doi:10.1016/j.gaitpost.2011.02.026

6

Aging induced loss of complexity and dedifferentiation: consequences for coordination dynamics within and between brain, muscular and behavioral levels

Rita Sleimen-Malkoun[1,2]*, **Jean-Jacques Temprado**[1] **and S. Lee Hong**[3]

[1] CNRS, Institut des Sciences du Mouvement UMR 7287, Aix-Marseille Université, Marseille, France
[2] Inserm, Institut de Neurosciences des Systèmes UMR_S 1106, Faculté de Médecine Timone, Aix-Marseille Université, Marseille, France
[3] Ohio Musculoskeletal and Neurological Institute, Ohio University, Athens, OH, USA

Edited by:
Sige Zou, National Institute on Aging, USA

Reviewed by:
Xiaopeng Zhao, University of Tennessee, USA
Thomas Arendt, Universität Leipzig, Germany

***Correspondence:**
Rita Sleimen-Malkoun, Inserm, Institut de Neurosciences des Systèmes UMR_S 1106, Faculté de Médecine Timone, Aix-Marseille Université, 27 BD Jean Moulin 13385, Marseille Cedex 05, France
e-mail: rita.sleimen-malkoun@univ-amu.fr

Growing evidence demonstrates that aging not only leads to structural and functional alterations of individual components of the neuro-musculo-skeletal system (NMSS) but also results in a systemic re-organization of interactions within and between the different levels and functional domains. Understanding the principles that drive the dynamics of these re-organizations is an important challenge for aging research. The present *Hypothesis and Theory* paper is a contribution in this direction. We propose that age-related declines in brain and behavior that have been characterized in the literature as *dedifferentiation* and the *loss of complexity* (LOC) are: (i) synonymous; and (ii) integrated. We argue that a causal link between the aforementioned phenomena exists, evident in the dynamic changes occurring in the aging NMSS. Through models and methods provided by a dynamical systems approach to coordination processes in complex living systems, we: (i) formalize operational hypotheses about the general principles of changes in cross-level and cross-domain interactions during aging; and (ii) develop a theory of the aging NMSS based on the combination of the frameworks of coordination dynamics (CD), dedifferentiation, and LOC. Finally, we provide operational predictions in the study of aging at neural, muscular, and behavioral levels, which lead to testable hypotheses and an experimental agenda to explore the link between CD, LOC and dedifferentiation within and between these different levels.

Keywords: aging, coordination dynamics, complexity, dedifferentiation, variability

INTRODUCTION

Understanding the mechanisms underlying age-related declines across multiple functional subsystems ranks highly on the agenda of science and society. To achieve this objective, the most commonly adopted approach in aging research has emphasized dividing the neuro-musculo-skeletal system (NMSS) into smaller and presumably, more tractable units. From this perspective, declines in neural, cognitive, sensori-motor and muscular functioning are generally considered as separate domains, each having its own evolution over time. During the last 30 years, this approach has considerably improved our understanding of how aging affects the different levels of observation and functional sub-systems of the organism. However, it has also made aging research a complicated intellectual puzzle, with pieces that do not necessarily fit together, hence limiting our understanding of the aging NMSS as a whole. Despite (or rather, because of) the proliferation of isolated theories and potential mechanisms operating at different levels (about 300 have been identified by Medvedev, 1990), aging research remains data rich and theoretically poor.

In contrast to classic research, a growing body of literature in both aging and biomedical research acknowledges the fact that the human NMSS is a complex system comprising many interacting (complex) component subsystems that are connected over a variety of different scales of space and time (Chauvet, 1995; Buchman, 1996; Yates, 2008). Accordingly, it is also becoming clear that aging is a "parallel distributed process". which not only affects the structures and functions of the individual subsystems but also the interactions between them. These changes alter the range of behaviors that the system can achieve, leading to impairments in behavioral adaptability (Lipsitz, 2002; Vaillancourt and Newell, 2002; Newell et al., 2006; Hong and Rebec, 2012). To better understand the coordination/coupling processes that occur during aging, both within and between the different subsystems and their consequences, an integrated framework—inspired by system biology and/or dynamical systems approach—is required (Haken, 1983; Kelso, 1995; Yates, 2008). The goal of the current paper is to develop a conceptual framework inspired by dynamical systems analysis to understand the general principles of age-related reorganization of the NMSS and its consequences on brain, behavioral and muscular dynamics. In the following, firstly, we review the literature on two phenomena that characterize the aging NMSS, namely, *dedifferentiation* and *loss of complexity* (LOC). We argue in this respect that these phenomena could actually be closely related. Indeed, although they seem to refer to different facets of aging, they both reflect both systemic and systematic reorganizations in the NMSS. Then, using the theory of coordination dynamics (CD; Kelso, 1995, 2009), we attempt to explain how dedifferentiation and LOC affect variability of system outputs and patterns dynamics at the levels of brain, muscles and behavior. Finally, we present hypotheses and empirical predictions that could be tested experimentally.

THE DEDIFFERENTIATION HYPOTHESIS

Dedifferentiation can be defined as "*a process by which structures, mechanisms of behavior that were specialized for a given function lose their specialization and become simplified, less distinct or common to different functions*" (modified from Baltes and Lindenberger, 1997). Historically, the concept of dedifferentiation was introduced by Baltes and colleagues (Baltes, 1980; Baltes et al., 1998) to account for age-related increases in the correlation between levels of performance on different cognitive tasks. Dedifferentiation suggests the existence of a common cause of cognitive declines in aging (e.g., a general slowing of information processing; Birren, 1965; Birren et al., 1980; Cerella, 1985, 1991, 1994; Bashore, 1994; Salthouse, 1996), arising from reduced distinctiveness of mental representations and/or increased neural noise (e.g., a deficit in catecholaminergic modulation; Li et al., 2001). Both cross-sectional and longitudinal studies show that performance on sensory, cognitive and motor tasks are more correlated in the elderly, supporting the existence of *cognitive-motor dedifferentiation* (Lindenberger and Baltes, 1994; Baltes and Lindenberger, 1997; Lindenberger and Ghisletta, 2009). The following sections review existing evidence on dedifferentiation in brain and muscles.

DEDIFFERENTIATION IN BRAIN FUNCTION

Numerous brain-imaging studies have shown that the aging brain accommodates anatomical and physiological changes by reorganizing activation patterns between neural ensembles (Cabeza, 2002; Reuter-Lorenz, 2002; Ward, 2006; Serrien et al., 2007; see Park and Reuter-Lorenz, 2009 for review and theoretical account; Seidler et al., 2010). Specifically, in addition to stronger activation in dedicated regions, older adults generally exhibit activation of additional areas of the brain not observed (or only marginally) in young participants. For instance, it has been shown that brain dedifferentiation manifests in a shift from unilateral to bilateral activation (Cabeza, 2002; Cabeza et al., 2002; Ward, 2006) and/or an increase in activation of prefrontal areas (Heuninckx et al., 2005, 2008; Serrien et al., 2007).

During motor tasks, dedifferentiation takes the form of an increase in activation of neural structures presumably dedicated to cognitive processes (Heuninckx et al., 2005, 2008; Serrien et al., 2007; Park and Reuter-Lorenz, 2009; Seidler et al., 2010). This expanded activation is generally more pronounced with increasing motor task complexity, presumably reflecting greater involvement of executive control processes (Mattay et al., 2002; Ward and Frackowiak, 2003; Heuninckx et al., 2005). This hypothesis is supported by dual-task studies that have shown cognitive permeation of the motor domain i.e., interdependencies between sensorimotor and cognitive processes, becomes accentuated during aging (Li and Lindenberger, 2002; Schäfer et al., 2006; Schaefer and Schumacher, 2010). Dedifferentiated activation is also not limited to performance-based contexts. Comparable effects of aging have also been described during learning (i.e., dedifferentiation between explicit and implicit learning; Dennis and Cabeza, 2011), visual processing (i.e., dedifferentiation between pathways involved in faces, places and objects recognition; Park et al., 2004) and memory functions (i.e., between episodic and working memory; Papenberg et al., 2011).

DEDIFFERENTIATION IN MUSCLE STRUCTURE AND FUNCTION

One of the primary effects of aging on human musculature is a change in muscle fiber composition. Specifically, as reviewed in Lexell (1995), and recently demonstrated by Nilwik et al. (2013), the loss of muscle mass in aging (i.e., sarcopenia) is dominated by declines in the size of the fast-twitch fibers. While young adults have a nearly even ratio of fast- (type II) and slow (type I)-twitch muscle fibers, the elderly exhibit a higher proportion of slow-twitch fibers (see Table 2 from Lexell, 1995, for a summary). In addition, apart from atrophy of the type II fibers, aging also results in "clustering" or "grouping" of muscle fibers. In the young, fast- and slow-twitch fibers are almost evenly distributed or scattered in a muscle cross-section. With aging, muscle fibers form clusters as type I fibers form visibly distinct groups from type II fibers (see Andersen, 2003 for a review).

While not often discussed, it is important to note that "hybrid" muscle fibers also exist (see Pette and Staron, 2000, for a review), leading to altered contractile properties that fall between exclusively type I and type II fibers (Hilber et al., 1999). Aging leads to an increase in the proportion of hybrid fibers within a muscle (Monemi et al., 1999; Pette and Staron, 2000). These morphological changes would lead to dedifferentiation in muscle function, as aged muscles will exhibit a high level of homogeneity in contractile rate and force generation capacity. Effectively, as muscle fiber structure and function is homogenized, their ability to contract at different speeds and generate different force levels is restricted, hence narrowing their functional range. The dedifferentiation in muscle structure and function would leave them in a state where they are limited to acting on narrower scales of space and time.

LOSS OF COMPLEXITY

The LOC hypothesis was introduced 30 years ago in biomedical research by the pioneering work of Lipsitz and Goldberger (1992) on heart rate variability (HRV). Using nonlinear time series analysis (i.e., approximate entropy, ApEn but see Costa et al., 2002; Peng et al., 2009; Bravi et al., 2011, for reviews of the different methods), these authors observed a tendency toward more regular fluctuations in HRV (i.e., "less complex patterns" of variability) during aging and disease, which remained undetected by variance-based measures (coefficient of variation, SD). These changes have been interpreted as a LOC, which is currently considered as a generic driving principle of aging in a wide range of functional systems. LOC has even been hypothesized to be an indicator of the transition from normal aging to frailty (Lipsitz, 2002, 2004; Lang et al., 2009). However, increased behavioral variability is widely viewed as a hallmark of aging (Hultsch et al., 2008). Greater magnitudes of intra-individual variability in cognitive and motor performance are commonly attributed to increased levels of Gaussian noise produced at anatomical, functional and neuro-modulatory levels of the central nervous system (CNS; see MacDonald et al., 2009b for a review). However, there is further evidence that the magnitude and structure of variability may change independently of one another during aging (Slifkin and Newell, 1999; Sosnoff et al., 2006). This suggests that "variability" (amplitude) and "complexity" (pattern) of fluctuations stem from different origins and might have different functional significance (Sosnoff et al., 2006; McIntosh et al., 2010; Balasubramaniam and Torre, 2012).

The LOC hypothesis has been supported in studies of physiological, cognitive, and motor systems (see Vaillancourt and Newell, 2002; Newell et al., 2006; Rey-Robert et al., 2011). Yet, the effects of aging on the complexity of behavioral output fluctuations have been shown to depend on the functional system under investigation and/or the task being performed (Vaillancourt and Newell, 2002). This raised the proposal that aging impairs behavioral adaptability by restricting the ability to alter levels of behavioral complexity (Vaillancourt and Newell, 2002). Thus, a critical property of the system seems to be its capability to reorganize the interactions between its components (i.e., its functional degrees of freedom) to adjust the degree of unpredictability of behavioral fluctuations to meet task demands (Vaillancourt and Newell, 2002), leading to a proposal of the *Change in Complexity Hypothesis* by some of the authors of this article (CICH; Rey-Robert et al., 2011).

Changes in complexity have also been investigated in brain aging research. In resting state EEG studies where the subject is not engaged in any type of cognitive or motor task (i.e., under the instruction to relax), the elderly exhibit higher levels of brain signal complexity (Anokhin et al., 1996; Pierce et al., 2000, 2003; Müller and Lindenberger, 2012). Similar findings were also reported using fMRI (Yang et al., 2013). Conversely, task-driven brain activation signals seem to express a smaller complexity reduction in older subjects in comparison to the young (Müller and Lindenberger, 2012). Additionally, age-related changes of brain signal complexity appear to be scale-dependent. Using Multiscale entropy (MSE), McIntosh et al. (2014) found that, the elderly possess less complex brain signals at coarse time-scales, and more complex signaling at fine time-scales in comparison to the young. fMRI studies show an age-related decrease in brain signal variance as measured by the standard deviation of BOLD activity, and this was reported in both resting and task-driven states (Garrett et al., 2011, 2013; however, see Yang et al., 2013 for a conflicting result).

Altogether these findings support the systemic nature of age-related changes in the complexity of behavioral and brain signals. However, the direction of these changes (increase versus decrease) and the in-between level mapping is not straightforward and deserves further investigation.

LINKING LOSS OF COMPLEXITY AND DEDIFFERENTIATION IN THE NEURO-MUSCULO-SKELETAL SYSTEM

Although LOC and dedifferentiation hypotheses have developed independently in the literature, there is evidence to indicate that they constitute two intertwined facets of the same underlying aging process. The systemic breakdown of the structure of fluctuations of behavioral outputs observed during aging are currently attributed to changes in coupling interactions (i.e., functional synergies) between the components of the different system over multiple temporal and spatial scales (Lipsitz, 2002; Vaillancourt and Newell, 2002; Newell et al., 2006). A plausible hypothesis is that LOC might arise, at least in part, from dedifferentiation occurring within and between the different subsystems.

At this juncture, an integrative theoretical framework that connects the LOCH and dedifferentiation hypotheses is needed. Four critical domains must be accounted for, namely: (1) *tasks*—classification of constraints and metrics of behavioral difficulty; (2) *structures*—anatomical and biochemical changes from organ to molecular level; (3) *function*—coordination of the individual structures and levels of organization; and (4) *behavior*—overt measures of systems outputs (i.e., pattern dynamics and behavioral output fluctuations). In this respect, we contend that principles of self-organization in complex systems identified by physics/dynamical systems theory (e.g., Glass and Mackey, 1988; Lipsitz, 2002, 2004; West, 2006) are essential. As a step in this direction, Vaillancourt and Newell (2002) proposed a standard approach to infer changes in the complexity of a system (independent of its nature) and its consequences on behavioral state and output fluctuations. They argued that a system's complexity depends on: (i) the number of independent variables that is needed to reproduce or predict the output of the system; (ii) the functional states of the different components; and (iii) noise present in the system. To our knowledge, no systematic exploration of the consequences of separate or concomitant changes in the different factors identified by Vaillancourt and Newell (2002) has been undertaken in the literature. To achieve this objective, the challenge is finding task protocols that are rich enough to capture the coupling mechanism and properties of the neuro-behavioral system, but not so complicated that it precludes modeling. We contend that it could be done through the use of the conceptual framework, task paradigms and the methods of analysis of *CD*.

COORDINATION DYNAMICS AS A CONCEPTUAL FRAMEWORK FOR THE STUDY OF THE NMSS

CD is a conceptual framework dedicated to the study of coordinative processes that occur within and between brain and behavioral levels in a wide range of tasks. It refers to set of principles developed to capture the formation and functional adaptation of synergies and coordination patterns to meet different demands (Kelso, 2009, 2012; Tognoli and Kelso, 2009). From this perspective, coupling and self-organization properties allow the adaptive assembly, stabilization and dismantling of synergies between functional components and subsystems. Coupling over multiple spatial and temporal scales also ensure efficient informational exchanges within the neurobehavioral system through feedback loops and regulation processes (Slifkin and Newell, 1999; West, 2006; West and Grigolini, 2010; McIntosh et al., 2014).

These coordinative processes are evident in the presence of multiple stable states in the neurobehavioral repertoire and the ability to switch between these stable states to adapt to task or environmental constraints. Whatever the level of observation or the system under consideration, pattern dynamics capture the time-evolution of collective variables characterizing the state of the system (order parameters) under the influence of a set of internal and external constraints of various origins (control parameters). These control parameters may trigger switching between the different spontaneous states of the system, without prescribing these states. At a more abstract level, CD can be conceived as an evolving landscape of "attractor" wells, which is best represented by a potential function (Haken, 1977, 1983): the deeper the wells of the landscape, the more stable the patterns and the more resistant these patterns will be to perturbations. Control parameters modulate the landscape of attractors, thereby leading to loss of stability of behavioral states and phase transitions between them.

BEHAVIORAL COORDINATION DYNAMICS

One of the most representative paradigms of CD in living systems is that using rhythmic bimanual movements (Kelso et al., 1981; Kelso, 1984; Haken et al., 1985; see Kelso, 1995, for an overview). In this task, the relative phase between the displacements of each limb is considered as the collective variable (order parameter), which captures the dynamics of coordination patterns (i.e., their evolution over time) under the effects of constraints of various origins. The neurobehavioral repertoire is characterized by the presence of two preferred stable patterns of coordination: in-phase and anti-phase (Kelso, 1984), which can be spontaneously produced when participants are instructed to move their arms rhythmically in synergy. The in-phase pattern involves symmetric motion of the hands in opposite directions, whereas the anti-phase pattern involves motion in the same direction (**Figure 1**).

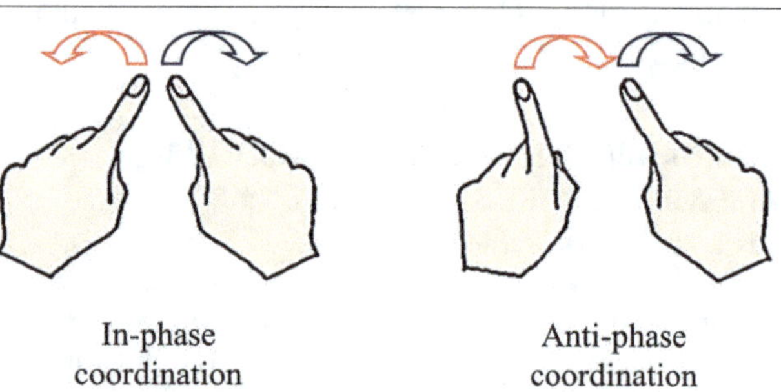

FIGURE 1 | Stable patterns of spontaneous bimanual coordination. The in-phase pattern consists in symmetric movements in opposite directions (0° of relative phase) involving the simultaneous activation of homologous muscles. The anti-phase pattern consists in parallel movements in the same directions (180° of relative phase) involving the simultaneous activation of antagonist muscles.

Stability and flexibility are salient features of CD that have been elucidated by driving the bimanual system toward a point of instability where a *phase transition* subsequently occurs (i.e., an abrupt switch in the order parameter). The anti-phase pattern is generally considered to be less stable than the in-phase pattern, as a spontaneous switch from the former to the latter occurs when oscillation frequency (control parameter) increased beyond a given critical value (Kelso, 1981, 1984). Phase transitions are preceded by a destabilization of the current pattern (anti-phase), resulting from decrease in coupling strength, assuming the presence of noise of constant magnitude (Schöner et al., 1986), evidenced by a dramatic increase in relative phase fluctuations. Such "critical fluctuations" decrease following the phase transition, once the in-phase pattern is adopted (Kelso et al., 1986). These spontaneous/intrinsic dynamics of bimanual coordination are formalized through a tripartite scheme (**Figure 2**) in which the dynamics of the relative phase arise from a low-energy (nonlinear) coupling function linking nonlinear oscillators that represent the limbs (Haken et al., 1985; see Kelso, 1995, 2009, for detailed developments).

The CD formalization of attractor landscape and pattern dynamics is not limited to spontaneous dynamics of bimanual coordination patterns. For one, it has been extended to the study of different movement tasks (e.g., Kelso et al., 1990; Bardy et al., 1999; Temprado and Laurent, 2004; Salesse and Temprado, 2005; Sleimen-Malkoun et al., 2012) and in different populations (e.g., Temprado et al., 2010; Sleimen-Malkoun et al., 2011, 2013). In addition, it has been applied to the study of how the spontaneous dynamics is shaped through cognitive factors as attention (Temprado et al., 1999; Monno et al., 2002), intention (Scholz and Kelso, 1990), and learning (Zanone and Kelso, 1992),

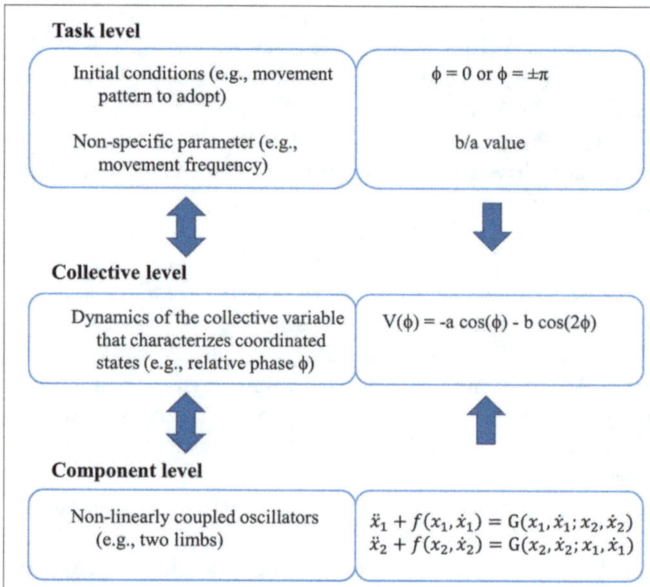

FIGURE 2 | The tripartite scheme (inspired from Kelso, 1995). It links the three phenomenological levels of description from the perspective of dynamic pattern theory.

sometimes termed "directed or goal-directed dynamics". Here, intention, attention and learning provide behavioral information that forms a continuous "force" to shape the dynamics of the collective variable. Intentionally switching from one pattern to another is an example in this regard (Scholz and Kelso, 1990). Selective attentional focus on an existing pattern (e.g., in-phase or anti-phase) generates behavioral information that does not compete with intrinsic tendencies, increases the stability of the coordination pattern (Lee et al., 1996; Temprado et al., 1999) and delays or even prevents the phase transition from occurring. In the case of learning, behavioral information may be perceptually specified by metronomes or memory, leading to greater stability of a previously unstable coordination pattern (Yamanishi et al., 1980; Zanone and Kelso, 1992). Although the information is different in both cases, visual feedback versus memorized information, similar modifications to the dynamics of bimanual coordination have been found (e.g., Schöner et al., 1992).

COORDINATION DYNAMICS IN BRAIN AND BEHAVIOR

The presence and the switching between multiple patterns of activity across neural ensembles have now been shown in the brain (Meyer-Lindenberg et al., 2002; Jantzen et al., 2009; see Fuchs and Jirsa, 2008, and Kelso, 2009, for reviews). Subsequently, a multi-level approach was developed to connect phenomenological findings at the behavioral level to underlying neural mechanisms (see Jirsa and Haken, 1996; Jirsa et al., 1998; Kelso et al., 1999, 2013). To that aim, functionally relevant (coupled) components were identified at the brain level as it was previously done for the behavioral level. Fuchs et al. (2000) proposed a model to capture the relationship between rhythmic finger movements and neuronal activation. The model accounts for the presence of two stable states at low movement frequencies and predicts the destabilization of the anti-phase at higher frequencies. Thus, CD allowed traversing the different scales of the neuro-behavioral system to connect neural and behavioral dynamics (see Kelso et al., 2013, for a recent overview), presented in **Figure 3**.

COORDINATION DYNAMICS AT MUSCULAR LEVEL

Whether and how neuro-muscular factors have a role in neuro-behavioral CD has led to considerable debate over the last decade (Carson et al., 2000; Mechsner et al., 2001; Temprado et al., 2003; Carson and Kelso, 2004; Mechsner, 2004). Initially (Kelso, 1981, 1984), phase transitions reflected a switch from simultaneous activation of non-homologous muscle groups (flexors-extensors) to activation of homologous muscles (flexor-flexor/extensor-extensor). These observations have been extended to wrist and upper limb oscillations, suggesting that the "default" output of brain CD was the activation of homologous muscles,

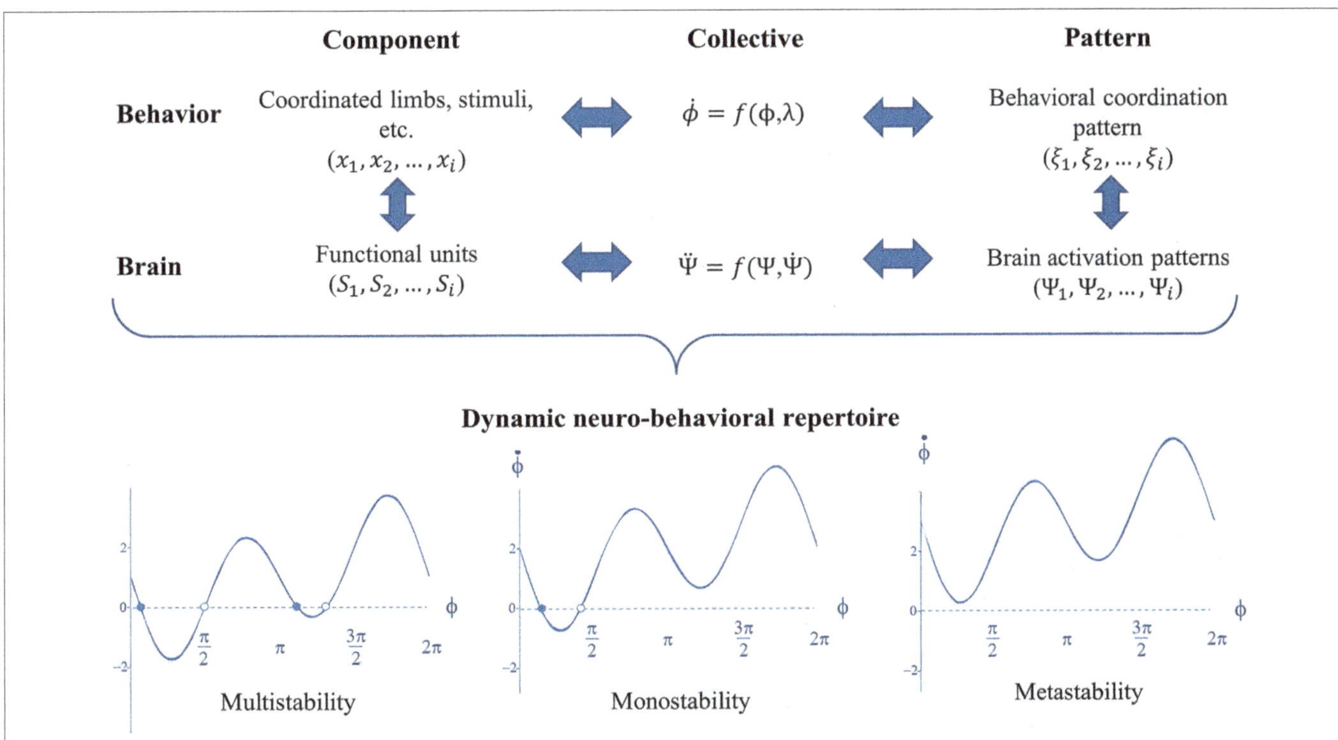

FIGURE 3 | Traversing scales of the neuro-behavioral system by virtue of shared dynamics. At each level of organization, e.g., brain and behavior, the complex dynamics is expressed through lower dimensional patterns that can be captured through the dynamics of the collective variable(s). Accordingly, the neurobehavioral system possesses a dynamic repertoire of attractor states, in which multiple stable attractors can coexist (multistability) or not (monostability). Attractors can also be virtually present as "ghost attractors" giving rise to both phase trapping and phase scattering dynamical flows (metastability).

forming the core of inter-limb CD in a wide range of different tasks.

However, a number of subsequent experiments have demonstrated that the intrinsic dynamics of behavioral patterns were relatively independent of neuro-muscular factors. For instance, in ipsilateral hand-foot coordination, Baldissera et al. (1982, 1991) showed that phase transition prominently depended on directional coupling, instead of muscular synergies. This hypothesis was confirmed in inter-personal coordination tasks: transitions from movements performed in opposite directions to patterns of iso-directional movements were systematically observed (e.g., Schmidt et al., 1990; Temprado and Laurent, 2004). These findings were interpreted as evidence supporting task-dependent informational coupling at the brain level. Mechsner et al. (2001) challenged the *neuro-muscular hypothesis* in bimanual finger coordination by showing that the bias of two-finger oscillations was towards perceptually-based spatial symmetry, irrespective of the muscles involved. Accordingly, they suggested that spontaneous bimanual coordination phenomena were perceptually driven (see also Mechsner, 2004). These debates about the role of intrinsic muscular synergies in inter-limb CD (e.g., Carson, 2004; Carson and Kelso, 2004), eventually converged on a consensus that behavioral CD result from a coalition of (task-dependent) constraints of various origins, including those arising from neuro-muscular factors (e.g., Temprado et al., 2003; Temprado and Salesse, 2004; Salesse and Temprado, 2005).

A COORDINATION DYNAMICS PERSPECTIVE ON NEURO-BEHAVIORAL AGING

The framework of CD has been scarcely applied in aging research (see Greene and Williams, 1996; Temprado et al., 2010; Sleimen-Malkoun et al., 2013, for noticeable exceptions). The above developments suggest however that it might constitute a conceptual framework to age-related adaptations of a complex neuro-behavioral system on fast and slow time-scales.

AGING[1] AS COMPLEX NEURO-BEHAVIORAL SYSTEM DYNAMICS

The description of the time-evolution of the whole neuro-behavioral system, which emerges from complex interactions, is a critical issue in aging research. Performance curves alone are not able to capture declines in behavioral adaptability as it demands the capacity to preserve two apparently contradictory properties, namely stability and flexibility. Stability is classically indexed by variability surrounding a behavioral pattern that is to be maintained and the ability to resist perturbations to this pattern. Flexibility is indexed by the number of intrinsic patterns in the repertoire (i.e., multi-stability) and the ability to switch between them (i.e., transitions). It should be noted that long-range correlations within a time-series are sometimes considered as an indirect marker of system flexibility (Lipsitz, 2002), although (to our knowledge) the empirical confirmation of this hypothesis through appropriate protocols (i.e., perturbation studies) is lacking in aging literature. Despite this lack of direct evidence, from a dynamical systems perspective, variability and pattern dynamics are markers of system's adaptability that should also be able to serve as indices of functional status in the aging NMSS.

THE DYNAMICS OF FUNCTIONAL STATUS DURING AGING

Although it is currently admitted that age-related LOC of the entire neuro-behavioral system may lead to nonlinear changes in functional status over time (Goldberger et al., 2002), a precise description of these states is lacking in the literature. This issue refers to whether and how many "biological ages" can be distinguished on the basis of specific markers, independent of chronological age. Frailty—a geriatric syndrome associated with increased vulnerability, higher rate of morbidity and loss of autonomy—might be heuristic in this respect. Indeed, frailty is viewed as the signature of the degradation of multiple subsystems that normally contribute, through their (weak) couplings, to flexible behavioral adaptations to stressors of various origins (see Clegg et al., 2013; Cesari et al., 2014, for overviews). Even if this general definition is widely accepted in the literature, true system views of frailty are scarce and there are few issues that remain a matter of debate, namely: (i) how frailty can be characterized systemically, if not as the sum of declines in individual parts; and (ii) how changes in levels of systemic (dys) function are detected during healthy aging, at the onset of frailty, and during its progression. Lipsitz (2002, 2004) hypothesized that frailty might be reflected in a global loss of physiological complexity (**Figure 4**). Unfortunately, there is no absolute measure of optimal complexity (i.e., only relative change is informative) and, consequently, precluding a definition of a critical threshold that determines the transition to frailty (e.g., Lipsitz, 2002, 2004; Vaillancourt and Newell, 2002; Newell et al., 2006).

The empirical focus on physiological or behavioral output complexity, however, did not provide concrete framework to describe the age-related changes in coordination processes operating within and between the different subsystems. Thus, at least, the general characterizations of functional status through variability/complexity analysis (i.e., long range correlated structures), at a system level, should be complemented by a precise description of the time-evolution of the behavioral repertoire during aging. In the ensuing sections we describe how pattern dynamics, as a marker of evolving stability and flexibility, evolve in aging.

THE DYNAMICS OF INTRINSIC PATTERNS OF THE BEHAVIORAL REPERTOIRE DURING AGING

At a general level, the aging NMSS can be addressed by studying: (i) the emergence of new patterns; (ii) the stabilization, destabilization and transitions between existing patterns; or even (iii) the loss of patterns of the behavioral repertoire. Landscapes of behavioral attractors can be used to represent these macroscopic dynamics (**Figure 5**). For instance, the epigenetic landscape initially introduced by Waddington (1942, 1957) has been subsequently popularized in development literature by Muchisky et al. (1996), and is now used in numerous domains (e.g., Aimetti, 2009; see Baedke (2013), for overview and discussion).

These landscapes allow one to envision the expression of aging in cognitive-motor skills (posture, locomotion, object manipulation, inter-limb coordination, etc.) as evolving behavioral

[1] Aging currently refers to changes that occur over life span. Here we use it to refer to the period from adulthood to old chronological age.

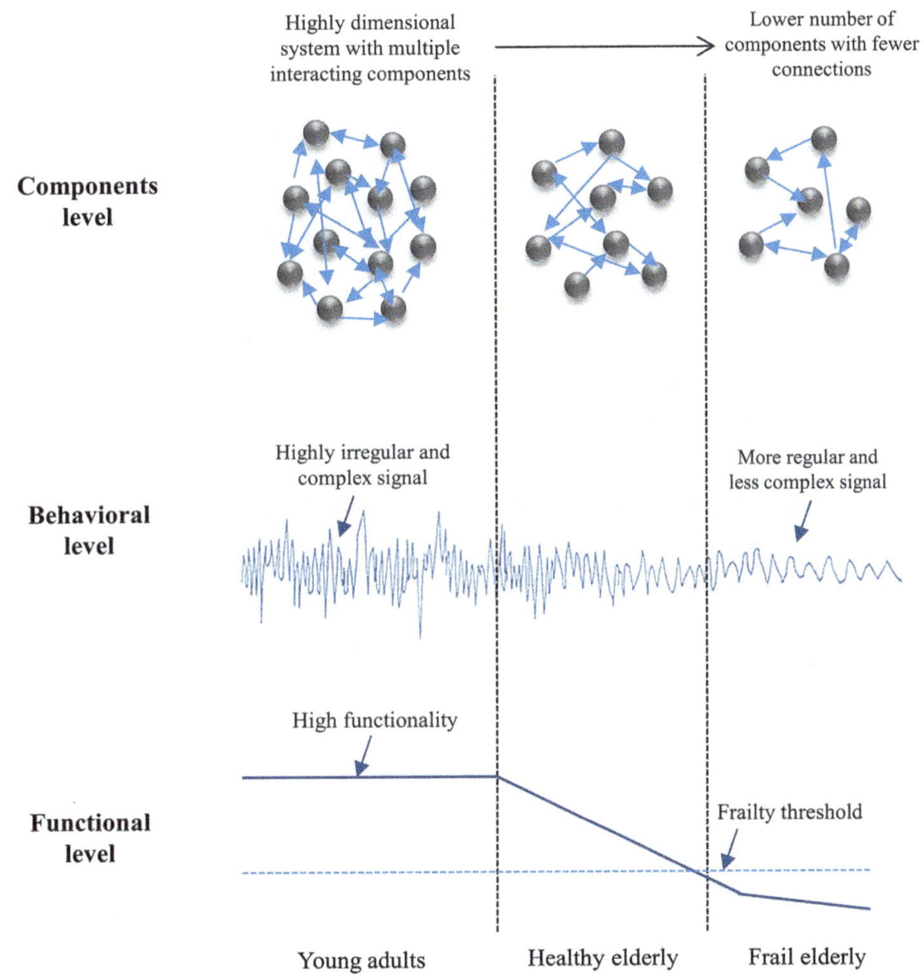

FIGURE 4 | Loss of complexity with age and frailty (inspired from Lipsitz, 2002). A representation of how the interacting sub-systems/components (system's inputs) produce highly complex dynamics (system's output) in young adults with high functionality, due to the richness of the underlying interactions; and as the number of components and the complexity of their interactions drop down, behavior becomes increasingly predictable and the organism loses its functionality (e.g., in elderly). The frailty threshold represents the critical level of function below which the organism can no longer adapt to stress.

(attractor) states. An increase in the number of wells represents the enrichment of the repertoire through a differentiation process, which can be formalized as pitchfork bifurcations. Smith and Thelen (2003) elegantly laid the ground for this idea by characterizing behavioral dynamics during development as a landscape with wells of different depths, i.e., varying stability (see also Newell et al., 2003, 2005). The framework of developmental epigenetic landscape can be extended to lifespan to account for emerging, modifying and dissolving behavioral patterns during aging as a result of the coalition of multiple (i.e., genetic, chemical, cellular, structural, environmental) underlying factors. A decrease in the number of wells can be considered a signature of dedifferentiation that could result from saddle-node bifurcations (old wells cease to exist by dead-ending) or from merging with another well.

Taking bimanual coordination as a representative illustration, we can envision age-related changes from the Haken-Kelso-Bunz model (HKB) potential function. We introduce the dimension of time (i.e., chronological age taken as a control parameter) to represent the deformation of the HKB potential landscape that mimics the changes in the spontaneous dynamics of bimanual patterns. At the most basic level of the HKB model: (i) only two terms are used, thus, only in-phase and anti-phase wells are present; and (ii) the attractor strengths are scaled in proportion to one another. What this means is that the healthy landscape comprises stronger and weaker attractors whose attractiveness is scaled in proportion to one another. Age can be hypothesized to drag the system to function in the middle where all wells tend to have lower and progressively more similar levels of attractiveness. The landscape would be dedifferentiated as all of the attractors would lose their scale-invariance, leading to greater similarity in strength as the highs and lows are no longer present. The result is a more evenly distributed landscape with attractors of equal or near-equal strength.

The complete dedifferentiation at the level of the collective variables (i.e., attractors on the landscape) would mean that the subcomponents are de-coupled from one another as any

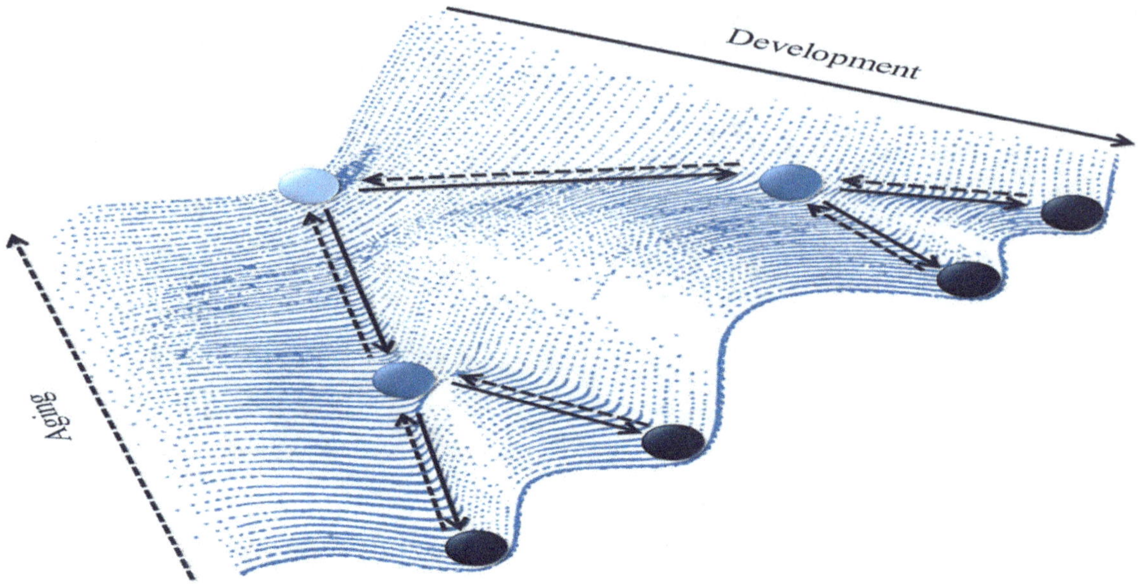

FIGURE 5 | Aging as a macro dynamic phenomenon on an epigenetic landscape (inspired by Waddington, 1942). A metaphoric representation of the life-span evolution of the landscape of behavioral attractors. During development, the number of attractor stable states (represented by wells in which a rolling ball can be trapped) increases through a differentiation process (filled lines arrows). Conversely, during aging (dashed lines arrows), the landscape goes through a dedifferentiation process leading to the disappearance or merging of some attractors.

dynamic relationship between any of them would be equally viable, leading to increased magnitude of variability. Correspondingly, the individual subcomponents would then return to their natural oscillations or intrinsic dynamics (Haken et al., 1985), or even cease to oscillate (Daido, 2008), leading to a LOC. At the most general level, such a deformation of the HKB model would represent a system in which the potential energy is not conserved, since the tradeoff between potential and the number of attractor wells is broken.[2] As Zanone and Kelso (1997) have demonstrated (in conjunction with the inherent properties of the HKB model), a solution for maintaining potential energy constant in the system is strengthening an existing attractor wells, at the expense of the other well. This perspective of aging-induced loss of multistability affords a different account from the dedifferentiation perspective, which was discussed above. Indeed, one could expect that during aging some attractors become deeper and stronger. Such changes would come at the expense of reduced strength at the other attractors or even their disappearance. This assumption is consistent with recent studies by some of us, in which we provided empirical evidence of age-related change in attractor landscape, namely, a decrease in pattern stability (Temprado et al., 2010) and a loss of existing patterns (Sleimen-Malkoun et al., 2013). From this perspective, one can envision the deformation of the HKB model as if the subject started with a higher level of b/a ratio and the decrease of lower, critical values. However, in the HKB model, b/a supposedly mimics the effect of frequency on coupling strength at task-related time scale. Consequently, the longer time dimension of aging should be rather added under the form of another extension that changes the initial stability of intrinsic patterns, decrease their stability over time or even leads to loss of attractor states (see Newell et al., 2008 for modeling the inverse tendency during development).

Age-related deformation of the HKB potential landscape that represents the dynamics of intrinsic patterns presumably influences the directed dynamics that is, how the behavioral repertoire is shaped, temporarily or durably, through cognitive factors as attention, intention and learning in older adults. This issue is of particular importance for aging research, according to the cognitive-motor dedifferentiation that occurs over time.

LINKING VARIABILITY AND COMPLEXITY OF NEURO-BEHAVIORAL OUTPUTS TO PATTERN DYNAMICS: AN ENTRY POINT FOR UNDERSTANDING AGE-RELATED REORGANIZATION IN THE NMSS

At this point in the paper, the question remains of how pattern dynamics give rise to the observed NMSS declines in aging. In addition, the role of noise must also be incorporated in the conceptualization which is frequently considered to be an explanation for increased variability in cognitive and motor tasks in aging (see MacDonald et al., 2009a). Empirically, attempts to describe changes in system's output variability (including structured fluctuations) and pattern dynamics using the same task have been scarce. In the following, we offer a dynamical system reading/interpretation of studies of relevance to this issue at behavioral, brain and mus-

[2]Indeed, the HKB model is founded on a Fourier series with a doubling process that increases the number of potential wells in the system. When the number of parameters is increased, the number of attractor wells increases, but their "attractiveness", is decreased.

cular levels, and that, in both young and aged NMSS. We also point out the directions that must be explored in future work.

VARIABILITY AND THE DYNAMICS OF BEHAVIORAL PATTERNS

Originally, fluctuations in rhythmic behavior were considered to be a product of random events (Wing and Kristofferson, 1973). Pioneering studies demonstrated long-range correlations structure of fluctuations of coordination patterns in finger tapping tasks (i.e., syncopation and synchronization, Chen et al., 1997; Ding et al., 2002) exhibiting that fluctuations in the tapping pattern were not random. In this type of task, participants must flex their index finger "on-" (synchronization) or "off-" a metronome beat (syncopation), at different frequencies. The synchronization (corresponding to in-phase pattern) and syncopation (i.e., anti-phase) patterns have been shown to follow the same dynamics as those described in bimanual coordination (see modeling efforts in Kelso et al., 1990; Kelso, 1995). In these experiments, the authors showed that correlated structures of fluctuations: (i) were different between syncopation and synchronization patterns; and (ii) depended on the cognitive strategy used to perform the task (e.g., finger extension on the beat instead of flexion off).

Torre and collaborators (Torre et al., 2007; Torre, 2010) extended these studies from one finger to bimanual coordination (see also Schmidt et al., 1991). They hypothesized that these fluctuations are indicative of the compromise between stability and flexibility of the neuro-behavioral system and thus, play a specific role in pattern dynamics. Their results provided evidence for $1/f$ noise in both in-phase and anti-phase patterns and showed a greater presence of long-range correlations in relative phase fluctuations were negatively correlated with the critical frequency of transition in young adults (Torre et al., 2007). From a LOC perspective, participants with more complex relative fluctuations were able to delay the phase transition to a higher critical frequency. In contrast, no relation was observed between the amplitude of variability (as measured by the signal variance) and critical frequency. This result suggests different and specific functional roles for structure and amplitude of variability.

Torre and Balasubramaniam (Torre and Balasubramaniam, 2011; Balasubramaniam and Torre, 2012) tested the potential relationship between magnitude and pattern of variability in bimanual coordination tasks. Their reasoning was that a positive correlation between magnitude and pattern of variability would create a "snowball effect", pushing relative phase away from its current value. Conversely, a negative correlation would have a conservative effect, thereby maintaining the pattern within its current boundaries. Their results confirmed this hypothesis as a negative correlation between amplitude and structure of variability was observed for the anti-phase pattern at high frequencies. However, how these phenomena are related to mechanisms underlying pattern dynamics (coupling strength, time delays, component-pattern relationship...) remains to be determined. Moreover, aging consequences have never been investigated in this context. One would suspect that if aging reduces the complexity of coordinated fluctuations, it would also reduce the maximal frequency at which a given pattern can be sustained.

VARIABILITY AND THE DYNAMICS OF BRAIN ACTIVITY

As it was recently argued by some of us (Hong and Rebec, 2012), variability and noise in brain activity serve a functional role (Ghosh et al., 2008; Deco et al., 2009, 2011; Garrett et al., 2011), making the ability to "shift" and distribute noise around the brain essential. Effectively, the healthy brain is able to modulate noise and variability depending on task demands and desired behavioral output (Hong and Rebec, 2012).

Network model studies showed how the interplay between brain structural connectivity, noise level and interaction delays shapes the functional dynamics (Ghosh et al., 2008; Deco et al., 2011). Specifically, they showed that neuro-anatomical connectivity gives rise to a dynamic multistable attractor landscape that is functionally relevant. Indeed, even in the absence of any task and any external stimulation (i.e., the resting-state of the brain), brain activity shows structured spatio-temporal patterns characterized by a latent multistable dynamics. As a critical property, the healthy brain is continuously exploring its dynamic repertoire of attractor states without getting trapped in a single state. In the brain aging literature, the most investigated aspect of the dynamics is related to brain signal fluctuations, their magnitude, structure and distribution over cerebral areas. Despite a number of discrepancies in available literature (e.g., in terms of used methods, task conditions and reported results), some guiding principles can still be extracted.

One recurrent observation is an inverted relation between age-related changes in resting-state and in task-evoked activity. Specifically, whereas at rest EEG signals show more complex fluctuations in older than in younger adults (i.e., less deterministic and with higher dimensionality—Anokhin et al., 1996; Pierce et al., 2000, 2003; Müller and Lindenberger, 2012), during task-relevant activity the tendency seems to be reversed: MSE decreases for coarse scales, as well as distributed entropy (McIntosh et al., 2014), whereas dimensional complexity reduction during task has a tendency to attenuate (Müller and Lindenberger, 2012). However, McIntosh et al. (2014) revealed the presence of temporal-scale dependency, according to which complexity values were higher in elderly at fine time-scales. On slow-time scales (i.e., in fMRI studies), brain activity was found to be less variable in elderly, in both fixation (no task) and different cognitive tasks (Garrett et al., 2011, 2013), with a greater increase from fixation to task in younger adults (Garrett et al., 2013). Specifically, young participants exhibited higher variability in 84% of brain areas, whereas, in the remaining 16% (mainly cerebellum and sub-cortical structures) older subjects were the more variable (Garrett et al., 2011).

In a similar vein, McIntosh et al. (2014) found that multi-scale entropy at fine scales (taken as an indicator of the amount of information processed locally) increased with aging, whereas distributed entropy (i.e., mutual information shared by two sources and linked to functional connectivity) and complexity at coarse time-scales decreased. Aging, in this context, leads to the spatial clustering of information processing, instead of transmitting information across the brain like the young subjects. Pierce et al. (2000, 2003) found that older subjects displayed a higher complexity of spatial distribution of EEG activity suggesting a decrease in the degree of coordination among cortical areas in the aged-brain. Garrett et al. (2011) showed that the elderly exhibited nearly indistinguishable levels of variability across brain structures (i.e., spatial dedifferentiation) while young adults had a 78% difference between the less (mainly sub-cortical) and more variable (cortical) structures. Interestingly, young subjects appear to modulate the magnitude and the spatial representation of the variability of their brain activation to a greater extent and in a more expansive set in region than older subjects do (Garrett et al., 2013). These findings converge to indicate that aging leads to a reduction in coordinated activity. The elderly seem to rely on localized information processing in a manner that is similar to the clustering of different muscle fiber types.

VARIABILITY AND THE INTERACTION BETWEEN BRAIN AND BEHAVIORAL LEVELS

Age-related increases in behavioral variability are currently considered to reflect the amount of neural noise, that is, the age-related increase in random background of activity in the CNS (Li et al., 2000; Li and Sikström, 2002). The presence of continually fluctuating background activity, random or not, is pervasive at all levels of the CNS, even at the most molecular level (see Faisal et al., 2008). Based on widely accepted declines in dopaminergic neurotransmission with aging, neuro-computational models predict a greater variability in neural signaling, and as a consequence, greater behavioral variability and loss of distinctiveness of mental representations (Li et al., 2001). Still, there is debate regarding whether there is truly random (white) noise in the NMSS (Sosnoff and Newell, 2011). This debate, however, is only pertinent if one assumes that neural noise must be: (i) white (i.e., flat power spectrum); and (ii) truly random and uncorrelated. Actually, the activity of neurons *in-vitro* is correlated, following a power law distribution known as the avalanche dynamic (Beggs and Plenz, 2003). Moreover, the relationship between dopamine and neural dynamics takes on an inverted U-shape, where correlations within the signal (i.e., lowest noise or least randomness) are achieved at the mid-range of dopamine levels (Stewart and Plenz, 2006). Either too much or too little dopamine leads to a breakdown in the internal correlations and a flattening of the neural activity distribution, which has consequence of reduced precision and consistency of the produced behavior, based on Li et al. (2000) computational model.

Whether brain signal variability could be taken as a performance predictor is yet another unsettled debate. A strong evidence for a positive correlation was provided by Garrett et al. (2011) by measuring SD of BOLD activity in young and older subjects in three cognitive tasks. In this study, the authors found that brain variability was highly correlated with age and performance: younger, faster (i.e., shorter reaction times) and more consistent (i.e., lower intra-individual standard deviations) participants exhibited greater levels of brain signal variability. Using similar task conditions, McIntosh et al. (2014) reported scale-dependent differences in brain signal (recorded with EEG and MEG) complexity between young and older participants, who displayed comparable accuracy but slower reaction times. Nevertheless, no direct correlation analyses were performed between behavioral (performance) and entropy (brain complexity) measures. In other studies, also investigating brain variability in the context of perceptual and cognitive tasks, the relation between brain fluctuations and performance was even less clear. For instance, Müller and Lindenberger (2012) found associations between perceptual speed performance and brain dynamics for only a few EEG electrodes. Another example can be seen in the Pierce et al. (2000) study in which significant correlations were found between complexity in the spatial distribution over time of EEG activity and only one measure amongst the twelve measures provided by the Visual and Auditory Continuous Performance Test. In particular, higher algorithmic complexity was associated with higher scores on the Consistency-Visual measure. It should be noted, however, that in this specific context, older adults performed significantly better than younger adults.

Strikingly, in all of the reviewed studies, none investigated movement tasks, thereby raising a number of open questions, which should be addressed in future research. One issue of great interest is the systematic exploration of age-related changes in magnitude and structure of fluctuations in both brain and behavior, along with the respective correspondences. A preliminary step would be determining how amplitude and structure of fluctuations relate to meta-stability/self-organizing criticality of activation patterns in the brain (Kelso, 2012). This constitutes an exciting entry point to explore whether and how the aging modifies of the functional relationship between amplitude and structure of variability first within the brain then, between the different levels of organization such as brain and behavior, but also muscular activation.

VARIABILITY AND THE DYNAMICS OF MUSCULAR ACTIVITY

It is striking that in most studies on brain-behavior relationships, the dynamics of muscular activity is omitted. However, since aging leads to significant structural and functional changes in the nervous system (NS), at both central and peripheral levels, muscular function should be subsequently affected (Manini et al., 2013).

Most studies carried out to explore age-related changes in muscular activity focused on the consequences of peripheral modifications on the variability of force production.[3] In this respect, structural changes in muscle composition are consistent with the findings of a LOC in force output in the elderly (see Morrison and Newell, 2012 for a recent review). Supposedly, the loss of range in muscle fiber contractility leads to a decreased number of time-scales along which force output can be modulated, hence, a less complex force output. With a reduction in capacity to alter force output on different time-scales and force amplitudes, the motor behavior of the elderly consistent with the LOCH would be expected. The literature is replete with evidence of narrowed functional ranges in motor behavior, where the LOC is observed across a variety of different functions, including gait, posture, tremor, and muscle force output (see Morrison and Newell, 2012 for a recent review). These findings support the hypothesis that there are commonalities between LOC and dedifferentiation.

[3]The relationship between kinematic and kinetic fluctuations remains to be elucidated.

Despite this, there is far less empirical evidence on the LOC in the musculature beyond motor behavior, that is, in terms of motor unit activity. Thus, experiments should be conducted to explore systematically the links between dedifferentiation, LOC in the musculature and behavioral dynamics (i.e., force outputs). As we reviewed earlier, one of the consequences of aging is a change in muscle fiber proportions, where there is a transition toward a greater proportion of slower, hybrid fibers. The consequence of dedifferentiation at this level would be to reduce the number of different time-scales of muscle contraction. Consequently, a decline in the ability to generate high and low forces (and consequently, fast and slow movements) is to be expected. Smoothness at high speeds would become difficult to achieve, as the necessary bell-shaped velocity profiles (see Harris and Wolpert, 1998) require large muscle forces both to initiate and terminate the movement. At low speeds (e.g., tai chi), jerky movements would still occur as all of the muscle contractions are occurring at a single rate. Thus, instead of a single, continuous movement arising from a combination of fast and slow contractions, the aged muscle would be restricted to a sequence of smaller movements, resulting in a jerky action. This phenomenon is identical to finding that the elderly have a reduced ability to generate smooth sinusoidal isometric force traces and difficulty in generating rapid corrections while attempting to maintain a constant force output (Vaillancourt and Newell, 2002).

Age-related alterations of central processes may also affect how the CNS generates patterns of muscle synergies (Carson, 2006) that is, how the large number of degrees of freedom of the musculoskeletal system is mastered to achieve goal-directed tasks (Bernstein, 1967). In this respect, the coordination problem encountered by the aging CNS at neuro-muscular level is fundamentally a dimensional reduction problem, consisting of the mapping of an infinite number of different task goals onto an infinite set of muscle patterns. A current efficient solution envisaged in the literature is that pre-assembled muscular synergies would be represented in the CNS under the form of a small set of discrete, time-varying muscle synergies, which are combined to generate muscle patterns (d'Avella and Tresch, 2002; d'Avella et al., 2003; Tresch and Jarc, 2009; Dominici et al., 2011). As a general adaptation principle, these synergies would be scaled in amplitude and time to achieve flexible goals in a wide variety of motor tasks (see d'Avella et al., 2003, for details). If one accepts this hypothesis, the question arises of how age-related dedifferentiation and LOC in the CNS: (i) modifies the repertoire of pre-assembled muscular synergies; and (ii) affects the scaling process, thereby impairing movement adaptability.

HYPOTHESES AND EXPERIMENTAL AGENDA

As developed above, using CD affords an unique opportunity to connect, within an integrative approach, the LOC and dedifferentiation hypotheses by focusing on uncovering the effects of aging on complementary aspects of the NMSS (i.e., variability and pattern dynamics) and studying functional ranges rather than single dimensions of brain, muscles and behavior, leading to the following hypotheses:

A. *Aging leads to a generalized intra-individual LOC and dedifferentiation in the different functional subsystems.* The LOC hypothesis arises from separate studies carried out with different groups of participants. Thus, an intra-individual comparison of changes in complexity occurring across the different physiological, cognitive and motor systems is lacking in the literature. The hypothesis of intra-individual LOC could be tested by measuring intra-individual variability (including complexity indexes) of behavioral outputs of cognitive, sensori-motor, physiologic, neural, etc. systems in specific tasks (reaction time, force control, postural control, gait, etc.). One would expect to observe a convergence in behavior complexity in older participants across all of the subsystems being examined. Such general tendency would represent a dedifferentiation of the different subsystems, which leads to a less complex NMSS overall. An interesting avenue would be to explore conditions under which young and older adults differentially modulate their levels of behavioral and brain signal complexity in response to task constraints. Indeed, the modulation of the levels of complexity (depending on the task and the environment) presumably reflects the ability of the NMSS to manage its multiple of degrees of freedom in an optimal manner. Experimentally, it requires testing the subjects under: (i) spontaneous or minimally constrained conditions, in which the system can freely express its complex dynamics (e.g., resting state, postural tremor, oscillation at a natural frequency); and (ii) complex task constraints requiring the system to significantly reduce its fluctuations (e.g., cognitive-motor task-evoked activity, constrained trajectory, force production levels, or frequency).

B. *Information transmission underlying the control of cognitive-motor tasks is altered as a result of age-related LOC of the neurobehavioral system.* To explore this hypothesis, one could exploit the Complexity Matching Principle (West and Grigolini, 2010), which predicts that when several coupled sub-systems exchange information within a complex system to perform a task, the most efficient information transmission occurs when complexity is optimal. This hypothesis could be tested through the use of a dual-task situation associating a force control paradigm and a RT task. In this type of situation, in addition to the complexity of force fluctuations, one can assess the efficiency and cost of information processing by specific variables (i.e., signal to noise ratio and RT, respectively, Slifkin and Newell, 1999). At a preferred level of force production, one expects to observe the highest level of complexity, associated with optimal information processing, a high signal to noise ratio and a low RT.

Another hypothesis is that when initially independent systems with different levels of output complexity, are coupled, the system with a lower output complexity will move toward the one generating the higher level of complexity (Stepp and Turvey, 2010; Marmelat and Delignières, 2012). This hypothesis could be tested in an inter-personal coordination task (see Temprado and Laurent, 2004; Oullier and Kelso, 2009; Riley et al., 2011) by comparing: (i) young-young; (ii) old-old; and (iii) young-old pairs of participants. One predicts that limb components would modify their individual dynamics when assembled/coupled to produce a stable synergy. Specifically, when young and older participants are paired, informational coupling should allow for a transfer of complexity from higher (young adult) to lower (old). Thus, the motor output of the elderly will be more complex when performed in tandem with the young if compared against a solo performance of a similar motor task. If affirmative, it would have theoretical and practical implications for the use dyadic intergenerational associations in complex motor tasks as a mode of motor rehabilitation.

C. As a result of dimensional reduction (i.e., decrease in functional degrees of freedom), aging leads to a narrowing the neurobehavioral repertoire and reduced adaptability to task demands. At the very general level of epigenetic landscape, one should observe a decrease in the number of behavioral patterns in the repertoire. To limit the analysis to a single dimension, one could examine the deformation of behavioral landscape using a bimanual task protocol (i.e., the scanning paradigm; Zanone and Kelso, 1992, 1997). In case of an age-related loss of multistability, destabilization of one of the existing states is expected, hence deforming the behavioral landscape toward monostability. The state to-be lost will exhibit a flatter potential, i.e., lower stability. Empirically, these changes should be observable in elderly through an increase in behavioral variability (measured by relative phase variability) and attentional cost (measured by RT in a dual-task) associated with the anti-phase pattern, as well as more frequent transitions toward the in-phase pattern starting at rather low movement frequencies. Conversely, if aging modifies the landscape towards greater similarity between attractors, coordination patterns will exhibit similar levels of stability and behavior would be more easily locked into a single pattern. Changes in the structure of behavioral fluctuations would also be expected revealing a loss of criticality in the system, i.e., an inability to seamlessly transition between behavioral states.

As a result of the modification of intrinsic dynamics of the behavioral repertoire, one also predicts to observe increasing difficulties in learning new behavioral patterns. To test this hypothesis, one could explore whether phase transitions from anti-phase to in-phase can be delayed by extensive practice that is, by stabilization of an already existing pattern in the intrinsic repertoire. One could also explore whether phase transitions from anti-phase to in-phase can be delayed by extensive practice that is, by stabilizing an already existing pattern. This issue is important since it might show that older adults are able to preserve adaptability of their repertoire of cognitive-motor skills through appropriate training procedures. It would also be of interest to explore whether learning capacity depends on the route adopted to acquire and stabilize a new pattern (Kostrubiec et al., 2012).

The loss of adaptability that would be observed at the behavioral level should be mirrored in brain dynamics and in brain signal variability. Accordingly, several issues should be investigated using brain activity recordings (fMRI, EEG, MEG): (i) changes in complexity at different spatial and temporal scales; and (ii) loss of multistability in the aged-dynamic repertoire; (iii) changes in terms of coupling strength; (iv) expression of metastability; and (v) the relative contribution of local and global connectivity.

D. Aging reduces the ability to resist and recover from perturbations. An example of the reduced capacity to recovery from perturbations in the elderly is the cardiovascular response to the tilt-table (Lipsitz, 2002). Similar tests can be conducted using sensory or mechanical perturbations to test this hypothesis in motor behavior. Transcranial magnetic stimulation provides an opportunity to perturb the CNS, allowing the effects on neural communication to be measured using EEG, for example. Based on this hypothesis, it would be predicted that the elderly: (i) are more easily displaced from a given coordination pattern; and (ii) require more time to recover their original pattern following the perturbation.

E. Dedifferentiation is accompanied by LOC in individual cognitive and sensorimotor functions and assembling of specific cognitive-motor synergies. Here, the hypothesis is that age-related changes in cognitive-motor interplay (dedifferentiation) should modify the assembling of synergies associating cognitive and sensorimotor processes. In addition, cognitive-motor synergies should allow preserving the internal complexity of the whole cognitive-motor systems (and its adaptability), while the complexity of individual cognitive/sensorimotor outputs should decrease. This hypothesis could be tested using classic dual-task paradigms (see Temprado et al., 1999; Pellecchia et al., 2005). Such experiments would contribute to the current and still unsettled debate about the adaptive/non adaptive function of cognitive-motor dedifferentiation (e.g., Mattay et al., 2002; Heuninckx et al., 2008). Specifically, they will permit the determination of whether increased coupling between cognitive and motor processes allows preserving the complexity of the whole cognitive-motor system by association of functional structures (Chauvet, 1995). Experiments could also be carried out to study the effects of aging on intentional switching from in-phase to anti-phase and vice-versa. One can predict that switching time would be influenced by age due to the differential strength of coupling between limb components.

F. The repertoire of pre-assembled muscular synergies should be reduced, thereby impairing movement adaptability. To our knowledge, these issues have not been addressed in the literature until now. In this context, it can be predicted that: (i) in each muscle system, the repertoire of synergies should be reduced toward intrinsic synergies or even a subset of intrinsic synergies, thereby limiting flexible adaptation of movements (i.e., similar to dedifferentiation); and (ii) central and peripheral changes that are at origin of loss of muscular strength (i.e., dynapenia/sarcopenia) should strongly constrain the assembling of synergies within which the muscles are activated. How changes in variability (amplitude and structure) of behavioral outputs (kinetic and kinematic) reflect the modifications of these coordinative processes underlying the formation of muscle synergies remain to be further explored and modeled.

G. Aging affects the interactions between behavioral dynamics, variability and complexity, and underlying large-scale neural network mechanisms. CD in brain and behavior have been previously studied using MEG (e.g., Kelso et al., 1992; Fuchs et al., 2000) and EEG (Wallenstein et al., 1995; Mayville et al., 1999; Banerjee et al., 2012). However, to our knowledge, the effects of aging on the re-organization of cortical networks underlying stable behavioral patterns, the resulting instabilities, and phase transitions that occur under changes in control parameter have never been explored. In particular, the question arises as to: (i) whether maintaining bimanual coordination patterns is associated with more recruitment of additional networks to those that control unimanual movements instead of simply a temporal modulation of these unimanual networks; and (ii) what are the consequences of such recruitment on correlated evolutions of variability/complexity at brain and behavioral levels. Although in young participants, maintaining stable bimanual patterns seems to result from temporal modulation (Banerjee et al., 2012), the hypothesis of additional recruitment in the elderly is consistent with the dedifferentiation hypothesis. It would reflect more age-related cognitive involvement in maintaining coordination patterns (Heuninckx et al., 2005, 2008). In addition, evidence supporting a small amount of additional recruitment at the vicinity of the transition from anti-phase to in-phase has been provided by Banerjee et al. (2012). One can hypothesize that such amount of recruitment could be larger in older adults.

The issue of correlated changes in variability/complexity indexes at brain and behavioral levels also deserves to be addressed. Indeed, it has been suggested that amplitude and structure of variability might play specific roles in behavioral pattern dynamics (see above). Thus, it should be determined how these two types of variability are correlated with those observed for pattern of neural activity. To our knowledge, no strict correspondences have been established yet between the amplitude and structure of variability in brain and behavior. Additionally, existing literature on aging is largely biased towards the study of cognitive performance. Indeed, sensori-motor aging is largely under-investigated, although the use of continuous movement tasks offers the possibility of conducting nonlinear analyses on time series recorded for both brain and behavioral levels.

SUMMARY AND CONCLUSION

The present paper offers an integrative theoretical framework that provides a broader perspective on the consequences of aging on coordination processes that occur within the NMSS. It affords a global picture of the age-related dimensional reduction of the neuro-behavioral system leading to loss of behavioral flexibility. This systems view diverges from the conventional viewpoint that aging is the sum of decline(s) in function(s) away from a youthful state. Instead, driven by complexity changes and dedifferentiation within and between the different functional subsystems, aging is viewed as a systemic re-organization of the whole NMSS. From this perspective, our general hypothesis is that the emergence of order within and between the different levels during aging obeys to general principles (LOC) and underlying mechanisms (dedifferentiation) independent of the level of observation (i.e., neural, muscular, behavioral). At a methodological level, variability and pattern dynamics are two key markers to follow the functional status of the NMSS during aging and frailty. Employing a systems approach to study aging, i.e., a view that transcends different sub-systems and functional domains, significantly adds to the currently dominant approach comprising the study of separate sub-systems. By understanding how many different components and their interactions change with the course of aging yields important insight into compensatory and adaptive processes that occur as we age. Such a level of understanding could lead to novel approaches to promote healthy aging and reduce levels of disability in the elderly.

ACKNOWLEDGMENTS

The present *Hypothesis and Theory* paper concretizes the motivation behind the *CoordAge* project that is currently funded by *Aix-Marseille University* foundation *A*MIDEX*. We thank the *CoordAge* team, in particular Viktor Jirsa and Frédérique Retornaz for many helpful exchanges on how to link complexity, changes in brain dynamic repertoire, aging and frailty.

REFERENCES

Aimetti, G. (2009). "Modelling early language acquisition skills: towards a general statistical learning mechanism," in *Proceedings of the 12th Conference of the European Chapter of the Association for Computational Linguistics: Student Research Workshop* (Athens, Greece: Association for Computational Linguistics).

Andersen, J. L. (2003). Muscle fibre type adaptation in the elderly human muscle. *Scand. J. Med. Sci. Sports* 13, 40–47. doi: 10.1034/j.1600-0838.2003.00299.x

Anokhin, A. P., Birbaumer, N., Lutzenberger, W., Nikolaev, A., and Vogel, F. (1996). Age increases brain complexity. *Electroencephalogr. Clin. Neurophysiol.* 99, 63–68. doi: 10.1016/0921-884x(96)95573-3

Baedke, J. (2013). The epigenetic landscape in the course of time: conrad hal Waddington's methodological impact on the life sciences. *Stud. Hist. Philos. Biol. Biomed. Sci.* 44, 756–773. doi: 10.1016/j.shpsc.2013.06.001

Baldissera, F., Cacallari, P., and Civashi, P. (1982). Preference coupling between voluntary movements of ipsilateral limbs. *Neurosci. Lett.* 34, 95–100. doi: 10.1016/0304-3940(82)90098-2

Balasubramaniam, R., and Torre, K. (2012). Complexity in neurobiology: perspectives from the study of noise in human motor systems. *Crit. Rev. Biomed. Eng.* 40, 459–470. doi: 10.1615/critrevbiomedeng.2013006841

Baldissera, F., Cavallari, P., Marini, G., and Tassone, G. (1991). Differential control of in-phase and anti-phase coupling of rhythmic movements of ipsilateral hand and foot. *Exp. Brain Res.* 83, 375–380. doi: 10.1007/bf00231161

Baltes, B. P. (1980). Integration versus differentiation of fluid/crystallized intelligence in old age. *Dev. Psychol.* 16, 625–635. doi: 10.1037//0012-1649.16.6.625

Baltes, B. P., Lindenberger, U., and Staudinger, U. M. (1998). "Life-span theory in developmental psychology," in *Theoretical Models of Human Development*, ed R. M. Lerner 5th Edn. (New York: Wiley), 1029–1143.

Baltes, P. B., and Lindenberger, U. (1997). Emergence of a powerful connection between sensory and cognitive functions across the adult life span: a new window to the study of cognitive aging? *Psychol. Aging* 12, 12–21. doi: 10.1037//0882-7974.12.1.12

Banerjee, A., Tognoli, E., Kelso, J. A., and Jirsa, V. K. (2012). Spatiotemporal reorganization of large-scale neural assemblies underlies bimanual coordination. *Neuroimage* 62, 1582–1592. doi: 10.1016/j.neuroimage.2012.05.046

Bardy, B. G., Marin, L., Stoffregen, T. A., and Bootsma, R. J. (1999). Postural coordination modes considered as emergent phenomena. *J. Exp. Psychol. Hum. Percept. Perform.* 25, 1284–1301. doi: 10.1037//0096-1523.25.5.1284

Bashore, T. R. (1994). Some thoughts on neurocognitive slowing. *Acta Psychol. (Amst)* 86, 295–325. doi: 10.1016/0001-6918(94)90006-x

Beggs, J. M., and Plenz, D. (2003). Neuronal avalanches in neocortical circuits. *J. Neurosci.* 23, 11167–11177.

Bernstein, N. A. (1967). *The Co-Ordination and Regulation of Movements.* Oxford: Pergamon Press.

Birren, J. E. (1965). "Age changes in speed of behavior: its central nature and physiological correlates," in *Behavior, Aging and the Nervous System*, eds A. T. Welford and J. E. Birren (Springfield, IL: Charles C. Thomas), 191–216.

Birren, J. E., Woods, A. M., and Williams, M. W. (1980). "Behavioral slowing with age: causes, organization and consequences," in *Aging in the 1980's*, ed L. W. Poon (Washington, DC: American Psychological Association), 293–308.

Bravi, A., Longtin, A., and Seely, A. (2011). Review and classification of variability analysis techniques with clinical applications. *Biomed. Eng. Online* 10:90. doi: 10.1186/1475-925X-10-90

Buchman, T. G. (1996). Physiologic stability and physiologic state. *J. Trauma* 41, 599–605. doi: 10.1097/00005373-199610000-00002

Cabeza, R. (2002). Hemispheric asymmetry reduction in older adults: the HAROLD model. *Psychol. Aging* 17, 85–100. doi: 10.1037/0882-7974.17.1.85

Cabeza, R., Anderson, N. D., Locantore, J. K., and Mcintosh, A. R. (2002). Aging gracefully: compensatory brain activity in high-performing older adults. *Neuroimage* 17, 1394–1402. doi: 10.1006/nimg.2002.1280

Carson, R. G. (2004). "Governing coordination: why do muscles matter," in *Coordination Dynamics: Issues and Trends*, eds V. K. Jirsa and J. A. S. Kelso (Berlin: Springer-Verlag), 141–154.

Carson, R. G. (2006). Changes in muscle coordination with training. *J. Appl. Physiol. (1985)* 101, 1506–1513. doi: 10.1152/japplphysiol.00544.2006

Carson, R. G., and Kelso, J. A. S. (2004). Governing coordination: behavioural principles and neural correlates. *Exp. Brain Res.* 154, 267–274. doi: 10.1007/s00221-003-1726-8

Carson, R. G., Riek, S., Smethurst, C. J., Parraga, J. F., and Byblow, W. D. (2000). Neuromuscular-skeletal constraints upon the dynamics of unimanual and bimanual coordination. *Exp. Brain Res.* 131, 196–214. doi: 10.1007/s002219900272

Cerella, J. (1985). Information processing rates in the elderly. *Psychol. Bull.* 98, 67–83. doi: 10.1037//0033-2909.98.1.67

Cerella, J. (1991). Age effects may be global, not local: comment on Fisk and Rogers (1991). *J. Exp. Psychol. Gen.* 120, 215–223. doi: 10.1037/0096-3445.120.2.215

Cerella, J. (1994). Generalized slowing in Brinley plots. *J. Gerontol.* 49, P65–P71. doi: 10.1093/geronj/49.2.p65

Cesari, M., Gambassi, G., van Kan, G. A., and Vellas, B. (2014). The frailty phenotype and the frailty index: different instruments for different purposes. *Age Ageing* 43, 10–12. doi: 10.1093/ageing/aft160

Chauvet, G. (1995). *La Vie dans la Matière: Le Rôle de L'espace en Biologie (Life in Material: The Role of Space in Biology).* Paris: Champs Flammarion.

Chen, Y. Q., Ding, M. Z., and Kelso, J. A. S. (1997). Long memory processes (1/f(alpha) type) in human coordination. *Phys. Rev. Lett.* 79, 4501–4504. doi: 10.1103/physrevlett.79.4501

Clegg, A., Young, J., Iliffe, S., Rikkert, M. O., and Rockwood, K. (2013). Frailty in elderly people. *Lancet* 381, 752–762. doi: 10.1016/S0140-6736(12)62167-9

Costa, M., Goldberger, A. L., and Peng, C. K. (2002). Multiscale entropy analysis of complex physiologic time series. *Phys. Rev. Lett.* 89:068102. doi: 10.1103/PhysRevLett.89.068102

Daido, H. (2008). Aging transition and disorder-induced coherence in locally coupled oscillators. *EPL* 84:10002. doi: 10.1209/0295-5075/84/10002

d'Avella, A., Saltiel, P., and Bizzi, E. (2003). Combinations of muscle synergies in the construction of a natural motor behavior. *Nat. Neurosci.* 6, 300–308. doi: 10.1038/nn1010

d'Avella, A., and Tresch, M. C. (2002). "Modularity in the motor system: decomposition of muscle patterns as combinations of time-varying synergies," in *Advances in Neural Information Processing Systems* 14, eds T. G. Dietterich, S. Becker and Z. Ghahramani (Cambridge, MA: MIT Press), 141–148.

Deco, G., Jirsa, V., Mcintosh, A. R., Sporns, O., and Kötter, R. (2009). Key role of coupling, delay and noise in resting brain fluctuations. *Proc. Natl. Acad. Sci. U S A* 106, 10302–10307. doi: 10.1073/pnas.0906701106

Deco, G., Jirsa, V. K., and McIntosh, A. R. (2011). Emerging concepts for the dynamical organization of resting-state activity in the brain. *Nat. Rev. Neurosci.* 12, 43–56. doi: 10.1038/nrn2961

Dennis, N. A., and Cabeza, R. (2011). Age-related dedifferentiation of learning systems: an fMRI study of implicit and explicit learning. *Neurobiol. Aging* 32, 2318.e17–2318.e30. doi: 10.1016/j.neurobiolaging.2010.04.004

Ding, M., Chen, Y., and Kelso, J. A. (2002). Statistical analysis of timing errors. *Brain Cogn.* 48, 98–106. doi: 10.1006/brcg.2001.1306

Dominici, N., Ivanenko, Y., Cappellini, G., d'avella, A., Mondı, V., Cicchese, M., et al. (2011). Locomotor primitives in newborn babies and their development. *Science* 334, 997–999. doi: 10.1126/science.1210617

Faisal, A. A., Selen, L. P. J., and Wolpert, D. M. (2008). Noise in the nervous system. *Nat. Rev. Neurosci.* 9, 292–303. doi: 10.1038/nrn2258

Fuchs, A., and Jirsa, V. K. (2008). *Coordination: Neural, Behavioral and Social Dynamics.* Heidelberg: Springer.

Fuchs, A., Jirsa, V. K., and Kelso, J. A. S. (2000). Theory of the relation between human brain activity (MEG) and hand movements. *Neuroimage* 11, 359–369. doi: 10.1006/nimg.1999.0532

Garrett, D. D., Kovacevic, N., Mcintosh, A. R., and Grady, C. L. (2011). The importance of being variable. *J. Neurosci.* 31, 4496–4503. doi: 10.1523/JNEUROSCI.5641-10.2011

Garrett, D. D., Kovacevic, N., Mcintosh, A. R., and Grady, C. L. (2013). The modulation of BOLD variability between cognitive states varies by age and processing speed. *Cereb. Cortex* 23, 684–693. doi: 10.1093/cercor/bhs055

Ghosh, A., Rho, Y., Mcintosh, A. R., Kötter, R., and Jirsa, V. K. (2008). Noise during rest enables the exploration of the brain's dynamic repertoire. *PLoS Comput. Biol.* 4:e1000196. doi: 10.1371/journal.pcbi.1000196

Glass, L., and Mackey, M. (1988). *From Clocks to Chaos: The Rythms of Life.* Princeton: Princeton University Press.

Goldberger, A. L., Amaral, L. A. N., Hausdorff, J. M., Ivanov, P. C., Peng, C.-K., and Stanley, H. E. (2002). Fractal dynamics in physiology: alterations with disease and aging. *Proc. Natl. Acad. Sci. U S A* 99(Suppl. 1), 2466–2472. doi: 10.1073/pnas.012579499

Greene, L. S., and Williams, H. G. (1996). "Aging and coordination from the dynamic pattern perspective," in *Advances in Psychology: Changes in Sensory Motor Behavior in Aging*, eds A.-M. Ferrandez and N. Teasdale (Amsterdam: Elsevier), 89–131.

Haken, H. (1977). *Synegetics.* Berlin: Springer.

Haken, H. (1983). *Synergetics: An Introduction.* Berlin: Springer-Verlag.

Haken, H., Kelso, J. A., and Bunz, H. (1985). A theoretical model of phase transitions in human hand movements. *Biol. Cybern.* 51, 347–356. doi: 10.1007/bf00336922

Harris, C. M., and Wolpert, D. M. (1998). Signal-dependent noise determines motor planning. *Nature* 394, 780–784. doi: 10.1038/29528

Heuninckx, S., Wenderoth, N., and Swinnen, S. P. (2008). Systems neuroplasticity in the aging brain: recruiting additional neural resources for successful motor performance in elderly persons. *J. Neurosci.* 28, 91–99. doi: 10.1523/JNEUROSCI.3300-07.2008

Heuninckx, S., Wenderoth, N., Debaere, F., Peeters, R., and Swinnen, S. P. (2005). Neural basis of aging: the penetration of cognition into action control. *J. Neurosci.* 25, 6787–6796. doi: 10.1523/jneurosci.1263-05.2005

Hilber, K., Galler, S., Gohlsch, B., and Pette, D. (1999). Kinetic properties of myosin heavy chain isoforms in single fibers from human skeletal muscle. *FEBS Lett.* 455, 267–270. doi: 10.1016/s0014-5793(99)00903-5

Hong, S. L., and Rebec, G. V. (2012). Biological sources of inflexibility in brain and behavior with aging and neurodegenerative diseases. *Front. Syst. Neurosci.* 6:77. doi: 10.3389/fnsys.2012.00077

Hultsch, D. F., Strauss, E., Hunter, M. A., and Macdonald, S. W. (2008). "Intraindividual variability, cognition and aging," in *The Handbook of Aging and Cognition*, eds F. I. M. Craik and T. A. Salthouse 3rd Edn. (New York, NY: Psychology Press), 491–556.

Jantzen, K. J., Steinberg, F. L., and Kelso, J. A. S. (2009). Coordination dynamics of large-scale neural circuitry underlying rhythmic sensorimotor behavior. *J. Cogn. Neurosci.* 21, 2420–2433. doi: 10.1162/jocn.2008.21182

Jirsa, V. K., Fuchs, A., and Kelso, J. A. (1998). Connecting cortical and behavioral dynamics: bimanual coordination. *Neural Comput.* 10, 2019–2045. doi: 10.1162/089976698300016954

Jirsa, V. K., and Haken, H. (1996). Field theory of electromagnetic brain activity. *Phys. Rev. Lett.* 77, 960–963. doi: 10.1103/physrevlett.77.960

Kelso, J. A. (1984). Phase transitions and critical behavior in human bimanual coordination. *Am. J. Physiol.* 246, R1000–R1004.

Kelso, J. A., Dumas, G., and Tognoli, E. (2013). Outline of a general theory of behavior and brain coordination. *Neural Netw.* 37, 120–131. doi: 10.1016/j.neunet.2012.09.003

Kelso, J. A., Holt, K. G., Rubin, P., and Kugler, P. N. (1981). Patterns of human interlimb coordination emerge from the properties of non-linear, limit cycle oscillatory processes: theory and data. *J. Mot. Behav.* 13, 226–261. doi: 10.1080/00222895.1981.10735251

Kelso, J. A. S. (1981). On the oscillatory basis of movement. *Bull. Psychon. Soc.* 18, 63.

Kelso, J. A. S. (1995). *Dynamic Patterns: The Self-Organization of Brain and Behavior.* Cambridge: MIT Press.

Kelso, J. A. S. (2009). Synergies: atoms of brain and behavior. *Adv. Exp. Med. Biol.* 629, 83–91. doi: 10.1007/978-0-387-77064-2_5

Kelso, J. A. S. (2012). Multistability and metastability: understanding dynamic coordination in the brain. *Philos. Trans. R. Soc. Lond. B Biol. Sci.* 367, 906–918. doi: 10.1098/rstb.2011.0351

Kelso, J. A. S., Bressler, S. L., Buchanan, S., Deguzman, G. C., Ding, M., Fuchs, A., et al. (1992). A phase transition in human brain and behavior. *Phys. Lett. A* 169, 134–144. doi: 10.1016/0375-9601(92)90583-8

Kelso, J. A. S., Delcolle, J., and Schöner, G. (1990). "Action-Perception as a pattern formation process," in *Attention and Performance XIII*, ed M. Jeannerod (Hillsdale, NJ: Erlbaum), 139–169.

Kelso, J. A. S., Fuchs, A., and Jirsa, V. (1999). "Traversing scales of brain and behavioral organization I: concepts and experiments," in *Analysis of Neurophysiological Brain Functioning*, ed C. Uhl (Berlin Heidelberg: Springer), 73–89.

Kelso, J. A. S., Scholz, J. P., and Schöner, G. (1986). Nonequilibrium phase transitions in coordinated biological motion: critical fluctuations. *Phys. Lett. A* 118, 279–284. doi: 10.1016/0375-9601(86)90359-2

Kostrubiec, V., Zanone, P. G., Fuchs, A., and Kelso, J. A. (2012). Beyond the blank slate: routes to learning new coordination patterns depend on the intrinsic dynamics of the learner-experimental evidence and theoretical model. *Front. Hum. Neurosci.* 6:222. doi: 10.3389/fnhum.2012.00222

Lang, P.-O., Michel, J.-P., and Zekry, D. (2009). Frailty syndrome: a transitional state in a dynamic process. *Gerontology* 55, 539–549. doi: 10.1159/000211949

Lee, T. D., Blandin, Y., and Proteau, L. (1996). Effects of task instructions and oscillation frequency on bimanual coordination. *Psychol. Res.* 59, 100–106. doi: 10.1007/bf01792431

Lexell, J. (1995). Human aging, muscle mass and fiber type composition. *J. Gerontol. A Biol. Sci. Med. Sci.* 50, 11–16. doi: 10.1093/gerona/50a.special_issue.11

Li, K. Z. H., and Lindenberger, U. (2002). Relations between aging sensory/sensorimotor and cognitive functions. *Neurosci. Biobehav. Rev.* 26, 777–783. doi: 10.1016/s0149-7634(02)00073-8

Li, S., Lindenberger, U., and Sikström, S. (2001). Aging cognition: from neuromodulation to representation. *Trends Cogn. Sci.* 5, 479–486. doi: 10.1016/s1364-6613(00)01769-1

Li, S. C., Lindenberger, U., and Frensch, P. A. (2000). Unifying cognitive aging: from neuromodulation to representation to cognition. *Neurocomputing* 32–33, 879–890. doi: 10.1016/s0925-2312(00)00256-3

Li, S. C., and Sikström, S. (2002). Integrative neurocomputational perspectives on cognitive aging, neuromodulation and representation. *Neurosci. Biobehav. Rev.* 26, 795–808. doi: 10.1016/s0149-7634(02)00066-0

Lindenberger, U., and Baltes, P. B. (1994). Sensory functioning and intelligence in old age: a strong connection. *Psychol. Aging* 9, 339–355. doi: 10.1037/0882-7974.9.3.339

Lindenberger, U., and Ghisletta, P. (2009). Cognitive and sensory declines in old age: gauging the evidence for a common cause. *Psychol. Aging* 24, 1–16. doi: 10.1037/a0014986

Lipsitz, L. A. (2002). Dynamics of stability: the physiologic basis of functional health and frailty. *J. Gerontol. A Biol. Sci. Med. Sci.* 57, B115–B125. doi: 10.1093/gerona/57.3.b115

Lipsitz, L. A. (2004). Physiological complexity, aging and the path to frailty. *Sci. Aging Knowledge Environ.* 2004:pe16. doi: 10.1126/sageke.2004.16.pe16

Lipsitz, L. A., and Goldberger, A. L. (1992). Loss of complexity and aging. Potential applications of fractals and chaos theory to senescence. *JAMA* 267, 1806–1809. doi: 10.1001/jama.1992.03480130122036

MacDonald, S. W. S., Cervenka, S., Farde, L., Nyberg, L., and Bäckman, L. (2009a). Extrastriatal dopamine D2 receptor binding modulates intraindividual variability in episodic recognition and executive functioning. *Neuropsychologia* 47, 2299–2304. doi: 10.1016/j.neuropsychologia.2009.01.016

MacDonald, S. W. S., Li, S.-C., and Bäckman, L. (2009b). Neural underpinnings of within-person variability in cognitive functioning. *Psychol. Aging* 24, 792–808. doi: 10.1037/a0017798

Manini, T. M., Hong, S. L., and Clark, B. C. (2013). Aging and muscle: a neuron's perspective. *Curr. Opin. Clin. Nutr. Metab. Care* 16, 21–26. doi: 10.1097/MCO.0b013e32835b5880

Marmelat, V., and Delignières, D. (2012). Strong anticipation: complexity matching in interpersonal coordination. *Exp. Brain Res.* 222, 137–148. doi: 10.1007/s00221-012-3202-9

Mattay, V. S., Fera, F., Tessitore, A., Hariri, A. R., Das, S., Callicott, J. H., et al. (2002). Neurophysiological correlates of age-related changes in human motor function. *Neurology* 58, 630–635. doi: 10.1212/wnl.58.4.630

Mayville, J. M., Bressler, S. L., Fuchs, A., and Kelso, J. A. (1999). Spatiotemporal reorganization of electrical activity in the human brain associated with a timing transition in rhythmic auditory-motor coordination. *Exp. Brain Res.* 127, 371–381. doi: 10.1007/s002210050805

McIntosh, A. R., Kovacevic, N., Lippe, S., Garrett, D., Grady, C., and Jirsa, V. (2010). The development of a noisy brain. *Arch. Ital. Biol.* 148, 323–337.

McIntosh, A. R., Vakorin, V., Kovacevic, N., Wang, H., Diaconescu, A., and Protzner, A. B. (2014). Spatiotemporal dependency of age-related changes in brain signal variability. *Cereb. Cortex* 24, 1806–1817. doi: 10.1093/cercor/bht030

Mechsner, F. (2004). "A perceptual-cognitive approach to bimanual coordination," in *Coordination Dynamics: Issues and Trends*, eds V. K. Jirsa and J. A. S. Kelso (Berlin: Springer), 177–195.

Mechsner, F., Kerzel, D., Knoblich, G., and Prinz, W. (2001). Perceptual basis of bimanual coordination. *Nature* 414, 69–73. doi: 10.1038/35102060

Medvedev, Z. A. (1990). An attempt at a rational classification of theories of ageing. *Biol. Rev. Camb. Philos. Soc.* 65, 375–398. doi: 10.1111/j.1469-185x.1990.tb01428.x

Meyer-Lindenberg, A., Ziemann, U., Hajak, G., Cohen, L., and Berman, K. F. (2002). Transitions between dynamical states of differing stability in the human brain. *Proc. Natl. Acad. Sci. U S A* 99, 10948–10953. doi: 10.1073/pnas.162114799

Monemi, M., Eriksson, P. O., Kadi, F., Butler-Browne, G. S., and Thornell, L. E. (1999). Opposite changes in myosin heavy chain composition of human masseter and biceps brachii muscles during aging. *J. Muscle Res. Cell Motil.* 20, 351–361. doi: 10.1023/A:1005421604314

Monno, A., Temprado, J.-J., Zanone, P.-G., and Laurent, M. (2002). The interplay of attention and bimanual coordination dynamics. *Acta Psychol. (Amst)* 110, 187–211. doi: 10.1016/s0001-6918(02)00033-1

Morrison, S., and Newell, K. M. (2012). Aging, neuromuscular decline and the change in physiological and behavioral complexity of upper-limb movement dynamics. *J. Aging Res.* 2012:891218. doi: 10.1155/2012/891218

Muchisky, M., Gershkoff-Stowe, L., Cole, E., and Thelen, E. (1996). "The epigenetic landscape revisited: a dynamic interpretation," in *Advances in Infancy Research*, ed C. Rovee-Collier (Norwood, NJ: Ablex), 121–159.

Müller, V., and Lindenberger, U. (2012). Lifespan differences in nonlinear dynamics during rest and auditory oddball performance. *Dev. Sci.* 15, 540–556. doi: 10.1111/j.1467-7687.2012.01153.x

Newell, K. M., Liu, Y.-T., and Mayer-Kress, G. (2003). A dynamical systems interpretation of epigenetic landscapes for infant motor development. *Infant Behav. Dev.* 26, 449–472. doi: 10.1016/j.infbeh.2003.08.003

Newell, K. M., Liu, Y.-T., and Mayer-Kress, G. (2005). Learning in the brain-computer interface: insights about degrees of freedom and degeneracy in a landscape model of motor learning. *Cognit. Process.* 6, 37–47. doi: 10.1007/s10339-004-0047-6

Newell, K. M., Liu, Y.-T., and Mayer-Kress, G. (2008). "Landscapes beyond the HKB model," in *Coordination: Neural, Behavioral and Social Dynamics*, eds A. Fuchs and V. K. Jirsa (Berlin: Springer Verlag), 27–44.

Newell, K., Vaillancourt, D., and Sosnoff, J. (2006). "Aging, complexity and motor performance," in *Handbook of the Psychology of Aging*, eds J. E. Birren and K. W. Schaie (London, UK: Elsevier Academic Press), 163–178.

Nilwik, R., Snijders, T., Leenders, M., Groen, B. B., Van Kranenburg, J., Verdijk, L. B., et al. (2013). The decline in skeletal muscle mass with aging is mainly attributed to a reduction in type II muscle fiber size. *Exp. Gerontol.* 48, 492–498. doi: 10.1016/j.exger.2013.02.012

Oullier, O., and Kelso, J. A. S. (2009). "Coordination from the perspective of social coordination dynamics," in *The Encyclodedia of Complexity and Systems Science*, ed R. A. Meyer (Heideberg: Springer), 8198–8213.

Papenberg, G., Backman, L., Chicherio, C., Nagel, I. E., Heekeren, H. R., Lindenberger, U., et al. (2011). Higher intraindividual variability is associated with more forgetting and dedifferentiated memory functions in old age. *Neuropsychologia* 49, 1879–1888. doi: 10.1016/j.neuropsychologia.2011.03.013

Park, D. C., Polk, T. A., Park, R., Minear, M., Savage, A., and Smith, M. R. (2004). Aging reduces neural specialization in ventral visual cortex. *Proc. Natl. Acad. Sci. U S A* 101, 13091–13095. doi: 10.1073/pnas.0405148101

Park, D. C., and Reuter-Lorenz, P. (2009). The adaptive brain: aging and neurocognitive scaffolding. *Annu. Rev. Psychol.* 60, 173–196. doi: 10.1146/annurev.psych.59.103006.093656

Pellecchia, G. L., Shockley, K., and Turvey, M. T. (2005). Concurrent cognitive task modulates coordination dynamics. *Cogn. Sci.* 29, 531–557. doi: 10.1207/s15516709cog0000_12

Peng, C.-K., Costa, M., and Goldberger, A. L. (2009). Adaptative data analysis of complex fluctuations in physiologic time series. *Adv. Adapt. Data Anal.* 1, 61–70. doi: 10.1142/s1793536909000035

Pette, D., and Staron, R. S. (2000). Myosin isoforms, muscle fiber types and transitions. *Microsc. Res. Tech.* 50, 500–509. doi: 10.1002/1097-0029(20000915)50:6<500::aid-jemt7>3.3.co;2-z

Pierce, T. W., Kelly, S. P., Watson, T. D., Replogle, D., King, J. S., and Pribram, K. H. (2000). Age differences in dynamic measures of EEG. *Brain Topogr.* 13, 127–134. doi: 10.1023/A:1026659102713

Pierce, T. W., Watson, T. D., King, J. S., Kelly, S. P., and Pribram, K. H. (2003). Age differences in factor analysis of EEG. *Brain Topogr.* 16, 19–27. doi: 10.1023/A:1025654331788

Reuter-Lorenz, P. A. (2002). New visions of the aging mind and brain. *Trends Cogn. Sci.* 6, 394–400. doi: 10.1016/s1364-6613(02)01957-5

Rey-Robert, B., Temprado, J.-J., and Berton, E. (2011). Aging and changes in complexity in the neurobehavioral system. *Medicina (Kaunas)* 47, 1–10.

Riley, M. A., Richardson, M. J., Shockley, K., and Ramenzoni, V. C. (2011). Interpersonal synergies. *Front. Psychol.* 2:38. doi: 10.3389/fpsyg.2011.00038

Salesse, R., and Temprado, J. J. (2005). The effect of visuo-motor transformations on hand-foot coordination: evidence in favor of the incongruency hypothesis. *Acta Psychol. (Amst)* 119, 143–157. doi: 10.1016/j.actpsy.2004.12.002

Salthouse, T. A. (1996). The processing-speed theory of adult age differences in cognition. *Psychol. Rev.* 103, 403–428. doi: 10.1037/0033-295x.103.3.403

Schaefer, S., and Schumacher, V. (2010). The interplay between cognitive and motor functioning in healthy older adults: findings from dual-task studies and suggestions for intervention. *Gerontology* 57, 239–246. doi: 10.1159/000322197

Schäfer, S., Huxhold, O., and Lindenberger, U. (2006). Healthy mind in healthy body? A review of sensorimotor–cognitive interdependencies in old age. *Eur. Rev. Aging Phys. Act.* 3, 45–54. doi: 10.1007/s11556-006-0007-5

Schmidt, R. C., Beek, P. J., Treffner, P. J., and Turvey, M. T. (1991). Dynamical substructure of coordinated rhythmic movements. *J. Exp. Psychol. Hum. Percept. Perform.* 17, 635–651. doi: 10.1037//0096-1523.17.3.635

Schmidt, R. C., Carello, C., and Turvey, M. T. (1990). Phase transitions and critical fluctuations in the visual coordination of rhythmic movements between people. *J. Exp. Psychol. Hum. Percept. Perform.* 16, 227–247. doi: 10.1037/0096-1523.16.2.227

Scholz, J. P., and Kelso, J. A. (1990). Intentional switching between patterns of bimanual coordination depends on the intrinsic dynamics of the patterns. *J. Mot. Behav.* 22, 98–124. doi: 10.1080/00222895.1990.10735504

Schöner, G., Haken, H., and Kelso, J. A. (1986). A stochastic theory of phase transitions in human hand movement. *Biol. Cybern.* 53, 247–257. doi: 10.1007/bf00336995

Schöner, G., Zanone, P. G., and Kelso, J. A. (1992). Learning as change of coordination dynamics: theory and experiment. *J. Mot. Behav.* 24, 29–48. doi: 10.1080/00222895.1992.9941599

Seidler, R. D., Bernard, J. A., Burutolu, T. B., Fling, B. W., Gordon, M. T., Gwin, J. T., et al. (2010). Motor control and aging: links to age-related brain structural, functional and biochemical effects. *Neurosci. Biobehav. Rev.* 34, 721–733. doi: 10.1016/j.neubiorev.2009.10.005

Serrien, D. J., Ivry, R. B., and Swinnen, S. P. (2007). The missing link between action and cognition. *Prog. Neurobiol.* 82, 95–107. doi: 10.1016/j.pneurobio.2007.02.003

Sleimen-Malkoun, R., Temprado, J. J., and Berton, E. (2013). Age-related changes of movement patterns in discrete Fitts' task. *BMC Neurosci.* 14:145. doi: 10.1186/1471-2202-14-145

Sleimen-Malkoun, R., Temprado, J. J., Huys, R., Jirsa, V., and Berton, E. (2012). Is Fitts' law continuous in discrete aiming? *PLoS One* 7:e41190. doi: 10.1371/journal.pone.0041190

Sleimen-Malkoun, R., Temprado, J.-J., Thefenne, L., and Berton, E. (2011). Bimanual training in stroke: how do coupling and symmetry-breaking matter? *BMC Neurol.* 11:11. doi: 10.1186/1471-2377-11-11

Slifkin, A. B., and Newell, K. M. (1999). Noise, information transmission and force variability. *J. Exp. Psychol. Hum. Percept. Perform.* 25, 837–851. doi: 10.1037//0096-1523.25.3.837

Smith, L. B., and Thelen, E. (2003). Development as a dynamic system. *Trends Cogn. Sci.* 7, 343–348. doi: 10.1016/S1364-6613(03)00156-6

Sosnoff, J. J., and Newell, K. M. (2011). Aging and motor variability: a test of the neural noise hypothesis. *Exp. Aging Res.* 37, 377–397. doi: 10.1080/0361073x.2011.590754

Sosnoff, J. J., Valantine, A. D., and Newell, K. M. (2006). Independence between the amount and structure of variability at low force levels. *Neurosci. Lett.* 392, 165–169. doi: 10.1016/j.neulet.2005.09.010

Stepp, N., and Turvey, M. T. (2010). On strong anticipation. *Cogn. Syst. Res.* 11, 148–164. doi: 10.1016/j.cogsys.2009.03.003

Stewart, C. V., and Plenz, D. (2006). Inverted-U profile of dopamine-NMDA-mediated spontaneous avalanche recurrence in superficial layers of rat prefrontal cortex. *J. Neurosci.* 26, 8148–8159. doi: 10.1523/jneurosci.0723-06.2006

Temprado, J.-J., and Laurent, M. (2004). Attentional load associated with performing and stabilizing a between-persons coordination of rhythmic limb movements. *Acta Psychol. (Amst)* 115, 1–16. doi: 10.1016/j.actpsy.2003.09.002

Temprado, J. J., and Salesse, R. (2004). Interlimb coordination: real constraints and false dichotomies. *J. Mot. Behav.* 36, 398–400, 402–407; discussion 408–417.

Temprado, J. J., Swinnen, S. P., Carson, R. G., Tourment, A., and Laurent, M. (2003). Interaction of directional, neuromuscular and egocentric constraints on the stability of preferred bimanual coordination patterns. *Hum. Mov. Sci.* 22, 339–363. doi: 10.1016/s0167-9457(03)00049-6

Temprado, J. J., Vercruysse, S., Salesse, R., and Berton, E. (2010). A dynamic systems approach to the effects of aging on bimanual coordination. *Gerontology* 56, 335–344. doi: 10.1159/000262445

Temprado, J. J., Zanone, P. G., Monno, A., and Laurent, M. (1999). Attentional load associated with performing and stabilizing preferred bimanual patterns. *J. Exp. Psychol. Hum. Percept. Perform.* 25, 1579–1594. doi: 10.1037/0096-1523.25.6.1579

Tognoli, E., and Kelso, J. A. S. (2009). Brain coordination dynamics: true and false faces of phase synchrony and metastability. *Prog. Neurobiol.* 87, 31–40. doi: 10.1016/j.pneurobio.2008.09.014

Torre, K. (2010). The correlation structure of relative phase variability influences the occurrence of phase transition in coordination. *J. Mot. Behav.* 42, 99–105. doi: 10.1080/00222890903507891

Torre, K., and Balasubramaniam, R. (2011). Disentangling stability, variability and adaptability in human performance: focus on the interplay between local variance and serial correlation. *J. Exp. Psychol. Hum. Percept. Perform.* 37, 539–550. doi: 10.1037/a0020556

Torre, K., Delignieres, D., and Lemoine, L. (2007). 1/f (beta) fluctuations in bimanual coordination: an additional challenge for modeling. *Exp. Brain Res.* 183, 225–234. doi: 10.1007/s00221-007-1035-8

Tresch, M. C., and Jarc, A. (2009). The case for and against muscle synergies. *Curr. Opin. Neurobiol.* 19, 601–607. doi: 10.1016/j.conb.2009.09.002

Vaillancourt, D. E., and Newell, K. M. (2002). Changing complexity in human behavior and physiology through aging and disease. *Neurobiol. Aging* 23, 1–11. doi: 10.1016/s0197-4580(01)00247-0

Waddington, C. H. (1942). The epigenotype. *Endeavour* 1, 18–20.

Waddington, C. H. (1957). *The Strategy of the Genes; a Discussion of Some Aspects of Theoretical Biology.* London: Allen and Unwin.

Wallenstein, G. V., Kelso, J. A. S., and Bressler, S. L. (1995). Phase transitions in spatiotemporal patterns of brain activity and behavior. *Phys. D* 84, 626–634. doi: 10.1016/0167-2789(95)00056-a

Ward, N. S. (2006). Compensatory mechanisms in the aging motor system. *Ageing Res. Rev.* 5, 239–254. doi: 10.1016/j.arr.2006.04.003

Ward, N. S., and Frackowiak, R. S. J. (2003). Age-related changes in the neural correlates of motor performance. *Brain* 126, 873–888. doi: 10.1093/brain/awg071

West, B. J. (2006). *Where Medicine Went Wrong: Rediscovering the Path to Complexity, Studies of Nonlinear Phenomena in Life Science (Vol. 11).* Teaneck, NJ: World Scientific.

West, B. J., and Grigolini, P. (2010). The living matter way to exchange information. *Med. Hypotheses* 75, 475–478. doi: 10.1016/j.mehy.2010.04.028

Wing, A. M., and Kristofferson, A. B. (1973). Response delays in the timing of discrete motor responses. *Percept. Psychophys.* 14, 5–12. doi: 10.3758/bf03198607

Yamanishi, J., Kawato, M., and Suzuki, R. (1980). Two coupled oscillators as a model for the coordinated finger tapping by both hands. *Biol. Cybern.* 37, 219–225. doi: 10.1007/bf00337040

Yang, A. C., Huang, C. C., Yeh, H. L., Liu, M. E., Hong, C. J., Tu, P. C., et al. (2013). Complexity of spontaneous BOLD activity in default mode network is correlated with cognitive function in normal male elderly: a multiscale entropy analysis. *Neurobiol. Aging* 34, 428–438. doi: 10.1016/j.neurobiolaging.2012.05.004

Yates, F. E. (2008). Homeokinetics/Homeodynamics: a physical Heuristic for life and complexity. *Ecol. Psychol.* 20, 148–179. doi: 10.1080/10407410801977546

Zanone, P. G., and Kelso, J. A. (1992). Evolution of behavioral attractors with learning: nonequilibrium phase transitions. *J. Exp. Psychol. Hum. Percept. Perform.* 18, 403–421. doi: 10.1037//0096-1523.18.2.403

Zanone, P. G., and Kelso, J. A. S. (1997). Cooordination dynamics of learning and transfer: collective and component levels. *J. Exp. Psychol. Hum. Percept. Perform.* 23, 1454–1480. doi: 10.1037//0096-1523.23.5.1454

7

Benefits of physical exercise on basic visuo-motor functions across age

Marika Berchicci[1], Giuliana Lucci[2], Rinaldo Livio Perri[1,3], Donatella Spinelli[1,2] and Francesco Di Russo[1,2]*

[1] Department of Human Movement, Social and Health Sciences, University of Rome "Foro Italico," Rome, Italy
[2] Neuropsychological Unit, IRCCS Santa Lucia Foundation, Rome, Italy
[3] Department of Psychology, University of Rome "La Sapienza," Rome, Italy

Edited by:
S. Lee Hong, Ohio University, USA

Reviewed by:
Rita Sleimen-Malkoun, Aix-Marseille Université, France
Ross Andel, University of South Florida, USA

***Correspondence:**
Francesco Di Russo, Dipartimento di Scienze Motorie, Umane e della Salute, Università Degli Studi di Roma "Foro Italico," Piazza Lauro De Bosis, Roma 15, Italy
e-mail: francesco.dirusso@uniroma4.it

Motor performance deficits of older adults are due to dysfunction at multiple levels. Age-related differences have been documented on executive functions; motor control becomes more reliant on cognitive control mechanisms, including the engagement of the prefrontal cortex (PFC), possibly compensating for age-related sensorimotor declines. Since at functional level the PFC showed the largest age-related differences during discriminative response task, we wonder whether those effects are mainly due to the cognitive difficulty in stimulus discrimination or they could be also detected in a much easier task. In the present study, we measured the association of physical exercise with the PFC activation and response times (RTs) using a simple response task (SRT), in which the participants were asked to respond as quickly as possible by manual key-press to visual stimuli. Simultaneous behavioral (RTs) and electroencephalographic (EEG) recordings were performed on 84 healthy participants aged 19–86 years. The whole sample was divided into three cohorts (young, middle-aged, and older); each cohort was further divided into two equal sub-cohorts (exercise and not-exercise) based on a self-report questionnaire measuring physical exercise. The EEG signal was segmented in epochs starting 1100 prior to stimulus onset and lasting 2 s. Behavioral results showed age effects, indicating a slowing of RTs with increasing age. The EEG results showed a significant interaction between age and exercise on the activities recorded on the PFC. The results indicates that: (a) the brain of older adults needs the PFC engagement also to perform elementary task, such as the SRT, while this activity is not necessary in younger adults, (b) physical exercise could reduce this age-related reliance on extra cognitive control also during the performance of a SRT, and (c) the activity of the PFC is a sensitive index of the benefits of physical exercise on sensorimotor decline.

Keywords: simple response task, response time, event-related potential, prefrontal cortex, lifespan

INTRODUCTION

The proportion of adults over the age of 65 is expected to increase over the years. With advancing age, structural and functional deterioration occurs in most physiological systems, even in the absence of overt disease, including the central and peripheral nervous systems, as well as the neuromuscular system. A significant amount of new evidence has accumulated regarding the benefits of regular physical activity and exercise for older healthy adults (see Miller et al., 2012; Hayes et al., 2013, for reviews). Regular physical activity increases average life expectancy through its influence on sensorimotor control and functioning, and represents a low-cost, large-scale behavioral intervention that may slow the progression of physiological age-related cognitive and motor decline in healthy older adults.

In the last few years, neuroimaging studies have provided support for a positive correlation between cardiorespiratory fitness and cerebral structures and functions in humans (Colcombe et al., 2003; Gordon et al., 2008; Erickson et al., 2010; Bugg and Head, 2011; Weinstein et al., 2012), showing that brain structures, in particular the hippocampus and frontal and parietal areas mediate the positive association between fitness and cognition with particular emphasis on the executive functions of older adults. Intervention studies confirmed that aerobic exercise positively impacts the abovementioned brain structures (Colcombe et al., 2006; Erickson et al., 2011; Ruscheweyh et al., 2011; Voss et al., 2012). Other studies linked physical fitness to enhanced cognitive performance, which was mediated by the activity in most of the aforementioned areas in high-fit older adults (Colcombe et al., 2004; Godde and Voelcker-Rehage, 2010; Rosano et al., 2010; McGregor et al., 2011; Prakash et al., 2011; Smith et al., 2011; Voelcker-Rehage et al., 2011).

Despite the extensive neuroimaging literature on the effects of physical activity on brain health and cognitive functions, there is less electrophysiological evidence to date. It is well known that aging is associated with slowing of speed processing (Salthouse, 2000). The behavioral variable most frequently used to measure processing speed is the response time (RT) that is the interval between the onset of an external stimulus (e.g., visual, acoustic, etc.) and the manual response, such as key-press; when the RTs are recorded simultaneously to electroencephalographic (EEG) recordings, very rich information can be derived. The event-related potentials (ERPs) provide a description at high-temporal resolution of the various stages of motor preparation and information processing. ERPs represent a powerful tool to investigate the temporal dynamic of neural processing and, thus, provide clues to understand the neural basis of age-related slowing, and the cognitive strategy adopted by older adults. Differential slowing of separable ERP components can be linked to specific decline at sensory, motor, or cognitive level (see Daffner et al., 2013; Li et al., 2013; Stothart et al., 2013; Wiegand et al., 2013, for more details); this subtle discrimination is not possible using neuroimaging techniques. Some ERP studies focused on the brain activities preceding the stimulus onset during the motor preparation process. The results indicated that older adults were slower to react, because the pre-response processing were slowed and/or enhanced rather than perceptual processing (Yordanova et al., 2004; Roggeveen et al., 2007; Wild-Wall et al., 2007). However, fewer studies have investigated the relationship between physical fitness and electrophysiological activity in older adults. Hillman et al. (2004) recorded the ERPs during a visuo-motor discrimination task, and showed that physically active elderly have faster stimulus-related cognitive processing (as indicated by the latency of the parietal activity, measured by means of the well-known P3 component) and faster RTs than their sedentary peers. In our previous work, we reported that older adults engaged more prefrontal cortex (PFC) resources than middle-aged and young adults during response preparation in a visuo-motor discrimination task; this enable them to reach the same task accuracy as their younger counterparts, while their response speed was slower (Berchicci et al., 2012). We also showed that the participation at physical exercise programs could slow down the age-related cognitive decline from 35 to 40 years of age onward (Berchicci et al., 2013). In particular, we observed that physical activity was linked to enhanced executive performance during a go/no-go task mediated by decreased activity in prefrontal regions during movement preparation.

These findings indicate that increased age is associated with slower performance and enhanced recruitment of prefrontal areas in visuo-motor discrimination tasks; moreover, physical exercise could slow down this age-related cognitive decline. Since at functional level, the PFC, supporting executive control (Ridderinkhof et al., 2004), showed the largest age-related differences, we wonder whether the observed effects of physical activity were detectable only for difficult tasks, such as discriminative tasks, or they could also be detected in a much easier task not requiring discrimination. In the present study, we measured the relationship between physical exercise and both PFC activity and RTs using a simple response task (SRT). Based on previous findings, we expected to not observe exercise-related differences in cortical and behavioral measures of young adults; in contrast, the effects of physical exercise could be found in older adults. The investigation of middle-aged and older adults will tell us whether the PFC hyperactivity emerges also in a SRT; if this holds true, as reported by Berchicci et al. (2012), we could disconfirm the cognitive difficulty explanation reported in the literature (Yordanova et al., 2004) and consider the PFC hyperactivity as a generalized effect of aging. Further, if physical exercise could favor a decreased engagement of higher-order cortical structures also in a simple task, this could support the view that physical exercise is a non-pharmacological intervention able to reduce the age-related reliance on cognitive control. Finally, if the benefits of physical exercise in a SRT were confirmed at the PFC level but not at the level of pre-motor regions, then we can suggest that the PFC activity is a more sensitive electrophysiological index of motor decline with age.

MATERIALS AND METHODS

PARTICIPANTS

A total of 84 participants volunteered. They were distributed across the following three adult age classes: younger ($n = 30$, 10 females, mean age = 24 years, age range: 19–35), middle-aged ($n = 32$, 12 females, mean age = 49 years, age range: 40–63), and older ($n = 22$, 14 females, mean age = 73 years, age range: 65–86). Education levels were similar in the two older groups (16.2 ± 2.1 and 16.0 ± 2.9 years of study for middle-aged and older, respectively) and slightly lower for younger adults (14.9 ± 1.6 years). Based on the self-report questionnaire about physical exercise (see below), the whole sample was equally divided into sub-cohorts: young adults who exercise (mean age: 24 ± 2.9 years) and do not exercise (mean age: 24 ± 5.4 years); middle-aged adults who exercise (mean age: 48 ± 3.8 years) and do not exercise (mean age: 51 ± 5.5 years); older adults who exercise (mean age: 74 ± 3.4 years) and do not exercise (mean age: 72 ± 4.2 years). To control potential confounds regarding gender and education level, the six sub-cohorts were preliminarily statistically compared. Results yielded not significant differences, indicating that they are matched for those factors. Furthermore, to control potential confounds regarding physical and mental health, only healthy people were included in the sample.

The general cognitive state of older participants was assessed using the mini-mental state examination (MMSE; Folstein et al., 1975). Older participants were not cognitively impaired, with an average MMSE score of 29 out of 30 (range: 28–30). All of the participants were healthy and without history of neurological, psychiatric, or chronic somatic problems. They were not taking psychoactive or vasoactive medication and had normal or corrected-to-normal vision. All of the participants were fully right-handed (Edinburgh Handedness Inventory; Oldfield, 1971). The older groups were recruited among friends of the authors and through the *Vitattiva Association* in Rome, the middle-aged participants were recruited among friends of the authors and among the employers of the University of Rome "Foro Italico," and the younger participants were recruited from the local student population. The study received prior approval by the ethical committee of the IRCCS Santa Lucia Foundation. Written informed consent was obtained according to the Declaration of Helsinki from each participant.

PHYSICAL ACTIVITY ASSESSMENT

Participants were asked to fill in a self-report questionnaire about physical exercise daily performed defined by the level of intensity in accordance with the American college of sport medicine guidelines (Chodzko-Zajko et al., 2009): moderate activity between three and six metabolic equivalent of tasks (METs) and vigorous activity greater than six METs. One MET is defined as the energy expenditure for sitting quietly, which, for the average adult, approximates 3.5 ml of oxygen uptake per kilogram of body weight per minute. Six METs was the threshold used to split the sample into not-exercise and exercise cohorts. The participants who reported general physical activities greater than six METs were also involved in regular physical exercise programs and sports at least 3 days/week, 1 h/session (i.e., swimming, running, martial arts, fencing, low- and high-impact exercise). Although the questionnaire approach may lead to omissions, inaccuracies, and bias, evidence has been reported about correlation between the results of subjective measures of physical activity and objective maximal oxygen consumption values (Bowles et al., 2004). Furthermore, the effects of physical fitness on cognitive and neural measures in older adults are consistent across different assessment methods (McAuley et al., 2011).

APPARATUS AND PROCEDURE

The participants were tested after a 64-channel EEG active-cap was mounted on their scalp; they were seated in a darkened room in front of a screen placed 114 cm from their eyes. The visual stimuli were four squared configurations made by vertical and horizontal bars subtending $4° \times 4°$ presented on a dark gray background; one of these stimuli was randomly displayed for 260 ms with equal probability ($p = 0.25$). The inter-stimulus interval varied randomly from 1 to 2 s in order to maintain uncertainty of the RT. The order of presentation was randomized within blocks. The duration of each run was 2.5 min with a pause interleaved; five runs allowed us to obtain 500 trials. A yellow circle (diameter 0.15° of visual angle) placed at the center of the screen and set at the participant's eye level was the fixation point. Participants were asked to respond as fast as possible to all of the stimuli by pressing a button with the right index finger avoiding anticipations. Stimulus presentation and behavioral data acquisition were performed by Presentation™ software.

BEHAVIORAL DATA ANALYSIS

Accuracy was measured by the percentage of anticipations (i.e., responses shorter than 100 ms or responses issued before the stimulus onset). The RTs' medians for correct trials were calculated for each participant; the medians were used because the RTs' means distributions are usually positively skewed, and the median is the appropriate measure under such conditions as long as RT differences are relevant (Baayen and Milin, 2010). The median RTs of each subject were then averaged using the mean for each sub-cohort. Factorial (3×2) ANOVAs were separately performed on the RTs and accuracy using the following factors: age (younger vs. middle-aged vs. older) and physical exercise (not-exercise vs. exercise). *Post hoc* comparisons were conducted using Tukey's HSD test. The overall alpha level was fixed at 0.05 after the Geisser–Greenhouse correction.

ELECTROPHYSIOLOGICAL RECORDING AND ANALYSIS

The continuous EEG was recorded using the BrainVision™ system with 64 active (ActiCap™) electrodes (BrainProducts GmbH, Munich, Germany) mounted according to the 10–10 International System, which were referenced to the left mastoid. The EEG was digitized at 250 Hz, amplified (bandpass of 0.01–80 Hz, including a 50 Hz notch filter), and stored for off-line averaging. Off-line analysis was performed utilizing the BrainVision™ analyzer 2.0.1 software (Brain Products GmbH, Munich, Germany). Raw EEG data were visually inspected to identify and discard epochs contaminated with artifacts prior to the signal averaging. The first trial of each block was discarded from further analysis. The trials with artifacts (e.g., blinks or gross movements) and amplitude exceeding threshold of $\pm 120\,\mu V$ were automatically excluded from the averaging, whereas eye movement artifacts were corrected using the Gratton et al. (1983) algorithm. Horizontal eye movements (electro-oculogram, EOG) were monitored with bipolar recordings from electrodes at the left and right outer canthi. The blinks and vertical eye movements were recorded with an electrode below the left eye, which was referenced to site Fp1. The participants were required to concentrate on the task performance and minimize distractions as much as possible. Possible sources of distraction and noise were minimized.

To comprehensively study the brain activity related to both response preparation and stimulus perception, EEG recordings were separately segmented and averaged into non-overlapping 2000-ms epochs that were measured from 1100 ms before to 900 ms after the stimulus onset. To further reduce high-frequency noise, the time EEG grand-averages were low-pass filtered at 25 Hz. The baseline was derived from the mean amplitude over the initial 200 ms of the averaged epochs. This approach allows investigating not only the post-stimulus ERP components [i.e., P1, prefrontal positivity (Pp), N1, P2, and P3], but also the pre-stimulus components related to the movement preparation [i.e., Bereitschaftspotential (BP) and prefrontal negativity (pN)], since the baseline was calculated from more than 1 s before the stimulus onset and not 100–200 ms right before the stimulus onset, as usually done. The mean amplitude in the −500/0 ms time window, reflecting activity during the pre-stimulus preparation stage, has been selected for further analysis on the following electrodes: Cz (roughly overlaying pre-motor and motor areas) for the BP component; Fp1 and Fp21 (over the PFC) for the pN component. After stimulus onset, peak amplitudes and latencies of the major ERP components were calculated for each subject in the following standard time windows: P1: 80–150 ms; pP: 80–120 ms; N1: 130–200 ms; P2: 180–300 ms; and P3: 250–700 ms. The electrodes selection was based on the scalp topography which allowed identifying the greatest activity for a given component at the group level (i.e., the P1 and P2 on PO7 or PO8, the pP on Fp1 or Fp2, the N1 on O1 or O2, the P3 on Pz) and on previous reports (e.g., Shibasaki and Hallett, 2006; Berchicci et al., 2012).

Factorial (3×2) ANOVAs were separately performed on the mean amplitude in the −500/0 ms time windows (pN and BP components) and on the peak latency and amplitude of the aforementioned post-stimulus components. Factors were: age (younger vs. middle-aged vs. older) and physical exercise (not-exercise vs. exercise). *Post hoc* comparisons were conducted using Tukey's HSD test. The overall alpha level was fixed at 0.05 after the Geisser–Greenhouse correction. The correlation coefficients (Pearson's r coefficients) were separately computed for exercise and not-exercise cohorts between the RTs and mean activity preceding the stimulus onset over central (BP component) and prefrontal (pN component) derivations. The significance was set at 0.05 (two-tailed) for all of the analyses.

To visualize the voltage topography of the ERP components, spline interpolated three-dimensional maps were constructed using the BESA 2000 software (MEGIS Software GmbH, Gräfelfing, Germany).

RESULTS

BEHAVIORAL RESULTS

The accuracy and mean response times for the sub-cohorts are presented in **Table 1**. Older adults responded significantly slower than middle-aged and younger adults did, while not committing a greater number of anticipations (anticipation rates were below 1% and not differed between cohorts; all $ps > 0.05$). The factorial ANOVA did not reveal a significant age × physical exercise effect interaction ($F_{2,78} = 0.03$, $p = 0.968$, $\eta^2 = 0.000$). There was a main effect of age on the RTs ($F_{2,78} = 17.18$, $p < 0.0001$, $\eta^2 = 0.305$). Younger participants were on average 22 ms faster than middle-aged ($p = 0.004$) and 47 ms faster ($p = 0.0001$) than older participants, who were on average 25 ms slower ($p = 0.002$) than middle-aged. The RTs during this SRT were not significantly affected by physical exercise habits ($F_{2,78} = 2.54$, $p = 0.114$, $\eta^2 = 0.031$); however, **Table 1** indicates that, on average, exercise cohorts were 10 ms faster than not-exercise cohorts.

Table 1 | Mean and standard deviation (Mean ± SD) of the response times (RT) and anticipations (An) for each sub-cohort.

Cohorts	Not-exercise		Exercise	
	RT (ms)	An (%)	RT (ms)	An (%)
Young	211 ± 19	0.31 ± 0.07	200 ± 20	0.21 ± 0.06
Middle-aged	233 ± 38	0.15 ± 0.04	221 ± 32	0.18 ± 0.05
Older	256 ± 31	0.30 ± 0.04	248 ± 30	0.22 ± 0.09

ELECTROPHYSIOLOGICAL RESULTS

Figure 1 shows the grand-averaged ERP waveforms at the representative prefrontal (Fp2) and central (Cz) sites, where the pN and BP components were maximal. Waveforms of the three age groups were superimposed and separately displayed for not-exercise and exercise cohorts. The activity over prefrontal sites was modulated by both age and exercise. Vertical dotted lines represent the RTs in each cohort. Within the not-exercise cohorts, the waveform of the young adults was slightly positive before the stimulus onset, whereas those of the middle-aged and older adults showed a slow rising negativity (pN), which began very early in the older cohort. Within the exercise cohorts, the pN of the three age groups was absent (did not differ from baseline). After stimulus onset, another main component over the PFC was detectable: the pP. The peak latency was approximately 196 ms in all of the cohorts independently from physical exercise, whereas pP amplitude increased with age. The BP component was very similar in all of the cohorts over the central derivation (Cz). This component showed the typical slow rising negativity that reflects motor preparation. This negativity reached the peak at approximately 100 ms after the stimulus onset.

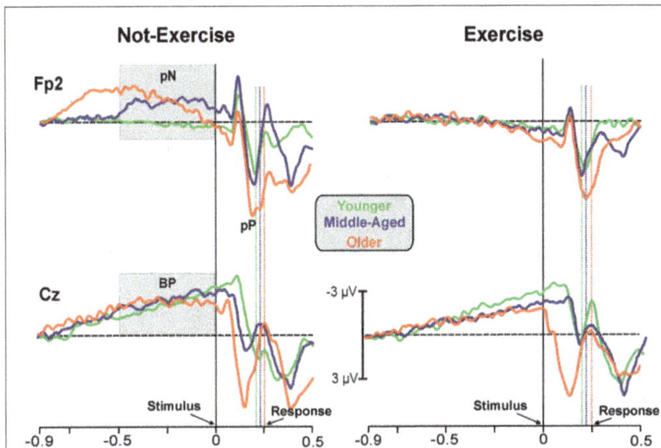

FIGURE 1 | Grand-average ERP waveforms at the prefrontal (Fp2) and central (Cz) electrodes. The age groups are superimposed with different colors (see the legend in the figure) and divided between not-exercise (left) and exercise (right) cohorts. The time zero represents the stimulus appearance; the vertical dotted lines represent the response emissions for each cohort, based on the color of the ERP waveforms.

Statistical analysis of the pN amplitude showed a main effect of physical exercise ($F_{1,78} = 6.17$, $p = 0.015$, $\eta^2 = 0.073$). The ANOVA did reveal a significant age × physical exercise effect interaction ($F_{2,78} = 3.12$, $p = 0.045$, $\eta^2 = 0.074$). *Post hoc* analysis showed that the participants who exercise did not recruit the PFC to accomplish this SRT regardless of the age group, whereas the older ($-2.23 \pm 0.9\,\mu V$) and middle-aged adults ($-1.86 \pm 0.6\,\mu V$) with a more sedentary lifestyle needed the intervention of the PFC control also in this very easy task. ANOVA on the pP amplitude did not reveal a significant age × physical exercise effect interaction, but there was a main effect of age ($F_{2,78} = 6.59$, $p = 0.002$, $\eta^2 = 0.172$), with larger pP amplitude in older ($6.43 \pm 0.5\,\mu V$) than middle-aged ($4.32 \pm 0.4\,\mu V$) and younger ($4.04 \pm 0.4\,\mu V$) adults. Physical exercise did not significantly affect the pP amplitude ($F_{1,78} = 1.38$, $p > 0.05$, $\eta^2 = 0.016$), even thought the exercise cohorts showed lower amplitude ($4.81 \pm 0.3\,\mu V$) than not-exercise ($5.48 \pm 0.3\,\mu V$) cohorts. The pP latency was not different across cohorts. Statistical analysis of the BP amplitude did not yield significant results. Similarly, analysis on the P1, N2, and P2 peak latency and amplitude were not significant. ANOVA on the P3 latency showed a main effect of age ($F_{2,78} = 8.059$, $p = 0.006$, $\eta^2 = 0.120$), with later P3 in older (417 ± 75.80 ms) than middle-aged (363 ± 77.68 ms) and younger (356 ± 87.65 ms) adults. The physical exercise effect and the interaction were not significant. Not significant effects were found on the P3 amplitude.

Figure 2 shows the scatter plot of the correlations between the RTs and the pN component on Fp2, which was the most representative site, for both exercise and not-exercise cohorts. A significant negative correlation was found in the not-exercise cohort (continuous line in the figure; $R = -0.48$; $p = 0.001$), whereas no correlation was observed in the participants that exercise (dashed line in the figure; $R = -0.17$; $p = 0.277$). Removing the two outliers (filled squares RTs: 332 and 348 ms) from middle-aged and older adults that do not exercise, the correlation was even stronger ($R = -0.55$; $p = 0.001$). No correlation was found between RTs and the BP component parameters.

TOPOGRAPHICAL MAPS

Three-dimensional topographical maps of the grand-averaged data for the pN and the pP components are displayed in **Figure 3**. The maps of younger, middle-aged, and older participants are displayed from the left to the right for not-exercise cohorts (a) and exercise cohorts (b). The top row maps show the negative activity over the PFC in the −500/0 ms time window, which was present only in the older not-exercise adults. The bottom row maps show the topography of the pP when it was maximal. The positivity was very large in older adults, but it was also visible in middle-aged and younger adults that do not exercise. The maps of the physical exercise cohorts show the smaller pP than not-exercise in all of the age groups.

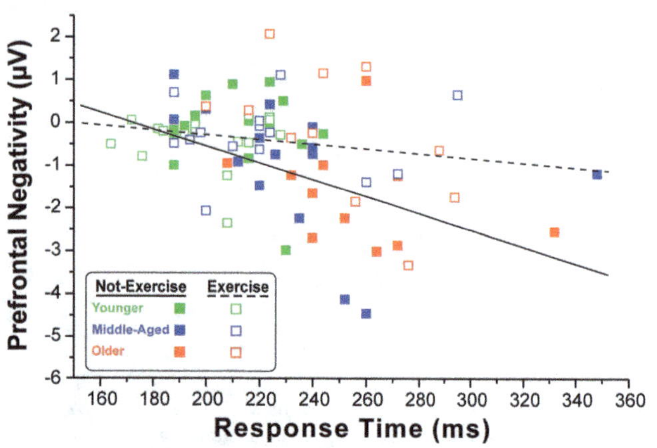

FIGURE 2 | Scatter plot of the correlation between the RTs and pN component in the two cohorts of exercise and not-exercise participants. The dashed line represents the linear fit of the exercise cohort, whereas the solid line refers to the not-exercise cohort. Only the former is significant, showing that larger is the PFC activity and slower is the RT.

DISCUSSION

This study examined the effects of active lifestyle on PFC activity and RTs across ages using a simple response task. The results indicate that: (a) the PFC control is needed also for a very simple task in older adults, while it is not necessary in younger adults, (b) physical exercise could reduce this age-related reliance on additional cognitive control, (c) age-related decline and physical exercise did not affect the activity of pre-motor and visual areas, and (d) as known, parietal areas were affected by age (delay of the P3 component), but not by physical exercise.

Task difficulty is a confounding factor in studies investigating sensorimotor changes with advancing age. Indeed, discrimination increases task difficulty, as indicated by errors increment and, remarkably, much longer RTs than in the SRT in all of the age groups (Berchicci et al., 2012). There is abundant evidence for a decreased efficiency of motor neuron recruitment in elderly that can be compensated by increased involvement of prefrontal cortical resources as a function of task difficulty, because the same task tend to be more demanding for older than younger adults (Stewart et al., 2013). Thus, older adults use compensatory mechanisms in order to maintain a performance level comparable to their younger counterparts (Reuter-Lorenz and Cappell, 2008) except for the slowing of RTs. However, present and past studies (Berchicci et al., 2012) showed a prefrontal hyperactivity also when the discrimination factor was excluded.

A study combining ERP and fMRI measures localized this preparatory prefrontal activity in the inferior frontal gyrus (iFg) of both hemispheres (Di Russo et al., 2013). Other fMRI studies using a SRT confirmed enhanced activity of prefrontal regions in elderly compared with younger participants (Sailer et al., 2000; Davis et al., 2008). Transcranial magnetic stimulation (TMS) studies

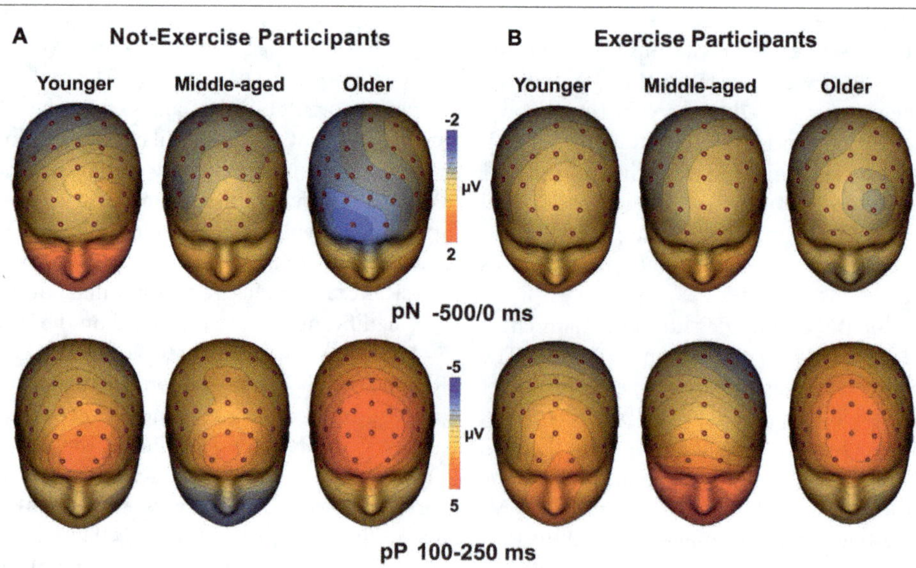

FIGURE 3 | Topographical maps of the pN (up) and pP (bottom) components. The maps for young, middle-aged, and older adults are displayed from the left to the right for not-exercise **(A)** and exercise **(B)** cohorts.

showed that the excitability of corticospinal pathways of older adults is tuned in advance to speed up response generation and enhance the response threshold of the ipsilateral cortex (Levin et al., 2011); this preparatory strategy could increase the readiness for fast and accurate response (Sinclair and Hammond, 2009). In the present study, although the task difficulty was minimal, older adults were slower than younger and middle-aged adults. Note also the remarkable difference in the RTs between young and middle-aged adults, confirming that the slowing of processing is detectable already in middle-aged, compromising activities of daily living (such as driving, crossing the street, grasping an object that is falling down, etc.), social interactions, decision making and learning (Birren and Fisher, 1995). Further, the RTs of the participants that have a more physically active life style tend to be shorter than their less active counterparts (see **Table 1**), although the difference did not reach significant level. Interestingly, in not-exercise cohort, we found a negative correlation between the RTs and pN amplitude, likely mediated by the iFg and reflecting the cognitive preparation of the response. The recruitment of the iFg increases with age, as well as the RTs: the larger the activity in prefrontal structures before the stimulus onset, the slower was the RT. On the other hand, the physical exercise reduced the age-related recruitment of the iFg and this was associated with faster RTs.

Another prefrontal activity characterized by positive polarity (the pP component) started about 100 ms after stimulus onset and reached the peak concomitantly to the key-press in young adults and few milliseconds before the response in older adults. The pP was localized in the anterior Insula and was considered as a process of sensory evidence accumulation up to reaching a threshold for motor response (Di Russo et al., 2013). The pP was larger in older than younger adults, but it was not modified in a significant way by physical exercise, although the topographical maps suggest this trend. Considering this activity as a process of sensory evidence accumulation for response execution, older people, and in part also middle-aged adults, need more time than younger adults to reach the response threshold, with a concomitant slowing in processing speed: this could make the person (i.e., elderly and sedentary) behaviorally slow, according to the literature on age-related slowing of nerve conduction (Macaluso and De Vito, 2004), and would explain the greater engagement of the brain structures involved. This conclusion is in line with other studies, showing a greater insular activation with increased task difficulty (Philiastides and Sajda, 2007) and aging (Williamson et al., 1999).

The activity in pre-motor and visual regions during this SRT was affected neither by age nor by physical exercise. As previously found (e.g., Berchicci et al., 2012), the age-related delay in response emission and categorization (indexed by the parietal P3) was confirmed, but no effects of physical exercise were found. This latter result is only partially in line with previous studies, because Hillman et al. (2004) showed that the P3 latency was modulated by physical exercise. However, they found differences in the P3 latency only between high physically active older adults and the other groups (moderate and low active participants); in the present study there are only two groups, and this methodological difference could explain the lack of differences between exercise and not-exercise cohorts. It is worth noting that one limitation of the present study is the size of the sample, which is relatively small especially for the older cohorts. Indeed, lack of significance on the P3 latency and at behavioural level could also be explained by the small size of the sub-cohorts analysed.

Meta-analyses of physical activity interventions confirmed that the effect of exercise on cognitive functions is both general and specific (Erickson et al., 2013). It is general because different cognitive domains are positively affected by exercise, regardless of the physical activity and fitness assessment used (Liu-Ambrose et al., 2012). It is specific because the executive functions are more improved by exercise interventions than other functions (Colcombe and Kramer, 2003; Hillman et al., 2008). This suggests that brain regions and networks supporting executive functions might be more sensitive to the effects of exercise than other brain areas. Changes in the frontal cortical areas cause the decline of cognitive processes associated with executive and attentional functioning, while other cognitive processes which do not rely on these brain areas, such as implicit memory, verbal ability, and word knowledge, remain relatively stable across lifespan (Ballesteros et al., 2013); these latter functions are also less affected by physical exercise. One possible explanation is that the PFC is more plastic than other brain regions (Van Praag et al., 2005; Kempermann et al., 2010). The ability to mitigate age-related motor and cognitive decline is critical for a successful aging (Seidler et al., 2010) and the physical exercise interventions hold great promise in this regard (Miller et al., 2012). Present findings expand previous studies, demonstrating that the beneficial effects of physical exercise are detectable at brain level also during an extremely simple response task, but were not indeed evident at behavioral level. This kind of task could be a handy tool suitable to investigate the effectiveness of training programs and to verify the outcomes of rehabilitation interventions, because it allows to assess both behavioral and cortical age-related changes with physical exercise. In particular, the behavioral variables are sensitive to sensorimotor age-related decline, but are not completely responsive to the exercise-related changes, which could be well disclosed using ERPs analysis. Furthermore, future studies using self-paced paradigms would also improve our knowledge about the exercise-induced modulation on spontaneous actions which are not activated by external events.

REFERENCES

Baayen, R. H., and Milin, P. (2010). Analyzing reaction times. *Int. J. Psychol. Res. (Medellin)* 3, 12–28.

Ballesteros, S., Mayas, J., and Reales, J. M. (2013). Does physically active lifestyle attenuate decline in all cognitive functions in old age? *Curr. Aging Sci.* 6, 189–198. doi:10.2174/18746098112059990001

Berchicci, M., Lucci, G., and Di Russo, F. (2013). The benefits of physical exercise on the aging brain: the role of the prefrontal cortex. *J. Gerontol. A Biol. Sci. Med. Sci.* 68, 1337–1341. doi:10.1093/gerona/glt094

Berchicci, M., Lucci, G., Pesce, C., Spinelli, D., and Di Russo, F. (2012). Prefrontal hyperactivity in older people during motor planning. *Neuroimage* 62, 1750–1760. doi:10.1016/j.neuroimage.2012.06.031

Birren, J. E., and Fisher, L. M. (1995). Aging and speed behavior: possible consequences for psychological functioning. *Annu. Rev. Psychol.* 46, 329–353. doi:10.1146/annurev.ps.46.020195.001553

Bowles, H. R., Fitzgerald, S. J., Morrow, J. R. Jr., Jackson, A. W., and Blair, S. N. (2004). Construct validity of self-reported historical physical activity. *Am. J. Epidemiol.* 160, 279–286. doi:10.1093/aje/kwh209

Bugg, J. M., and Head, D. (2011). Exercise moderates age-related atrophy of the medial temporal lobe. *Neurobiol. Aging* 32, 506–514. doi:10.1016/j.neurobiolaging.2009.03.008

Chodzko-Zajko, W. J., Proctor, D. N., Singh, M. A. F., Minson, C. T., Nigg, C. R., Salem, G. J., et al. (2009). Exercise and physical activity in older adults. *Med. Sci. Sports Sci.* 41, 1510–1530.

Colcombe, S. J., Erickson, K. I., Raz, N., Webb, A. G., Cohen, N. J., McAuley, E., et al. (2003). Aerobic fitness reduces brain tissue loss in aging humans. *J. Gerontol. A Biol. Sci. Med. Sci.* 58, 176–180. doi:10.1093/gerona/58.2.M176

Colcombe, S. J., Erickson, K. I., Scalf, P. E., Kim, J. S., Prakash, R., McAuley, E., et al. (2006). Aerobic exercise training increases brain volume in aging humans. *J. Gerontol. A Biol. Sci. Med. Sci.* 61, 1166–1170. doi:10.1093/gerona/61.11.1166

Colcombe, S. J., and Kramer, A. F. (2003). Fitness effects on the cognitive function of older adults: a meta-analytic study. *Psychol. Sci.* 13, 125–130. doi:10.1111/1467-9280.t01-1-01430

Colcombe, S. J., Kramer, A. F., Erickson, K. I., Scalf, P., McAuley, E., Cohen, N. J., et al. (2004). Cardiovascular fitness, cortical plasticity, and aging. *Proc. Natl. Acad. Sci. U.S.A.* 101, 3316–3321. doi:10.1073/pnas.0400266101

Daffner, K. R., Haring, A. E., Alperin, B. R., Zhuravleva, T. Y., Mott, K. K., and Holcomb, P. J. (2013). The impact of visual acuity on age-related differences in neural markers of early visual processing. *Neuroimage* 67, 127–136. doi:10.1016/j.neuroimage.2012.10.089

Davis, S. W., Dennis, N. A., Daselaar, S. M., Fleck, M. S., and Cabeza, R. (2008). Qué PASA? The posterior-anterior shift in aging. *Cereb. Cortex* 18, 1201–1209. doi:10.1093/cercor/bhm155

Di Russo, F., Lucci, G., Sulpizio, V., Berchicci, M., Spinelli, D., Pitzalis, S., et al. (2013). Spatiotemporal mapping of response inhibition in the prefrontal cortex. *Neuropsychol. Trends* 79.

Erickson, K. I., Gildengers, A. G., and Butters, M. A. (2013). Physical activity and brain plasticity in late adulthood. *Dialogues Clin. Neurosci.* 15, 99–108.

Erickson, K. I., Raji, C. A., Lopez, O. L., Becker, J. T., Rosano, C., Newman, A. B., et al. (2010). Physical activity predicts gray matter volume in late adulthood: the Cardiovascular Health Study. *Neurology* 75, 1415–1422. doi:10.1212/WNL.0b013e3181f88359

Erickson, K. I., Voss, M. W., Prakash, R. S., Basak, C., Szabo, A., Chaddock, L., et al. (2011). Exercise training increases size of hippocampus and improves memory. *Proc. Natl. Acad. Sci. U.S.A.* 108, 3017–3022. doi:10.1073/pnas.1015950108

Folstein, M. F., Folstein, S. E., and McHugh, P. R. (1975). "Mini-mental state." A practical method for grading the cognitive state of patients for the clinician. *J. Psychiatr. Res.* 12, 189–198. doi:10.1016/0022-3956(75)90026-6

Godde, B., and Voelcker-Rehage, C. (2010). More automation and less cognitive control of imagined walking movements in high- versus low-fit older adults. *Front. Aging Neurosci.* 2:139. doi:10.3389/fnagi.2010.00139

Gordon, B. A., Rykhlevskaia, E. I., Brumback, C. R., Lee, Y., Elavsky, S., Konopack, J. F., et al. (2008). Neuroanatomical correlates of aging, cardiopulmonary fitness level, and education. *Psychophysiology* 45, 825–838. doi:10.1111/j.1469-8986.2008.00676.x

Gratton, G., Coles, M. G. H., and Donchin, E. (1983). A new method for off-line removal of ocular artifact. *Electroencephalogr. Clin. Neurophysiol.* 55, 468–484. doi:10.1016/0013-4694(83)90135-9

Hayes, S. M., Hayes, J. P., Cadden, M., and Verfaellie, M. (2013). A review of cardiorespiratory fitness-related neuroplasticity in the aging brain. *Front. Aging Neurosci.* 5:31. doi:10.3389/fnagi.2013.00031

Hillman, C. H., Belopolsky, A. V., Snook, E. M., Kramer, A. F., and McAuley, E. (2004). Physical activity and executive control: implications for increased cognitive health during older adulthood. *Res. Q. Exerc. Sport* 75, 176–185. doi:10.1080/02701367.2004.10609149

Hillman, C. H., Erickson, K. I., and Kramer, A. F. (2008). Be smart, exercise your heart: exercise effects on brain and cognition. *Nat. Rev. Neurosci.* 9, 58–65. doi:10.1038/nrn2298

Kempermann, G., Fabel, K., Ehninger, D., Babu, H., Leal-Galicia, P., Garthe, A., et al. (2010). Why and how physical activity promotes experience-induced brain plasticity. *Front. Neurosci.* 4:189. doi:10.3389/fnins.2010.00189

Levin, O., Cuypers, K., Netz, Y., Thijs, H., Nuttin, B., Helsen, W. F., et al. (2011). Age-related differences in human corticospinal excitability during simple reaction time. *Neurosci. Lett.* 487, 53–57. doi:10.1016/j.neulet.2010.09.072

Li, L., Gratton, C., Fabiani, M., and Knight, R. T. (2013). Age-related frontoparietal changes during the control of bottom-up and top-down attention: an ERP study. *Neurobiol. Aging* 34, 477–488. doi:10.1016/j.neurobiolaging.2012.02.025

Liu-Ambrose, T., Nagamatsu, L. S., Voss, M. W., Khan, K. M., and Handy, T. C. (2012). Resistance training and functional plasticity of the aging brain: a 12-month randomized controlled trial. *Neurobiol. Aging* 33, 1690–1698. doi:10.1016/j.neurobiolaging.2011.05.010

Macaluso, A., and De Vito, G. (2004). Muscle strength, power and adaptations to resistance training in older people. *Eur. J. Appl. Physiol.* 91, 450–472. doi:10.1007/s00421-003-0991-3

McAuley, E., Szabo, A. N., Mailey, E. L., Erickson, K. I., Voss, M., White, S. M., et al. (2011). Non-exercise estimated cardiorespiratory fitness: associations with brain structure, cognition, and memory complaints in older adults. *Ment. Health Phys. Act.* 4, 5–11. doi:10.1016/j.mhpa.2011.01.001

McGregor, K. M., Zlatar, Z., Kleim, E., Sudhyadhom, A., Bauer, A., Phan, S., et al. (2011). Physical activity and neural correlates of aging: a combined TMS/fMRI study. *Behav. Brain Res.* 222, 158–168. doi:10.1016/j.bbr.2011.03.042

Miller, D. I., Taler, V., Davidson, P. S. R., and Messier, C. (2012). Measuring the impact of exercise on cognitive aging: methodological issues. *Neurobiol. Aging* 33, .e29–.e622. doi:10.1016/j.neurobiolaging.2011.02.020

Oldfield, R. C. (1971). The assessment and analysis of handedness: the Edinburgh inventory. *Neuropsychologia* 104, 199–206.

Philiastides, M. G., and Sajda, P. (2007). EEG-informed fMRI reveals spatiotemporal characteristics of perceptual decision making. *J. Neurosci.* 27, 13082–13091. doi:10.1523/JNEUROSCI.3540-07.2007

Prakash, R. S., Voss, M. W., Erickson, K. I., Lewis, J., Chaddock, L., Malkowski, E., et al. (2011). Cardiorespiratory fitness and attentional control in the aging brain. *Front. Hum. Neurosci.* **4**:229. doi:10.3389/fnhum.2010.00229

Reuter-Lorenz, P. A., and Cappell, K. A. (2008). Neurocognitive aging and the compensation hypothesis. *Curr. Dir. Psychol. Sci.* 17, 177–182. doi:10.1111/j.1467-8721.2008.00570.x

Ridderinkhof, K. R., van den Wildenberg, W. P. M., Segalowitz, S. J., and Carter, C. S. (2004). Neurocognitive mechanisms of cognitive control: the role of prefrontal cortex in action selection, response inhibition, performance monitoring, and reward-based learning. *Brain Cogn.* 56, 129–140. doi:10.1016/j.bandc.2004.09.016

Roggeveen, A. B., Prime, D. J., and Ward, L. M. (2007). Lateralized readiness potentials reveal motor slowing in the aging brain. *J. Gerontol. B Psychol. Sci. Soc. Sci.* 62, 78–84. doi:10.1093/geronb/62.2.P78

Rosano, C., Venkatraman, V. K., Guralnik, J., Newman, A. B., Glynn, N. W., Launer, L., et al. (2010). Psychomotor speed and functional brain MRI 2 years after completing a physical activity treatment. *J. Gerontol. A Biol. Sci. Med. Sci.* 65, 639–647. doi:10.1093/gerona/glq038

Ruscheweyh, R., Willemer, C., Kruger, K., Duning, T., Warnecke, T., Sommer, J., et al. (2011). Physical activity and memory functions: an interventional study. *Neurobiol. Aging* 32, 1304–1319. doi:10.1016/j.neurobiolaging.2009.08.001

Sailer, A., Dichgans, J., and Gerloff, C. (2000). The influence of normal aging on the cortical processing of a simple motor task. *Neurology* 55, 979–985. doi:10.1212/WNL.55.7.979

Salthouse, T. A. (2000). Aging and measures of processing speed. *Biol. Psychol.* 54, 35–54. doi:10.1016/S0301-0511(00)00052-1

Seidler, R. D., Bernard, J. A., Burutolu, T. B., Fling, B. W., Gordon, M. T., Gwin, J. T., et al. (2010). Motor control and aging: links to age-related brain structural, functional, and biochemical effects. *Neurosci. Biobehav. Rev.* 34, 721–733. doi:10.1016/j.neubiorev.2009.10.005

Shibasaki, H., and Hallett, M. (2006). What is bereitschaftspotential? *Clin. Neurophysiol.* 117, 2341–2356. doi:10.1016/j.clinph.2006.04.025

Sinclair, C., and Hammond, G. R. (2009). Excitatory and inhibitory processes in primary motor cortex during the fore period of a warned reaction time task are unrelated to response expectancy. *Exp. Brain Res.* 194, 103–113. doi:10.1007/s00221-008-1684-2

Smith, J. C., Nielson, K. A., Woodard, J. L., Seidenberg, M., Verber, M. D., Durgerian, S., et al. (2011). Does physical activity influence semantic memory activation in amnestic mild cognitive impairment? *Psychiatry Res.* 193, 60–62. doi:10.1016/j.pscychresns.2011.04.001

Stewart, J. C., Tran, X., and Cramer, S. C. (2013). Age-related variability in performance of a motor action selection task is related to differences in brain function and structure among older adults. *Neuroimage* 14, 1635–1643. doi:10.2217/pgs.13.152

Stothart, G., Tales, A., and Kazanina, N. (2013). Evoked potentials reveal age-related compensatory mechanisms in early visual processing. *Neurobiol. Aging* 34, 1302–1308. doi:10.1016/j.neurobiolaging.2012.08.012

Van Praag, H., Shubert, T., Zhao, C., and Gage, F. H. (2005). Exercise enhances learning and hippocampal neurogenesis in aged mice. *J. Neurosci.* 25, 8680–8685. doi:10.1523/JNEUROSCI.1731-05.2005

Voelcker-Rehage, C., Godde, B., and Staudinger, U. M. (2011). Cardiovascular and coordination training differentially improve cognitive performance and neural processing in older adults. *Front. Hum. Neurosci.* 5:26. doi:10.3389/fnhum.2011.00026

Voss, M. W., Heo, S., Prakash, R. S., Erickson, K. I., Alves, H., Chaddock, L., et al. (2012). The influence of aerobic fitness on cerebral white matter integrity and cognitive function in older adults: results of a one-year exercise intervention. *Hum. Brain Mapp.* 34, 2972–2985. doi:10.1002/hbm.22119

Weinstein, A. M., Voss, M. W., Prakash, R. S., Chaddock, L., Szabo, A., White, S. M., et al. (2012). The association between aerobic fitness and executive function is mediated by prefrontal cortex volume. *Brain Behav. Immun.* 26, 811–819. doi:10.1016/j.bbi.2011.11.008

Wiegand, I., Finke, K., Muller, H. J., and Tollner, T. (2013). Event-related potentials dissociate perceptual from response-related age effects in visual search. *Neurobiol. Aging* 34, 973–985. doi:10.1016/j.neurobiolaging.2012.08.002

Wild-Wall, N., Hohnsbein, J., and Falkenstein, M. (2007). Effects of ageing on cognitive task preparation as reflected by event-related potentials. *Clin. Neurophysiol.* 118, 558–569. doi:10.1016/j.clinph.2006.09.005

Williamson, J. W., McColl, R., Matheus, D., Ginsburg, M., and Mitchell, J. H. (1999). Activation of the insular cortex is affected by the intensity of exercise. *J. Appl. Physiol.* 87, 1213–1219.

Yordanova, J., Kolev, V., Hohnsbein, J., and Falkenstein, M. (2004). Sensorimotor slowing with ageing is mediated by a functional dysregulation of motor-generation processes: evidence from high-resolution event-related potentials. *Brain* 127, 351–362. doi:10.1093/brain/awh042

8

The neuromuscular junction: aging at the crossroad between nerves and muscle

Marta Gonzalez-Freire[1,2]*, Rafael de Cabo[1], Stephanie A. Studenski[1,2] and Luigi Ferrucci[1,2]

[1] Translational Gerontology Branch, National Institute on Aging, Intramural Research Program, National Institutes of Health, Baltimore, MD, USA
[2] Longitudinal Studies Section, Baltimore Longitudinal Study of Aging, National Institute on Aging, National Institutes of Health, Baltimore, MD, USA

Edited by:
Brian C. Clark, Ohio University, USA

Reviewed by:
David J. Clark, Malcom Randall VA Medical Center, USA
David W. Russ, Ohio University, USA
Michael R. Deschenes, College of William and Mary, USA

***Correspondence:**
Marta Gonzalez-Freire, Translational Gerontology Branch, National Institute on Aging, BRC Room 09C506, 251 Bayview Blvd Baltimore, MD 21224, USA
e-mail: marta.gonzalezfreire@nih.gov

Aging is associated with a progressive loss of muscle mass and strength and a decline in neurophysiological functions. Age-related neuromuscular junction (NMJ) plays a key role in musculoskeletal impairment that occurs with aging. However, whether changes in the NMJ precede or follow the decline of muscle mass and strength remains unresolved. Many factors such as mitochondrial dysfunction, oxidative stress, inflammation, changes in the innervation of muscle fibers, and mechanical properties of the motor units probably perform an important role in NMJ degeneration and muscle mass and strength decline in late life. This review addresses the primary events that might lead to NMJ dysfunction with aging, including studies on biomarkers, signaling pathways, and animal models. Interventions such as caloric restriction and exercise may positively affect the NMJ through this mechanism and attenuate the age-related progressive impairment in motor function.

Keywords: aging, denervation, motor unit, neuromuscular junction, sarcopenia

INTRODUCTION

Autopsy studies in persons who died of acute trauma while relatively healthy have shown that aging is associated with a gradual loss of motor neurons (Valdez et al., 2010; Rowan et al., 2012). The mechanism that leads to neuronal loss with aging is still unclear and may involve both impaired trophic signaling from the central nervous system (CNS), local degeneration, and feedback from dysfunctional muscle. Indeed, individuals over 65 years of age exhibit reduced activity in motor brain areas, increased oxidative stress in motor neurons and impaired energetic metabolism in muscle fibers (Deschenes et al., 2010; Ferrucci et al., 2012; Reid et al., 2012, 2014; Manini et al., 2013). However, there is evidence that this decrease in muscle energetic metabolism is not solely affected by aging but also by the levels of physical activity, suggesting that energetic changes are more likely to be a function of activity, and not time (Tevald et al., 2010; Russ and Lanza, 2011).

Regardless of the cause, when a motor neuron is lost, fibers previously innervated by that neuron, globally defined as a motor unit, are no longer controlled by the nervous system and fail to contribute to the force generated during a volitional muscle contraction. In the attempt to counteract the functional consequence of this process, denervated orphan fibers express proteins and produce chemotactic signals that stimulate the sprouting of new dendrites from residual motor neurons. This process leads re-innervation by the expansion of pre-existing motor units and is aimed at returning to function previously denervated muscle fibers. This dynamic denervation–re-innervation cycle successfully compensates for neuronal loss, with little decline in global strength and only slightly reduced control. However, there is evidence that this compensatory mechanism starts failing with aging. Some denervated fibers are not successfully re-innervated, become apoptotic, and are not replaced by new fibers. It is hypothesized that this phenomenon contributes to a progressive decline in muscle mass and strength with aging.

The reason for a progressive impairment of the re-innervation process with aging is unknown, but some lines of evidence point to changes that occur with aging in the neuromuscular junction (NMJ), which is the synaptic interface between a branch of a motor neuron and muscle cells. The NMJ is composed of three elements: pre-synaptic (motor nerve terminal), intrasynaptic (synaptic basal lamina), and post-synaptic part (muscle fiber and muscle membrane) (Punga and Ruegg, 2012). When an action potential reaches the pre-synaptic element, voltage-dependent calcium channels open allowing calcium to enter the neuron and trigger the delivery of acetylcholine (ACh) in the synaptic cleft. Acetylcholine triggers nicotin acetylcholine receptors (nAChR) located in the post-synaptic membrane to produce an action potential, which in turn, activates voltage-gated dihydropyridine receptors (DHPRs) located in the sarcolemma and by induction, ryanodine receptors (RyRs). Of note, the post-synaptic membrane presents folds that expand its area. Calcium released from the sarcoplasmic reticulum through the RyRs binds to troponin C and allows cross-bridge cycling and force production (**Figure 1**).

Over the last decade, age-associated degeneration of the NMJ has been reported. It has been proposed that such changes may be causally related to the decline in muscle mass and function that occurs in most aging individuals. However, whether changes in the NMJ precede or follow the decline of muscle mass and strength remains unresolved. Understanding whether the primary event in the pathway to sarcopenia is muscle denervation, NMJ fragmentation or muscle fiber degeneration is important because the identification of the source of the primary event influences strategies to delay the onset of age-related muscle dysfunction. In this report, we review our current understanding of the events that lead to NMJ dysfunction with aging, including studies on biomarkers,

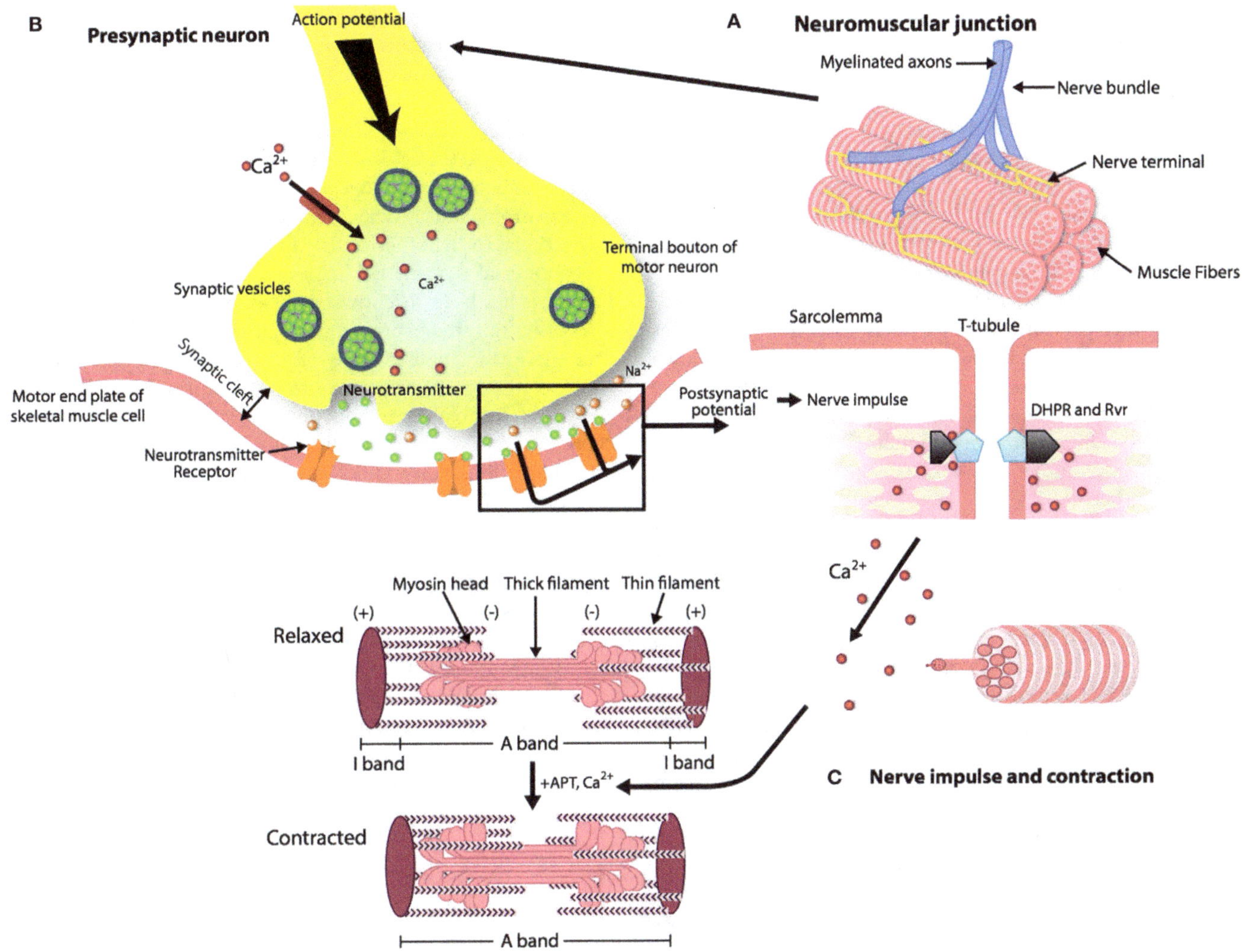

FIGURE 1 | The architecture of a neuromuscular junction (NMJ). **(A, B)** The NMJ is composed of three elements: pre-synaptic (motor nerve terminal), intrasynaptic (synaptic basal lamina), and post-synaptic component (muscle fiber and muscle membrane) (Punga and Ruegg, 2012). When the action potential reaches the motor nerve terminal the calcium channels open and the calcium enters in the neuron and delivers ACh in the synaptic cleft. **(C)** AChR activates the DHPRs located in the sarcolemma and by induction the RyRs. Calcium released from the sarcoplasmic reticulum through the RyRs binds to troponin C and allows cross-bridge cycling and force production.

signaling pathways, and animal models. We propose that interventions aimed at preventing the deterioration of the NMJ should be aimed at reversing the mechanisms that lead to NMJ degeneration with aging. It is important to underline that our comprehension of the global mechanism that lead to NJM impairment with aging is still patchy. Some of the elements emerging in the literature will be described and their relationship with aging explored. However, it is worth noticing that how these different parts participate and interact within a unique global mechanism and cause NMJ dysfunction with aging is not understood.

THE AGED NEUROMUSCULAR JUNCTION

CHANGES THAT OCCUR WITH AGING IN THE NMJ

The structure of the NMJ varies depending on the muscle fiber innervated and potentially on the level of muscle activity (Smith and Rosenheimer, 1982; Rosenheimer and Smith, 1985; Arrowsmith, 2007). There is strong evidence that changes in end-plate morphology and NMJ remodeling occur with aging and precede loss of fast motor units. Morphologically, both the nerve terminal area and the number of post-synaptic folds are reduced leading to a functional impairment in the post-synaptic response of the NMJ (i.e., motor nerve conduction velocity becomes slower and the amplitude of compound muscle action potential (CMAP) decreases) (Kurokawa et al., 1999). Mitochondria in the plaque region are numerically reduced and tend to show signs of degeneration. In particular, some authors have described dramatic alterations in mitochondrial morphology in axon terminals, including cristae disruption, swelling, and formation of megamitochondria due to multiple fusions between adjacent mitochondria (Garcia et al., 2013). Studies of pre-synaptic plaque changes with aging have found high levels of oxidative damage, decreased number of synaptic vesicles, and lower quantities of neurotransmitter released during depolarization (**Figure 2**). These changes have been correlated with denervation of muscle fibers and muscle atrophy occurring in a fiber dependent manner (Banker et al., 1983; Jang and Van Remmen, 2011; Rowan et al., 2012). Hypothesized mechanisms include (1) progressively reduced capacity of motor neurons to re-innervate muscle fibers that are denervated or regenerating; (2) impaired excitation–contraction coupling; and (3) age-associated decline in satellite cell proliferation (Clark and Fielding, 2012; Rosso et al., 2013) (**Figure 3**). In particular, Clark and Fielding (2012) suggest that the NMJ activation of muscle agonists is impaired in some older adults in whom weakness is more prominent than reduced muscle mass.

As mentioned previously, some studies (Li et al., 2011) suggest that in mice, NMJ changes follow degeneration and regeneration of individual muscle fibers, while others suggest that muscle denervation might be a consequence of high energetic demand in skeletal muscle fibers, as found in human mutant SOD1 (mSOD1) mice who develop amyotrophy and muscle denervation (Dupuis et al., 2004, 2009, 2011).

Mitochondrial dysfunction and oxidative stress in NMJ dysfunction

Mitochondria play a critical role in regulating energy production, metabolism, signal transduction, and apoptosis and are also the primary source of oxygen free radicals generated by the dislocation of electrons traveling across the respiratory chain (Peterson et al., 2012). The numerous mitochondria in the axon not only provide energy but also buffer the large calcium ion loads which are essential for excite–contraction coupling (Barrett et al., 2011). Decline in number and function of mitochondria as well as frequent modification of their morphological structure with aging has been described in many tissues, including skeletal muscle. Dysfunctional mitochondria are often found with aging, characterized by increased levels of oxidation and nitrosylation products and decreased enzymatic activity. It has been hypothesized that the diffusion of mitochondrial nitric oxide (NO) and hydrogen peroxide (H_2O_2) to the cytosol is decreased in the aged brain and may impair mitochondrial biogenesis (Navarro and Boveris, 2009). Since neurons and muscle fibers are highly metabolically active, it is rational to hypothesize that they are affected by even minor mitochondrial dysfunction (Li et al., 2013; Baines et al., 2014). Indeed, it has been recently shown in sarcopenic rats with NMJ disruption that the expression of genes implicated in mitochondrial energy metabolism is down regulated (Ibebunjo et al., 2013). However, the role of oxidative stress in peripheral nervous system aging and pathology remains poorly understood (Lin and Beal, 2006; Garcia et al., 2013). Reduced ATP production and impaired calcium buffering in the subsarcolemmal mitochondria located near the NMJ may impair both neurotransmission and vesicular recycling (Deschenes, 2011).

Changes in the innervation of muscle fibers and motor units

Neuron loss (cell death) that occurs with aging is progressive and, as far as we know, irreversible. Loss of motor units in young adults results in re-innervation of denervated fibers by sprouting from other motor neurons and in death of fibers that are not successfully re-innervated. The details of this process have been studied mostly in animal models. Chai et al. (2011) have shown that in mice, while the size and number of alpha motor neurons in the

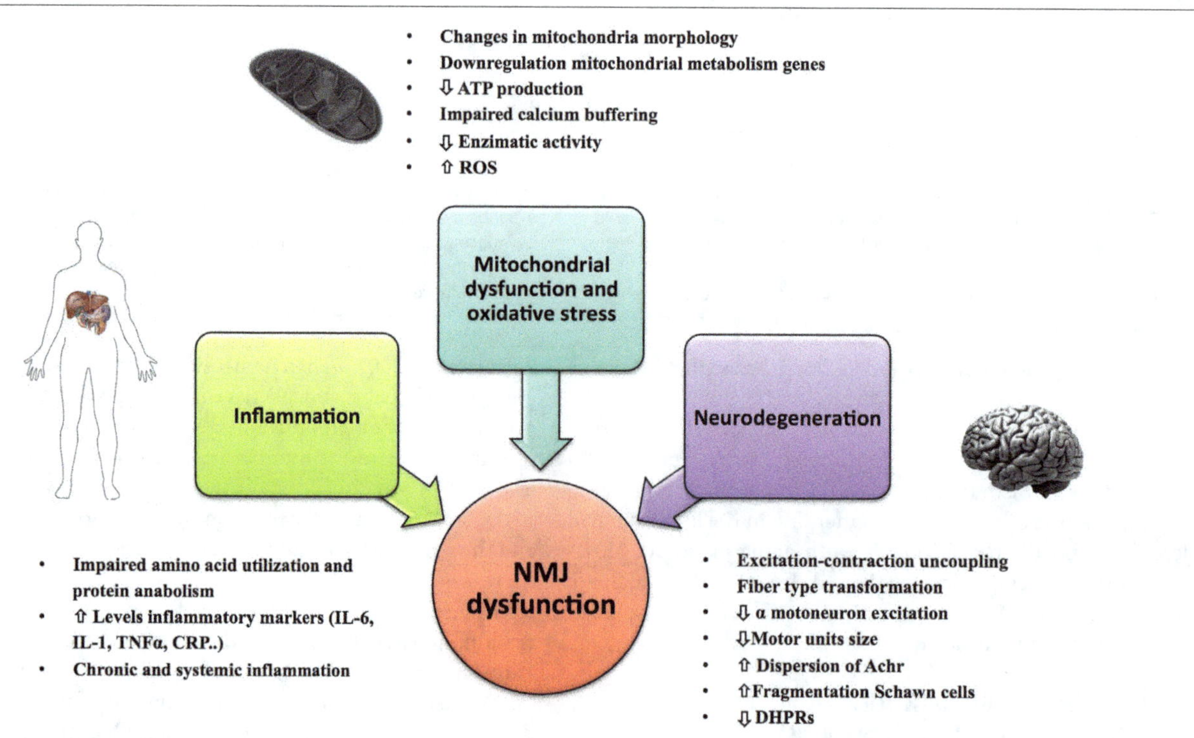

FIGURE 2 | Primary causes of NMJ dysfunction during aging. Factors such as mitochondrial dysfunction, oxidative stress, inflammation, and changes in the innervation of muscle fiber and mechanical properties of the motor units could play an important role in the NMJ degeneration and development of sarcopenia.

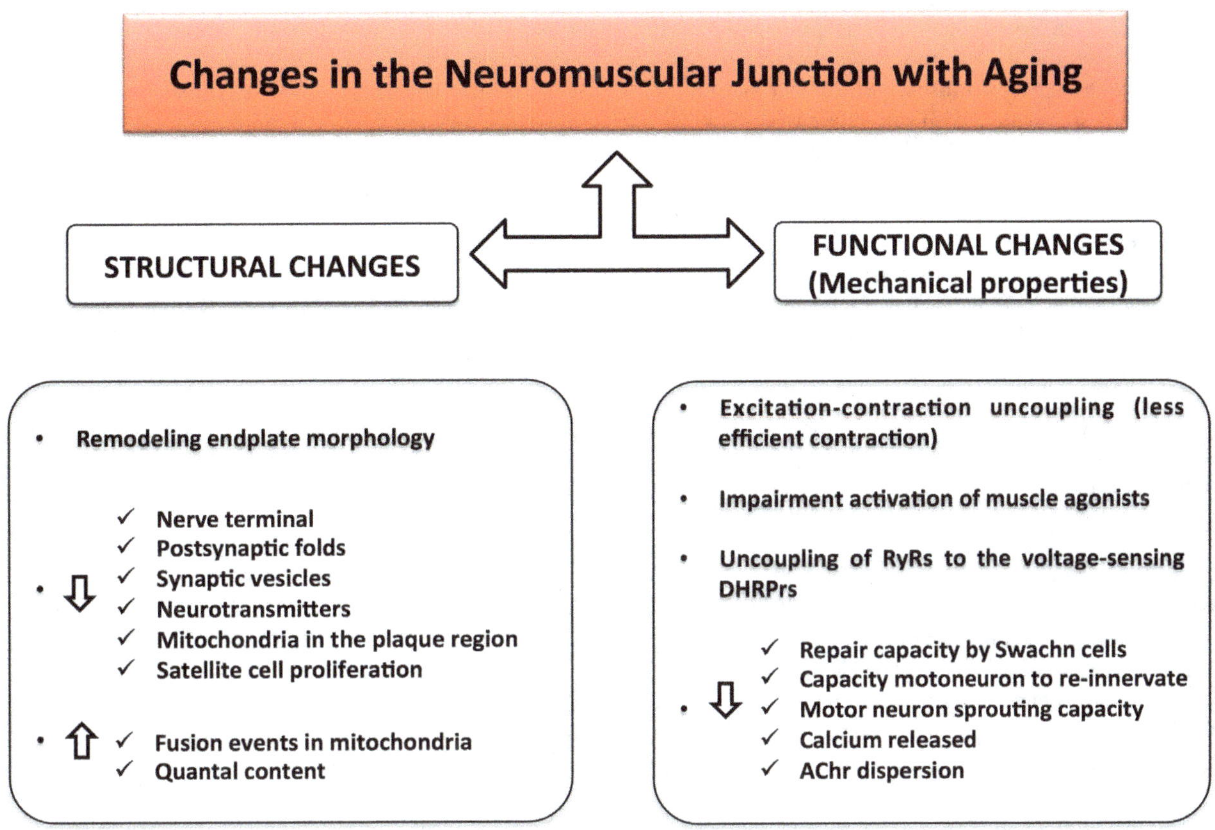

FIGURE 3 | Changes in the neuromuscular junction with aging. Structural changes together with functional alterations result in a NMJ impairment during aging. The excitation–contraction uncoupling leads to a loss of communication between the nervous and muscular system, causing a decline in skeletal muscle strength and muscle mass.

spinal cord do not change until very late in life, profound earlier change is observed at the NMJ. In very late life, motor neurons show impaired capacity to sprout and re-innervate denervated fibers, and as a consequence, larger motor units become smaller, and more fatigable and there is a considerable atrophy of muscle fibers (Luff, 1998; Roubenoff, 2000; Glass and Roubenoff, 2010). Macroscopic age-associated muscle atrophy is due to a combination of individual fiber atrophy and a decrease in the total number of type II fibers (fast and glycolytic muscle fibers) (Lexell, 1995, 1997; Andersen, 2003; Suetta et al., 2012). These alterations in morphologic remodeling in the aged NMJ result in more dispersed AChR, with greater spatial uncoupling between ACh vesicle clusters and receptor clusters. These events together induce physiological adaptations (i.e., changes of a quantal level) in the aged NMJ that have been extensively reviewed by Deschenes (2011).

According to current views, Schwann cells (cells that myelinate axons) play an critical role in synaptic repair following denervation, through their ability to direct axonal regrowth, remyelinate, and allow functional recovery by secreting trophic and growth factors (Rangaraju et al., 2009; Rangaraju and Notterpek, 2011; Kim et al., 2013). Impairment in these cells, such as increased fragmentation, damage, or denervation may contribute to ineffective re-innervation and neuromuscular dysfunction in aging (Verge et al., 1996; Kawabuchi et al., 2001, 2011; Gordon et al., 2009).

Changes that occur at the NMJ with aging are paralleled by a progressive uncoupling of the excitation–contraction in the skeletal muscle (Delbono et al., 1995, 1997; Delbono, 2003). It has been hypothesized that age-related muscle uncoupling is due to a mismatch between DHPR and RyR. In particular RyR would be more numerous than DHPR. This uncoupling reduces calcium release after an action potential, resulting in less efficient contraction (Wang et al., 2004; Shear and Martyn, 2009). It has been shown that insulin-like growth factor-I (IGF-1) could prevent the age-related decline in the number of DHPRs, therefore preventing the changes in nerve terminal and NMJ (Delbono, 2000, 2003; Zheng et al., 2002). These findings suggest that overexpression of IGF-1 may have a role in preventing muscle strength decline with aging.

Inflammation in aging (inflammaging)

Aging is characterized by high circulating levels of inflammatory markers such as interleukin 6 (IL-6), interleukin 1 (IL-1), tumor necrosis factor alpha (TNF-alpha), and C-reactive protein (CRP) in blood and tissues, often without a clear cause. This chronic low-grade inflammation in older persons has been defined by

Franceschi et al. (2007) as "inflammaging." Epidemiological studies have consistently demonstrated that "inflammaging" is a risk factor for accelerated decline of muscle mass and strength with aging, and that these changes in muscle performance may be a critical mediating step in the causal pathway between "inflammaging" and mobility disability (Ferrucci et al., 1999, 2005). In addition, medical conditions characterized by chronic overt inflammation often cause muscle wasting and weakness (Saini et al., 2007, 2009; Degens, 2010; Ferrucci et al., 2013). The mild pro-inflammatory state of aging may affect muscle performance and maintenance in many ways. For example, Schwann cell senescence has been associated with overexpression of IL-6, suggesting a role of inflammation in the age-related alterations in axonal regeneration (Saheb-Al-Zamani et al., 2013). Chronic inflammation down regulates the production of IGF-1 and blunts its biological activity. Inflammation is associated with impaired amino acid (Aa) utilization and protein anabolism, especially in critical periods such as after a meal or after a bout of exercise.

BIOMARKERS OF NMJ IN AGING AND SIGNALING PATHWAYS

The direct study of the NMJ in human beings presents challenges that are almost insurmountable. The NMJ is seldom detected in muscle needle biopsies and requires open surgery biopsies that are only done for diagnostic purposes. Newly emerging neurophysiological techniques may be used in the future to study the NMJ but they are still at an early stage of development. One of the most promising areas of investigation and perhaps the one with the strongest translational potential is the study of circulating biomarkers, such as neurotrophic factors, muscle anabolic hormones, and growth factors that are known to have a role in NMJ dysfunction. Although most of the biomarkers addressed in this section are known to change with aging, whether they modulate the causal pathway from aging to NMJ impairment with aging is not fully established. Nevertheless, correlational studies may provide knowledge that in the future may help reconstructing a general model of the mechanism leading to NMJ degeneration with aging.

NEUROTROPHIC FACTORS

Neurotrophins are a family of proteins implicated in neural development, maintenance, and maturation that also play a role in neurotransmission. Changes in production and response to neurotrophins with aging may contribute to reduced axonal regeneration, and dysfunction at multiple levels, including motor axons, post-synaptic membrane, and Schwann cells. One of the most studied neurotrophic factors is brain-derived neurotrophic factor (BDNF), which plays a critical role in neural plasticity and facilitates synaptic function by increasing pre-synaptic depolarization at the NMJ (Seeburger and Springer, 1993; Springer et al., 1995; Huang and Reichardt, 2001; Lipsky and Marini, 2007; Jiang et al., 2008; Gomez-Pinilla, 2011) and maintaining AChR clustering in the NMJ (Gomez-Pinilla et al., 2002; Peng et al., 2003). Interestingly, there is some initial evidence that production of glia cell-derived neurotrophic factor (GDNF) declines with aging (Li et al., 1995). Denervation leads to an up regulation of GDNF in rat and human skeletal muscle (Lie and Weis, 1998). Consistently, *in vitro* studies have found that GDNF is a potent trophic factor for motor neuron survival and a potent regulator of pre- and post-synaptic plasticity (Lin et al., 1993; Nguyen et al., 1998). Moreover, GDNF protein content in aged rat skeletal muscle might be controlled by stretching the muscle and the membrane depolarization of AChR acts to decrease GDNF protein content (McCullough et al., 2011).

There is evidence that short-term exercise increases levels of GDNF in the skeletal muscle and spinal cord of young and old rats (McCullough et al., 2013). Gyorkos et al. (2014) found increased GDNF protein levels at the end plate in the soleus and extensor digitorum longus muscles following training, supporting the idea that GDNF is activity dependent. Different models of exercise type and intensity could have varying effects on GDNF protein content in slow- and fast-twitch muscle fibers. The authors concluded that GDNF may play a role in remodeling of the NMJ in slow and fast-twitch muscle fibers.

INSULIN-LIKE GROWTH FACTOR 1

Insulin-like growth factor 1 is a pleiotropic growth factor with many functions, including a neutrotrophic effect, promotion of motor neuron survival, maintenance of muscle mass and strength, and protection from oxidative stress (Yuan et al., 2000; Maggio et al., 2006, 2013; Apel et al., 2010). Many studies have found that circulating IGF-1 declines with aging and such decline may contribute to NMJ degeneration and motor unit denervation (Delbono, 2003; Messi and Delbono, 2003). In accordance with this hypothesis, in mouse models, the overexpression of muscle-specific IGF-1 reverses sarcopenia (Musaro et al., 2001), prevents the age-dependent decrease in type IIB and increase in type IIA fibers (Messi and Delbono, 2003), and also leads to improved nerve regeneration by acting on axons, Schwann cells, and the NMJ. Systemic administration of IGF-1 decreased motor neuron cell death and promoted muscle re-innervation after injury in young animals, suggesting that the decline in IGF-1 with aging may impair the ability of aging animals to repair and maintain the integrity of NMJ (Vergani et al., 1998). IGF-1 sensitivity may not decrease with age, so that IGF-1 could promote regeneration after nerve injury even in older individuals. Overexpression of muscle-specific IGF-1 in mice increases the size of NMJ without substantial changes in muscle fiber size suggesting that preservation of specific force in aged animals overexpressing IGF-1 in muscle is achieved, in part, by improved motor neurons-muscle coupling (Payne et al., 2006).

AGRIN-MuSK SIGNALING PATHWAY

Acetylcholine receptors clustering on the post-synaptic membrane is a main event in the differentiation of NMJ. This process requires the presence of neural agrin, a basal lamina proteoglycan that activates a muscle-specific kinase (MuSK), which is essential for AChR clustering.

Agrin is transported along the axons and finally released into synaptic basal lamina where it is inactivated by cleavage from neurotrypsin, a synaptic protease, which produces a soluble 22 kDa C-terminal agrin fragment (CAF). Importantly, CAF can be easily detected and measured in human serum (Bolliger et al., 2010; Butikofer et al., 2011). The destabilization of the NMJ by proteolysis of agrin results in precocious sarcopenia (Drey et al.,

2013; Hettwer et al., 2013). This is consistent with findings in experiments with transgenic mice overexpressing neurotrypsin in spinal motoneurons that shown the full sarcopenia phenotype (Butikofer et al., 2011).

Wnt SIGNALING PATHWAY

There is wide evidence, both in animals models and in humans, the Wnt signaling pathway is down regulated with aging and contributes to the progressive reduction in muscle regeneration and repair capacity (Conboy and Rando, 2012). Wnt proteins are a large family (19 members in humans) of secreted glycoproteins that are highly evolutionary conserved. Wnt signaling modulates the formation and the function of synapses and is involved in maintenance and function of many tissues including muscle and nerve. Wnt deregulation produces many neurodegenerative and mental diseases (Okerlund and Cheyette, 2011; Mulligan and Cheyette, 2012; Stamatakou and Salinas, 2013).

The role of WNT signaling on the NMJ is complex. Canonical and non-canonical Wnt pathways exert opposite effects on the formation of the vertebrate NMJ (Korkut and Budnik, 2009). The non-canonical Wnt cascade has a positive role on post-synaptic development. In contrast, activation of the canonical Wnt pathway has a negative effect on NMJ formation. Thus, while the role of Wnt signaling on NMJ development and in muscle regeneration impairment with aging is well established, evidence for a direct effect of Wnt on NMJ plasticity, maintenance, and repair is lacking and requires further investigation.

VOLTAGE-GATED SODIUM CHANNEL: $Na_V1.5$

The Na_V channel gene family ($Na_V1.1$–$Na_V1.9$, NaVX) codes for voltage-gated sodium channels (NaChs), which are essential for the initiation and propagation of action potentials in both nerve and muscle (Young and Caldwell, 2005). Adult skeletal muscle expresses two isoforms of Nav (Nav1.4 and Nav1.5) (Rannou et al., 2011; Kraner et al., 2012). The isoform $Na_V1.5$ is particularly relevant to aging because it is mainly expressed in adult muscle following denervation (Kallen et al., 1990; Morel et al., 2010). Consistently, fibers positive for tetrodotoxin resistant (TTX-R) $Na_V1.5$ channels are more prevalent in muscles from old compared with young mice, suggesting a potential biomarker for muscle denervation during aging (Wang et al., 2005; Rowan et al., 2012).

PEROXISOME PROLIFERATOR-ACTIVATED RECEPTOR GAMMA COACTIVATOR 1-ALPHA (PGC-1α)

Peroxisome proliferator-activated receptor gamma coactivator 1-alpha (PGC-1α) is a transcription factor that promotes mitochondrial biogenesis. Studies have consistently shown that PGC-1α decline with aging and in many age-related chronic diseases suggesting that such decline may explain the progressive mitochondrial dysfunction with aging.

Recent studies using muscle-specific PGC-1α knockout and PGC-1α overexpressing mice have suggested that PGC-1α is a key protein involved in NMJ integrity, and the decline in PGC-1α may cause NMJ degeneration with aging by a mechanism that is separate from the effect of PGC-1α on mitochondrial biogenesis (Handschin et al., 2007; Wenz et al., 2009; Liang et al., 2011; Gouspillou et al., 2013). There is recent strong evidence that elevated activity of the co-activator PGC-1α in skeletal muscle contributes to the efficient pre- and post-synaptic remodeling of the NMJ (Arnold et al., 2014).

Gouspillou et al. (2013) hypothesized that the denervation and innervation cycle observed with aging is under the control of PGC-1α expression and proposed that the aging-related decline in PGC-1α may be a central mechanism promoting instability of the NMJ and consequently aging-related alterations of myofiber innervation in sarcopenia. Interestingly, the decline in muscle PGC-1α levels with aging is attenuated by caloric restriction (CR) and exercise (Derbre et al., 2012; Garcia-Valles et al., 2013).

PROTEIN DEGRADATION PATHWAYS: MAFbx AND MuRF1

The ubiquitin–proteasome and the autophagic-lysosomal pathways are activated during disease-related muscle atrophy and, perhaps, during the development of age-related sarcopenia. The ubiquitin–proteasome system is required to remove sarcomeric proteins, either because they are damaged or in response to decline in muscle activity. Two main enzymes at the core of this system, the ubiquitin ligases muscle atrophy f-box (Atrogin1/MAFbx) and muscle ring finger-1 (MuRF1), increase significantly in muscular atrophy, in part due to enhanced expression of tumor necrosis factor alpha (TNF-α). Mice lacking both are resistant to atrophy induced by denervation (Bodine et al., 2001; Lecker et al., 2004; Nordquist et al., 2007; Furlow et al., 2013). There is some evidence that MuRF1 could play a role in NMJ control by regulating AChR lifetime, implicating a role of MuRF1 in membrane protein turnover during aging (Rudolf et al., 2013; Franke et al., 2014; Khan et al., 2014).

THE STUDY OF NMJ IN AGING: ANIMALS MODELS

The NMJ is the best model to study synaptogenesis, because, at least in animals, it is experimentally accessible in a living organism. The mechanisms that lead to differentiation and maturation of the NMJ have been studied extensively while changes that occur with aging and lead to impairment of the NMJ are not fully understood. Most of the studies conducted in this field focused on early development (i.e., the KO mice for synaptic regulators such as rapsyn, agrin, MuSK, and AChR) (Yampolsky et al., 2010; Witzemann et al., 2013). Mouse models that were originally developed to study neuromuscular diseases [i.e., amyotrophic lateral sclerosis (ALS)] could be used to explore the effect of aging on the NMJ. The prototype of these models is the $Sod1^{-/-}$ mice.

$Sod1^{-/-}$ MICE

The homozygous deletion of Cu/Zn superoxide dismutase (Cu/Zn SOD) leads to age-dependent muscle atrophy with alterations in NMJ similar to, but more severe than aging-related muscle atrophy (Sakellariou et al., 2011, 2014). This model is of great interest because the main function of SOD is to scavenge free oxygen radicals, being the oxidative stress, one of the landmarks of aging.

The $Sod1^{-/-}$ mice were originally created to study ALS and addresses pathological events in the spinal cord, peripheral axons, and muscle. However, the neuromuscular sarcopenic phenotypes exhibited by this mouse share several characteristics with age-related sarcopenia, namely shift from fast to slow fiber type, mitochondrial dysfunction, and increased mitochondrial ROS generation (Jang and Van Remmen, 2009, 2011). In particular, the mitochondrial dysfunction might contribute to early motor terminal death in these mice (Muller et al., 2007). Rocha et al. (2013) have shown that the $Sod1^{-/-}$ mice undergo cycles of denervation/re-innervation by mixed NMJ populations (Sod1a, Sod1b) supporting morphological evidence for two populations of motor units in $Sod1^{-/-}$ mice (Schaefer et al., 2005). All together these data suggest that the impairment in neuromuscular transmission follows post-synaptic changes.

MRF4-NULL MICE

Muscle regulatory factor 4 (MRF4) is a member of the family of myogenic transcription factors (MyoD, myogenin, and myf-5) necessary for the differentiation of skeletal muscle (Weis et al., 2000). MRF4-null mice express genes encoding nAChR subunits and contractile proteins at normal levels, but express myogenin at dramatically increased levels. These mice have normal morphology and fiber-type composition (Zhang et al., 1995) and reduced expression of the Na_V 1.4 NaCh (Snow et al., 2005). Denervation leads to a rapid increase of MRF4 protein in myofiber and satellite cell nuclei in all muscle fiber types, suggesting that MRF4 might mediates the earliest responses to denervation and muscle damage (Weis et al., 2000). The NMJs in these mice at older age show higher levels of synaptic vesicle glycoprotein 2B (SV2B) a marker of synaptic vesicles and a decrease in MRF4 expression, suggesting an age-related loss of vesicles in the pre-synaptic terminal of MRF4-null mice that could lead to NMJ dysfunction (Wang et al., 2011). These authors propose MRF4 as a good therapeutic target to restoring and maintaining NMJ in aging and diseases.

INTERVENTIONS TO IMPROVE NMJ DYSFUNCTION IN AGING

Caloric restriction and exercise attenuate age-related declines in most physiological systems including the neuromuscular system (McKiernan et al., 2004; Gillette-Guyonnet and Vellas, 2008; Valdez et al., 2010; Mercken et al., 2012; Chistiakov et al., 2014). It has been shown that CR, but not exercise, blunts age-related loss of motor neurons and muscle fibers (Deschenes, 2011). Aging '*per se*' limits the capacity of a person to adapt to an exercise training program since muscle plasticity is reduced with aging (Degens, 2010). Because the NMJ could be impaired during aging, with a reduced capacity to adapt to fatigue, CR and exercise are candidate interventions to delay the onset of age-related NMJ dysfunction and sarcopenia.

CALORIC RESTRICTION

Caloric restriction has long been shown to be the most effective, non-genetic intervention to extend lifespan and delay the onset of age-related diseases (McCay et al., 1935; Fontana et al., 2010; Anderson and Weindruch, 2012; Gouspillou and Hepple, 2013). Valdez et al. (2010) found that CR from 4 to 24 months of age led to sparing of many NMJs in the tibialis anterior (TA) muscle in mice. The frequencies of fragmented and denervated post-synaptic sites were all significantly lower in these calorically restricted mice than in controls. The authors concluded that CR reduced the incidence of axonal atrophy and attenuated the deleterious effects of age on the structure of the NMJ. Other authors have found that dietary restriction (40% of *ad libitum* fed diet) attenuates age-associated muscle atrophy by lowering oxidative stress in $Sod1^{-/-}$ mice and up-regulating manganese superoxide dismutase (MnSOD), the main mitochondrial antioxidant enzyme responsible for scavenging superoxide produced by the mitochondrial electron transport chain (ETC). These data suggest that the CR model may be useful to identify mechanisms and targets for interventions aimed at preservation of NMJ with aging (Jang et al., 2012). Furthermore, Mayhew et al. (1998) propose that CR preserves the mechanical properties of aging skeletal muscles in rats through an increased expression of DHPRs.

EXERCISE

Voluntary physical activity declines with aging in humans and in most other animal species. The consequent reduction in fitness leads to reduced resistance to fatigue, lower muscle strength, and increased risk of frailty (Degens and Alway, 2006; Ferrucci et al., 2008; Afilalo et al., 2014). Neuromuscular fatigue (progressively impaired transduction of action potentials through the NMJ during exercise) has been identified as a factor constraining exercise intensity and duration, and a contributor to reduced response to exercise training during aging (Belluardo et al., 2001; Deschenes, 2011). A recent review highlighted the beneficial effects of exercise on the maintenance and regeneration of NMJs (Nishimune et al., 2014). Exercise induces NMJ hypertrophy and improves recovery from peripheral nerve injuries, while decreased physical activity results in NMJ degeneration and nerve terminal sprouting (Wilson and Deschenes, 2005; Nishimune et al., 2012, 2014). Clark et al. (2013) suggest that voluntary neuromuscular activation declines with advancing age, contributing to a reduction in power production, and precedes the decline of mobility function. Aging limit the capacity of NMJ to adapt to endurance training (Deschenes et al., 2010; Valdez et al., 2010). These findings suggest that in the presence of mitochondrial DNA (mtDNA) mutation induced by ROS, strength training (ST) can reverse the loss of muscle function and altered muscle morphology associated with age and can promote the normalization of dysfunctional mitochondria (Hurley et al., 2011). Voluntary running exercise begun in late middle-age is sufficient to preserve much of the endplate nerve terminal area (Cheng et al., 2013). In mice, endurance training reduced muscle fiber size in young adults even as NMJ size increased (Deschenes, 2011). Also, in mice, Fahim (1997) showed that if the exercise training is introduced during old age, the age-related expansion of NMJ is minimized and modulated at a lower level compared with sedentary controls, indicating that the mouse NMJ undergoes a process of physiological and morphological remodeling during aging, and such plasticity could be modulated differently by endurance exercise.

CONCLUSION AND FUTURE DIRECTIONS

Age-related NMJ dysfunction seems to be a key to understanding musculoskeletal impairment during aging. Morphological changes together with physiological alterations result in a remodeling of the motor unit and in a decline of the number of motor neurons, particularly the type II muscle fiber. These changes lead to excitation–contraction uncoupling, and a loss of communication between the nervous and muscular system, causing a decline in skeletal muscle strength and muscle mass. Despite the extensive evidence about muscle denervation in older persons, because the direct study of NMJ in humans remains extremely challenging, it remains unclear whether denervation precedes sarcopenia or vice versa. Understanding the molecular basis of NMJ dysfunction is essential and the study of biomarker is essential both to make scientific progress in this area and translating such research in search for new treatment. Not only new structural and molecular studies, but also novel animal models to clarify what really happens to this key connection between brain and muscle are needed.

ACKNOWLEDGMENTS

This review was supported entirely by the Intramural Research Program of the NIH, National Institute on Aging.

REFERENCES

Afilalo, J., Alexander, K. P., Mack, M. J., Maurer, M. S., Green, P., Allen, L. A., et al. (2014). Frailty assessment in the cardiovascular care of older adults. *J. Am. Coll. Cardiol.* 63, 747–762. doi:10.1016/j.jacc.2013.09.070

Andersen, J. L. (2003). Muscle fibre type adaptation in the elderly human muscle. *Scand. J. Med. Sci. Sports* 13, 40–47. doi:10.1034/j.1600-0838.2003.00299.x

Anderson, R. M., and Weindruch, R. (2012). The caloric restriction paradigm: implications for healthy human aging. *Am. J. Hum. Biol.* 24, 101–106. doi:10.1002/ajhb.22243

Apel, P. J., Ma, J., Callahan, M., Northam, C. N., Alton, T. B., Sonntag, W. E., et al. (2010). Effect of locally delivered IGF-1 on nerve regeneration during aging: an experimental study in rats. *Muscle Nerve* 41, 335–341. doi:10.1002/mus.21485

Arnold, A. S., Gill, J., Christe, M., Ruiz, R., McGuirk, S., St-Pierre, J., et al. (2014). Morphological and functional remodelling of the neuromuscular junction by skeletal muscle PGC-1alpha. *Nat Commun* 5, 3569. doi:10.1038/ncomms4569

Arrowsmith, J. E. (2007). The neuromuscular junction. *Surgery* (Oxford) 25, 105–111. doi:10.1016/j.mpsur.2007.02.001

Baines, H. L., Turnbull, D. M., and Greaves, L. C. (2014). Human stem cell aging: do mitochondrial DNA mutations have a causal role? *Aging Cell* 13, 201–205. doi:10.1111/acel.12199

Banker, B. Q., Kelly, S. S., and Robbins, N. (1983). Neuromuscular transmission and correlative morphology in young and old mice. *J. Physiol.* 339, 355–377.

Barrett, E. F., Barrett, J. N., and David, G. (2011). Mitochondria in motor nerve terminals: function in health and in mutant superoxide dismutase 1 mouse models of familial ALS. *J. Bioenerg. Biomembr.* 43, 581–586. doi:10.1007/s10863-011-9392-1

Belluardo, N., Westerblad, H., Mudo, G., Casabona, A., Bruton, J., Caniglia, G., et al. (2001). Neuromuscular junction disassembly and muscle fatigue in mice lacking neurotrophin 4. *Mol. Cell. Neurosci.* 18, 56–67. doi:10.1006/mcne.2001.1001

Bodine, S. C., Latres, E., Baumhueter, S., Lai, V. K., Nunez, L., Clarke, B. A., et al. (2001). Identification of ubiquitin ligases required for skeletal muscle atrophy. *Science* 294, 1704–1708. doi:10.1126/science.1065874

Bolliger, M. F., Zurlinden, A., Luscher, D., Butikofer, L., Shakhova, O., Francolini, M., et al. (2010). Specific proteolytic cleavage of agrin regulates maturation of the neuromuscular junction. *J. Cell Sci.* 123(Pt 22), 3944–3955. doi:10.1242/jcs.072090

Butikofer, L., Zurlinden, A., Bolliger, M. F., Kunz, B., and Sonderegger, P. (2011). Destabilization of the neuromuscular junction by proteolytic cleavage of agrin results in precocious sarcopenia. *FASEB J.* 25, 4378–4393. doi:10.1096/fj.11-191262

Chai, R. J., Vukovic, J., Dunlop, S., Grounds, M. D., and Shavlakadze, T. (2011). Striking denervation of neuromuscular junctions without lumbar motoneuron loss in geriatric mouse muscle. *PLoS ONE* 6:e28090. doi:10.1371/journal.pone.0028090

Cheng, A., Morsch, M., Murata, Y., Ghazanfari, N., Reddel, S. W., and Phillips, W. D. (2013). Sequence of age-associated changes to the mouse neuromuscular junction and the protective effects of voluntary exercise. *PLoS ONE* 8:e67970. doi:10.1371/journal.pone.0067970

Chistiakov, D. A., Sobenin, I. A., Revin, V. V., Orekhov, A. N., and Bobryshev, Y. V. (2014). Mitochondrial Aging and Age-Related Dysfunction of Mitochondria. *BioMed. Res. Int.* 2014, 238463. doi:10.1155/2014/238463

Clark, D. J., and Fielding, R. A. (2012). Neuromuscular contributions to age-related weakness. *J Gerontol A. Biol. Sci. Med. Sci.* 67, 41–47. doi:10.1093/gerona/glr041

Clark, D. J., Pojednic, R. M., Reid, K. F., Patten, C., Pasha, E. P., Phillips, E. M., et al. (2013). Longitudinal decline of neuromuscular activation and power in healthy older adults. *J. Gerontol.* 68, 1419–1425. doi:10.1093/gerona/glt036

Conboy, I. M., and Rando, T. A. (2012). Heterochronic parabiosis for the study of the effects of aging on stem cells and their niches. *Cell Cycle (Georgetown, Tex.)* 11, 2260–2267. doi:10.4161/cc.20437

Degens, H. (2010). The role of systemic inflammation in age-related muscle weakness and wasting. *Scand. J. Med. Sci. Sports* 20, 28–38. doi:10.1111/j.1600-0838.2009.01018.x

Degens, H., and Alway, S. E. (2006). Control of muscle size during disuse, disease, and aging. *Int. J. Sports Med.* 27, 94–99. doi:10.1055/s-2005-837571

Delbono, O. (2000). Regulation of excitation contraction coupling by insulin-like growth factor-1 in aging skeletal muscle. *J. Nutr. Health Aging* 4, 162–164.

Delbono, O. (2003). Neural control of aging skeletal muscle. *Aging Cell* 2, 21–29. doi:10.1046/j.1474-9728.2003.00011.x

Delbono, O., O'Rourke, K. S., and Ettinger, W. H. (1995). Excitation-calcium release uncoupling in aged single human skeletal muscle fibers. *J. Memb. Biol.* 148, 211–222. doi:10.1007/BF00235039

Delbono, O., Renganathan, M., and Messi, M. L. (1997). Excitation-Ca2+ release-contraction coupling in single aged human skeletal muscle fiber. *Muscle Nerve Suppl.* 5, S88–S92. doi:10.1002/(SICI)1097-4598(1997)5+<88::AID-MUS21>3.0.CO;2-U

Derbre, F., Gomez-Cabrera, M. C., Nascimento, A. L., Sanchis-Gomar, F., Martinez-Bello, V. E., Tresguerres, J. A., et al. (2012). Age associated low mitochondrial biogenesis may be explained by lack of response of PGC-1alpha to exercise training. *Age* (Dordr) 34, 669–679. doi:10.1007/s11357-011-9264-y

Deschenes, M. R. (2011). Motor unit and neuromuscular junction remodeling with aging. *Curr Aging Sci* 4, 209–220. doi:10.2174/1874609811104030209

Deschenes, M. R., Roby, M. A., Eason, M. K., and Harris, M. B. (2010). Remodeling of the neuromuscular junction precedes sarcopenia related alterations in myofibers. *Exp. Gerontol.* 45, 389–393. doi:10.1016/j.exger.2010.03.007

Drey, M., Sieber, C. C., Bauer, J. M., Uter, W., Dahinden, P., Fariello, R. G., et al. (2013). C-terminal agrin fragment as a potential marker for sarcopenia caused by degeneration of the neuromuscular junction. *Exp. Gerontol.* 48, 76–80. doi:10.1016/j.exger.2012.05.021

Dupuis, L., Gonzalez de Aguilar, J.-L., Echaniz-Laguna, A., Eschbach, J., Rene, F., Oudart, H., et al. (2009). Muscle mitochondrial uncoupling dismantles neuromuscular junction and triggers distal degeneration of motor neurons. *PLoS ONE* 4:e5390. doi:10.1371/journal.pone.0005390

Dupuis, L., Oudart, H., Rene, F., Gonzalez de Aguilar, J. L., and Loeffler, J. P. (2004). Evidence for defective energy homeostasis in amyotrophic lateral sclerosis: benefit of a high-energy diet in a transgenic mouse model. *Proc. Natl. Acad. Sci. U S A.* 101, 11159–11164. doi:10.1073/pnas.0402026101

Dupuis, L., Pradat, P. F., Ludolph, A. C., and Loeffler, J. P. (2011). Energy metabolism in amyotrophic lateral sclerosis. *Lancet Neurol.* 10, 75–82. doi:10.1016/S1474-4422(10)70224-6

Fahim, M. A. (1997). Endurance exercise modulates neuromuscular junction of C57BL/6NNia aging mice. *J. Appl. Physiol.* 83, 59–66.

Ferrucci, L., Baroni, M., Ranchelli, A., Lauretani, F., Maggio, M., Mecocci, P., et al. (2014). Interaction between bone and muscle in older persons with mobility limitations. *Curr. Pharm. Des.* 20, 3178–3197. doi:10.2174/13816128113196660690

Ferrucci, L., Corsi, A., Lauretani, F., Bandinelli, S., Bartali, B., Taub, D. D., et al. (2005). The origins of age-related proinflammatory state. *Blood* 105, 2294–2299. doi:10.1182/blood-2004-07-2599

Ferrucci, L., de Cabo, R., Knuth, N. D., and Studenski, S. (2012). Of Greek heroes, wiggling worms, mighty mice, and old body builders. *J Gerontol. A. Biol. Sci. Med. Sci.* 67, 13–16. doi:10.1093/gerona/glr046

Ferrucci, L., Giallauria, F., and Schlessinger, D. (2008). Mapping the road to resilience: novel math for the study of frailty. *Mech. Ageing Dev.* 129, 677–679. doi:10.1016/j.mad.2008.09.007

Ferrucci, L., Harris, T. B., Guralnik, J. M., Tracy, R. P., Corti, M. C., Cohen, H. J., et al. (1999). Serum IL-6 level and the development of disability in older persons. *J. Am. Geriatr. Soc.* 47, 639–646.

Fontana, L., Partridge, L., and Longo, V. D. (2010). Extending healthy life span – from yeast to humans. *Science* 328, 321–326. doi:10.1126/science.1172539

Franceschi, C., Capri, M., Monti, D., Giunta, S., Olivieri, F., Sevini, F., et al. (2007). Inflammaging and anti-inflammaging: a systemic perspective on aging and longevity emerged from studies in humans. *Mech Ageing Dev* 128, 92–105. doi:10.1016/j.mad.2006.11.016

Franke, B., Gasch, A., Rodriguez, D., Chami, M., Khan, M. M., Rudolf, R., et al. (2014). Molecular basis for the fold organization and sarcomeric targeting of the muscle atrogin MuRF1. *Open Biol.* 4, 130172. doi:10.1098/rsob.130172

Furlow, J. D., Watson, M. L., Waddell, D. S., Neff, E. S., Baehr, L. M., Ross, A. P., et al. (2013). Altered gene expression patterns in muscle ring finger 1 null mice during denervation- and dexamethasone-induced muscle atrophy. *Physiol. Genomics* 45, 1168–1185. doi:10.1152/physiolgenomics.00022.2013

Garcia, M. L., Fernandez, A., and Solas, M. T. (2013). Mitochondria, motor neurons and aging. *J. Neurol. Sci.* 330, 18–26. doi:10.1016/j.jns.2013.03.019

Garcia-Valles, R., Gomez-Cabrera, M. C., Rodriguez-Manas, L., Garcia-Garcia, F. J., Diaz, A., Noguera, I., et al. (2013). Life-long spontaneous exercise does not prolong lifespan but improves health span in mice. *Longev. Healthspan* 2, 14. doi:10.1186/2046-2395-2-14

Gillette-Guyonnet, S., and Vellas, B. (2008). Caloric restriction and brain function. *Curr. Opin. Clin. Nutr. Metab. Care* 11, 686–692. doi:10.1097/MCO.0b013e328313968f

Glass, D., and Roubenoff, R. (2010). Recent advances in the biology and therapy of muscle wasting. *Ann. N Y Acad. Sci.* 1211, 25–36. doi:10.1111/j.1749-6632.2010.05809.x

Gomez-Pinilla, F. (2011). The combined effects of exercise and foods in preventing neurological and cognitive disorders. *Prev. Med.* 52(Suppl. 1), S75–S80. doi:10.1016/j.ypmed.2011.01.023

Gomez-Pinilla, F., Ying, Z., Roy, R. R., Molteni, R., and Edgerton, V. R. (2002). Voluntary exercise induces a BDNF-mediated mechanism that promotes neuroplasticity. *J. Neurophysiol.* 88, 2187–2195. doi:10.1152/jn.00152.2002

Gordon, T., Udina, E., Verge, V. M. K., and de Chaves, E. I. P. (2009). Brief electrical stimulation accelerates axon regeneration in the peripheral nervous system and promotes sensory axon regeneration in the central nervous system. *Motor Control* 13, 412–441.

Gouspillou, G., and Hepple, R. T. (2013). Facts and controversies in our understanding of how caloric restriction impacts the mitochondrion. *Exp. Gerontol.* 48, 1075–1084. doi:10.1016/j.exger.2013.03.004

Gouspillou, G., Picard, M., Godin, R., Burelle, Y., and Hepple, R. T. (2013). Role of peroxisome proliferator-activated receptor gamma coactivator 1-alpha (PGC-1alpha) in denervation-induced atrophy in aged muscle: facts and hypotheses. *Longev. Healthspan* 2, 13. doi:10.1186/2046-2395-2-13

Gyorkos, A. M., McCullough, M. J., and Spitsbergen, J. M. (2014). Glial cell line-derived neurotrophic factor (GDNF) expression and NMJ plasticity in skeletal muscle following endurance exercise. *Neuroscience* 257, 111–118. doi:10.1016/j.neuroscience.2013.10.068

Handschin, C., Kobayashi, Y. M., Chin, S., Seale, P., Campbell, K. P., and Spiegelman, B. M. (2007). PGC-1alpha regulates the neuromuscular junction program and ameliorates Duchenne muscular dystrophy. *Genes Dev.* 21, 770–783. doi:10.1101/gad.1525107

Hettwer, S., Dahinden, P., Kucsera, S., Farina, C., Ahmed, S., Fariello, R., et al. (2013). Elevated levels of a C-terminal agrin fragment identifies a new subset of sarcopenia patients. *Exp. Gerontol.* 48, 69–75. doi:10.1016/j.exger.2012.03.002

Huang, E. J., and Reichardt, L. F. (2001). Neurotrophins: roles in neuronal development and function. *Ann. Rev. Neurosci.* 24, 677–736. doi:10.1146/annurev.neuro.24.1.677

Hurley, B. F., Hanson, E. D., and Sheaff, A. K. (2011). Strength training as a countermeasure to aging muscle and chronic disease. *Sports Med.* 41, 289–306. doi:10.2165/11585920-000000000-00000

Ibebunjo, C., Chick, J. M., Kendall, T., Eash, J. K., Li, C., Zhang, Y., et al. (2013). Genomic and proteomic profiling reveals reduced mitochondrial function and disruption of the neuromuscular junction driving rat sarcopenia. *Mol. Cel. Biol.* 33, 194–212. doi:10.1128/MCB.01036-12

Jang, Y. C., Liu, Y., Hayworth, C. R., Bhattacharya, A., Lustgarten, M. S., Muller, F. L., et al. (2012). Dietary restriction attenuates age-associated muscle atrophy by lowering oxidative stress in mice even in complete absence of CuZnSOD. *Aging Cell* 11, 770–782. doi:10.1111/j.1474-9726.2012.00843.x

Jang, Y. C., and Van Remmen, H. (2009). The mitochondrial theory of aging: insight from transgenic and knockout mouse models. *Exp. Gerontol.* 44, 256–260. doi:10.1016/j.exger.2008.12.006

Jang Y. C., and Van Remmen, H. (2011). Age-associated alterations of the neuromuscular junction. *Exp. Gerontol.* 46, 193–198. doi:10.1016/j.exger.2010.08.029

Jiang, X., Tian, F., Du, Y., Copeland, N. G., Jenkins, N. A., Tessarollo, L., et al. (2008). BHLHB2 controls Bdnf promoter 4 activity and neuronal excitability. *J. Neurosci.* 28, 1118–1130. doi:10.1523/JNEUROSCI.2262-07.2008

Kallen, R. G., Sheng, Z. H., Yang, J., Chen, L. Q., Rogart, R. B., and Barchi, R. L. (1990). Primary structure and expression of a sodium channel characteristic of denervated and immature rat skeletal muscle. *Neuron* 4, 233–242. doi:10.1016/0896-6273(90)90098-Z

Kawabuchi, M., Tan, H., and Wang, S. (2011). Age affects reciprocal cellular interactions in neuromuscular synapses following peripheral nerve injury. *Ageing Res. Rev.* 10, 43–53. doi:10.1016/j.arr.2010.10.003

Kawabuchi, M., Zhou, C. J., Wang, S., Nakamura, K., Liu, W. T., and Hirata, K. (2001). The spatio temporal relationship among Schwann cells, axons and post-synaptic acetylcholine receptor regions during muscle reinnervation in aged rats. *Anat. Rec.* 264, 183–202. doi:10.1002/ar.1159

Khan, M. M., Strack, S., Wild, F., Hanashima, A., Gasch, A., Brohm, K., et al. (2014). Role of autophagy, SQSTM1, SH3GLB1, and TRIM63 in the turnover of nicotinic acetylcholine receptors. *Autophagy* 10, 123–136. doi:10.4161/auto.26841

Kim, H. A., Mindos, T., and Parkinson, D. B. (2013). Plastic fantastic: Schwann cells and repair of the peripheral nervous system. *Stem Cells Transl. Med.* 2, 553–557. doi:10.5966/sctm.2013-0011

Korkut, C., and Budnik, V. (2009). WNTs tune up the neuromuscular junction. *Nat. Rev. Neurosci.* 10, 627–634. doi:10.1038/nrn2681

Kraner, S. D., Novak, K. R., Wang, Q., Peng, J., and Rich, M. M. (2012). Altered sodium channel-protein associations in critical illness myopathy. *Skelet. Muscle* 2, 17. doi:10.1186/2044-5040-2-17

Kurokawa, K., Mimori, Y., Tanaka, E., Kohriyama, T., and Nakamura, S. (1999). Age-related change in peripheral nerve conduction: compound muscle action potential duration and dispersion. *Gerontology* 45, 168–173. doi:10.1159/000022081

Lecker, S. H., Jagoe, R. T., Gilbert, A., Gomes, M., Baracos, V., Bailey, J., et al. (2004). Multiple types of skeletal muscle atrophy involve a common program of changes in gene expression. *FASEB J.* 18, 39–51.

Lexell, J. (1995). Human aging, muscle mass, and fiber type composition. *J Gerontol. A. Biol. Sci. Med. Sci.* 50 Spec No, 11–16.

Lexell, J. (1997). Evidence for nervous system degeneration with advancing age. *J. Nutr.* 127, 1011S–1013S.

Li, H., Kumar Sharma, L., Li, Y., Hu, P., Idowu, A., Liu, D., et al. (2013). Comparative bioenergetic study of neuronal and muscle mitochondria during aging. *Free Rad. Biol. Med.* 63, 30–40. doi:10.1016/j.freeradbiomed.2013.04.030

Li, L., Wu, W., Lin, L. F., Lei, M., Oppenheim, R. W., and Houenou, L. J. (1995). Rescue of adult mouse motoneurons from injury-induced cell death by glial cell line-derived neurotrophic factor. *Proc. Natl. Acad. Sci. U S A* 92, 9771–9775. doi:10.1073/pnas.92.21.9771

Li, Y., Lee, Y. I., and Thompson, W. J. (2011). Changes in aging mouse neuromuscular junctions are explained by degeneration and regeneration of muscle fiber segments at the synapse. *J. Neurosci.* 31, 14910–14919. doi:10.1523/JNEUROSCI.3590-11.2011

Liang, H., Ward, W. F., Jang, Y. C., Bhattacharya, A., Bokov, A. F., Li, Y., et al. (2011). PGC-1alpha protects neurons and alters disease progression in an amyotrophic lateral sclerosis mouse model. *Muscle Nerve* 44, 947–956. doi:10.1002/mus.22217

Lie, D. C., and Weis, J. (1998). GDNF expression is increased in denervated human skeletal muscle. *Neurosci. Lett.* 250, 87–90. doi:10.1016/S0304-3940(98)00434-0

Lin, L. F., Doherty, D. H., Lile, J. D., Bektesh, S., and Collins, F. (1993). GDNF: a glial cell line-derived neurotrophic factor for midbrain dopaminergic neurons. *Science* 260, 1130–1132. doi:10.1126/science.8493557

Lin, M. T., and Beal, M. F. (2006). Mitochondrial dysfunction and oxidative stress in neurodegenerative diseases. *Nature* 443, 787–795. doi:10.1038/nature05292

Lipsky, R. H., and Marini, A. M. (2007). Brain-derived neurotrophic factor in neuronal survival and behavior-related plasticity. *Ann. NY Acad. Sci* 1122, 130–143. doi:10.1196/annals.1403.009

Luff, A. R. (1998). Age-associated changes in the innervation of muscle fibers and changes in the mechanical properties of motor units. *Ann. N. Y. Acad. Sci.* 854, 92–101. doi:10.1111/j.1749-6632.1998.tb09895.x

Maggio, M., Ble, A., Ceda, G. P., and Metter, E. J. (2006). Decline in insulin-like growth factor-I levels across adult life span in two large population studies. *J. Gerontol. A Biol. Sci. Med. Sci.* 61, 182–183. doi:10.1093/gerona/61.2.182

Maggio, M., De Vita, F., Lauretani, F., Butto, V., Bondi, G., Cattabiani, C., et al. (2013). IGF-1, the cross road of the nutritional, inflammatory and hormonal pathways to frailty. *Nutrients* 5, 4184–4205. doi:10.3390/nu5104184

Manini, T. M., Hong, S. L., and Clark, B. C. (2013). Aging and muscle: a neuron's perspective. *Curr. Opin. Clin. Nutr. Metab. Care* 16, 21–26. doi:10.1097/MCO.0b013e32835b5880

Mayhew, M., Renganathan, M., and Delbono, O. (1998). Effectiveness of caloric restriction in preventing age-related changes in rat skeletal muscle. *Biochem. Biophys. Res. Commun.* 251, 95–99. doi:10.1006/bbrc.1998.9438

McCay, C. M., Crowell, M. F., and Maynard, L. A. (1935). The effect of retarded growth upon the length of life span and upon the ulti- mate body size. *J. Nutr.* 10, 63–79.

McCullough, M. J., Gyorkos, A. M., and Spitsbergen, J. M. (2013). Short-term exercise increases GDNF protein levels in the spinal cord of young and old rats. *Neuroscience* 240, 258–268. doi:10.1016/j.neuroscience.2013.02.063

McCullough, M. J., Peplinski, N. G., Kinnell, K. R., and Spitsbergen, J. M. (2011). Glial cell line-derived neurotrophic factor protein content in rat skeletal muscle is altered by increased physical activity in vivo and in vitro. *Neuroscience* 174, 234–244. doi:10.1016/j.neuroscience.2010.11.016

McKiernan, S. H., Bua, E., McGorray, J., and Aiken, J. (2004). Early-onset calorie restriction conserves fiber number in aging rat skeletal muscle. *FASEB J.* 18, 580–581.

Mercken, E. M., Carboneau, B. A., Krzysik-Walker, S. M., and de Cabo, R. (2012). Of mice and men: the benefits of caloric restriction, exercise, and mimetics. *Ageing Res. Rev.* 11, 390–398. doi:10.1016/j.arr.2011.11.005

Messi, M. L., and Delbono, O. (2003). Target-derived trophic effect on skeletal muscle innervation in senescent mice. *J. Neurosci.* 23, 1351–1359.

Morel, J., Rannou, F., Talarmin, H., Giroux-Metges, M. A., Pennec, J. P., Dorange, G., et al. (2010). Sodium channel Na(V)1.5 expression is enhanced in cultured adult rat skeletal muscle fibers. *J. Membr. Biol.* 235, 109–119. doi:10.1007/s00232-010-9262-5

Muller, F. L., Song, W., Jang, Y. C., Liu, Y., Sabia, M., Richardson, A., et al. (2007). Denervation-induced skeletal muscle atrophy is associated with increased mitochondrial ROS production. *Am. J. Physiol. Regul. Integr. Comp. Physiol.* 293, R1159–R1168. doi:10.1152/ajpregu.00767.2006

Mulligan, K. A., and Cheyette, B. N. R. (2012). Wnt signaling in vertebrate neural development and function. *J. Neuroimmune Pharmacol.* 7, 774–787. doi:10.1007/s11481-012-9404-x

Musaro, A., McCullagh, K., Paul, A., Houghton, L., Dobrowolny, G., Molinaro, M., et al. (2001). Localized IGF-1 transgene expression sustains hypertrophy and regeneration in senescent skeletal muscle. *Nat. Genet.* 27, 195–200. doi:10.1038/84839

Navarro, A., and Boveris, A. (2009). Brain mitochondrial dysfunction and oxidative damage in Parkinson's disease. *J. Bioenerg. Biomembr* 41, 517–521. doi:10.1007/s10863-009-9250-6

Nguyen, Q. T., Parsadanian, A. S., Snider, W. D., and Lichtman, J. W. (1998). Hyperinnervation of neuromuscular junctions caused by GDNF overexpression in muscle. *Science* 279, 1725–1729. doi:10.1126/science.279.5357.1725

Nishimune, H., Numata, T., Chen, J., Aoki, Y., Wang, Y., Starr, M. P., et al. (2012). Active zone protein Bassoon co-localizes with presynaptic calcium channel, modifies channel function, and recovers from aging related loss by exercise. *PLoS ONE* 7:e38029. doi:10.1371/journal.pone.0038029

Nishimune, H., Stanford, J. A., and Mori, Y. (2014). Role of exercise in maintaining the integrity of the neuromuscular junction. *Muscle & Nerve* 49, 315–324. doi:10.1002/mus.24095

Nordquist, J., Hoglund, A. S., Norman, H., Tang, X., Dworkin, B., and Larsson, L. (2007). Transcription factors in muscle atrophy caused by blocked neuromuscular transmission and muscle unloading in rats. *Mol. Med.* 13, 461–470. doi:10.2119/2006-00066

Okerlund, N. D., and Cheyette, B. N. (2011). Synaptic Wnt signaling; a contributor to major psychiatric disorders? *J. Neurodev. Disord.* 3, 162–174. doi:10.1007/s11689-011-9083-6

Payne, A. M., Zheng, Z., Messi, M. L., Milligan, C. E., Gonzalez, E., and Delbono, O. (2006). Motor neurone targeting of IGF-1 prevents specific force decline in ageing mouse muscle. *J. Physiol.* 570(Pt 2), 283–294. doi:10.1113/jphysiol.2005.100032

Peng, H. B., Yang, J. F., Dai, Z., Lee, C. W., Hung, H. W., Feng, Z. H., et al. (2003). Differential effects of neurotrophins and Schwann cell-derived signals on neuronal survival/growth and synaptogenesis. *J. Neurosci.* 23, 5050–5060.

Peterson, C. M., Johannsen, D. L., and Ravussin, E. (2012). Skeletal muscle mitochondria and aging: a review. *J. Aging Res.* 2012, 194821. doi:10.1155/2012/194821

Punga, A. R., and Ruegg, M. A. (2012). Signaling and aging at the neuromuscular synapse: lessons learnt from neuromuscular diseases. *Curr. Opin. Pharmacol.* 12, 340–346. doi:10.016/j.coph.2012.02.002

Rangaraju, S., Hankins, D., Madorsky, I., Madorsky, E., Lee, W. H., Carter, C. S., et al. (2009). Molecular architecture of myelinated peripheral nerves is supported by calorie restriction with aging. *Aging Cell* 8, 178–191. doi:10.1111/j.1474-9726.2009.00460.x

Rangaraju, S., and Notterpek, L. (2011). Autophagy aids membrane expansion by neuropathic Schwann cells. *Autophagy* 7, 238–239. doi:10.4161/auto.7.2.14278

Rannou, F., Pennec, J.-P., Morel, J., Gueret, G., Leschiera, R., Droguet, M., et al. (2011). Na v1.4 and Na v1.5 are modulated differently during muscle immobilization and contractile phenotype conversion. *J. Appl. Physiol.* 111, 495–507. doi:10.1152/japplphysiol.01136.2010

Reid, K. F., Doros, G., Clark, D. J., Patten, C., Carabello, R. J., Cloutier, G. J., et al. (2012). Muscle power failure in mobility-limited older adults: preserved single fiber function despite lower whole muscle size, quality and rate of neuromuscular activation. *Eur J. Appl. Physiol.* 112, 2289–2301. doi:10.1007/s00421-011-2200-0

Reid, K. F., Pasha, E., Doros, G., Clark, D. J., Patten, C., Phillips, E. M., et al. (2014). Longitudinal decline of lower extremity muscle power in healthy and mobility-limited older adults: influence of muscle mass, strength, composition, neuromuscular activation and single fiber contractile properties. *Eur. J. Appl. Physiol.* 114, 29–39. doi:10.1007/s00421-013-2728-2

Rocha, M. C., Pousinha, P. A., Correia, A. M., Sebastiao, A. M., and Ribeiro, J. A. (2013). Early changes of neuromuscular transmission in the SOD1(G93A) mice model of ALS start long before motor symptoms onset. *PLoS ONE* 8:e73846. doi:10.1371/journal.pone.0073846

Rosenheimer, J. L., and Smith, D. O. (1985). Differential changes in the end-plate architecture of functionally diverse muscles during aging. *J. Neurophysiol.* 53, 1567–1581.

Rosso, A. L., Studenski, S. A., Chen, W. G., Aizenstein, H. J., Alexander, N. B., Bennett, D. A., et al. (2013). Aging, the central nervous system, and mobility. *J Gerontol. A. Biol. Sci. Med. Sci.* 68, 1379–1386. doi:10.1093/gerona/glt089

Roubenoff, R. (2000). Sarcopenia and its implications for the elderly. *Eur. J. Clin. Nutr.* 54(Suppl. 3), S40–S47. doi:10.1038/sj.ejcn.1601024

Rowan, S. L., Rygiel, K., Purves-Smith, F. M., Solbak, N. M., Turnbull, D. M., and Hepple, R. T. (2012). Denervation causes fiber atrophy and myosin heavy chain co-expression in senescent skeletal muscle. *PLoS ONE* 7:e29082. doi:10.1371/journal.pone.0029082

Rudolf, R., Bogomolovas, J., Strack, S., Choi, K. R., Khan, M. M., Wagner, A., et al. (2013). Regulation of nicotinic acetylcholine receptor turnover by MuRF1 connects muscle activity to endo/lysosomal and atrophy pathways. *Age (Dordr)* 35, 1663–1674. doi:10.1007/s11357-012-9468-9

Russ, D. W., and Lanza, I. R. (2011). The impact of old age on skeletal muscle energetics: supply and demand. *Curr. Aging Sci.* 4, 234–247. doi:10.2174/1874609811104030234

Saheb-Al-Zamani, M., Yan, Y., Farber, S. J., Hunter, D. A., Newton, P., Wood, M. D., et al. (2013). Limited regeneration in long acellular nerve allografts is associated with increased Schwann cell senescence. *Exp. Neurol.* 247, 165–177. doi:10.1016/j.expneurol.2013.04.011

Saini, A., Faulkner, S., Al-Shanti, N., and Stewart, C. (2009). Powerful signals for weak muscles. *Ageing Res. Rev.* 8, 251–267. doi:10.1016/j.arr.2009.02.001

Saini, A., Nasser, A. S., and Stewart, C. E. (2007). Waste management – cytokines, growth factors and cachexia. *Cytokine Growth Factor Rev.* 17, 475–486. doi:10.1016/j.cytogfr.2006.09.006

Sakellariou, G. K., Davis, C. S., Shi, Y., Ivannikov, M. V., Zhang, Y., Vasilaki, A., et al. (2014). Neuron-specific expression of CuZnSOD prevents the loss of muscle mass and function that occurs in homozygous CuZnSOD-knockout mice. *FASEB J.* 28, 1666–1681. doi:10.1096/fj.13-240390

Sakellariou, G. K., Pye, D., Vasilaki, A., Zibrik, L., Palomero, J., Kabayo, T., et al. (2011). Role of superoxide-nitric oxide interactions in the accelerated age-related loss of muscle mass in mice lacking Cu,Zn superoxide dismutase. *Aging Cell* 10, 749–760. doi:10.1111/j.1474-9726.2011.00709.x

Schaefer, A. M., Sanes, J. R., and Lichtman, J. W. (2005). A compensatory subpopulation of motor neurons in a mouse model of amyotrophic lateral sclerosis. *J. Comparat. Neurol.* 490, 209–219. doi:10.1002/cne.20620

Seeburger, J. L., and Springer, J. E. (1993). Experimental rationale for the therapeutic use of neurotrophins in amyotrophic lateral sclerosis. *Exp. Neurol.* 124, 64–72. doi:10.1006/exnr.1993.1176

Shear, T. D., and Martyn, J. A. J. (2009). Physiology and biology of neuromuscular transmission in health and disease. *J. Crit. Care* 24, 5–10. doi:10.1016/j.jcrc.2008.08.002

Smith, D. O., and Rosenheimer, J. L. (1982). Decreased sprouting and degeneration of nerve terminals of active muscles in aged rats. *J. Neurophysiol.* 48, 100–109.

Snow, L. M., McLoon, L. K., and Thompson, L. V. (2005). Adult and developmental myosin heavy chain isoforms in soleus muscle of aging Fischer Brown Norway rat. *Anat. Rec. A. Discov. Mol. Cell. Evol. Biol.* 286, 866–873. doi:10.1002/ar.a.20218

Springer, J. E., Seeburger, J. L., He, J., Gabrea, A., Blankenhorn, E. P., and Bergman, L. W. (1995). cDNA sequence and differential mRNA regulation of two forms of glial cell line-derived neurotrophic factor in Schwann cells and rat skeletal muscle. *Exp. Neurol.* 131, 47–52. doi:10.1016/0014-4886(95)90006-3

Stamatakou, E., and Salinas, P. C. (2013). Postsynaptic assembly: a role for Wnt signaling. *Dev. Neurobiol.* doi:10.1002/dneu.22138

Suetta, C., Frandsen, U., Jensen, L., Jensen, M. M., Jespersen, J. G., Hvid, L. G., et al. (2012). Aging affects the transcriptional regulation of human skeletal muscle disuse atrophy. *PLoS ONE* 7:e51238. doi:10.1371/journal.pone.0051238

Tevald, M. A., Foulis, S. A., Lanza, I. R., and Kent-Braun, J. A. (2010). Lower energy cost of skeletal muscle contractions in older humans. *Am. J. Physiol. Regul. Integr. Comp. Physiol.* 298, R729–R739. doi:10.1152/ajpregu.00713.2009

Valdez, G., Tapia, J. C., Kang, H., Clemenson, G. D., Gage, F. H., Lichtman, J. W., et al. (2010). Attenuation of age-related changes in mouse neuromuscular synapses by caloric restriction and exercise. *Proc. Natl. Acad. Sci.* U S A 107, 14863–14868. doi:10.1073/pnas.1002220107

Vergani, L., Di Giulio, A. M., Losa, M., Rossoni, G., Muller, E. E., and Gorio, A. (1998). Systemic administration of insulin-like growth factor decreases motor neuron cell death and promotes muscle reinnervation. *J. Neurosci. Res.* 54, 840–847. doi:10.1002/(SICI)1097-4547(19981215)54:6<840::AID-JNR12>3.3.CO;2-C

Verge, V. M., Gratto, K. A., Karchewski, L. A., and Richardson, P. M. (1996). Neurotrophins and nerve injury in the adult. *Philos. Trans. R. Soc. Lond. B. Biol. Sci.* 351, doi:10.1098/rstb.1996.0038

Wang, Q., Hebert, S. L., Rich, M. M., and Kraner, S. D. (2011). Loss of synaptic vesicles from neuromuscular junctions in aged MRF4-null mice. *Neuroreport* 22, 185–189. doi:10.1097/WNR.0b013e328344493c

Wang, X., Engisch, K. L., Li, Y., Pinter, M. J., Cope, T. C., and Rich, M. M. (2004). Decreased synaptic activity shifts the calcium dependence of release at the mammalian neuromuscular junction in vivo. *J. Neurosci.* 24, 10687–10692. doi:10.1523/JNEUROSCI.2755-04.2004

Wang, Z. M., Zheng, Z., Messi, M. L., and Delbono, O. (2005). Extension and magnitude of denervation in skeletal muscle from ageing mice. *J. Physiol.* 565(Pt 3), 757–764. doi:10.1113/jphysiol.2005.087601

Weis, J., Kaussen, M., Calvo, S., and Buonanno, A. (2000). Denervation induces a rapid nuclear accumulation of MRF4 in mature myofibers. *Dev. Dyn.* 218, 438–451. doi:10.1002/1097-0177(200007)

Wenz, T., Rossi, S. G., Rotundo, R. L., Spiegelman, B. M., and Moraes, C. T. (2009). Increased muscle PGC-1alpha expression protects from sarcopenia and metabolic disease during aging. *Proc. Natl. Acad. Sci.* U S A. 106, 20405–20410. doi:10.1073/pnas.0911570106

Wilson, M. H., and Deschenes, M. R. (2005). The neuromuscular junction: anatomical features and adaptations to various forms of increased, or decreased neuromuscular activity. *Int. J. Neurosci.* 115, 803–828. doi:10.1080/00207450590882172

Witzemann, V., Chevessier, F., Pacifici, P. G., and Yampolsky, P. (2013). The neuromuscular junction: selective remodeling of synaptic regulators at the nerve/muscle interface. *Mech. Dev.* 130, 402–411. doi:10.1016/j.mod.2012.09.004

Yampolsky, P., Pacifici, P. G., and Witzemann, V. (2010). Differential muscle-driven synaptic remodeling in the neuromuscular junction after denervation. *Eur. J. Neurosci.* 31, 646–658. doi:10.1111/j.1460-9568.2010.07096.x

Young, K. A., and Caldwell, J. H. (2005). Modulation of skeletal and cardiac voltage-gated sodium channels by calmodulin. *J. Physiol.* 565(Pt 2), 349–370. doi:10.1113/jphysiol.2004.081422

Yuan, Q., Wu, W., So, K. F., Cheung, A. L., Prevette, D. M., and Oppenheim, R. W. (2000). Effects of neurotrophic factors on motoneuron survival following axonal injury in newborn rats. *Neuroreport* 11, 2237–2241. doi:10.1097/00001756-200007140-00035

Zhang, W., Behringer, R. R., and Olson, E. N. (1995). Inactivation of the myogenic bHLH gene MRF4 results in up-regulation of myogenin and rib anomalies. *Genes Dev.* 9, 1388–1399. doi:10.1101/gad.9.11.1388

Zheng, Z., Wang, Z. M., and Delbono, O. (2002). Insulin-like growth factor-1 increases skeletal muscle dihydropyridine receptor alpha1s transcriptional activity by acting on the camp-response element-binding protein element of the promoter region. *J. Biol. Chem.* 277, 50535–50542. doi:10.1074/jbc.M210526200

9

Increased bilateral interactions in middle-aged subjects

Jolien Heetkamp*[1,2], *Tibor Hortobágyi*[2,3] and *Inge Zijdewind*[1]

[1] Department of Neuroscience, University Medical Center Groningen, University of Groningen, Groningen, Netherlands
[2] Center for Human Movement Sciences, University Medical Center Groningen, University of Groningen, Groningen, Netherlands
[3] Faculty of Health and Life Sciences, Northumbria University, Newcastle Upon Tyne, UK

Edited by:
Brian C. Clark, Ohio University, USA

Reviewed by:
Julia B. Pitcher, The University of Adelaide, Australia
Minoru Shinohara, Georgia Institute of Technology, USA

****Correspondence:***
Inge Zijdewind, Department of Neuroscience, University Medical Center Groningen, University of Groningen, Hanzeplein 1, HPC FB43, Groningen 9700 AV, Netherlands
e-mail: c.a.t.zijdewind@umcg.nl

A hallmark of the age-related neural reorganization is that old versus young adults execute typical motor tasks by a more diffuse neural activation pattern including stronger ipsilateral activation during unilateral tasks. Whether such changes in neural activation are present already at middle age and affect bimanual interactions is unknown. We compared the amount of associated activity, i.e., muscle activity and force produced by the non-task hand and motor evoked potentials (MEPs) produced by magnetic brain stimulation between young (mean 24 years, $n = 10$) and middle-aged (mean 50 years, $n = 10$) subjects during brief unilateral (seven levels of % maximal voluntary contractions, MVCs) and bilateral contractions (4×7 levels of % MVC combinations), and during a 120-s-long MVC of sustained unilateral index finger abduction. During the force production, the excitability of the ipsilateral (iM1) or contralateral primary motor cortex (cM1) was assessed. The associated activity in the "resting" hand was ~2-fold higher in middle-aged (28% of MVC) versus young adults (11% of MVC) during brief unilateral MVCs. After controlling for the background muscle activity, MEPs in iM1 were similar in the two groups during brief unilateral contractions. Only at low (bilateral) forces, MEPs evoked in cM1 were 30% higher in the middle-aged versus young adults. At the start of the sustained contraction, the associated activity was higher in the middle-aged versus young subjects and increased progressively in both groups (30 versus 15% MVC at 120 s, respectively). MEPs were greater at the start of the sustained contraction in middle-aged subjects but increased further during the contraction only in young adults. Under these experimental conditions, the data provide evidence for the reorganization of neural control of unilateral force production as early as age 50. Future studies will determine if the altered neural control of such inter-manual interactions are of functional significance.

Keywords: fatigue, associated muscle activity, middle-aged, bimanual interactions, ipsilateral corticospinal excitability

INTRODUCTION

The contralateral primary motor cortex (M1) is the main controller of unimanual voluntary movements. However, evidence shows that especially when a task is more complex or requires a strong effort, the ipsilateral M1 (iM1) becomes increasingly active (Hess et al., 1986; Ugawa et al., 1993; Stedman et al., 1998; Tinazzi and Zanette, 1998; Hortobagyi et al., 2003; Zijdewind et al., 2006; van Duinen et al., 2007; Perez and Cohen, 2009; Post et al., 2009b). These excitatory ipsilateral effects can be so strong that contralateral, homologous muscles become active (Curshmann, 1906; Cernacek, 1961; Armatas et al., 1994; Zijdewind and Kernell, 2001; Cincotta and Ziemann, 2008; Post et al., 2009b). Compared with isolated strong muscle contractions, activation of ipsilateral cortical motor areas is even more pronounced during a sustained fatiguing contraction (Liu et al., 2003; Post et al., 2009b) and is accompanied by increased levels of associated contralateral muscle activity (Zijdewind and Kernell, 2001; Post et al., 2009a). This associated activity results in behavioral changes because subjects start to perform overt, associated movements with the hand contralateral to the target hand.

With advancing age, ipsilateral motor areas – including iM1 – become functionally more relevant (Talelli et al., 2008a; Fling et al., 2011; Boudrias et al., 2012; Fling and Seidler, 2012). One prediction could be that performing a unimanual sustained voluntary contraction would generate higher levels of excitability in the iM1 of old when compared with young adults, resulting in a greater contralateral associated activity. Because imaging studies across the lifespan suggest the appearance of anatomical changes in the motor brain already in late midlife (Haug and Eggers, 1991; Marner et al., 2003; Madden et al., 2004; Seidler et al., 2010; Taki et al., 2013; Zhou et al., 2013), it is reasonable to expect that neurophysiological changes in M1 and iM1 are also present. Therefore, the purpose of the present study was to determine if middle-aged compared with young adults execute unilateral motor tasks with higher iM1 excitability and with higher levels of associated contralateral activity. An additional question is whether a sustained contraction would further increase the already elevated ipsilateral activation and associated activity in middle-aged subjects. In other words, would middle-aged subjects who already demonstrate associated activity at the start of the contraction increase this associated activity even more during a fatiguing contraction or do they just start at higher levels and end up producing the same amount of associated activity as young subjects? Data in older adults (>65 years) provide evidence for this latter scenario (Shinohara et al., 2003). However, if increased cortical activation is required to maintain appropriate voluntary drive to the relevant muscles, as is suggested by data of McNeil et al. (2009, 2011a), one would expect that the increase would be similar in all participants, independent of the starting point. A decrease or a smaller increase in cortical activation would otherwise result in diminished activation of the target muscles. Thus, if ipsilateral activation in the middle-aged subjects reflects the amount of effort added upon increased ipsilateral activation (due to age-related changes), one would expect a progressive increase in associated activity during a sustained contraction.

MATERIALS AND METHODS

SUBJECTS

Twenty right-handed volunteers (10 females) were subdivided into two age groups, young adults ($n = 10$, age 24 years, 2 SD, range 21–27; 5 females) and middle-aged adults ($n = 10$, age 50 years, 3 SD, range 46–53, 5 females). Prior to the experiment, a checklist was issued to exclude subjects with migraine, neurologic or muscle diseases, or epileptic episodes. All subjects signed an informed consent, approved by the local ethics committee. Right handedness was confirmed with the Handedness Questionnaire (Brainmapping.org. adapted from Oldfield, 1971; mean laterality index: 89.8, range 65–100). All subjects performed the experiment twice, 1 week apart. In one experiment, transcranial magnetic brain stimulation (TMS) targeted the right hand and in the other experiment, the left hand. The order of the experiments was alternated between subjects. In the methods, we describe the set-up for the experiment in which TMS was given to the left motor cortex (see **Figure 1**).

EXPERIMENTAL SET-UP

Subjects sat in a height-adjustable chair with both arms resting on a table instrumented with force transducers. With the elbows flexed at 135°, both forearms were clamped in a vertical position halfway between pronation and supination. The wrists and hands were kept in a vertical position with pressure plates. The

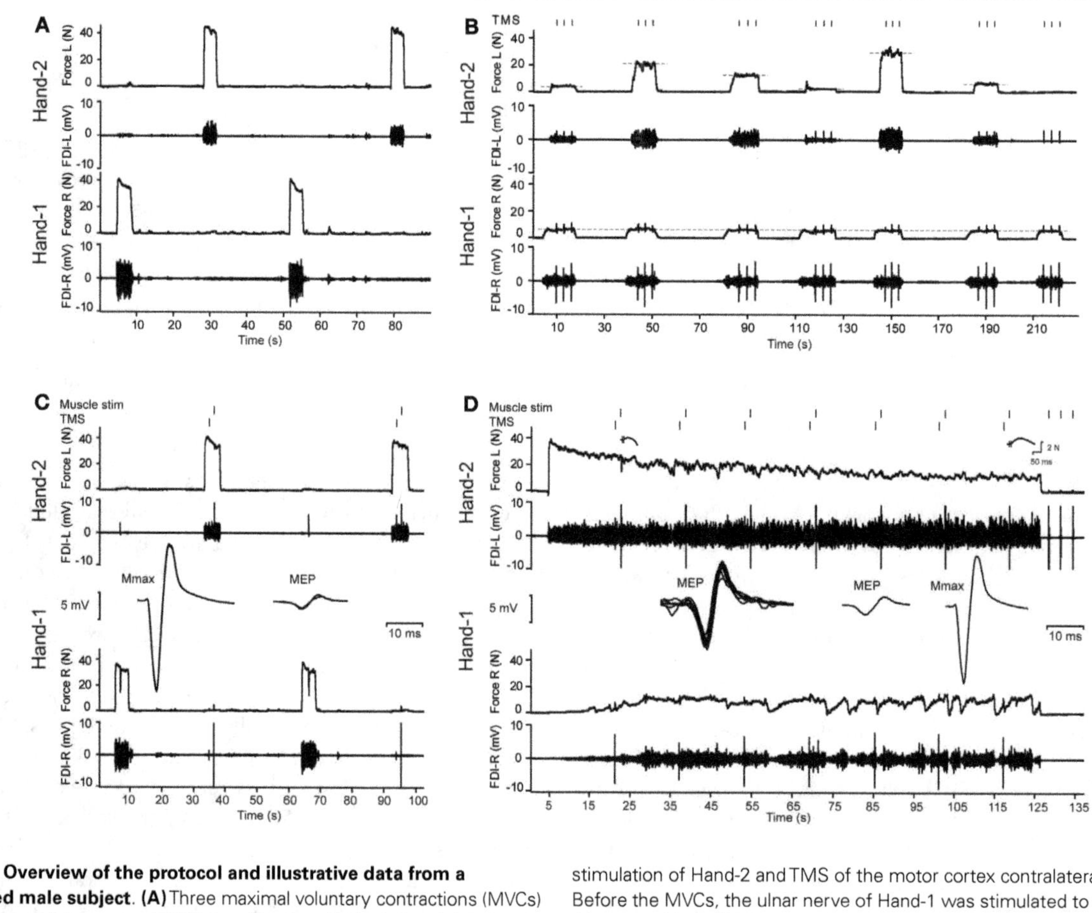

FIGURE 1 | Overview of the protocol and illustrative data from a middle-aged male subject. (A) Three maximal voluntary contractions (MVCs) of the first dorsal interosseus (FDI) intermittently with the left and right hand (only two MVCs are presented in this figure). **(B)** Example of the bilateral contractions. The subject started with Hand-1 (in this figure the right hand) followed by Hand-2 (in this figure the left hand). During the contractions, three transcranial magnetic stimuli (TMS) were given to the motor cortex contralateral to Hand-1. Feedback of the target and actual produced forces were presented to the subject on-line. **(C)** MVCs combined with muscle stimulation of Hand-2 and TMS of the motor cortex contralateral to Hand-1. Before the MVCs, the ulnar nerve of Hand-1 was stimulated to evoke maximal M-waves (M_{max}). **(C)** Shows an overlay of five M_{max} responses, followed by an overlay of three MEPs (recorded in the right hand) obtained during MVCs of the left hand. **(D)** Two-minute contraction with Hand-2. During the contractions, MEPs were evoked in Hand-1; an overlay of all MEPs during the fatigue test is presented together with the MEP during a brief contraction of the left hand and M_{max} ($n = 5$) obtained after the fatiguing task. Note the increase in associated activity in Hand-1.

middle, ring, and little fingers were mechanically isolated from the index finger using a small plastic plate. The thumb was slightly stretched toward extension with a strap. Both index fingers were inserted into snugly fitting rings around the proximal interphalangeal joint, and connected to a force transducer (Zijdewind and Kernell, 1994), which was adjustable in height to keep the index fingers in a slightly abducted position.

EMG recordings

Surface electromyographic (EMG) activity was recorded from the first dorsal interosseus (FDI) muscle of both hands. For the right FDI, one electrode (Ag–AgCl, 4 mm, *in vivo* metrics, Gainesville, FL, USA) was placed over the muscle belly and a second electrode close to on the metacarpophalangeal joint of the index finger. For the left FDI, one adhesive electrode was placed on the proximal border of FDI muscle, in between the first and second metacarpal bones. The second electrode was placed on the distal border of the FDI (see Zijdewind et al., 1998). This set of electrodes was also used to electrically stimulate the left FDI muscle (see "Muscle stimulation"). Adhesive grounding electrodes were strapped around each wrist.

Force and EMG data were amplified and sampled at 2000, 5000, and 500 Hz for EMG, motor evoked potentials (MEPs), and force recordings, respectively (CED 1401 plus interface, Cambridge Electronic Design, UK). Data were stored on a personal computer for off-line analysis.

STIMULATION

Electrical nerve stimulation

Adhesive electrodes were placed on the skin at the wrist above the ulnar nerve. The ulnar nerve of the right side was stimulated with increasing current (5 mA steps, Digitimer DS7, UK) to obtain maximal M-waves (M_{max}). During the experiment, the ulnar nerve was stimulated at 130% of the intensity to obtain M_{max}.

Muscle stimulation

To estimate voluntary drive, we superimposed twitches on maximal voluntary contractions (MVCs) of the left FDI (twitch superimposition technique, Merton, 1954; Allen et al., 1995; Zijdewind et al., 1998). The stimulation consisted of two 200-μs-long pulses with an inter-pulse interval of 10 ms. We used the same electrodes for EMG recording and electrical stimulation of the left FDI (see "EMG Recordings"). The stimulating current was increased in steps of 5 mA until maximal force was evoked. Throughout the experiment, the current that produced the maximal twitch force was used for the muscle stimulation. The force evoked by the paired-pulse stimulation is referred to as doublet force.

Transcranial magnetic stimulation

A figure-of-eight branding iron coil (diameter 50 mm) connected to a TMS stimulator (Magstim 200 rapid, Dyfed, UK) was used to elicit MEPs in the contralateral FDI muscle. Subjects wore a tight fitting cap and the location on the head where the biggest response in the contralateral FDI could be evoked was marked. Because the rapid stimulator produces a biphasic pulse, both coil current directions were examined in a subject as suggested by the manufacturer. In all subjects and in both hemispheres, lower stimulation thresholds were found with the current in the coil in an anterio-posterior position. Resting motor threshold (RMT) was defined as the lowest stimulation intensity required for eliciting MEPs in the contralateral FDI muscle at rest of at least 50 μV in at least three out of five consecutive trials (Rossini et al., 1994). During the experiment, 110% of the RMT was used.

EXPERIMENTAL TASKS

The experiment was conducted twice in each subject with at least 1 week apart, preferably on the same day of the week but always at the same time. If during the first experiment MEPs and M-waves were evoked in the right FDI and superimposed twitches in the left FDI, then in the second experiment MEPs and M-waves were evoked in the left FDI and superimposed twitches in the right FDI. Half of the subjects started with TMS and M-waves in the right FDI, the other half with the left FDI.

The experiment consisted of four tasks. Continuous feedback of the index finger abduction force produced by the left and right FDI with the lines for the target forces being displayed in real-time on a computer screen in front of the subject (see **Figure 1**).

Maximal voluntary contractions

Subjects produced three MVCs with the left and right FDI with 1-min of rest between consecutive contractions, alternating between the two sides (**Figure 1A**). During the MVCs, maximal force and RMS-EMG (100 ms around the maximal peak force) was determined during each contraction, as well as the maximal force and RMS-EMG (100 ms around peak force) produced by the contralateral FDI.

Unilateral and bilateral sub-maximal contractions with MEPs

After the MVCs, subjects produced an abduction force with their right index finger (Hand-1) at four force levels (0, 5, 15, or 30% of MVC). When the subject reached the required force level, they were requested to produce a concurrent force with their left index finger abductor (Hand-2). Subjects received continuous feedback of the target and the produced forces.

During a set of contractions, the force level of Hand-1 was fixed at one of the four levels, whereas the force levels of Hand-2 was varied between 0, 5, 10, 15, 30, 50, and 70% of MVC (**Figure 1B**). Subjects were instructed to maintain the required force levels until the delivery of three TMS pulses was complete. A contraction lasted about 20 s and the subject received at least 30 s of rest between the contractions. One set of seven contractions lasted about 6 min.

In total, all subjects performed unilateral contractions with the FDI of Hand-1 (5, 15, or 30% of MVC) and Hand-2 (5, 10, 15, 30, 50, and 70% of MVC) and bilateral contractions consisting of 18 force combinations (Hand-1: 5, 15, or 30% of MVC and Hand-2: 5, 10, 15, 30, 50, and 70% of MVC). The MEPs were always evoked in the FDI of Hand-1, i.e., the hand that started the bilateral contraction.

Maximal voluntary contraction with twitch interpolation

After finishing the sub-maximal force task, we repeated the MVC measurements combined with different forms of stimulation (**Figure 1C**). During the MVCs of Hand-1 (right hand), the subject received a TMS stimulus over the (left) motor cortex contralateral to the contracting FDI. During MVCs with Hand-2 (left hand), a TMS stimulus was given over the (left) motor cortex ipsilateral to the contracting FDI, followed by an electrical stimulus to the contracting (left) FDI muscle (twitch superimposition; inter-stimulus interval between TMS pulse and electrical simulation, 1.5 s).

Sustained, fatiguing maximal contraction

Subjects produced a 2-min sustained contraction with the FDI of Hand-2 (left hand, i.e., the FDI muscle that received the muscle stimulation). The instruction to the subjects was to produce maximal abduction force with the left index finger for 2 min; no further instructions were given regarding their contralateral hand. Subjects were verbally encouraged to give maximum effort throughout the sustained contraction. During the 2 min, TMS was applied seven times to the (left) hemisphere ipsilateral to the fatiguing muscle (i.e., the Hand-2 FDI) followed by electrical muscle stimulation of the (left) fatiguing FDI (i.e., Hand-2 FDI). The interval between each pair of stimulating pulses (the TMS and electrical muscle stimulation) was 17 s and the interval between TMS and muscle stimulation was 1.5 s (**Figure 1D**). After 2 min, subjects relaxed the index finger abductor and muscle stimulation was applied three times within 5 s after the end of the fatiguing contraction, which was immediately followed by a brief MVC with the Hand-1 FDI (right non-fatigued FDI) during which TMS was applied and a brief MVC with Hand-2 FDI (left fatigued FDI) during which TMS and muscle stimulation was applied. To finish the protocol, ulnar nerve stimulation was applied five times in the Hand-1 FDI (right hand).

In the second experiment, the TMS and muscle stimulation were delivered to the contralateral side. The fatiguing task was also performed with the contralateral muscle.

DATA ANALYSIS

Maximal voluntary contractions

During the MVCs, the maximal force and RMS-EMG (100 ms time window around peak force) was determined. The maximal force value during the MVCs was considered as the "true" MVC and force values obtained during voluntary and associated contractions were expressed as a percentage of this MVC value. The maximal RMS-EMG value obtained during MVCs was used to normalize all EMG values (both voluntary contractions and associated activity). The RMS-EMG and force values during the associated contractions of the contralateral FDI during the MVCs were averaged over the three MVC-trials.

The MVC and associated activity was analyzed with repeated measures mixed design ANOVA with Hand (left and right) as within-subject factors, and Age-group (young and middle-aged) and sex (male and female) as between-subject factors.

Unilateral and bilateral sub-maximal contractions

When the subjects reached their force targets, the mean index finger abduction force was measured for a 1-s time window before the TMS stimulus. The three 1-s values obtained during one contraction were averaged. For the same time window, the mean RMS-EMG values were determined for both FDI muscles. Additionally, the mean RMS-EMG in the Hand-1 FDI was assessed 100 ms before the TMS stimulus. All force and EMG values were expressed as percentage of the MVC values. The amplitude and area of the MEPs were expressed as a percentage of the M-wave. To quantify performance on the bilateral task, we calculated the force difference with the following Eq. (1):

$$\text{Bilateral force difference} = \sqrt{\begin{aligned}&\big((\text{target force}_{\text{Hand}-1} - \text{produced force}_{\text{Hand}-1})^2\\ &+ (\text{target force}_{\text{Hand}-2} - \text{produced force}_{\text{Hand}-2})\big)^2\end{aligned}}$$

To investigate the effect of a contraction on the ipsilateral motor cortex excitability, we choose to analyze the force, MEP, and EMG values obtained during unilateral and bilateral contractions separately. During the unilateral contractions, changes in force, MEP amplitude and area, and background RMS-EMG were statistically analyzed with a repeated measures mixed design ANOVA. As within-subject factors were identified, force of Hand-1 (Force-H1: 5, 15, and 30% of MVC) or force of Hand-2 (Force-H2: 5, 10, 15, 30, 50, and 70% of MVC) and Hand (left and right); Age-group (young and middle-aged) was assigned as a between-subject factors.

During the bilateral contractions, we analyzed force difference, MEP, and EMG values. The mixed design repeated measures ANOVA that was used consisted of Force-H1 (5, 15, and 30% of MVC), Force-H2 (5, 10, 15, 30, 50, and 70% of MVC) and Hand (left and right) as within-subject factors, and Age-group (young and middle-aged) as a between-subject factors. For unilateral and bilateral contractions, *post hoc* analysis (least significant difference, LSD) in which we compared the data obtained at 5% of MVC versus data obtained at higher force levels (for Hand-1: 15 and 30% of MVC, and Hand-2: 10, 15, 30, 50, and 70% of MVC) were performed to break down significant effects where appropriate.

Fatigue task

Mean force and RMS-EMG values were obtained for 2-s time periods during the sustained contraction. Epochs in which TMS stimuli or muscle stimuli were given (7 × 4 s-periods) were excluded from the analysis. This resulted in 46 epochs of 2 s. The mean force and RMS-EMG data were expressed as a percentage of the pre-fatigue MVC values. The forces evoked by the muscle stimulation were measured and expressed as a percentage of the potentiated doublet-force obtained before the fatiguing contractions. The amplitude and area of the MEP was measured and expressed as a percentage of the M-wave.

Changes in force and EMG values (% MVC) during the sustained maximal contraction were analyzed with a repeated measures mixed design ANOVA (2 × 46 × 2) with Hand (left and right) and Time (1–46 periods of 2 s) as within-subjects factors; Age-group was included as a between-subject factor.

Some of the doublet-forces evoked during the sustained contraction could not be analyzed due to fast variations in voluntary background force. It was then impossible to decide which part of the force increase was due to voluntary activation and which part was due to the evoked twitch. Instead of using a fixed time interval to determine the evoked force, we excluded this data point and analyzed the twitch forces with a multilevel analysis. The multilevel analysis is less affected by missing data points (in contrast to the repeated measures ANOVA; Snijders and Bosker, 1999). We also used the multilevel analysis for the MEPs evoked during unilateral contractions of Hand-2. During these contractions (especially at higher forces), some subjects could not completely relax Hand-1 and EMG activity was visible before the TMS stimulus. These MEPs were excluded from the analysis. Because this resulted in missing data points in some subjects, we choose to perform multilevel statistical tests.

Associations between the relevant parameters (MVC, amount of associated activity, fatigability) obtained in the two sessions were determined with linear regression analysis. Similar statistics were used to explore associations between values of associated activity and bimanual interference.

Statistical significance was set at $\alpha = 0.05$; if violation of sphericity of the data occurred, degrees of freedom were corrected using Huynh–Feldt estimates of sphericity.

RESULTS

Table 1 shows the main characteristics of the subjects. There was no difference in the intensity used for muscle, nerve, and cortical stimulation between the two experiments and age-groups ($p > 0.1$). During the sustained contraction, the force recording in one subject and the EMG recording in another subject could not be used due to technical problems. There was some noise interference (>10 μV) in 20% of the EMG recordings. This noise could be due to having both the electrical stimulator and the EMG amplifier simultaneously connected to the electrodes. Although the noise was small, the noise occurred more often in the middle-aged subjects than in the younger subjects. Therefore, we analyzed in those cases, both the non-filtered and notch-filtered EMG signals (IRR 50 Hz filter). In the text, we present the notch-filtered EMG data, if the analysis shows differences between the non-filtered and notch-filtered data, we present both results.

Table 1 | Subject characteristics displayed in mean ± SD.

	Young adults ($n = 10$)	Middle-aged adults ($n = 10$)	Total
Age (years)	23.6 (2.3)	49.8 (2.5)	36.7 (13.6)
Laterality index	86.5 (14.3)	93.0 (10.9)	89.8 (12.8)
RMT (% max stimulator output)	55.1 (6.6)	59.5 (8.5)	57.5 (7.9)
Muscle stimulation (mA)	36.2 (9.9)	38.7 (9.1)	37.6 (9.4)
Nerve stimulation (mA)	36.1 (9.8)	41.8 (8.7)	38.7 (9.1)
M-wave (mV)	24.5 (6.0)	24.6 (5.7)	24.5 (5.3)
Rest MEP[a] (mV)	0.6 (0.4)	0.7 (0.5)	0.7 (0.4)

Age in years, laterality index, RMT in percentage of maximum stimulator output, muscle and nerve stimulation in mA.

[a] Rest MEP at 100% resting motor threshold.

MAXIMAL VOLUNTARY CONTRACTIONS ARE SIMILAR IN THE TWO AGE GROUPS

Males (45.2 *N*, 7.3 SD) had a higher maximal index finger abduction force than females [33.6 *N*, 6.8 SD; $F_{(1,16)} = 19.10, p < 0.001$]. The MVC force was not significantly different between the two age groups (young adults: 41.6 *N*, 8.7 SD; middle age adults: 37.2 *N*, 9.2 SD; $p = 0.12$), neither between the left (39.0 *N*, 9.0 SD) and right hand (39.7 *N*, 9.4 SD; $p = 0.67$), nor between the two experiments ($p = 0.67$). No interaction effects between Sex, Experiment, Age-group, or Hand were found ($p > 0.25$, for all interactions). For the MVC force in both the left and right hand, there was an association between the two experiments and there was an association between the MVC force of the left and right hand of the participants [$F_{(1,38)} = 123.20$, $R^2 = 0.76$ and $F_{(1,38)} = 39.10$, $R^2 = 0.51$, respectively; both $p < 0.001$].

AMOUNT OF ASSOCIATED ACTIVITY DIFFERS BETWEEN THE TWO AGE GROUPS

During the MVCs, most subjects showed some amount of contralateral activity. Statistical analysis demonstrated main effects of Experiment [force: $F_{(1,16)} = 5.04$, $p = 0.04$] and Age-group [force: $F_{(1,16)} = 4.43$, $p = 0.05$; EMG: $F_{(1,16)} = 5.23$, $p = 0.04$]. In addition, there was an Age-group by Experiment by Sex interaction for both the associated force [$F_{(1,16)} = 6.76$, $p = 0.02$] and associated EMG activity [$F_{(1,16)} = 4.58$, $p = 0.05$]. Associated activity was higher in middle-aged subjects (force: 28.9 and 11.5% MVC, for middle-aged and young subjects, respectively), and higher in females (force: 26.7 and 18.7% MVC, EMG: 22.4 and 15.7% MVC; for Experiments 1 and 2, respectively) compared with males (force: 14.4 and 12.8% MVC, EMG: 11.7 and 11.1% MVC; for Experiments 1 and 2, respectively) in Experiment 1. The amount of associated activity in Experiments 1 and 2, and also in left and right hands were positively associated [$F_{(1,38)} = 49.68$, $R^2 = 0.57$ and $F_{(1,38)} = 47.33$, $R^2 = 0.55$, for EMG and force between the two experiments, respectively; $F_{(1,38)} = 82.38$, $R^2 = 0.68$ and $F_{(1,38)} = 67.48$, $R^2 = 0.64$, for EMG and force of the left and right hand, respectively; $p < 0.001$ in all cases].

UNILATERAL CONTRACTIONS WITH TMS OF THE CONTRALATERAL M1

To investigate possible differences between the age groups in the effect of muscle activation on the MEPs, participants performed unilateral contractions with their FDI (Hand-1) at three different force levels (5, 15, and 30% MVC) and were instructed to keep their contralateral FDI (Hand-2) relaxed. During the contraction, the contralateral motor cortex was stimulated three times (inter-stimulus interval >3 s).

All subjects performed the task as expected. The force data showed an Age-group by Hand by Force interaction for Force difference [$F_{(1.7,30.6)} = 3.60, p = 0.05$] because young subjects produced a marginally larger force with their left FDI at high force levels than middle-aged subjects (Force difference left FDI: young: +0.29% MVC and middle-aged: −1.3% MVC at 30% MVC target; $p = 0.05$). The evoked MEPs increased with increasing force and EMG levels [**Figures 2A,B**, right side; $F_{(2,36)} = 36.76$, $p < 0.001$; larger MEPs at 15% ($p = 0.001$) and 30% of MVC ($p < 0.001$)] without a difference between the two Age-groups ($p = 0.49$).

UNILATERAL CONTRACTIONS WITH TMS OF THE IPSILATERAL M1

The purpose of these runs was to determine: (a) the age-related differences in iM1 activation and (b) the magnitude of associated force and EMG activity in the resting hand. Participants performed unilateral contractions with their FDI of Hand-2 (ipsilateral to the cortex receiving TMS) at six different force levels (5, 10, 15, 30, 50,

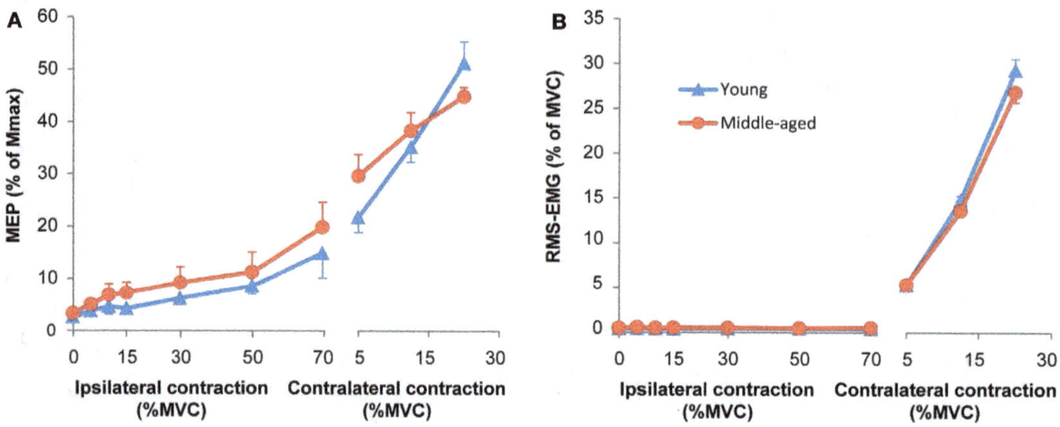

FIGURE 2 | (A) Mean and standard error of motor evoked potentials (MEPs) during unilateral force production for young (blue) and middle-aged subjects (red). The left side of the panel shows MEPs obtained during an ipsilateral contraction at increasing force levels. Only MEPs were included that were not preceded by any voluntary activity; all MEPs of 8 out of 40 experiments (seven subjects: five middle-aged, two young adults) were excluded because more than half of the MEPs at high force levels showed small signs of EMG activity. The right side of the panel the MEPs obtained during a contralateral contraction (only for the MEPs of the same subjects as included in the ipsilateral contraction). The MEPs increased with ipsilateral and contralateral force without significant difference between young and middle-aged subjects. **(B)** Mean and standard error of RMS-EMG (100 ms before MEP) upon which the MEPs were evoked at increasing force levels of the hand ipsilateral to the motor cortex receiving the TMS pulse (left panel) and the contralateral hand (right panel) for young (blue) and middle-aged subjects (red). The background RMS-EMG was close to zero during the ipsilateral contraction and increased proportional with the force during the contralateral contraction. No differences were observed between young and middle-aged subjects.

and 70% of MVC). They were instructed to keep their contralateral hand relaxed (i.e., the hand in which MEPs were evoked). However, if subjects forcefully contracted the FDI of Hand-2, the FDI of Hand-1 also became activated [force: $F_{(1.2,21.5)} = 4.37, p = 0.04$; RMS-EMG: $F_{(1.3,23.1)} = 5.20$, $p = 0.03$, **Figure 4A**; larger force in Hand-1 when ipsilateral hand contracted at 50% ($p = 0.02$) and a trend toward significance at 70% of MVC ($p = 0.06$); larger RMS-EMG in Hand-1 when the ipsilateral hand contracted at 70% of MVC ($p = 0.03$)].

As expected from the changes in force and EMG in Hand-1, the MEPs evoked in the FDI of Hand-1 increased together with the activation of the FDI in Hand-2 [$F_{(2.4,43.9)} = 34.73$, $p < 0.001$; from 4.4% of M_{max} (0.6 SD) at 5% MVC force to 6.4 of M_{max} at 30% ($p = 0.02$), 9.8% of M_{max} (1.2 SD) at 50% MVC ($p < 0.001$), and to 17.5% of M_{max} (2.2 SD) at 70% MVC ($p < 0.001$)]. To correct for the increase in background EMG, we excluded all MEPs from the statistical analysis that were preceded by EMG (100 ms before the TMS stimulus). In eight experiments (seven subjects, five middle-aged subjects), no MEPs at force levels above 30% of MVC remained after rejection of trials with background EMG. We therefore excluded all of the data for these subjects from the statistical analyses. To be able to perform the analysis despite missing data points, we analyzed the MEPs with multilevel analysis. The analysis showed a relationship between the RMS-EMG in Hand-2 FDI and the MEPs [$F_{(1,31.14)} = 31.14$, $p < 0.001$; **Figure 2A**, left side], no main or interaction effect of Age-group was found.

BILATERAL CONTRACTIONS

The purpose of these runs was to determine the effects of age on bilateral interaction. We parametrically increased the contraction intensity (5, 10, 15, 30, 50, and 70% of MVC) in one FDI (Hand-2) and measured the corticospinal excitability in the other FDI while contracting at three low intensities (5, 15, or 30% of MVC; Hand-1, **Figures 1** and **4**). During these contractions, three magnetic stimuli were given to evoke MEPs in the FDI of Hand-1.

To quantify the performance in the bilateral task, we used Eq. 1 to calculate the difference between the target force and the force subjects actually produced. The force difference showed significant main effects for the force levels of Hand-1 [$F_{(2,34)} = 26.68$, $p < 0.001$; 5 versus 15%, $p = 0.03$, versus 30% $p < 0.001$], Hand-2 [$F_{(1.8,29.8)} = 40.63$, $p < 0.01$; 5 versus 50 and 70%, both $p < 0.001$], and an interaction effect for Hand-1 by Hand-2 [$F_{(6.4,108.3)} = 4.14$, $p = 0.001$; see **Figure 3** for contrasts] with the force difference being larger at higher force levels of Hand-1 (**Figure 3**). There was an Age-group by Hand interaction in the force difference [$F_{(1,17)} = 7.4$, $p = 0.01$]; the force difference was smaller when the left hand started the contraction in the young subjects. Overall, the force difference was larger for middle-aged subjects than for young subjects [$F_{(1,17)} = 4.56$, $p = 0.05$].

The EMG values in Hand-1 (both the 1-s as well as the 100-ms before the TMS stimulus data) showed a main effect of the force in Hand-1 [$F_{(1.2,21.9)} = 312.18$ and 284.70 for 1-s and 100 ms epochs, both $p < 0.001$; 5 versus 15 and 30% $p < 0.001$] and the force in Hand-2 [$F_{(3.4,62.1)} = 7.51$ and 6.51, both $p < 0.001$; 5% versus all force levels $p < 0.05$ for 1-s, 5% versus force $> 15\%$ $p < 0.05$ for 100 ms epoch]. In addition, there was an Age-group by Hand-1 interaction [$F_{(1.2,21.9)} = 5.19$ and 4.65, both $p < 0.03$ for 1-s and 100-ms epochs] because the middle-aged compared with young subjects had lower EMG activity at 30% MVC (26.9 and 33.4% RMS-MVC; **Figure 4D**; only significant effect for 100 ms epoch). The EMG in Hand-2 was modulated with the force level of Hand-2 [$F_{(2.5,45.7)} = 628.60$, $p < 0.001$]. No further main or interaction effects occurred.

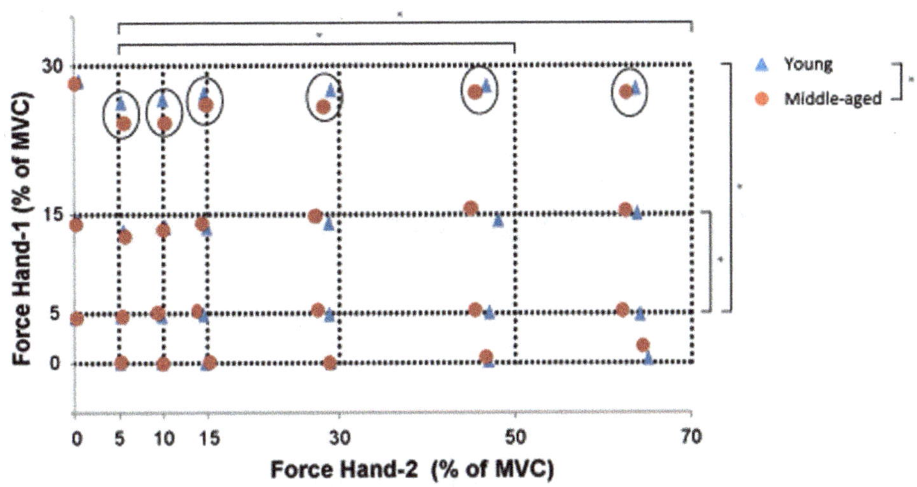

FIGURE 3 | The combination of bimanual forces produced by young (blue) and middle-aged subjects (red). The crossing of the interrupted lines represents the target force combination for Hand-1 (*y*-axis) and Hand-2 (*x*-axis). The measure of bilateral performance (force difference) is calculated as the Euclidean distance between the requested force combination and the produced force combination (see Eq. 1). Significant differences in force difference across bilateral force combinations are indicated by an asterisk (unilateral contractions were not included in the statistical analysis; main effect of Hand-1 and -2). The circles point to an Age-group effect on the amplitude of the force difference at high force levels in Hand-1. Overall, the force difference was larger for the middle-aged than for the young participants.

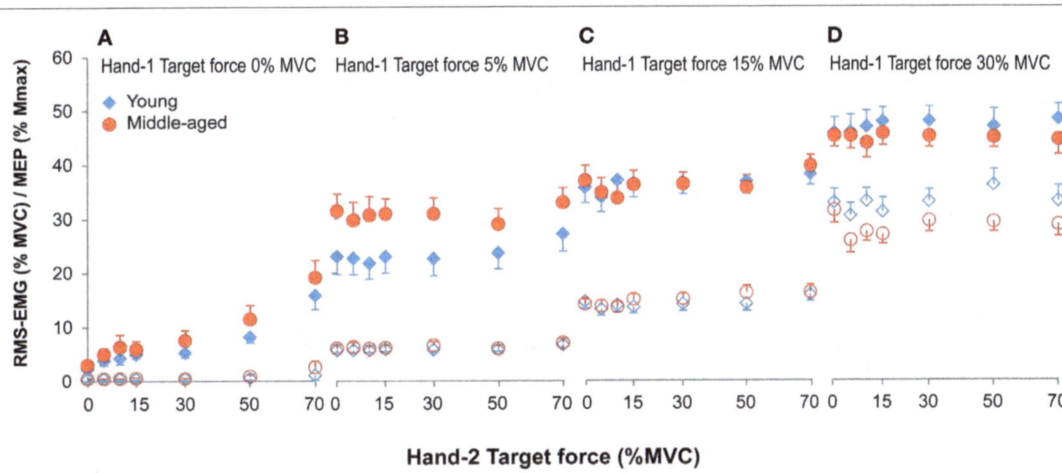

FIGURE 4 | Mean and standard error of RMS-EMG (100 ms, open symbols, bottom row) and MEPs (closed symbols, top row) during unilateral **(A)** and bilateral **(B–D)** forces at different force combinations for young (blue) and middle-aged (red) subjects. Hand-1 is the hand in which the MEPs in the FDI were evoked and the hand that started the contraction during the bilateral contractions. For the values presented in **(A)** and the unilateral contractions (force Hand-2 equals 0) in **(B–D)** all MEPs were included for calculating the mean values. **(A)** Shows a small but significant increase in RMS-EMG and an increase in MEP amplitude with increasing ipsilateral force. **(B–D)** Shows that the RMS-EMG and the MEPs in Hand-1 were affected by both the force production of Hand-1 and -2. At low force levels (5% MVC) MEPs were larger in middle-aged participants, whereas at high force levels (30% MVC) middle-aged participants had lower EMG values compared to young participants.

The MEPs were affected by both the force produced by Hand-1 [$F_{(1.7,30.6)} = 74.09$, $p < 0.001$] and the force produced by Hand-2 [$F_{(4.7,84.9)} = 4.18$, $p = 0.002$]. In addition, there was an Age-group by Hand-1 interaction [$F_{(1.7,30.64)} = 5.29$, $p = 0.014$]. In contrast to the RMS-EMG, the MEPs at 5% MVC were larger in the middle-aged subjects (30% of M_{max}) than in young subjects (23% of M_{max}; **Figure 4B**; 5 versus 15%, $p = 0.006$; 5 versus 30%, $p = 0.02$).

SUSTAINED CONTRACTION INDUCED MORE ASSOCIATED ACTIVITY IN MIDDLE-AGED SUBJECTS

Voluntary activity

During the sustained contraction, the index finger abduction force progressively decreased from 86% MVC (7.0 SD) to 36% MVC (11 SD). The statistical analysis showed a significant decline over time [$F_{(45,765)} = 196.27$, $p < 0.001$; **Figures 1D**, **5**, and **6A**] but no Hand nor Age-group effects. The RMS-EMG values showed a

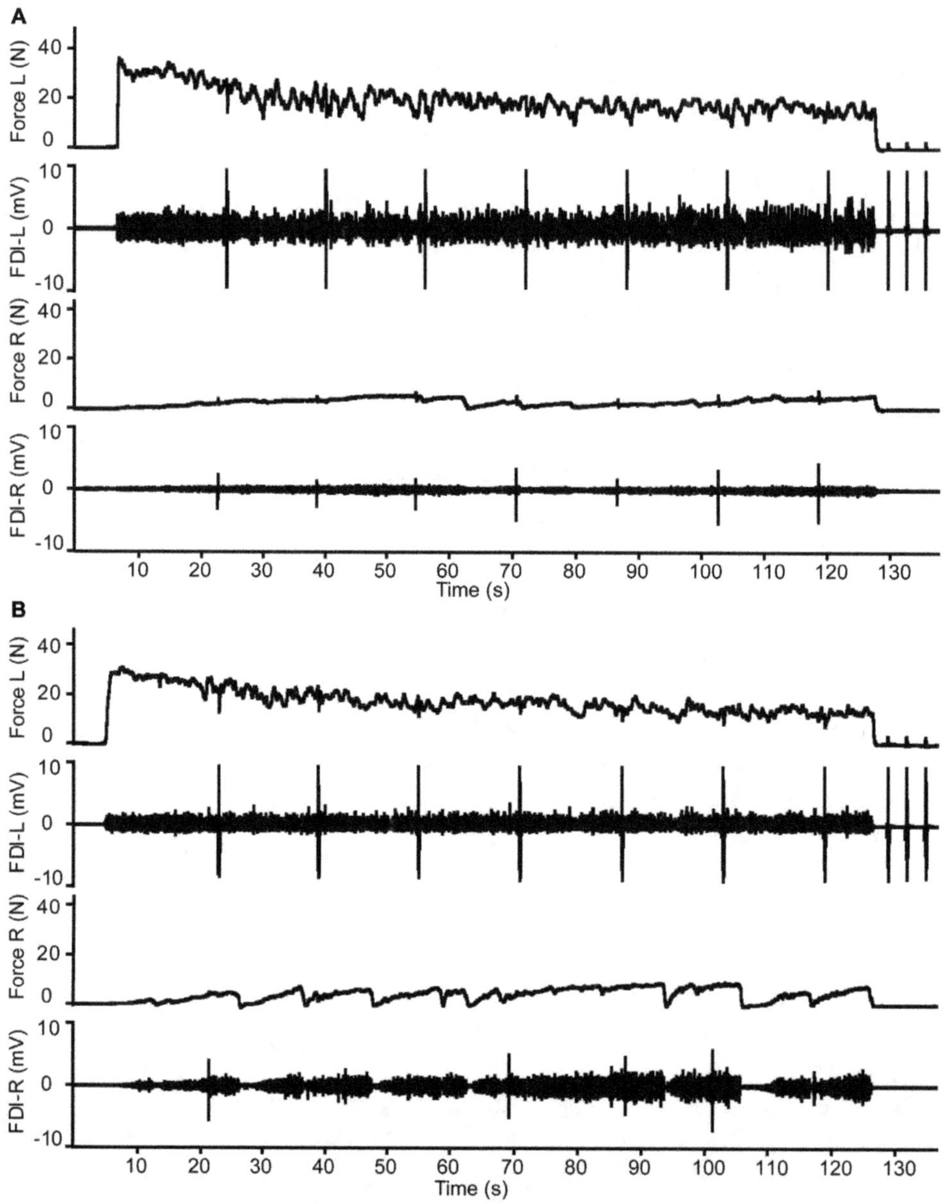

FIGURE 5 | Example of the changes in target and associated force and electromyography during the 2-min contraction with the FDI muscle of Hand-2 (left) in a young male (A) and middle-aged female participant (B). Please note the stronger activity in right hand (Hand-1) in the middle-aged participant.

more variable time course during the sustained task (**Figure 6B**), revealing a main effect of Time [$F_{(45,765)} = 2.49, p < 0.001$], and a Time by Hand interaction [$F_{(13.72,233.16)} = 2.12, p = 0.012$)]. The general trend was a decline in RMS-EMG in the left hand and a smaller change in the right hand.

During the sustained contraction, the FDI that performed the fatiguing task was stimulated seven times. The evoked force was used to estimate the voluntary drive during the sustained contraction. During the fatiguing task, the evoked doublet-force increased significantly (suggesting a decrease in voluntary drive) ($F = 3.22$, $p = 0.005$; **Figure 6E**); no main or interaction effects with Age-group were found.

Associated activity

During the sustained contraction, the amount of associated force and EMG increased significantly [force: $F_{(45,810)} = 9.58, p < 0.001$; RMS-EMG: $F_{(45,810)} = 10.97$, $p < 0.001$]. The amount of associated activity was significantly different between the Age-groups (**Figures 5** and **6A,B**). The associated force increased from 6.2 to 29.7% of MVC in the middle-aged subjects and from 2.7 to 15.2%MVC in the young subjects [Age-group: $F_{(1,18)} = 7.05$, $p = 0.016$]. The RMS-EMG showed a similar pattern; increase from 9.8 to 39.7% of MVC in the middle-aged subjects and from 3.8 to 18.4% of MVC for the young subjects [Age-group $F_{(1,18)} = 5.99, p = 0.025$].

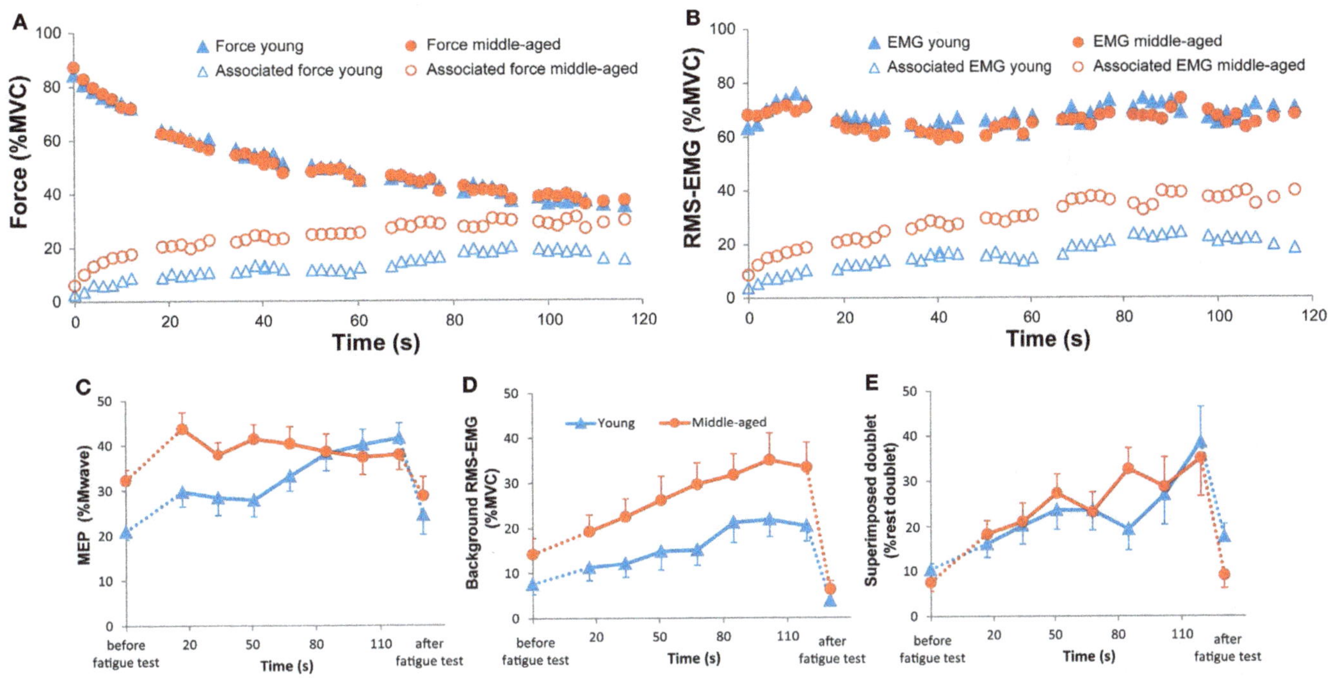

FIGURE 6 | Changes in mean force [(A), closed symbols] and RMS-EMG [2 s-values; **(B)**, closed symbols] expressed as % MVC, and mean associated force [**(A)**, open symbols] and RMS-EMG [2 s-values; **(B)**, open symbols] expressed as % MVC **(A,B)** during the sustained 2 min contraction for young (blue) and middle-aged subjects (red). During the test, stimuli are given to the cortex ipsilateral to the target muscle, and to the target (fatiguing) muscle. During the stimuli, no average force or RMS-EMG is calculated. Therefore, short time periods are missing in the graphs. **(C)** Changes in mean MEP amplitude (and standard error) during the sustained contraction for young (blue) and middle-aged (red) subjects separately. The first value shows the mean MEP during the contralateral MVC before the sustained contraction. The last values show MEP during the contralateral MVC after the sustained contraction. The analysis demonstrated a Time by Age group interaction ($p = 0.006$), revealing a decrease in MEP difference between the two Age groups with time. **(D)** Changes in mean (and standard error) RMS-EMG 100 ms before the TMS pulse. First and last values are the values obtained during the contralateral MVC. Note that the background RMS-EMG is associated activity. In contrast to the MEPs, the amount of ipsilateral activity increased progressively during the sustained contraction of young and middle-aged subjects ($p < 0.001$). **(E)** Changes in the mean (and standard error) superimposed doublet-force evoked in the FDI muscle that produces the maximal force during the sustained contraction. The doublet twitch increased throughout the sustained contraction reflecting a progressive decline in voluntary drive ($p = 0.005$), without a difference between the two Age-groups.

Evoked potentials

During the sustained contraction, MEPs were evoked in the FDI showing the associated activity. **Figure 6C** shows the Time by Age-group interaction for the MEP amplitude [MEP peak: $F_{(5.2,94.4)} = 3.53$, $p = 0.006$; MEP area: $F_{(5.2,94.4)} = 3.19$, $p = 0.009$]. The first MEP during the sustained contraction increased in comparison with the control MVC before the sustained contraction (young: from 20.9 to 29.7% of M_{max}, middle-aged: from 32.3 to 43.7% of M_{max}). During the sustained contraction, the MEP in the middle-aged participants started at a higher value (44% of M_{max}) than the MEP in the younger subjects and slowly decreased to 38% of M_{max}, whereas in the young participants the MEP progressively increased (from 30 to 41% of M_{max}) during the sustained contraction. As it was expected from the overall EMG measurement, the amount of background EMG upon which the MEP was evoked increased progressively during the fatiguing task [$F_{(8,144)} = 12.45, p < 0.001$; **Figure 6D**]. Overall, the EMG activity at the time of the TMS was higher in the middle-aged than younger subjects [$F_{(1,18)} = 4.50$, $p = 0.06$; **Figures 6B,D**]. Thus, the increase in MEP reflected the increase in background EMG in the young but not in the middle-aged subjects.

FATIGUE-RELATED CHANGES AFTER THE SUSTAINED CONTRACTIONS

The MVC of the fatigued FDI immediately after the fatiguing contraction decreased significantly to 67.2% of the pre-fatigue MVC [10.2 SD; $F_{(1,38)}$, 43.40, $p < 0.001$], without an Age-group effect. The MVC of the non-fatigued FDI also showed a small decline in force to 92.2% of MVC (SD 10.5); this decline was larger in the right (88.1% of MVC, 10.4 SD) than in the left FDI (95.1% of MVC, 10.3 SD, $p = 0.003$); no main or interaction effects were found for Age-group. The doublet-force evoked in the fatigued FDI declined to 47.3% compared to the control values in both age groups ($p = 0.22$).

The amplitude and area of the MEPs evoked during contralateral MVCs did not change after the fatiguing task (106.7%, 38.2 SD of pre-fatigue values), whereas the background (associated) EMG was smaller but similar in the two age groups after the fatiguing contraction [pre-fatigue: 10.9% of RMS-MVC and post-fatigue: 4.9% of RMS-MVC; $F_{(1,12)} = 12.41$, $p = 0.02$].

There was a main effect of Time [$F_{(1,33)} = 4.79$, $p = 0.05$] for the doublet-force superimposed on the MVC before and after the fatiguing contraction. The evoked force was larger after the fatiguing contraction (pre-fatigue: 7.8% versus post-fatigue:

12.2% doublet force at rest), suggesting a decline in voluntary activation after the fatiguing task. No interaction effect with Age-group was found.

WEAK ASSOCIATION BETWEEN BILATERAL PERFORMANCE AND ASSOCIATED ACTIVITY

The data demonstrated a weak but significant association between the measure of bilateral performance, i.e., force difference and the amount of associated activity during the MVCs for the left and right FDI (RMS-EMG: $R^2 = 0.17$, $p = 0.008$; force: $R^2 = 0.15$, $p = 0.015$; see **Figure 7**). Force difference was not significantly associated with the average amount of associated activity during the fatiguing sustained contraction ($p > 0.5$ for both average RMS-EMG and average force).

DISCUSSION

We compared the amount of associated activity and ipsilateral corticospinal excitability between young and middle-aged subjects during isometric contractions. We observed that the associated activity was ~2-fold higher in middle-aged (28% of MVC) when compared with young adults (11% of MVC) during brief as well as sustained MVCs (at 120 s: 15 versus 30% of MVC, for the young and middle-aged subjects). After carefully selecting MEPs that were not preceded by background EMG activity, no difference in ipsilateral corticospinal excitability was found between middle-aged versus young subjects during sub-maximal contractions. During the sustained contraction, MEPs were greater at the start of the contraction but there was no further increase *during* the contraction in middle-aged compared with young adults.

ASSOCIATED ACTIVITY DURING BRIEF MAXIMAL CONTRACTIONS IS HIGHER IN MIDDLE-AGED SUBJECTS

The increased levels of associated activity in middle-aged subjects during strong contractions confirm previous data obtained in elderly subjects [Bodwell et al., 2003 (65–85 years); Shinohara et al., 2003 (65–85 years); Baliz et al., 2005 (60–70 years); Addamo et al., 2009 (60–80 years); Fling and Seidler, 2012 (65–76 years)]. In a previous study, we demonstrated that the spinal motoneurons responsible for the associated contractions were activated via the contralateral corticospinal pathways; that is, the motor cortex ipsilateral to the target muscle (Zijdewind et al., 2006). Thus, our data demonstrate an additional increase in activity of these corticospinal pathways (ipsilateral to the target muscles) in middle-aged subjects during strong voluntary contractions. On basis of the present study, we cannot conclude whether these changes are present on cortical, spinal, or at both levels.

During a unilateral contraction, a MEP evoked in the ipsilateral motor cortex becomes facilitated (Hess et al., 1986; Ugawa et al., 1993; Stedman et al., 1998; Tinazzi and Zanette, 1998; Muellbacher et al., 2000; Liepert et al., 2001; Perez and Cohen, 2008, 2009). The larger MEPs during activation of the ipsilateral muscle are probably due to subliminal activation of the motor cortex contralateral to the target hemisphere. We did not find a significant difference in the ipsilateral MEPs between the two age groups during the sub-maximal contractions. It is possible that intra- and inter-cortical processes affect associated activity and ipsilateral excitability differently or we missed the increase in ipsilateral MEPs. The facilitation of the ipsilateral MEPs is more pronounced at high contralateral force levels (Hess et al., 1986; Ugawa et al., 1993; Stedman et al., 1998; Tinazzi and Zanette, 1998; Muellbacher et al., 2000; Liepert et al., 2001; Perez and Cohen, 2008, 2009) and since subjects were less able to prevent associated activation at higher force levels (see also Zijdewind and Kernell, 2001), hardly any MEPs at relatively high contralateral force levels remained.

Associated activity can be induced if the net excitation is above the spike-generating threshold for cortical neurons. Thus, the observation that middle-aged compared to young subjects more often show associated activity during strong contractions, suggests that the inhibition to the ipsilateral motor cortex is smaller or that the amount of excitation it receives is larger. It is often reported that intracortical inhibition (Peinemann et al., 2001; Hortobagyi et al., 2006; however, see Oliviero et al., 2006; Smith et al., 2009; McGinley et al., 2010), length of the silent period (Sale and Semmler, 2005) and interhemispheric inhibition (Talelli et al., 2008a,b; McGregor et al., 2011, 2013; Davidson and Tremblay, 2013) declines with age. However, one would expect to find an additional increase

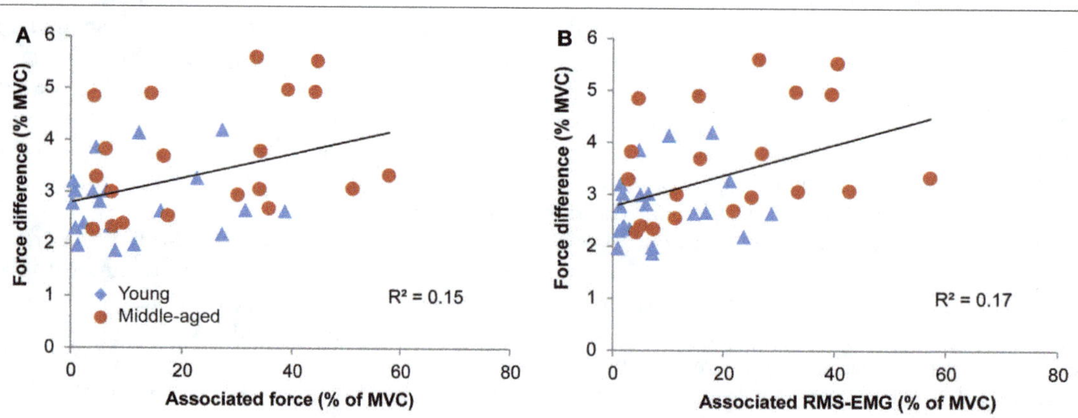

FIGURE 7 | Relationships between associated activity [EMG and force, in (A,B), respectively] and the measure of bilateral performance, i.e., force difference for young (blue triangle) and middle-aged subjects (red circles). Participants with high levels of associated activity tended to have an inferior bilateral performance.

in ipsilateral MEPs (see Perez and Cohen, 2008). On the other hand, Perez and Cohen (2008) showed that the ipsilateral MEPs did correlate with changes in short-latency intracortical inhibition but less with changes in interhemispheric inhibition. So, maybe the increased associated activity during strong contractions does reflect differences in interhemispheric inhibition between the two age groups (Talelli et al., 2008a,b; Fling and Seidler, 2012). One other possible explanation could be a reduction in synchronized *I*-waves in middle-aged subjects (see also *larger MEPs during low contralateral activation*). A TMS stimulus can evoke both direct (*D*) and a series of indirect (*I*) waves (Kernell and Chien-Ping, 1967; Amassian et al., 1987). At low stimulation intensities, the contribution of *I*-waves to the excitation of corticospinal pathways is more important than the contribution from *D*-waves. A decrease in synchronized *I*-waves would thus result in smaller MEPs (see also discussion of Pitcher et al., 2003). Small changes in synchronization will probably have less effect during voluntary (or associated) activation. Hence, this could explain the higher level of associated activity during strong contractions without an increase in ipsilateral MEP size at rest.

The increase in associated activity in middle-aged subjects during effortful contractions is consistent with fMRI data that showed higher blood oxygenation level dependent (BOLD) activation of ipsilateral motor areas during motor tasks in old compared with young adults [Hutchinson et al., 2002 (54–76 years); Ward and Frackowiak, 2003 (26–80 years); Heuninckx et al., 2005 (62–71 years); Wu and Hallett, 2005 (57–73 years); Naccarato et al., 2006 (18–79 years); Riecker et al., 2006 (58–82 years); Talelli et al., 2008a (19–78 years); McGregor et al., 2011 (60–85 years)]. Yet, in most of these studies the authors claim that no associated activity was present. Still, the BOLD response in fMRI is more sensitive to a change in input, and processing of this input in a certain area, than to the actual output of this area (Logothetis, 2002) and thus subliminal activation of the ipsilateral primary motor cortex would show up during fMRI even if no associated muscle activity is observed. Only if the ipsilateral activity results in an increase in the corticofugal output that is strong enough to activate motoneurons, associated activity is seen. Nevertheless, even before associated movement is seen small motor unit potentials can be seen in the EMG resulting in a small change in EMG activity (often smaller than 25 μV). We expected that this increase in (subliminal) ipsilateral activation would show up as an increase in MEP. However after carefully selecting the MEPs without background EMG activity, we found no difference in MEP size between young and middle-aged subjects.

The relevance of the ipsilateral activation and the probably related associated activity is still unclear but better motor performance seemed to be associated with higher ipsilateral activation (Mattay et al., 2002). However, not all studies confirm the functional importance of the age-related increase in cortical activity. For example, Riecker et al. (2006) showed increased activation in elderly subjects (58–82 years) during a tapping task but with no further age-related increase in activity with increasing frequency. Additionally, recent data obtained in middle-aged (McGregor et al., 2011) and older subjects (McGregor et al., 2011) showed that increased iM1 activation was related to shorter ipsilateral silent periods and decreased motor function. On the other hand, in a recent study, Zimerman et al. (2012) demonstrated reduced motor learning in older subjects after cathodal DC-stimulation of the ipsilateral motor cortex. Cathodal DC-stimulation induces a reduction in excitability of the stimulated cortex (for reviews, see Nitsche and Paulus, 2011; Jacobson et al., 2012). Hence, their data suggest that the ipsilateral cortex is more important for motor learning in older compared with younger subjects (Zimerman et al., 2012). Our data showed a weak but significant association between the amount of associated activity and bimanual interference (as measured by the difference between target force and actual produced force), suggesting that high levels of associated activity could be detrimental for bimanual control (cf. McGregor et al., 2013). Again, the mechanisms underlying associated activity and ipsilateral activation could be different and probably, the relationship between these two variables is task-dependent.

ASSOCIATED ACTIVITY DURING SUSTAINED CONTRACTIONS IS HIGHER IN MIDDLE-AGED SUBJECTS

The present study showed that, similarly to previous data in old adults [Shinohara et al., 2003 (66–80 years)], middle-aged compared with young subjects demonstrated higher associated activity already at the start of the voluntary muscle contraction. In the present experiment, this difference in associated activity was maintained throughout the sustained contraction and at the end of the 2-min contraction, the middle-aged compared with young subjects demonstrated a twofold larger level of associated activity. In the only other study that investigated associated activity during fatiguing contractions (Shinohara et al., 2003), the difference in associated activity between young and older subjects became progressively smaller as the contractions progressed. It is possible that this difference is due to age-differences; our middle-aged group was younger than the older subjects used by Shinohara et al. (2003) or to a difference in contraction type (anisometric contraction in Shinohara et al., 2003 versus isometric contractions in the present study).

During a sustained contraction, changes in excitability occur at different levels of the neuromuscular system. For instance, the excitability of the active motoneurons starts to decline as soon as 20 s after the start of the contraction (McNeil et al., 2009, 2011b). To maintain sufficient force production, the voluntary drive to motoneurons has to increase. This increase in drive is seen as an increase in activation of the contralateral primary motor cortex, as demonstrated by fMRI experiments (Dettmers et al., 1995; Liu et al., 2003; van Duinen et al., 2007; Post et al., 2009b). Furthermore, this increase in activity is accompanied by an increase in activity in the ipsilateral primary motor cortex (Dettmers et al., 1995; Liu et al., 2003; van Duinen et al., 2007; Post et al., 2009b), which could generate an increase in associated activity (see also Sehm et al., 2010). If the increase in voluntary drive is indeed reflected as an increase in associated activity, one would expect a progressive increase in associated activation during a sustained contraction. Since Shinohara et al. (2003) did not measure the voluntary drive, it is possible that during the sustained contraction the elderly subjects did not increase their drive similar to the young subjects and therefore did not increase their associated activity further as young subjects did. In the present experiment, both young and middle-aged subjects showed some decline in voluntary activation, as measured with the twitch superimposition technique, but we did not find a difference between the two age groups (see also Hunter et al., 2008).

AGE-RELATED DIFFERENCES IN IPSILATERAL CORTICOSPINAL EXCITABILITY DURING A SUSTAINED CONTRACTION

During a fatiguing task, the associated EMG progressively increases (Post et al., 2008). Despite the increase in background EMG in both groups, the MEPs remained unchanged in the middle-aged compared with young adults in whom the MEPs and the background EMG increased in parallel. The MEPs were comparable to the maximal MEPs obtained by Devanne et al., 1997; 45% M_{max}) in the FDI muscle with different levels of background activity and stimulation intensity. The relationship between background EMG and MEP amplitude in the FDI muscle is not linear but the MEP peaks between 25 and 50% MVC (Devanne et al., 1997; Martin et al., 2006; Perez and Cohen, 2009). At higher background EMG levels, the MEP starts to decline. This reduction in MEP amplitude starts at relatively low force levels in the FDI muscle compared to for instance, the biceps brachii muscle (Martin et al., 2006). The main reason seems to be a change in the balance between two mechanisms of force control, recruitment gradation, and rate modulation. In the FDI muscle, only a few additional motor units become activated at force levels at or higher than 50% MVC, whereas in the biceps brachii muscle recruitment of new motor units continues up to 80% MVC (Milner-Brown et al., 1973; Kukulka and Clamann, 1981). Thus, at higher force levels, the FDI hand muscle completely relies on rate gradation.

After activation of a motoneuron, the motoneuron displays a refractory period followed by afterhyperpolarization (AHP). The time course of the AHP shows an exponential decline until the resting membrane potential (Matthews, 1996; Kernell, 2006). With increasing firing rates, the chance that a TMS pulse reaches a motoneuron during the refractory period or at the initial part of the AHP increases. During this period, the motoneuron is less likely to be activated by the TMS pulse. If smaller number of motoneurons are activated, this will result in a smaller TMS evoked muscle response. During the sustained contraction, the amount of associated activity increased from 20 to 35% of max RMS-EMG in the middle-aged subjects and 12–20% of max RMS-EMG. Thus, for the younger subjects the MEP still has more potential to grow during the sustained contraction, whereas in the middle-aged subjects the MEPs will be closer to their maximal value. Furthermore, there are indications that during a sustained (sub)maximal contraction the intrinsic properties of the motoneuron change to lower excitability levels (McNeil et al., 2011b). This would also result in smaller MEPs especially at higher firing rates. Thus, the lack of increase in MEPs in middle-aged subjects is probably due to fatigue-related changes on a spinal level, but these changes can be accompanied by time-related changes on cortical levels. In young subjects, the excitability changes at spinal levels are partly compensated by an increase in cortical activity, accompanied by increased ipsilateral activity (Post et al., 2008, 2009b). It is not known whether the increase in cortical activity is similar in young and middle-aged subjects but our data did not show any indication that the voluntary drive in the middle-aged subjects was smaller or the voluntary drive changed differently during the sustained contraction. Furthermore, the increase in the amount of associated activity suggests that also the ipsilateral motor cortex increases its activity with time.

NO DIFFERENCE IN FATIGUE BETWEEN YOUNG AND MIDDLE-AGED SUBJECTS

During the fatiguing maximal contraction, there were no age-related differences in the amount of fatigue as indexed by force loss, voluntary activation, and twitch force. Previous studies showed inconsistent data with respect to muscle fatigability of hand muscles in young and older subjects (see for review Allman and Rice, 2002). We are unaware of other studies reporting age-related differences in voluntary activation in the FDI but data in the upper arm muscles suggest that older subjects have a comparable but more variable voluntary activation [Hunter et al., 2008 (67–78 years)]. During their fatiguing task, the voluntary activation decreased as subjects repeated the 22-s-long MVCs. Both, their and our data showed a progressive but similar decline in voluntary activation in the two age groups (Hunter et al., 2008). The decline in voluntary activation was, however, larger than expected (Zijdewind et al., 1998). It is possible that the TMS-response in the ipsilateral motor cortex induced a short ipsilateral silent period resulting in a small decline in force 1.5 s before the muscle stimulation. We looked for ipsilateral silent periods but they were rarely visible (but cf. Fling and Seidler, 2012) and the duration of the reduced EMG was much shorter, but still the stimulation could have affected the attention of the subjects, resulting in a small extra decline in their voluntary activation. After the sustained contraction, the force decline in the fatigued and non-fatigued FDI (see also Post et al., 2008) was not different for the two groups.

GREATER MEPs AT LOW FORCES DURING BILATERAL CONTRACTIONS IN MIDDLE-AGED SUBJECTS

At rest, there is evidence that with age the relationship between stimulus intensity and MEP size (the stimulus-response curve) shifts to the right without a change in the RMT (Pitcher et al., 2003). This observation demonstrates that with age, higher stimulus intensities are needed to obtain maximal MEPs. The most likely explanation for this shift in stimulus–response curve is reduced synchronization of I-waves (indirect activation of corticospinal neurons via interneurons) or changes in recruitment spacing in the motoneuron pool (e.g., due to loss of cortico-motoneurons, see Pitcher et al., 2003). In the present experiment, we used relatively low stimulus intensities, i.e., 110% RMT. It is therefore possible that with the TMS pulse we activated different portions of the corticospinal pathway in young or middle-aged subjects. However, we would expect to activate a smaller portion in the middle-aged subjects, resulting in smaller MEPs. At low force levels, the MEPs were larger in the middle-aged compared with young subjects (with similar background EMG). Although we only found a significant differential effect of background force and MEP size with age in the bilateral condition, the trend in the unilateral condition ($p = 0.097$) suggests that the effect was probably not confined to the bilateral condition.

The maximal rate at which motor units discharge action potentials declines with age (Kamen et al., 1995; Connelly et al., 1999). In hand muscles, all motor units are recruited at low force levels (below 50% MVC; Milner-Brown et al., 1973; Kukulka and Clamann, 1981). Thus, in hand muscles, high forces are extremely susceptible to changes in maximal firing rate and furthermore, these changes will affect the balance between recruitment and rate gradation. The change in balance between the two mechanisms of force control could be responsible for the larger MEP amplitude at low compared to high forces in middle-aged subjects. However, this possibility will require further confirmation in more detailed experiments.

In summary, our data show changes in associated activity during effortful contralateral contractions already in middle-aged subjects. Future experiments will have to determine if such changes in motor control at middle age are functionally relevant. Considering the widespread and increasing use of electronic devices that require high levels of bimanual coordination at work, the observed changes in corticospinal activity and bimanual control at middle age may have implications for screening individuals for such tasks and for designing interventions studies that modulate the levels of associated activity and improve motor function.

REFERENCES

Addamo, P. K., Farrow, M., Hoy, K. E., Bradshaw, J. L., and Georgiou-Karistianis, N. (2009). The influence of task characteristics on younger and older adult motor overflow. *Q. J. Exp. Psychol. (Hove)* 62, 239–247. doi:10.1080/17470210802269217

Allen, G. M., Gandevia, S. C., and McKenzie, D. K. (1995). Reliability of measurements of muscle strength and voluntary activation using twitch interpolation. *Muscle Nerve* 18, 593–600. doi:10.1002/mus.880180605

Allman, B. L., and Rice, C. L. (2002). Neuromuscular fatigue and aging: central and peripheral factors. *Muscle Nerve* 25, 785–796. doi:10.1002/mus.10116

Amassian, V. E., Stewart, M., Quirk, G. J., and Rosenthal, J. L. (1987). Physiological basis of motor effects of a transient stimulus to cerebral cortex. *Neurosurgery* 20, 74–93. doi:10.1097/00006123-198701000-00022

Armatas, C. A., Summers, J. J., and Bradshaw, J. L. (1994). Mirror movements in normal adult subjects. *J. Clin. Exp. Neuropsychol.* 16, 405–413. doi:10.1080/01688639408402651

Baliz, Y., Armatas, C., Farrow, M., Hoy, K. E., Fitzgerald, P. B., Bradshaw, J. L., et al. (2005). The influence of attention and age on the occurrence of mirror movements. *J. Int. Neuropsychol. Soc.* 11, 855–862. doi:10.1017/S1355617705051003

Bodwell, J. A., Mahurin, R. K., Waddle, S., Price, R., and Cramer, S. C. (2003). Age and features of movement influence motor overflow. *J. Am. Geriatr. Soc.* 51, 1735–1739. doi:10.1046/j.1532-5415.2003.51557.x

Boudrias, M. H., Goncalves, C. S., Penny, W. D., Park, C. H., Rossiter, H. E., Talelli, P., et al. (2012). Age-related changes in causal interactions between cortical motor regions during hand grip. *Neuroimage* 59, 3398–3405. doi:10.1016/j.neuroimage.2011.11.025

Cernacek, J. (1961). Contralateral motor irradiation – cerebral dominance. Its changes in hemiparesis. *Arch. Neurol.* 4, 165–172. doi:10.1001/archneur.1961.00450080047005

Cincotta, M., and Ziemann, U. (2008). Neurophysiology of unimanual motor control and mirror movements. *Clin. Neurophysiol.* 119, 744–762. doi:10.1016/j.clinph.2007.11.047

Connelly, D. M., Rice, C. L., Roos, M. R., and Vandervoort, A. A. (1999). Motor unit firing rates and contractile properties in tibialis anterior of young and old men. *J. Appl. Physiol.* 87, 843–852.

Curshmann, H. (1906). Beitrage zur Psysiologie und Pathologie der kontralateralen mitbewegungen. *Dtsch. Z. Nervenheilkd.* 31, 1–52. doi:10.1007/BF01668345

Davidson, T., and Tremblay, F. (2013). Age and hemispheric differences in transcallosal inhibition between motor cortices: an ispsilateral silent period study. *BMC Neurosci.* 14:62. doi:10.1186/1471-2202-14-62

Dettmers, C., Fink, G. R., Lemon, R. N., Stephan, K. M., Passingham, R. E., Silbersweig, D., et al. (1995). Relation between cerebral activity and force in the motor areas of the human brain. *J. Neurophysiol.* 74, 802–815.

Devanne, H., Lavoie, B. A., and Capaday, C. (1997). Input-output properties and gain changes in the human corticospinal pathway. *Exp. Brain Res.* 114, 329–338. doi:10.1007/PL00005641

Fling, B. W., Peltier, S. J., Bo, J., Welsh, R. C., and Seidler, R. D. (2011). Age differences in interhemispheric interactions: callosal structure, physiological function, and behavior. *Front. Neurosci.* 5:38. doi:10.3389/fnins.2011.00038

Fling, B. W., and Seidler, R. D. (2012). Fundamental differences in callosal structure, neurophysiologic function, and bimanual control in young and older adults. *Cereb. Cortex* 22, 2643–2652. doi:10.1093/cercor/bhr349

Haug, H., and Eggers, R. (1991). Morphometry of the human cortex cerebri and corpus striatum during aging. *Neurobiol. Aging* 12, 336–338; discussion 352–355. doi:10.1016/0197-4580(91)90013-A

Hess, C. W., Mills, K. R., and Murray, N. M. (1986). Magnetic stimulation of the human brain: facilitation of motor responses by voluntary contraction of ipsilateral and contralateral muscles with additional observations on an amputee. *Neurosci. Lett.* 71, 235–240. doi:10.1016/0304-3940(86)90565-3

Heuninckx, S., Wenderoth, N., Debaere, F., Peeters, R., and Swinnen, S. P. (2005). Neural basis of aging: the penetration of cognition into action control. *J. Neurosci.* 25, 6787–6796. doi:10.1523/JNEUROSCI.1263-05.2005

Hortobagyi, T., del Olmo, M. F., and Rothwell, J. C. (2006). Age reduces cortical reciprocal inhibition in humans. *Exp. Brain Res.* 171, 322–329. doi:10.1007/s00221-005-0274-9

Hortobagyi, T., Taylor, J. L., Petersen, N. T., Russell, G., and Gandevia, S. C. (2003). Changes in segmental and motor cortical output with contralateral muscle contractions and altered sensory inputs in humans. *J. Neurophysiol.* 90, 2451–2459. doi:10.1152/jn.01001.2002

Hunter, S. K., Todd, G., Butler, J. E., Gandevia, S. C., and Taylor, J. L. (2008). Recovery from supraspinal fatigue is slowed in old adults after fatiguing maximal isometric contractions. *J. Appl. Physiol.* 105, 1199–1209. doi:10.1152/japplphysiol.01246.2007

Hutchinson, S., Kobayashi, M., Horkan, C. M., Pascual-Leone, A., Alexander, M. P., and Schlaug, G. (2002). Age-related differences in movement representation. *Neuroimage* 17, 1720–1728. doi:10.1006/nimg.2002.1309

Jacobson, L., Koslowsky, M., and Lavidor, M. (2012). tDCS polarity effects in motor and cognitive domains: a meta-analytical review. *Exp. Brain Res.* 216, 1–10. doi:10.1007/s00221-011-2891-9

Kamen, G., Sison, S. V., Du, C. C., and Patten, C. (1995). Motor unit discharge behavior in older adults during maximal-effort contractions. *J. Appl. Physiol.* 79, 1908–1913.

Kernell, D. (2006). *The Motoneurone and Its Muscle Fibres.* Oxford: Oxford University Press.

Kernell, D., and Chien-Ping, W. U. (1967). Responses of the pyramidal tract to stimulation of the baboon's motor cortex. *J. Physiol.* 191, 653–672.

Kukulka, C. G., and Clamann, H. P. (1981). Comparison of the recruitment and discharge properties of motor units in human brachial biceps and adductor pollicis during isometric contractions. *Brain Res.* 219, 45–55. doi:10.1016/0006-8993(81)90266-3

Liepert, J., Dettmers, C., Terborg, C., and Weiller, C. (2001). Inhibition of ipsilateral motor cortex during phasic generation of low force. *Clin. Neurophysiol.* 112, 114–121. doi:10.1016/S1388-2457(00)00503-4

Liu, J. Z., Shan, Z. Y., Zhang, L. D., Sahgal, V., Brown, R. W., and Yue, G. H. (2003). Human brain activation during sustained and intermittent submaximal fatigue muscle contractions: an FMRI study. *J. Neurophysiol.* 90, 300–312. doi:10.1152/jn.00821.2002

Logothetis, N. K. (2002). The neural basis of the blood-oxygen-level-dependent functional magnetic resonance imaging signal. *Philos. Trans. R. Soc. Lond. B Biol. Sci.* 357, 1003–1037. doi:10.1098/rstb.2002.1114

Madden, D. J., Whiting, W. L., Huettel, S. A., White, L. E., MacFall, J. R., and Provenzale, J. M. (2004). Diffusion tensor imaging of adult age differences in cerebral white matter: relation to response time. *Neuroimage* 21, 1174–1181. doi:10.1016/j.neuroimage.2003.11.004

Marner, L., Nyengaard, J. R., Tang, Y., and Pakkenberg, B. (2003). Marked loss of myelinated nerve fibers in the human brain with age. *J. Comp. Neurol.* 462, 144–152. doi:10.1002/cne.10714

Martin, P. G., Gandevia, S. C., and Taylor, J. L. (2006). Output of human motoneuron pools to corticospinal inputs during voluntary contractions. *J. Neurophysiol.* 95, 3512–3518. doi:10.1152/jn.01230.2005

Mattay, V. S., Fera, F., Tessitore, A., Hariri, A. R., Das, S., Callicott, J. H., et al. (2002). Neurophysiological correlates of age-related changes in human motor function. *Neurology* 58, 630–635. doi:10.1212/WNL.58.4.630

Matthews, P. B. (1996). Relationship of firing intervals of human motor units to the trajectory of post-spike after-hyperpolarization and synaptic noise. *J. Physiol.* 492, 597–628.

McGinley, M., Hoffman, R. L., Russ, D. W., Thomas, J. S., and Clark, B. C. (2010). Older adults exhibit more intracortical inhibition and less intracortical facilitation than young adults. *Exp. Gerontol.* 45, 671–678. doi:10.1016/j.exger.2010.04.005

McGregor, K. M., Nocera, J. R., Sudhyadhom, A., Patten, C., Manini, T. M., Kleim, J. A., et al. (2013). Effects of aerobic fitness on aging-related changes of interhemispheric inhibition and motor performance. *Front. Aging Neurosci.* 5:66. doi:10.3389/fnagi.2013.00066

McGregor, K. M., Zlatar, Z., Kleim, E., Sudhyadhom, A., Bauer, A., Phan, S., et al. (2011). Physical activity and neural correlates of aging: a combined TMS/fMRI study. *Behav. Brain Res.* 222, 158–168. doi:10.1016/j.bbr.2011.03.042

McNeil, C. J., Giesebrecht, S., Gandevia, S. C., and Taylor, J. L. (2011a). Behaviour of the motoneurone pool in a fatiguing submaximal contraction. *J. Physiol.* 589, 3533–3544. doi:10.1113/jphysiol.2011.207191

McNeil, C. J., Giesebrecht, S., Khan, S. I., Gandevia, S. C., and Taylor, J. L. (2011b). The reduction in human motoneurone responsiveness during muscle fatigue is not prevented by increased muscle spindle discharge. *J. Physiol.* 589, 3731–3738. doi:10.1113/jphysiol.2011.210252

McNeil, C. J., Martin, P. G., Gandevia, S. C., and Taylor, J. L. (2009). The response to paired motor cortical stimuli is abolished at a spinal level during human muscle fatigue. *J. Physiol.* 587, 5601–5612. doi:10.1113/jphysiol.2009.180968

Merton, P. A. (1954). Interaction between muscle fibres in a twitch. *J. Physiol.* 124, 311–324.

Milner-Brown, H. S., Stein, R. B., and Yemm, R. (1973). The orderly recruitment of human motor units during voluntary isometric contractions. *J. Physiol.* 230, 359–370.

Muellbacher, W., Facchini, S., Boroojerdi, B., and Hallett, M. (2000). Changes in motor cortex excitability during ipsilateral hand muscle activation in humans. *Clin. Neurophysiol.* 111, 344–349. doi:10.1016/S1388-2457(99)00243-6

Naccarato, M., Calautti, C., Jones, P. S., Day, D. J., Carpenter, T. A., and Baron, J. C. (2006). Does healthy aging affect the hemispheric activation balance during paced index-to-thumb opposition task? An fMRI study. *Neuroimage* 32, 1250–1256. doi:10.1016/j.neuroimage.2006.05.003

Nitsche, M. A., and Paulus, W. (2011). Transcranial direct current stimulation – update 2011. *Restor. Neurol. Neurosci.* 29, 463–492. doi:10.3233/RNN-2011-0618

Oldfield, R. C. (1971). The assessment and analysis of handedness: the Edinburgh inventory. *Neuropsychologia* 9, 97–113. doi:10.1016/0028-3932(71)90067-4

Oliviero, A., Profice, P., Tonali, P. A., Pilato, F., Saturno, E., Dileone, M., et al. (2006). Effects of aging on motor cortex excitability. *Neurosci. Res.* 55, 74–77. doi:10.1016/j.neures.2006.02.002

Peinemann, A., Lehner, C., Conrad, B., and Siebner, H. R. (2001). Age-related decrease in paired-pulse intracortical inhibition in the human primary motor cortex. *Neurosci. Lett.* 313, 33–36. doi:10.1016/S0304-3940(01)02239-X

Perez, M. A., and Cohen, L. G. (2008). Mechanisms underlying functional changes in the primary motor cortex ipsilateral to an active hand. *J. Neurosci.* 28, 5631–5640. doi:10.1523/JNEUROSCI.0093-08.2008

Perez, M. A., and Cohen, L. G. (2009). Scaling of motor cortical excitability during unimanual force generation. *Cortex* 45, 1065–1071. doi:10.1016/j.cortex.2008.12.006

Pitcher, J. B., Ogston, K. M., and Miles, T. S. (2003). Age and sex differences in human motor cortex input-output characteristics. *J. Physiol.* 546, 605–613. doi:10.1113/jphysiol.2002.029454

Post, M., Bakels, R., and Zijdewind, I. (2009a). Inadvertent contralateral activity during a sustained unilateral contraction reflects the direction of target movement. *J. Neurosci.* 29, 6353–6357. doi:10.1523/JNEUROSCI.0631-09.2009

Post, M., Steens, A., Renken, R., Maurits, N. M., and Zijdewind, I. (2009b). Voluntary activation and cortical activity during a sustained maximal contraction: an fMRI study. *Hum. Brain Mapp.* 30, 1014–1027. doi:10.1002/hbm.20562

Post, M., Bayrak, S., Kernell, D., and Zijdewind, I. (2008). Contralateral muscle activity and fatigue in the human first dorsal interosseous muscle. *J. Appl. Physiol.* 105, 70–82. doi:10.1152/japplphysiol.01298.2007

Riecker, A., Groschel, K., Ackermann, H., Steinbrink, C., Witte, O., and Kastrup, A. (2006). Functional significance of age-related differences in motor activation patterns. *Neuroimage* 32, 1345–1354. doi:10.1016/j.neuroimage.2006.05.021

Rossini, P. M., Barker, A. T., Berardelli, A., Caramia, M. D., Caruso, G., Cracco, R. Q., et al. (1994). Non-invasive electrical and magnetic stimulation of the brain, spinal cord and roots: basic principles and procedures for routine clinical application. Report of an IFCN committee. *Electroencephalogr. Clin. Neurophysiol.* 91, 79–92. doi:10.1016/0013-4694(94)90029-9

Sale, M. V., and Semmler, J. G. (2005). Age-related differences in corticospinal control during functional isometric contractions in left and right hands. *J. Appl. Physiol.* 99, 1483–1493. doi:10.1152/japplphysiol.00371.2005

Sehm, B., Perez, M. A., Xu, B., Hidler, J., and Cohen, L. G. (2010). Functional neuroanatomy of mirroring during a unimanual force generation task. *Cereb. Cortex* 20, 34–45. doi:10.1093/cercor/bhp075

Seidler, R. D., Bernard, J. A., Burutolu, T. B., Fling, B. W., Gordon, M. T., Gwin, J. T., et al. (2010). Motor control and aging: links to age-related brain structural, functional, and biochemical effects. *Neurosci. Biobehav. Rev.* 34, 721–733. doi:10.1016/j.neubiorev.2009.10.005

Shinohara, M., Keenan, K. G., and Enoka, R. M. (2003). Contralateral activity in a homologous hand muscle during voluntary contractions is greater in old adults. *J. Appl. Physiol.* 94, 966–974. doi:10.1152/japplphysiol.00836.2002

Smith, A. E., Ridding, M. C., Higgins, R. D., Wittert, G. A., and Pitcher, J. B. (2009). Age-related changes in short-latency motor cortex inhibition. *Exp. Brain Res.* 198, 489–500. doi:10.1007/s00221-009-1945-8

Snijders, T., and Bosker, R. (1999). *Multilevel Analysis: An Introduction to Basic and Advanced Multilevel Modeling.* London: Sage Publications Inc.

Stedman, A., Davey, N. J., and Ellaway, P. H. (1998). Facilitation of human first dorsal interosseous muscle responses to transcranial magnetic stimulation during voluntary contraction of the contralateral homonymous muscle. *Muscle Nerve* 21, 1033–1039. doi:10.1002/(SICI)1097-4598(199808)21:8<1033::AID-MUS7>3.0.CO;2-9

Taki, Y., Thyreau, B., Kinomura, S., Sato, K., Goto, R., Wu, K., et al. (2013). A longitudinal study of age- and gender-related annual rate of volume changes in regional gray matter in healthy adults. *Hum. Brain Mapp.* 34, 2292–2301. doi:10.1002/hbm.22067

Talelli, P., Ewas, A., Waddingham, W., Rothwell, J. C., and Ward, N. S. (2008a). Neural correlates of age-related changes in cortical neurophysiology. *Neuroimage* 40, 1772–1781. doi:10.1016/j.neuroimage.2008.01.039

Talelli, P., Waddingham, W., Ewas, A., Rothwell, J. C., and Ward, N. S. (2008b). The effect of age on task-related modulation of interhemispheric balance. *Exp. Brain Res.* 186, 59–66. doi:10.1007/s00221-007-1205-8

Tinazzi, M., and Zanette, G. (1998). Modulation of ipsilateral motor cortex in man during unimanual finger movements of different complexities. *Neurosci. Lett.* 244, 121–124. doi:10.1016/S0304-3940(98)00150-5

Ugawa, Y., Hanajima, R., and Kanazawa, I. (1993). Interhemispheric facilitation of the hand area of the human motor cortex. *Neurosci. Lett.* 160, 153–155. doi:10.1016/0304-3940(93)90401-6

van Duinen, H., Renken, R., Maurits, N., and Zijdewind, I. (2007). Effects of motor fatigue on human brain activity, an fMRI study. *Neuroimage* 35, 1438–1449. doi:10.1016/j.neuroimage.2007.02.008

Ward, N. S., and Frackowiak, R. S. (2003). Age-related changes in the neural correlates of motor performance. *Brain* 126, 873–888. doi:10.1093/brain/awg071

Wu, T., and Hallett, M. (2005). The influence of normal human ageing on automatic movements. *J. Physiol.* 562, 605–615. doi:10.1113/jphysiol.2004.076042

Zhou, D., Lebel, C., Evans, A., and Beaulieu, C. (2013). Cortical thickness asymmetry from childhood to older adulthood. *Neuroimage* 83, 66–74. doi:10.1016/j.neuroimage.2013.06.073

Zijdewind, I., Butler, J. E., Gandevia, S. C., and Taylor, J. L. (2006). The origin of activity in the biceps brachii muscle during voluntary contractions of the contralateral elbow flexor muscles. *Exp. Brain Res.* 175, 526–535. doi:10.1007/s00221-006-0570-z

Zijdewind, I., and Kernell, D. (1994). Index finger position and force of the human first dorsal interosseus and its ulnar nerve antagonist. *J. Appl. Physiol.* 77, 987–997.

Zijdewind, I., and Kernell, D. (2001). Bilateral interactions during contractions of intrinsic hand muscles. *J. Neurophysiol.* 85, 1907–1913.

Zijdewind, I., Zwarts, M. J., and Kernell, D. (1998). Influence of a voluntary fatigue test on the contralateral homologous muscle in humans? *Neurosci. Lett.* 253, 41–44. doi:10.1016/S0304-3940(98)00609-0

Zimerman, M., Heise, K. F., Gerloff, C., Cohen, L. G., and Hummel, F. C. (2012). Disrupting the ipsilateral motor cortex interferes with training of a complex motor task in older adults. *Cereb. Cortex.* doi:10.1093/cercor/bhs385

10

Aging interferes central control mechanism for eccentric muscle contraction

Wan X. Yao[1]*, Jinqi Li[2], Zhiguo Jiang[3,4], Jia-Hong Gao[5], Crystal G. Franklin[2], Yufei Huang[1], Jack L. Lancaster[2] and Guang H. Yue[3]*

[1] *Department of Kinesiology, Health, and Nutrition, College of Education and Human Development, The University of Texas at San Antonio, San Antonio, TX, USA*
[2] *Research Imaging Institute, The University of Texas Health Science Center at San Antonio, San Antonio, TX, USA*
[3] *Human Performance and Engineering Laboratory, Kessler Foundation Research Center, West Orange, NJ, USA*
[4] *Department of Biomedical Engineering, New Jersey Institute of Technology, Newark, NJ, USA*
[5] *IDG/McGovern Institute for Brain Research, Peking University, Beijing, China*

Edited by:
Brian C. Clark, Ohio University, USA

Reviewed by:
Kentaro Oki, Ohio University, USA
Sheng Li, University Texas-Houston, USA

***Correspondence:**
Wan X. Yao, Department of Kinesiology, Health, and Nutrition, College of Education and Human Development, The University of Texas at San Antonio, San Antonio, TX 78249, USA
e-mail: wanxiang.yao@utsa.edu;
Guang H. Yue, Human Performance and Engineering Laboratory, Kessler Foundation Research Center, 1199 Pleasant Valley Way, West Orange, NJ 07052, USA
e-mail: gyue@kesslerfounation.org

Previous studies report greater activation in the cortical motor network in controlling eccentric contraction (EC) than concentric contraction (CC) despite lower muscle activation level associated with EC vs. CC in healthy, young individuals. It is unknown, however, whether elderly people exhibiting increased difficulties in performing EC than CC possess this unique cortical control mechanism for EC movements. To address this question, we examined functional magnetic resonance imaging (fMRI) data acquired during EC and CC of the first dorsal interosseous (FDI) muscle in 11 young (20–32 years) and 9 old (67–73 years) individuals. During the fMRI experiment, all subjects performed 20 CC and 20 EC of the right FDI with the same angular distance and velocity. The major findings from the behavioral and fMRI data analysis were that (1) movement stability was poorer in EC than CC in the old but not the young group; (2) similar to previous electrophysiological and fMRI reports, the EC resulted in significantly stronger activation in the motor control network consisting of primary, secondary and association motor cortices than CC in the young and old groups; (3) the biased stronger activation towards EC was significantly greater in the old than the young group especially in the secondary and association cortices such as supplementary and premotor motor areas and anterior cingulate cortex; and (4) in the primary motor and sensory cortices, the biased activation towards EC was significantly greater in the young than the old group. Greater activation in higher-order cortical fields for controlling EC movement by elderly adults may reflect activities in these regions to compensate for aging-related impairments in the ability to control complex EC movements. Our finding is useful for potentially guiding the development of targeted therapies to counteract age-related movement deficits and to prevent injury.

Keywords: brain activation, concentric contraction, eccentric contraction, fMRI, movement stability

INTRODUCTION

Our daily movements consist of shortening (concentric) and lengthening (eccentric) muscle contractions and it has well been documented that mechanical and neurophysiological characteristics of an eccentric contraction (EC) differ in many ways from those of a concentric contraction (CC) despite the fact that the two types of muscle activities are accomplished by the same muscle(s; See Duchateau and Enoka, 2008 for review). For example, after a period (30 min) of repetitive eccentric and concentric contractions at 50% maximal intensity, only those who performed eccentric exercise showed a significant reduction in mechanical stiffness and an increase in magnetic resonance imaging (MRI) T_2 relaxation time of the working muscle (Sesto et al., 2008). In addition, previous studies (Nardone et al., 1988; Howell et al., 1995) suggest that EC and CC may follow different motor-unit recruitment orders during non-fatigue muscle contractions [However, see Bawa and Jones (1999) and Kossev and Christova (1998) for contradictory findings]. Furthermore, compared to CC, EC had a smaller magnitude of electromyographic (EMG) signal against a given resistance, and depressed corticospinal neuron (Abbruzzese et al., 1994; Sekiguchi et al., 2001) and monosynaptic reflex (Moritani et al., 1988; Abbruzzese et al., 1994) excitability. Moritani et al. (1988) attributed the lower level of EMG for EC to fewer motor units being recruited and a lower discharge rate of the active motor units. Recent studies by Duclay and Martin (2005), Duclay et al. (2011) postulate that the differences in EMG activities between the two types of contractions are a result of differential modulations of motoneuron excitability at supraspinal and/or spinal levels and the modulation of the spinal motoneuron excitability by the supraspinal centers can be contraction-type specific (Duclay et al., 2009). T together, the aforementioned findings indicate a possible different neural control strategy for EC from the one for CC.

In an attempt to delineate potential differential central control mechanisms between voluntary EC and CC, Fang et al. (2001, 2004)conducted two studies to monitor electroencephalography (EEG) signals at submaxial and maximal intensity levels. They found that although the elbow flexor muscle activities (EMG) were lower during EC than CC, the magnitude of movement-related cortical potential (MRCP) derived from the EEG recordings was significantly greater for EC than CC at both intensity levels. They hypothesized that the greater cortical signal (MRCP) for EC might be due to greater effort in planning and programming the lengthening contractions that are more difficult to perform, prone to muscle tissue damage, and may possibly be involved with a different control strategy such as a reversed motor unit recruitment order. More recently, Kwon and Park (2011) examined brain activation patterns by quantifying functional MRI (fMRI) signals in the primary motor cortex, inferior parietal lobe, pre-supplementary area, anterior cingulate cortex, prefrontal cortex, and cerebellum in healthy young adults. They found that except in the right primary motor cortex, the EC resulted in greater fMRI signals than CC in all examined cortical areas. In summary, all three studies that directly monitored brain activities (Fang et al., 2001, 2004; Kwon and Park, 2011) reported a greater activation level in the cortical functional neural network in controlling eccentric than concentric muscle contractions despite a lower muscle activation level associated with EC than CC in healthy young individuals.

In the field of motor control research in aging, literature has consistently demonstrated that elderly individuals exhibit poorer movement stability or force steadiness during EC than CC (Laidlaw et al., 1999, 2002). Although movement stability during EC is also poorer than CC in young individuals, the magnitude of deficit is significantly larger in old than young age groups (Laidlaw et al., 1999, 2002), indicating force/movement control ability for EC is more affected in older adults and this poses greater risks for injury during EC activities. However, central control mechanisms between CC and EC in older adults have never been investigated. Given the expectation that poor control of EC by muscles such as quadriceps during walking downstairs may increase chances of falls, it is important to understand the central nervous systems (CNS) physiological factors contributing to a loss of EC control ability in later life. All findings from previous research seem to support the notion that differential central control mechanisms for EC and CC movements reflect activities of the CNS in dealing with unique strategies in recruiting motor units, altered means in producing force and power, and increased risks of tissue damage during EC. However, it is unknown whether old people exhibiting increased difficulties in performing EC than CC still possess the unique cortical control mechanism for EC like their younger counterparts. The purpose of the study was to address this question. It was hypothesized that the control mechanism (indicated by brain activation pattern) for EC and CC in an aging population would be different from the one adopted by young individuals based on the observation of different neuromuscular characteristics in aging including substantially worsened EC performance compared to young adults (Burnett et al., 2000; Hortobagyi et al., 2001; Laidlaw et al., 2002).

MATERIALS AND METHODS

SUBJECTS

Eleven young (4 males, 23.25 ± 4.09 years old, ranging from 20 to 32 years) and nine old (3 males, 68.72 ± 3.14 years old, ranging from 67 to 73) subjects participated in the study. All subjects were right-handed determined by the Edinburgh inventory (Oldfield, 1971) without neurological, neuromuscular, and musculoskeletal impairments. The study was approved by the Institutional Review Boards of the University of Texas at San Antonio and the University of Texas Health Science Center at San Antonio. Written informed consents were obtained from all the subjects prior to their participation.

TASKS AND EXPERIMENTAL SETUP

The subjects performed either concentric (muscle shortening, index finger moving towards the thumb) or eccentric (muscle lengthening, index finger passively moving away from the thumb) contractions of the first dorsal interosseous (FDI) muscle. Each type of contraction resulted in a 20-degree angular movement from the initial position against a constant load (30% of maximal isometric contraction of the FDI) with a constant speed (~10 degree/s or ~0.174 rad/s). After a practicing block of 20 concentric contractions (CC) and 20 eccentric contractions (EC), a total of 20 CC and 20 EC testing trials were performed while functional brain images were taken. During the practice and testing, CC and EC were performed alternately (e.g., CC → EC → CC...) while the subjects were lying supine in the MRI chamber with right arm and hand resting prone on a wooden board. The right arm was abducted 10° at shoulder joint with the elbow joint flexed to ~10°. The wrist, thumb, and the other three (middle, ring, and little) fingers of the right hand were constrained. The right index finger was fastened to a movable lever attached to a load (30% maximal) through a non-elastic cable and a pulley fixed on the wooden board. The subjects performed CC of the right FDI muscle from the initial position (IP) by lifting the weight to the end position (EP) and EC from the EP by "lowering" the weight to the IP. A 10-s rest was provided after each contraction during which the weight was supported by an external mechanism.

MEASUREMENTS AND DATA PROCESSING

Maximum voluntary contraction

Isometric maximum voluntary contraction (MVC) force was measured by requesting the subjects maximally abduct their right index figure against an unmovable force transducer (Sensotec, Columbus, OH, USA). Each subject performed two MVC trials and the trial with the higher peak force was chosen for further analysis. There was a 1-min rest between the two MVC trials.

Movement distance, speed and stability

A custom-built, MRI-compatible goniometer for measuring the angular/movement distance and speed of the finger was attached to the movable lever. The movement data for both CC and EC were trigger-averaged across the 20 trials for each subject with a trigger signal, which was generated when the finger moved 2° from the IP (10% of the movement distance) for CC and 2° from the EP (Fang et al., 2001, 2004). The movement speed was then derived from the trigger-averaged movement data. Standard deviation of the speed was taken to indicate stability of each movement.

Image acquisition

The fMRI procedures (Gao et al., 1996; Yue et al., 2000) are based on detecting changes in brain blood oxygenation – the so-called blood oxygenation level dependent (BOLD) signal changes. Functional images were acquired by a 3-T Magnetom Trio scanner (Siemens, Erlangen, Germany) with a 8-channel RF head coil using a single shot gradient echo EPI pulse sequence (TR = 2 s, TE = 30 ms, flip angle = 90°). The subjects were positioned supine on the sliding board of the scanner with his/her head positioned in the head coil. The head was stabilized by padded restraints. Subjects were told to remain as still as possible during the experiments. Both T1-weighted anatomical images and functional images were collected in the same transverse plane (aligned with a line connecting the anterior and posterior commissures). Each brain volume consisted of 21 slices (5 mm slice thickness and 1 mm inter slice gap) that covered the brain and cerebellum. (The collection of 1 brain volume was referred to as 1 scan hereafter.) The image field of view and matrix for the anatomical images were 256 × 256 mm and 256 × 256, respectively; and those for the function images were 256 × 256 mm and 128 × 128, yielding an in-plane spatial resolution of 1 × 1 mm for anatomical images and 2 × 2 mm for functional images. Pulse sequence for the anatomic image acquisition was TR/TE/flip angle = 2200 ms/2.83 ms/13°, non-selective inversion pulse, TI = 785 ms. All anatomical images were acquired after fMRI scans.

DATA ANALYSIS

The fMRI data were processed using FMRIB Software Library (FSL; Woolrich et al., 2009) and codes written in MATLAB (Math Works, Natick, MA). Image pre-processing procedures included skull stripping, motion correction, temporal filtering, and spatial smoothing with a Gaussian filter of 5 mm at FWHM. A non-linear Gaussian temporal filter was applied using a high-pass threshold of 100 s. Activation maps were generated using the general linear modeling (GLM) in the FEAT toolbox in FSL on a voxel-by-voxel basis and a threshold of $Z = 3.0$ ($p < 0.01$). All echo-planar images were co-registered first to each subject's corresponding anatomical images and then to the Collin brain, a high-resolution template (0.2 mm isotropic resolution) from a population-based, pseudo-Talairach space, before the activated volume and the subsequent group fMRI data were analyzed. A 2-way ANOVA (group × task) was employed to analyze movement parameters (speed and stability) and fMRI (volume passing activation threshold) results in each brain region showing CC- or EC-related activation. To better understand the relative activation level in each cortical area displaying strong activities during CC and EC, we calculated an EC-to-CC activation ratio in each area in each group. Independent *t*-test was employed to analyze the ratio data between the groups. Statistic significance level was set at $P = 0.05$ for all the analyses.

RESULTS

MVC

The mean MVC forces for the young and old groups were 48.9 ± 3.67 N and 40.3 ± 3.89 N, respectively. The independent *t*-test revealed a non-significant difference in MVC force between the two groups, $t(18) = 1.597$, $p = 0.128$.

MOVEMENT SPEED AND STABILITY

The mean speeds of EC and CC for the young group were 0.167 ± 0.015 rad/s and 0.174 ± 0.011 rad/s, respectively. For the old group, the speeds of EC and CC were 0.171 ± 0.020 rad/s and 0.170 ± 0.014 rad/s, respectively. The main effects for the age group and movement type analyzed by the 2-way ANOVA were not significant, $F(1,18) = 0.003$, $P = 0.96$, and $F(1,18) = 0.252$, $P = 0.622$, respectively; nor was the interaction between the two factors, $F(1,18) = 0.51$, $P = 0.484$. The standard deviations of the speed, representing movement stability, revealed a significant main effect for movement type but not group, $F(1,18) = 15.65$, $P = 0.001$, and $F(1,18) = 2.572$, $P = 0.126$, respectively. The interaction between the two factors on the movement stability was also significant, $F(1,18) = 5.896$, $P = 0.026$. The *post hoc* paired *t*-test on the movement stability was not significant between EC and CC for the young group, $t(10) = 1.299$, $P = 0.22$. In contrast; it was significant between the two movement types for the old group, $t(8) = 3.789$, $P < 0.01$ (**Figure 1**).

fMRI

The fMRI results revealed activation of a number of motor control-related cortical fields associated with the CC and EC in the left hemisphere contralateral to the performing (right) hand (see **Table 1** and **Figure 2**). For the young group, the activation was almost exclusively in the left hemisphere with the common threshold ($Z = 3.0$) set for activation detection in both groups. For the old group, the ipsilateral (right hemisphere) activation was stronger than young group but was still at a low level compared to the contralateral side (**Figures 2** and **3**). Since our primary interest was to learn potential brain activation difference between controlling CC and EC and the effect of aging on the differences and since the young group had almost no ipsilateral activation, our analysis was mainly focused on activation of the contralateral hemisphere

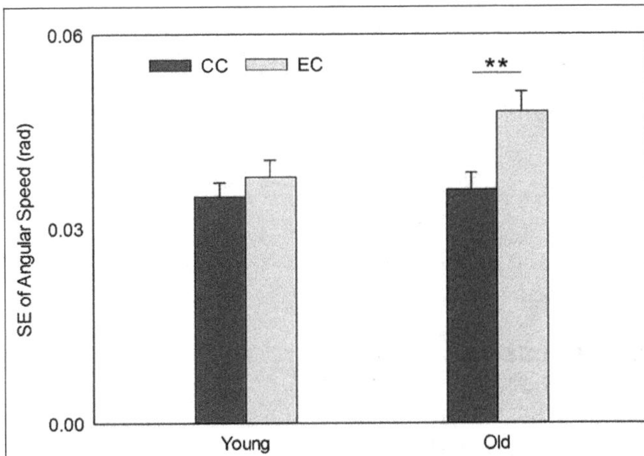

FIGURE 1 | Movement stability was poorer during EC (indicated by greater standard error [SE]) than CC in the old group but no such difference in the young group. $^{**}P < 0.01$.

Table 1 | The volume of brain areas activated during CC and EC.

		CC				EC				Volume (mm^3)	
		x	*y*	*z*	*Z*	*x*	*y*	*z*	*Z*	CC (M/SE)	EC (M/SE)
SMA	Young	3	−12	54	3.34	1	−12	54	4.13	533/86	1229/105
	Old	1	−13	52	3.23	2	−11	55	3.72	422/77	1635/167
ACC	Young	4	−6	44	3.41	−2	−10	43	3.27	301/35	457/64
	Old	−5	−10	42	3.26	4	−8	41	3.54	99/22	438/93
Lt. S1	Young	−40	−24	56	3.81	−28	−28	57	3.69	285/52	711/102
	Old	−41	−22	56	3.91	−27	−28	58	3.65	160/20	175/22
Rt. S1	Young	–	–	–	–	–	–	–	–	–	–
	Old	–	–	–	–	38	−28	56	3.05	–	136/22
Lt. PMC	Young	−24	−17	58	3.16	−21	−18	58	3.39	128/26	182/35
	Old	−23	−15	55	3.12	−22	−14	54	3.34	92/17	228/45
Lt. IPL	Young	−46	−33	52	3.45	−32	−38	52	3.21	249/29	278/31
	Old	−47	−32	52	3.56	−32	−37	53	3.61	196/23	265/62
Rt. IPL	Young	–	–	–	–	–	–	–	–	–	–
	Old	–	–	–	–	40	−43	44	3.41	186/23	192/48
Lt. M1	Young	−38	−23	57	3.46	−35	−22	57	3.42	129/35	748/114
	Old	−38	−21	55	3.12	−37	−26	56	3.70	98/18	443/76
Rt. M1	Young	–	–	–	–	–	–	–	–	–	–
	Old	–	–	–	–	20	−26	56	3.29	–	192/26
Rt. CBM	Young	28	−54	−26	3.06	30	−56	−20	3.32	108/7.6	178/14
	Old	33	−67	−21	3.27	32	−60	−20	3.20	188/36	172/23
Med. CBM	Young	–	–	–	–	–	–	–	–	–	–
	Old	8	−58	−28	3.12	16	−68	−24	3.02	90/12	330/27
Lt. Insula	Young	−47	−22	18	3.24	−40	−28	18	3.30	128/22	776/98
	Old	–	–	–	–	–	–	–	–	–	–
Lt. Sup Tem Gyri	Young	–	–	–	–	−46	−36	−14	3.07	–	784/116
	Old	–	–	–	–	–	–	–	–	–	–
Rt. Sup Tem Gyri	Young	–	–	–	–	−48	−45	−16	3.07	–	224/28
	Old	–	–	–	–	–	–	–	–	–	–
Lt. Putamen	Young	–	–	–	–	–	–	–	–	–	–
	Old	−22	3	−6	3.52	−22	−5	9	3.52	264/30	264/20
Rt. Putamen	Young	–	–	–	–	–	–	–	–	–	–
	Old	23	3	−6	3.17	21	−4	7	3.52	128/30	168/20

although ipsilateral activation results were also briefly reported and discussed.

ANOVA RESULTS

Medial BA6 (SMA)

Activation in the supplementary motor area (SMA) showed a significant main effect for movement type, $F(1,18) = 98.71$, $P < 0.0001$ but not for group, $F(1,18) = 2.07$, $P = 0.17$. There was a significant interaction between the two factors on the fMRI measure, $F(1,18) = 6.10$, $P = 0.024$. *Post hoc* independent t-test revealed a significantly greater activation for the elderly than young during EC but not during CC, $t(18) = 2.139$, $P = 0.046$, and $t(18) = 0.241$, $P = 0.81$, respectively (both **Figures 2** and **3** show SMA activation).

BA24 (anterior cingulate cortex)

Activation in the anterior cingulate cortex (ACC) showed a significant main effect for movement type, $F(1,18) = 24.95$, $P < 0.0001$ and a boarder-line significant main effect for group, $F(1,18) = 3.02$, $P = 0.099$. There was a significant interaction between the two factors on the fMRI signal, $F(1,18) = 4.46$, $P = 0.049$. *Post hoc* independent t-test demonstrated a significantly

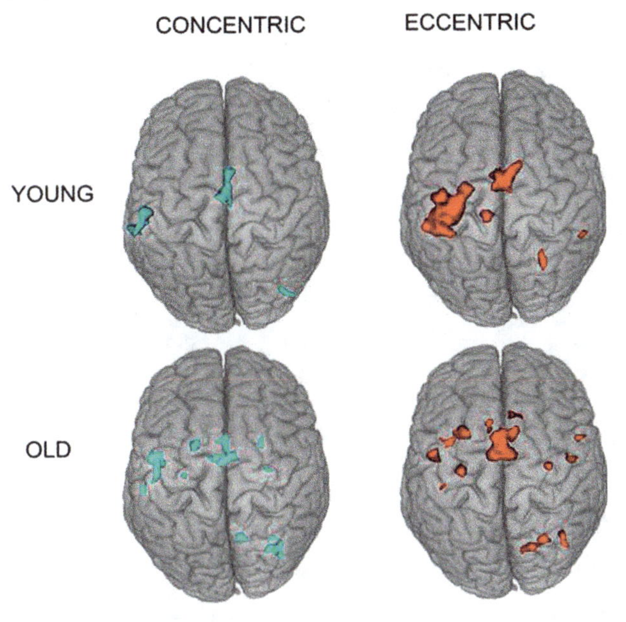

FIGURE 2 | Superior view of group activation during the two types of contractions in the two groups. It is clear that brain activation in young individuals are more localized in the contralateral (left) hemisphere but that in older adults are more distributed in the two hemispheres.

greater activation for the young than elderly during CC but not during EC, $t(18) = 4.94$, $P = 0.0001$, and $t(18) = 0.175$, $P = 0.86$, respectively (**Figure 3** shows ACC activation in both groups).

BA3,1,2 (primary sensory cortex)

Activation in the primary sensory cortex (S1) showed a significant main effect for both group and movement type, $F(1,18) = 22.07$, $P < 0.0001$ and $F(1,18) = 10.49$, $P < 0.005$, respectively. The interaction between the two factors was also significant, $F(1,18) = 11.01$, $P < 0.005$. *Post hoc* paired t-tests showed a significantly greater activation during EC than CC in the young group but not in the old group, $t(10) = 3.70$, $P = 0.004$, and $t(8) = 0.196$, $P = 0.849$, respectively.

BA4 (primary motor cortex)

Activation in the primary motor cortex (M1) showed a significant main effect for movement type, $F(1,18) = 53.10$, $P < 0.0001$ but not for group, $F(1,18) = 1.86$, $P = 0.19$; nor the interaction effect, $F(1,18) = 1.71$, $P = 0.21$.

Lateral BA6 (premotor cortex)

The premotor cortex (PMC) activation exhibited a significant main effect for movement type, $F(1,18) = 18.83$, $P < 0.0001$ but not for group, $F(1,18) = 2.05$, $P = 0.17$; nor the effect oFinteraction, $F(1,18) = 0.002$, $P = 0.97$.

BA40 (inferior parietal lobule)

Activation in the inferior parietal lobule (IPL) displayed a significant main effect for movement type, $F(1,18) = 4.74$, $P < 0.05$ but not for group, $F(1,18) = 0.70$, $P = 0.42$; nor the effect oFinteraction, $F(1,18) = 1.59$, $P = 0.22$.

Cerebellum

Activation in the cerebellum (CBM) showed a significant main effect for both movement type, $F(1,18) = 10.57$, $P < 0.01$ and group, $F(1,18) = 58.55$, $P < 0.001$. There was no significant interaction between the two factors on the fMRI signal, $F(1,18) = 2.90$, $P = 0.11$ (detailed activation results in all analyzed brain regions are listed in **Table 1**).

IPSILATERAL ACTIVATION AND ACTIVATION IN YOUNG OR OLD GROUP ONLY

Table 1 shows that ipsilateral (right) hemisphere activation during EC was only observed in S1, IPL and M1 in the elderly group. Only the old group had activation in both the left and right putamen during both CC and EC. Interestingly, only the young group demonstrated activation during EC in the left and right superior temporal gyri (Sup Tem Gyri) and during both CC and EC in the left insular cortex (**Table 1**).

EC-TO-CC RATIO RESULTS

The EC-to-CC activation ratio is a measure of relative cortical activation between the two types of contractions in a given brain region in a given subject or subject group. It is striking to see that all the seven regions in which activation occurred during both CC and EC in both groups showed a higher-than-1 ratio (greater activation during EC). In addition, three out of four higher-order cortical fields (SMA, ACC and PMC [except IPL]) exhibited a significantly higher EC-to-CC ratio in the old than the young group, $t(18) = 4.75$, $P < 0.001$; $t(18) = 4.36$, $P = 0.0001$; $t(18) = 3.96$, $P < 0.001$, respectively. The IPL and CBM although exhibited a higher EC-to-CC ratio in the old than the young group, the differences did not reach statistical significance, $t(18) = 1.15$, $P = 0.263$; $t(18) = 0.41$, $P = 0.687$, respectively. In contrast, the two primary motor and sensory cortices (M1 and S1) showed a reversed pattern: the EC-to-CC activation ratio was higher in the young than the old group, $t(18) = -3.86$, $P < 0.001$, and $t(18) = -5.01$, $P < 0.001$, respectively (**Table 2**).

DISCUSSION

The purpose of this study was to determine if older adults use different central nervous system (CNS) strategies to control concentric (CC, shortening) and eccentric (EC, lengthening) muscle contractions compared with young individuals. Gaining this knowledge is important as CC and EC comprise all of our daily movements. In addition, EC movements are more complex and difficult to control than CC especially for older adults, which poses increased chances of injuries such as falls during walking downstairs (EC of quadriceps) in elders. Knowing the mechanism could potentially help design more targeted therapeutic programs to prevent or reduce chances of such injuries. In general, the activation level (activation volume measured by fMRI) was higher during EC than CC in all cortical regions and cerebellum in both young and old groups, indicating that EC requires greater cortical resources to accomplish the movement. The finding of higher EC-to-CC activation ratio in a number of high-order cortical fields in the old than the young group suggests that the EC is even more difficult to perform in later life compared to early adulthood and this is supported by the poorer

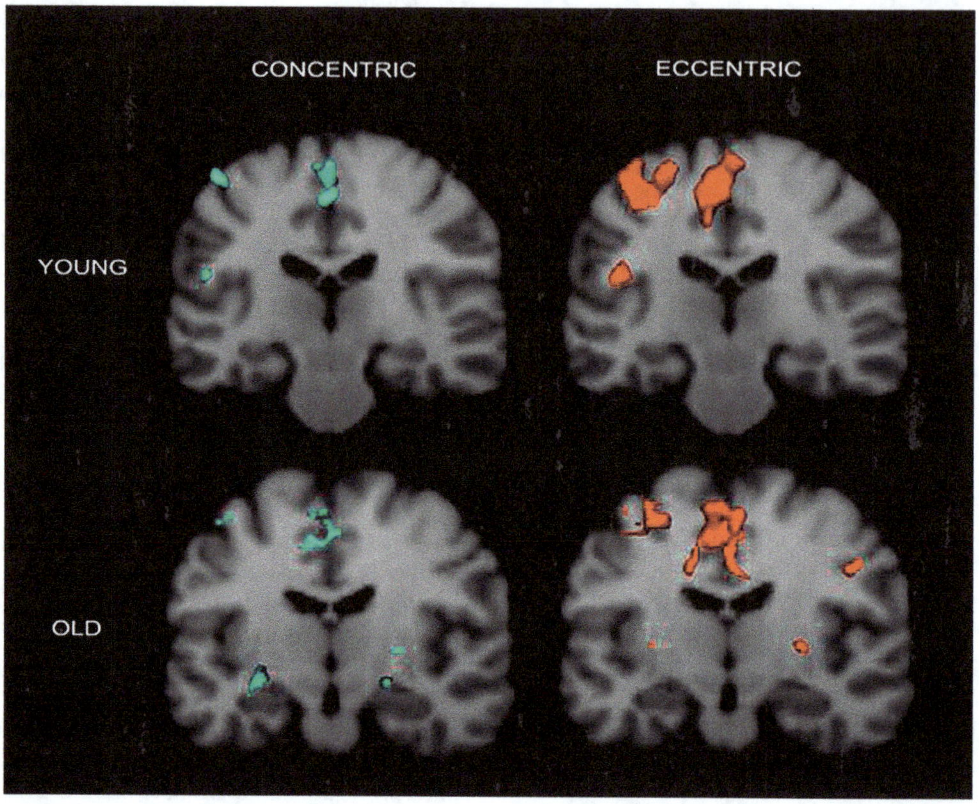

FIGURE 3 | Cronal view of group activation during the two types of contractions in the two groups. Again the figure shows that brain activation in young individuals are more localized in the contralateral (left) hemisphere but that in older adults are more distributed in the two hemispheres. Colored spots in the near-top central regions represent activated voxels in SMA and ACC.

Table 2 | EC-to-CC ratio in the cortical areas and cerebellum in young and old groups.

	SMA* (M/SE)	ACC* (M/SE)	S1* (M/SE)	PMC* (M/SE)	IPL (M/SE)	M1* (M/SE)	CBM (M/SE)
Young	2.31/0.21	1.52/0.23	2.49/0.29	1.42/0.10	1.12/0.04	5.80/0.24	1.65/0.12
Old	3.87/0.25	4.42/0.67	1.09/0.12	2.48/0.25	1.35/0.23	4.52/0.23	1.81/0.27

**t-test showing a significant difference in the ratio between young and old groups.*

movement stability during EC than CC in the old group (Laidlaw et al., 1999).

The general finding of greater cortical activation during EC than CC is consistent with all three previous studies that examined brain signals during the two types of muscle activities (Fang et al., 2001, 2004; Kwon and Park, 2011). The current study provides new evidence supporting the notion that a higher level of complexity of thè EC movement poses greater difficulties for one to perform, which demands additional planning, programming, sensorimotor integration and movement execution by the entire central control network. Compared to a CC, an EC is associated with greater movement variability (Laidlaw et al., 1999, 2002), causes more muscle damage especially at a high contraction intensity (Shellock et al., 1991), is possibly accomplished by a different motor unit recruitment strategy (Nardone et al., 1988; Howell et al., 1995), and produces greater force with a given neural signal (EMG; Fang et al., 2001, 2004). These characteristics of EC likely make EC movements more complex and difficult to control compared with CC movements.

Although in principal our fMRI findings are similar to fMRI results of Kwon and Park (2011), there is a substantial contradiction regarding activation in the primary motor cortex (M1). While we observed a larger activation volume in M1 during EC than CC in both groups (see **Tables 1** and **2**), they found that CC was associated with greater M1 activities than EC in young individuals. Kwon and Park (2011) argued that because M1 was traditionally considered to be responsible for movement execution rather than for planning/programming, it was reasonable to see more M1 activity during CC than EC as CC is involved with a higher level of EMG or greater motor unit activities (Fang et al., 2001, 2004). However, recent studies (Lemon, 2008; Kalaska, 2009) report that M1 is not only involved in executing a movement via its direct pathway to motor neuron pool in the spinal cord but also plays an important role in planning the movement. Possible explanations for the different observations regarding M1 activation during EC and CC between the two studies may be attributed to distinct muscles employed for the movements [FDI in our study and wrist extensors in Kwon and Park (2011)] and the load applied to the contractions (we applied 30% maximal load but the other study did not apply an external load). In addition, stronger brain activities found in M1 during EC in our study could be due to M1's engagement in planning the EC movements to deal with its high degree of movement difficulty. Further research is warranted to better delineate the role of M1 in controlling EC and CC contractions. The following discussion focuses on old and young comparisons especially in the secondary and association cortical areas linked to the EC and CC tasks.

Activation during EC vs. CC in secondary and association cortices

A major finding of the current study is that although both young and old groups exhibited greater cortical activation during EC than CC, this biased brain activation towards EC was more prominent in the old than the young group especially in the secondary and association cortices. For example, the old group showed a significantly higher EC-to-CC ratio in SMA, PMC and ACC than the young group (the EC-to-CC activation ratio in the IPL was also higher in the old than the young group but did not reach the significance level; **Table 2**). The ANOVA results revealed significantly stronger EC-than-CC activation in the old than the young groups in the SMA and ACC. The role of these higher-order cortical fields in motor control is well described in a standard neuroscience textbook (Part VI / Movement, Kandel et al., 2013). Among these higher-order control centers, the SMA and ACC demonstrated a significantly higher activation level by old than young adults during EC vs. CC shown by both the ANOVA and EC-to-CC ratio analyses, indicating that the two areas play an exceptionally important role in modulating EC movement in later life. It is well known that the SMA is a secondary motor area (consisted of SMA proper and pre-SMA) and is involved in controlling complex and coordinated motor acts (Rizzolatti and Strick, 2013). Given the complex nature of the EC (compared to CC) and its increased level of difficulty (poorer EC movement stability) in late adulthood, it is not surprising to see augmented activity in the SMA during EC in older adults. It has been known that the cingulate association cortex is a part of limbic system that controls emotion, motivation and other cognitive functions. Within the cingulate cortex, however, there exist distinct motor areas in ACC adjacent to the SMA with connections to the M1 and parietal association cortex, and they (SMA and ACC) are considered as an integrated motor control center (termed as medial premotor area) and shared similar functions in motor control (Rizzolatti and Strick, 2013).

In the sole study that compared brain activation patterns between CC and EC in healthy young individuals using fMRI, activation level in the SMA and ACC was seen to be significantly higher during EC than CC (Kwon and Park, 2011). Our study not only confirms this finding in young adulthood but also demonstrates that the biased activation in the SMA and ACC towards EC was even significantly more prominent in older adults than their younger counterparts. We postulate that the SMA and ACC play a special role in modulating EC performance in aging, perhaps by compensating for age-related degenerative adaptations in the motor control network that might have specially deteriorated the network's ability to control more complex EC movements. The PMC (lateral BA6 consisted of dorsal and ventral PMC, a secondary motor area) showed a significantly higher EC-to-CC activation ratio and the IPL (part of parietal association cortex) also exhibited a clearly higher EC-to-CC ratio (**Table 2**). The motor function of PMC (Rizzolatti and Kalaska, 2013; Rizzolatti and Strick, 2013) and IPL (Fogassi and Luppino, 2005) has been well described and the role of their prominent activation during EC during late life may be similar to that played by the SMA and ACC.

Cerebellum activation during EC vs. CC

The 2-way ANOVA analysis revealed significant main effects for both movement type and group and no significant effect for interaction which means that the cerebellar activation was greater during EC than CC for both groups and the old group exhibited a higher level of cerebellar activation than the young group. Kwon and Park (2011) reported similar results in young adults. They attributed it (greater cerebellar activity during EC) to the performance of EC movement as early stage learning of the motor skill by their subjects. Although we cannot exclude this possibility (i.e., early learning effect on cerebellar activation), the practice provided before the fMRI scan in our study diminished this likelihood. Thus, we attribute the stronger cerebellar activities observed in EC than CC to its role in dealing with a higher degree of difficulties associated with performing EC than CC movements. The higher activation level in the cerebellum in the old than the young group during both EC and CC movements reflects an increased functional load in the cerebellum for controlling the two types of movements. Previous studies have indicated that the cerebellum is involved in cognitive processes for problem solving (Kim et al., 1994), preparation of motor actions (Coffman et al., 2011), and balance control and movement error correction (Lisberger and Thach, 2013).

Activation in M1 and S1 during CC and EC

Unlike the secondary and association motor cortices that showed a higher EC-to-CC activation ratio in late adulthood, the primary motor and sensory cortices (M1, S1), however, exhibited a significantly higher such ratio in young than old individuals. It should be noted that the MVC force, movement speed, and movement stability between the young and the old groups did not differ significantly and thus, cannot explain the biased EC-to-CC activation in the M1 and S1in the young group. Instead, while older individuals may need to rely more on the secondary and association cortices to deal with more complex EC movements, the young adults are apt to use the primary motor and sensory areas to handle the more difficult EC. However, the validity of this age-specific brain site for motor planning needs to be further tested by future studies.

Ipsilateral activation and activation in young or old group only

The above discussion was focused on brain activation in the contralateral (to the performing hand) hemisphere. Besides the major findings in the contralateral side, the fMRI data have shown that ipsilateral (right) hemisphere activation was observed only during

EC in M1, S1 and IPL in the elderly group. In addition, only the elderly group had activation in both the left and right putamen in the basal ganglia during both CC and EC. These observations have never been made before and we do not yet know the appropriate explanations. A simple guess would be that these regions played a role in compensating for the worsened ability in the aging control network to manipulate EC movements as these ipsilateral activities were not seen in the young group. Many studies reported increased ipsilateral motor cortex and other region activation and reduced activation laterality during motor performance in healthy aging (e.g., Naccarato et al., 2006). Regarding the observation of bilateral activation in putamen during both CC and EC in the old group, we believe it might be a reflection of heavier use of basal ganglia-cerebellum-cerebral cortex motor control loop during voluntary motor action by older adults. Another interesting finding was that only the young group showed activation during EC in the left and right superior temporal gyri and during both CC and EC in the left insular cortex (**Table 1**). Little is known about the exact role of the temporal and insular cortices in control of CC and EC. In general, the superior temporal cortex is related to perceiving motion (Saygin, 2007) and visuomotor integration (Tanaka et al., 1986). Considering that our subjects performed the motor tasks with visual feedback, it is reasonable to expect activation in the superior temporal cortex. It is unclear though why only the young group showed the activity during the EC action. For activation in the insular cortex, it has been reported that the posterior part of the anterior insular cortex is dedicated for motor control of both upper and lower extremity movements (Mutschler et al., 2009). Again, it is yet to be determined the reason(s) underlying the lack of activation in the insular cortex in late life. Perhaps aging-related structural degeneration such as grey and white matter atrophy in these cortical regions prevented adequate activities in these specific areas.

SUMMARY

Both young and old individuals demonstrated stronger fMRI-measured activation during EC than CC in almost all cortical areas examined and this biased activation towards EC was more prominent in the old than young groups. Furthermore, all the secondary and association cortices and cerebellum engaged in the two types of muscle contractions exhibited higher EC- than-CC activation in old than young individuals especially in the supplementary motor area and anterior cingulate cortex. On the contrary, the two primary cortices (M1 and S1) showed stronger biased EC activation in young than old age groups. Greater activation in higher-order cortical fields for controlling EC movement in late life may reflect activities in these regions to compensate for impaired ability (perhaps in the primary sensorimotor cortices) to control complex EC movements. All these results associated with aging-related control of EC and CC movements are new and the special roles of the identified cortical fields in modulating EC in late life, especially those at higher levels of the control network justify further delineation by future studies.

ACKNOWLEDGMENT

The current study was partially supported by a grant from San Antonio Life Science Institutes. The authors are grateful to the reviewers' insightful suggestions and comments on this paper. We would also like to thank Dr. Michelle Stevenson and Ms. Deborah Silliman Wolfe for their useful comments and assistance in the preparation of the manuscript. This study was supported in part by San Antonio Life Science Institutes.

REFERENCES

Abbruzzese, G., Morena, M., Spadavecchia, L., and Schieppati, M. (1994). Response of arm flexor muscles to magnetic and electrical brain stimulation during shortening and lengthening tasks in man. *J. Physiol.* 481, 499–507.

Bawa, P., and Jones, K. E. (1999). Do lengthening contractions represent a case of reversal in recruitment order? *Prog. Brain Res.* 123, 215–220. doi: 10.1016/S0079-6123(08)62858-7

Burnett, R. A., Laidlaw, D. H., and Enoka, R. M. (2000). Coactivation of the antagonist muscle does not covary with steadiness in old adults. *J. Appl. Physiol.* 89, 61–71.

Coffman, K. A., Dum, R. P., and Strick, P. L. (2011). Cerebellar vermis is a target of projections from the motor areas in the cerebral cortex. *Proc. Natl. Acad. Sci. U.S.A.* 108, 16068–16073. doi: 10.1073/pnas.1107904108

Duchateau, J., and Enoka, R. M. (2008). Neural control of shortening and lengthening contractions: influence of task constraints. *J. Physiol.* 586, 5853–5864. doi: 10.1113/jphysiol.2008.160747

Duclay, J., and Martin, A. (2005). Evoked H-reflex and V-wave responses during maximal isometric, concentric, and eccentric muscle contraction. *J. Neurophysiol.* 94, 3555–3562. doi: 10.1152/jn.00348.2005

Duclay, J., Pasquet, B., Martin, A., and Duchateau, J. (2011). Specific modulation of corticospinal and spinal excitabilities during maximal voluntary isometric, shortening and lengthening contractions in synergist muscles. *J. Physiol.* 589, 2901–2916. doi: 10.1113/jphysiol.2011.207472

Duclay, J., Robbe, A., Pousson, M., and Martin, A. (2009). Effect of angular velocity on soleus and medial gastrocnemius H-reflex during maximal concentric and eccentric muscle contraction. *J. Electromyogr. Kinesiol.* 19, 948–956. doi: 10.1016/j.jelekin.2008.04.011

Fang, Y., Siemionow, V., Sahgal, V., Xiong, F., and Yue, G. H. (2001). Greater movement-related cortical potential during human eccentric versus concentric muscle contractions. *J. Neurophysiol.* 86, 1764–1772.

Fang, Y., Siemionow, V., Sahgal, V., Xiong, F., and Yue, G. H. (2004). Distinct brain activation patterns for human maximal voluntary eccentric and concentric muscle actions. *Brain Res.* 1023, 200–212. doi: 10.1016/j.brainres.2004.07.035

Fogassi, L., and Luppino, G. (2005). Motor functions of the parietal lobe. *Curr. Opin. Neurobiol.* 15, 626–631. doi: 10.1016/j.conb.2005.10.015

Gao, J. H., Parsons, L., Bower, J., Xiong, J., Li, J., and Fox, P. (1996). Cerebellum implicated in sensory acquisition and discrimination rather than motor control. *Science* 272, 545–547. doi: 10.1126/science.272.5261.545

Hortobagyi, T., Tunnel, D., Moody, J., Beam, S., and Devita, P. (2001). Low- or high-intensity strength training partially restores impaired quadriceps force accuracy and steadiness in aged adults. *J. Gerontol. A Biol. Sci. Med. Sci.* 56, B38–B47. doi: 10.1093/gerona/56.1.B38

Howell, J. N., Fuglevand, A. J., Walsh, M. L., and Bigland-Richie, B. (1995). Motor unit activity during isometric and concentric-eccentric contractions of the human first dorsal interosseus muscle. *J. Neurophysiol.* 74, 901–904.

Kalaska, J. F. (2009). From intention to action: motor cortex and the control of reaching movements. *Adv. Exp. Med. Biol.* 629, 139–178. doi: 10.1007/978-0-387-77064-2_8

Kandel, E. R., Schwartz, J. H., Jessell, T. M., Siegelbaum, S. A., and Hudspeth, A. J. (2013). *Principles of Neural Science*, 5th Edn. New York: McGraw-Hill.

Kim, S., Ugurbil, K., and Strick, P. (1994). Activation of a cerebellar output nucleus during cognitive processing. *Science* 265, 949–951. doi: 10.1126/science.8052851

Kossev, A., and Christova, P. (1998). Discharge pattern of human motor units during dynamic concentric and eccentric contractions. *Electroencephalogr. Clin. Neurophysiol.* 109, 245–255. doi: 10.1016/S0924-980X(98)00012-5

Kwon, Y. H., and Park, J. W. (2011). Different cortical activation patterns during voluntary eccentric and concentric muscle contractions: an fMRI study. *Neurorehabilitation* 29, 253–259. doi: 10.3233/NRE-2011-0701

Laidlaw, D. H., Hunter, S. K., and Enoka, R. M. (2002). Nonuniform activation of the agonist muscle does not covary with index finger acceleration in old adults. *J. Appl. Physiol.* 93, 1400–1410. doi: 10.1152/japplphysiol.00391.2002

Laidlaw, D. H., Kornatz, K. W., Keen, D. A., Suzuki, S., and Enoka, R. M. (1999). Strength training improves the steadiness of slow lengthening contractions performed by old adults. *J. Appl. Physiol.* 87, 1786–1795.

Lemon, R. N. (2008). Descending pathways in motor control. *Annu. Rev. Neurosci.* 31, 195–218. doi: 10.1146/annurev.neuro.31.060407.125547

Lisberger, S. G., and Thach, W. T. (2013). "The cerebellum," in *Principles of Neural Science*, 5th Edn, eds E. R. Kandel, J. H. Schwartz, T. M. Jessell, S. A. Siegelbaum and A. J. Hudspeth (New York: McGraw-Hill).

Moritani, T., Muramatsu, S., and Muro, M. (1988). Activity of motor units during concentric and eccentric contractions. *Am. J. Phys. Med.* 66, 338–350. doi: 10.1097/00002060-198812000-00003

Mutschler, I., Wieckhorst, B., Kowalevski, S., Derix, J., Wentlandt, J., Schulze-Bonhage, A., et al. (2009). Functional organization of the human anterior insular cortex. *Neurosci. Lett.* 457, 66–70. doi: 10.1016/j.neulet.2009.03.101

Naccarato, M., Calautti, C., Jones, P. S., Day, D. J., Carpenter, T. A., and Baron, J. C. (2006). Does healthy aging affect the hemispheric activation balance during paced index-to-thumb opposition task? An fMRI study. *Neuroimage* 32, 1250–1256. doi: 10.1016/j.neuroimage.2006.05.003

Nardone, A., Romano, C., and Schieppati, M. (1988). Selective recruitment of high-threshold human motor units during voluntary isotonic lengthening of active muscles. *J. Physiol. (Lond.)* 409, 451–471.

Oldfield, R. C. (1971). The assessment and analysis of handedness: the Edinburgh inventory. *Neuropsychologia* 9, 335–365. doi: 10.1016/0028-3932(71)90067-4

Rizzolatti, G., and Kalaska, J. F. (2013). "Voluntary movement: the parietal and premotor cortex," in *Principles of Neural Science*, 5th Edn, eds E. R. Kandel, J. H. Schwartz, T. M. Jessell, S. A. Siegelbaum, and A. J. Hudspeth (New York: McGraw-Hill).

Rizzolatti, G., and Strick, P. L. (2013). "Cognitive function of the premotor systems," in *Principles of Neural Science*, 5th Edn, eds E. R. Kandel, J. H. Schwartz, T. M. Jessell, S. A. Siegelbaum, and A. J. Hudspeth (New York: McGraw-Hill).

Saygin, A. P. (2007). Superior temporal and premotor brain areas necessary for biological motion perception. *Brain* 130, 2452–2461. doi: 10.1093/brain/awm162

Sekiguchi, H., Kimura, T., Yamanaka, K., and Nakazawa, K. (2001). Lower excitability of the corticospinal tract to transcranial magnetic stimulation during lengthening contractions in human elbow flexors. *Neurosci. Lett.* 312, 83–86. doi: 10.1016/S0304-3940(01)02197-8

Sesto, M. E., Chourasia, A. O., Block, W. F., and Radwin, R. G. (2008). Mechanical and magnetic resonance imaging changes following eccentric or concentric exertions. *Clin. Biomech.* 23, 961–968. doi: 10.1016/j.clinbiomech.2008.03.068

Shellock, F. G., Fukunaga, T., Mink, J. H., and Edgerton, V. R. (1991). Exertional muscle injury: evaluation of concentric versus eccentric actions with serial MR imaging. *Radiology* 179, 659–664.

Tanaka, K., Hikosaka, K., Saito, H., Yukie, M., Fukada, Y., and Iwai, E. (1986). Analysis of local and wide-field movements in the superior temporal visual areas of the macaque monkey. *J. Neurosci.* 6, 134–144.

Woolrich, M. W., Beckmann, C. F., Nichols, T. E., and Smith, S. M. (2009). *Statistical Analysis of fMRI Data, Neuromethods.* New York: Humana Press.

Yue, G. H., Liu, J. Z., Siemionow, V., Ranganathan, V. K., Ng, T. C., and Sahgal, V. (2000). Brain activation during human finger extension and flexion movements. *Brain Res.* 856, 291–300. doi: 10.1016/S0006-8993(99)02385-9

11

Safety margins in older adults increase with improved control of a dynamic object

Christopher J. Hasson[1]* and Dagmar Sternad[2]

[1] Neuromotor Systems Laboratory, Department of Physical Therapy, Movement and Rehabilitation Sciences, Northeastern University, Boston, MA, USA
[2] The Action Lab, Departments of Biology, Electrical and Computer Engineering, and Physics, Northeastern University, Boston, MA, USA

Edited by:
S. Lee Hong, Ohio University, USA

Reviewed by:
Matjaž Perc, University of Maribor, Slovenia
Hannah Justine Block, Indiana University, USA

***Correspondence:**
Christopher J. Hasson, Neuromotor Systems Laboratory, Department of Physical Therapy, Movement and Rehabilitation Sciences, Bouvé College of Health Sciences, Northeastern University, 360 Huntington Ave., 301 Robinson Hall, Boston, MA 02115-5005, USA
e-mail: c.hasson@neu.edu

Older adults face decreasing motor capabilities due to pervasive neuromuscular degradations. As a consequence, errors in movement control increase. Thus, older individuals should maintain larger safety margins than younger adults. While this has been shown for object manipulation tasks, several reports on whole-body activities, such as posture and locomotion, demonstrate age-related reductions in safety margins. This is despite increased costs for control errors, such as a fall. We posit that this paradox could be explained by the dynamic challenge presented by the body or also an external object, and that age-related reductions in safety margins are in part due to a decreased ability to control dynamics. To test this conjecture we used a virtual ball-in-cup task that had challenging dynamics, yet afforded an explicit rendering of the physics and safety margin. The hypotheses were: (1) When manipulating an object with challenging dynamics, older adults have smaller safety margins than younger adults. (2) Older adults increase their safety margins with practice. Nine young and 10 healthy older adults practiced moving the virtual ball-in-cup to a target location in exactly 2 s. The accuracy and precision of the timing error quantified skill, and the ball energy relative to an escape threshold quantified the safety margin. Compared to the young adults, older adults had increased timing errors, greater variability, and decreased safety margins. With practice, both young and older adults improved their ability to control the object with decreased timing errors and variability, and increased their safety margins. These results suggest that safety margins are related to the ability to control dynamics, and may explain why in tasks with simple dynamics older adults use adequate safety margins, but in more complex tasks, safety margins may be inadequate. Further, the results indicate that task-specific training may improve safety margins in older adults.

Keywords: aging, safety margin, human, dynamics, object manipulation, motor control, motor learning

INTRODUCTION

With aging comes an array of neuromuscular changes, such as weaker muscles, increased neural delays, and greater neuromuscular noise (Salthouse, 1996; Goodpaster et al., 2006), which together contribute to declines in motor function (Aoyagi and Shephard, 1992). Not only are the performance capabilities of older adults more limited than those of younger adults, the consequences of control errors are also more severe. This is particularly the case for locomotor activities, where a fall can cause life-threatening injuries (Berg et al., 1997). This combination of age-related neuromuscular degradations and greater costs of failure makes the maintenance of adequate safety margins a critical concern for older adults.

A common paradigm for studying safety margins is manipulation tasks, which often involve transporting a hand-held object. Here, the safety margin is typically defined as the difference between the grip force and the force required to prevent object slippage. Young adults are able to precisely regulate their grip force in response to varying object masses, staying just above the slip threshold (Johansson and Westling, 1984; Johansson and Cole, 1992). Young adults also modulate their grip force in response to load fluctuations during object acceleration (Flanagan and Wing, 1990, 1993). While older adults show similar patterns of adaptation, they generally produce higher grip forces compared to young adults (Cole, 1991; Cole and Beck, 1994; Gilles and Wing, 2003). This increases the safety margin against object slippage, which may be needed due to impaired control related to decrements in afferent function (Cole et al., 1999).

Although an age-related elevation in safety margins for object manipulation tasks is consistent with expectations, the opposite has been observed in whole-body activities, particularly locomotion and postural control. In locomotor tasks foot-obstacle clearance is critical. A small clearance implies a low safety margin against tripping. During level walking young and older adults maintain similar clearances (Winter et al., 1990). However, when the locomotor challenge is increased by adding different terrain features, older adults show reduced clearances. This includes when stepping over obstacles (McFadyen and Prince, 2002), stepping onto a raised platform (Begg and Sparrow, 2000), or descending stairs (Hamel et al., 2005). Older adults also show reduced safety margins in postural control. During upright standing older adults have reduced spatiotemporal margins of stability, which increases the risk of a fall (Slobounov et al., 1998; Van Wegen et al., 2002). Considering these observations, it appears paradoxical that in situations that warrant a larger safety margin due to more serious consequences of failure, e.g., falling, older adults use smaller, and not larger safety margins compared to young adults.

We posit that this paradox can be explained by the dynamic challenge presented by an activity or task. In grip force studies on age-related differences in object manipulation, the objects are usually rigid blocks with no further dynamics (Cole, 1991; Cole and Beck, 1994; Gilles and Wing, 2003). Changes in the load presented by the object are a linear function of the object's acceleration. On the other hand, in postural control and locomotion, the trajectory of the legs and center-of-mass are a complex function of inertial, ground reaction, and interaction forces between numerous body segments (Onyshko and Winter, 1980). In this case, older adults might be unable to control the dynamics of the body well enough to maintain adequate safety margins. In addition, in unpracticed tasks or novel dynamical experiences, individuals may be unable to utilize appropriate safety margins until sufficient skill is obtained. This is consistent with a report that in young adults improvements in performance on a virtual ball-in-a-cup transportation task are accompanied by increased safety margins (Hasson et al., 2012b).

We hypothesize that if safety margins depend on the ability to control object dynamics, then in a dynamically challenging task, older adults should have smaller safety margins than young adults (Hypothesis 1), but should increase their safety margins as their task performance improves with practice (Hypothesis 2). To test these hypotheses we used the task of moving a virtual ball-in-a-cup, representing a cup of coffee, to a target location (Hasson et al., 2012a,b; Sternad et al., 2014; Ye et al., 2014). This object has non-trivial dynamics and affords an explicit understanding of the object dynamics and a quantitative definition of the safety margin. The latter was defined as the ball energy relative to the energy needed to escape the cup. Young and older adults were asked to practice transporting the ball-and-cup to the target location in a time of exactly 2-s without letting the ball escape. This timing constraint prevented subjects from using a slowing strategy to increase safety margins but was still not fast enough to permit a range of movement strategies to achieve the task goal. Performance was assessed by the accuracy and precision of the timing error relative to the 2-s target time.

METHODS

PARTICIPANTS

Nine young subjects (21–35 years) and 10 healthy older adults (65–80 years) practiced moving a virtual cup and ball to a target point in 2 s. Data on the young subjects was previously reported in Hasson et al. (2012b). The older subjects were all community dwelling, ambulatory, independent, and had no major musculoskeletal problems affecting upper body control, and no major neurological problems. Prior to participating, subjects were given a mini-mental state exam to assess cognitive function (Folstein et al., 1975); all participants scored above 23 and were therefore eligible to participate (Tombaugh and McIntyre, 1992). Before participating, subjects were informed of all experimental procedures and read and signed an informed consent document approved by the Institutional Review Board at Northeastern University.

BALL AND CUP SIMULATION

The dynamics of the ball and cup object were based on that of a cart and pendulum system (**Figure 1A**). The cart and pendulum were haptically rendered with a robotic manipulandum (Haptic Master, Moog, Netherlands; Van der Linde and Lammertse, 2003). Details of the instrumentation are in Hasson et al. (2012b). A visual display on a rear-projection screen 2.4 m away showed the pendulum bob and a shallow "cup" drawn as an arc; the cart and the pendulum rod were not shown on the screen (**Figure 1B**). For subjects it appeared as if they were controlling a cup with a ball rolling inside, where the cup imposed an angular constraint on the ball. If the angle of the ball θ exceeded the maximum angle subtended by the cup, termed the escape angle θ_{ESC} ($\theta_{ESC} = 35°$), the ball escaped and visually "fell" out of the cup.

Subjects could manipulate the ball and cup object by applying horizontal forces to the manipulandum, which in turn accelerated the cart (cup) and the pendulum bob (ball). Forces could only be applied to the cup, and the moving ball exerted forces on the cup that subjects could feel through the manipulandum. The motion of the cup was confined to a horizontal line, and the ball could pivot about the pendulum axis of rotation, thus the system had two mechanical degrees of freedom. The cart and pendulum

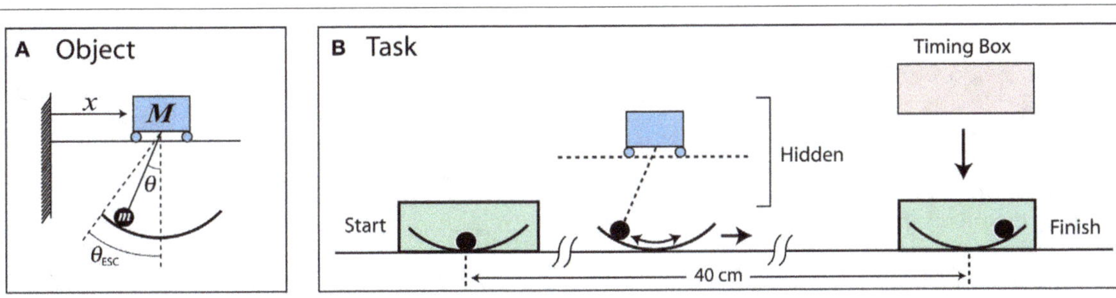

FIGURE 1 | (A) Model of the cart and pendulum system with variables and parameters. **(B)** Task implementation. The visual display showed the pendulum bob and an arc drawn for the cup; the cart and pendulum were not shown. The cart and pendulum were haptically rendered with a robotic manipulandum. Subjects applied forces to the manipulandum, which in turn accelerated the cart (cup) and pendulum bob (ball).

system behavior was governed by two equations of motion:

$$(m+M)\,\ddot{x} = F_A + F_B \tag{1}$$

and

$$\ddot{\theta} = \frac{\ddot{x}}{\ell}\cos\theta - \frac{g}{\ell}\sin\theta \tag{2}$$

where M is the cup mass ($M = 3.5$ kg), m is the ball mass ($m = 0.3$ kg), $\theta, \dot{\theta}$, and $\ddot{\theta}$ are the ball angle, angular velocity, and angular acceleration, respectively; $\ddot{x}$ is the cup's horizontal acceleration, ℓ is the pendulum length ($\ell = 0.35$ m), g is gravitational acceleration (9.81 m/s^2), F_A is an external horizontal force applied to the cup by a human actor, and F_B is the horizontal reaction force of the ball on the cup, given by

$$F_B = m\ell\ddot{\theta}\cos\theta - m\ell\dot{\theta}^2\sin\theta. \tag{3}$$

Details of the derivation of the equations of motion are in Hasson et al. (2012b).

TASK

Subjects were asked to transport the ball-and-cup to a spatial target located 0.4 m away in a target time of 2.0 s without letting the ball escape from the cup (**Figure 1B**). The 2.0 s movement time was a "comfortable" time for healthy young subjects. Because the task goal was not a limit performance, i.e., as fast as possible, a number of movement strategies could be used to complete the task in the target time; some strategies would be riskier than others, i.e., some would carry a greater risk of losing the ball. To prevent participants from spending a disproportional amount of time trying to keep the cup still in the goal region, the goal box was made "sticky" by applying a damping force $F_D = -26\dot{x}$ to the cup when both edges of the cup were inside the goal.

VISUAL FEEDBACK

Two filled green rectangles were displayed, one serving as the start box and one as the goal box. The timing error was signaled with a "timing box" that descended onto the spatial target with a constant velocity so that it passed through the target at a time of 2.0 s. The timing box stopped moving when the cup was brought to a stop ($\dot{x} < 0.02$ m/s). If the cup stopped too early (<2.0 s), the timing box was above the spatial target, if too late (>2.0 s), the timing box stopped below the spatial target. At the end of the trial, subjects were shown their temporal error in numeric form.

PROTOCOL

Data were collected while the participants practiced the transportation task in four blocks of 60 trials (240 total), with brief breaks between blocks.

ENERGY MARGIN

The "safety" or "riskiness" of a movement strategy was determined by computing the energy margin EM as

$$EM = (E_{ESC} - TE_{BALL})\,/E_{ESC} \tag{4}$$

where

$$E_{ESC} = mg\ell\,(1-\cos\theta_{ESC}) - m\,|\ddot{x}|\,\ell\sin\theta_{ESC} + m\,|\ddot{x}|\,\ell \tag{5}$$

and

$$TE_{BALL} = \frac{1}{2}m\left(\ell\dot{\theta}\right)^2 + mg\ell\,(1-\cos\theta) + PSE_{BALL} \tag{6}$$

where

$$PSE_{BALL} = \begin{cases} \ddot{x} \geq 0 & -m\ddot{x}\ell\sin\theta + m\ddot{x}\ell \\ \ddot{x} < 0 & -m\ddot{x}\ell\sin\theta - m\ddot{x}\ell \end{cases}. \tag{7}$$

The escape energy E_{ESC} defined the instantaneous energy threshold for ball escape. If the ball's total energy TE_{BALL} was below E_{ESC}, then the ball just oscillated within the cup and did not escape (assuming constant $\ddot{x}$). Otherwise, the ball would escape in the future (unless $\ddot{x}$ was changed). Note that E_{ESC} depended on $\ddot{x}$ and therefore changed during cup transportation.

The energy margin EM represented how close the current ball energy was to exceeding E_{ESC}. If EM was between 0 and 1, the ball did not escape. However, it would escape if EM was negative, assuming $\ddot{x}$ was not changed. It should be emphasized that EM extrapolated, i.e., it took the instantaneous energy of the ball and predicted whether the ball would escape in the future with constant $\ddot{x}$. Accordingly, E_{ESC} was not a "hard" constraint and could be exceeded for brief periods, provided an appropriate and timely correction was made before the ball reached the cup rim.

DEPENDENT VARIABLES

Manipulation ability was quantified with measures related to the goal of the task: the average and standard deviation of the absolute movement timing error across trials (MTE_{AVG} and MTE_{STD}, respectively). The timing error was the absolute value of the difference between subjects' movement time and the 2.0 s target time. A subject with high manipulation ability should be able to reach the goal accurately (small MTE_{AVG}) and reliability (small MTE_{STD}). The safety margin was quantified via the average energy margin EM_{AVG} and standard deviation of EM across multiple trials EM_{STD}. All measures (MTE_{AVG}, MTE_{STD}, EM_{AVG}, and EM_{STD}) were computed across the first 30 trials (excluding the first two trials) of Block 1 and the last 30 trials of Blocks 2–4.

DATA ANALYSIS

All data analysis was performed with MATLAB (R2012b, MathWorks, Natick, MA, USA). The raw data included time histories for $x, \dot{x}, \ddot{x}, \theta, \dot{\theta}, \ddot{\theta}$ and F_A, which were filtered with a dual-pass fourth-order low-pass Butterworth digital filter, and used to calculate the dependent variables (MTE_{AVG}, MTE_{STD}, EM_{AVG}, and EM_{STD}). Only trials in which the target location was reached and the ball was not dropped were analyzed. To facilitate averaging movement patterns across subjects for graphical presentation, time histories were normalized to a unitary movement time (0–100%) using linear interpolation.

STATISTICS

All statistical tests were performed with SPSS (Version 21, IBM Corporation, Armonk, NY, USA). A repeated-measures ANOVA was performed for each dependent variable with age as a between-subjects factor and practice block as a within-subjects factor. For all statistical tests, two subjects in the young group were identified as outliers and excluded. In contrast to the other seven subjects in the group, these subjects increased the variability of their movement patterns and used a different high-acceleration movement strategy (see Hasson et al., 2012b for more details). One subject in the older group was excluded due to excessively poor performance on the task. When appropriate, *post-hoc* comparisons were performed using Tukey's honestly significant difference test. Significance was set at $p < 0.05$ for all tests.

RESULTS

GENERAL TASK CHARACTERISTICS

The averaged ball and cup kinematics and kinetics for the young and older subjects in early and late practice are shown in **Figure 2A**. The ball and cup transit was divided into three phases. (1) Subjects applied a positive force to the cup, which accelerated the cup toward the spatial target and caused the ball to move backwards toward the rim of the cup (**Figure 2B**). These events caused the energy margin *EM* to rapidly decrease. If the force that accelerated the cup was too high, the *EM* could become negative and the ball may exceed the escape angle. (2) Subjects reduced their applied force as the cup reached the center of the workspace and the ball descended toward the center of the cup. (3) Subjects applied forces counter to the cup motion, which brought the cup to a stop at the spatial target; this was by far the riskiest part of the movement, highlighted by the rapid *EM* decrease. In early practice, the older adults applied more force to the ball at the start of each trial, causing the cup velocity to increase faster, the ball to move more, and consequently, the *EM* to decrease faster. In

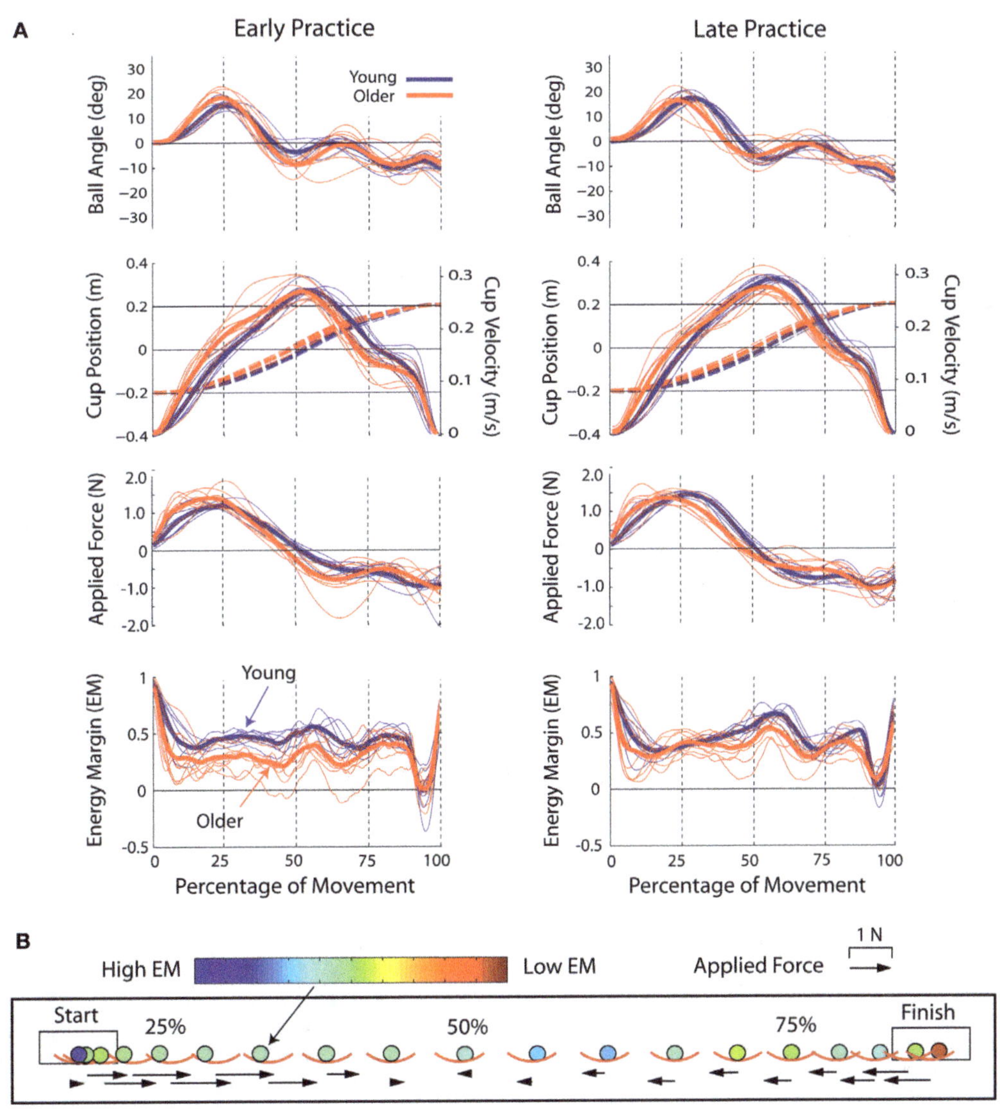

FIGURE 2 | (A) Ball angle, cup position (dashed lines), and velocity, applied force, and energy margin for the young (blue) and older (red) subjects. Individual subjects are shown as thin lines, group averages are the thick lines. **(B)** Example of a representative ball and cup transit of an older subject in late practice [shown in **(A)**]. Images are at 5% increments of the total movement time. The color of the ball represents the energy margin; dark blue represents a high energy margin ("safe") and dark red represents a low energy margin ("unsafe"). The arrows scale with the force applied to the cup. The size of the ball was enlarged for clarity.

early practice, the ball oscillation amplitudes remained larger in the older adults until the last quarter of the movement. In contrast, in late practice, the older adults reduced these amplitudes to be similar to the young adults, and therefore the *EM* was raised.

FAILURES

Overall the older adults had a higher failure rate, i.e., lost the ball more frequently, compared to young adults [main effect $F_{(1, 15)} = 6.8$; $p < 0.021$; **Figure 3A**]. Both groups decreased their failure rate with practice [main effect $F_{(3, 45)} = 5.7$; $p < 0.007$], but this decrease did not differ between the groups (i.e., no interaction; $p = 0.392$). For both young and old subjects, the point at which the ball was most likely to escape from the cup was when arriving at the goal (**Figure 3B**).

TASK PERFORMANCE

Performance was quantified with measures of timing accuracy and precision. Both young and older subjects decreased their average timing error MTE_{AVG} with practice [main effect $F_{(3, 45)} = 20.2$; $p < 0.001$; **Figure 4A**]. MTE_{AVG} in block 1 was higher than in blocks 2–4 ($p = 0.001$), errors in block 2 were higher than block 3 ($p = 0.034$), but not different from block 4 ($p = 0.546$). Blocks 3 and 4 were not different ($p = 0.195$). The young subjects had smaller MTE_{AVG} compared to older subjects [main effect $F_{(1, 15)} = 29.9$; $p < 0.001$]. There was no MTE_{AVG} interaction between the two factors practice and age ($p = 0.662$). The trial-to-trial variability of the timing error MTE_{STD} decreased with practice [main effect $F_{(3, 45)} = 15.7$; $p < 0.001$; **Figure 4B**]. MTE_{STD} in block 1 was higher than in blocks 2–4 ($p < 0.001$), but blocks 2–4 were not different from each other ($p > 0.759$ for all comparisons). The young subjects had smaller MTE_{STD} compared to older subjects [main effect $F_{(1, 15)} = 37.5$; $p < 0.001$]. There was no MTE_{STD} interaction between the factors practice and age ($p = 0.558$).

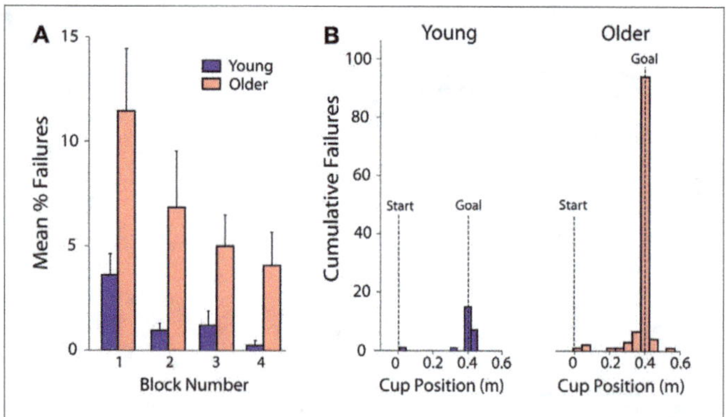

FIGURE 3 | (A) Both young and older subjects decreased their failure rate with practice, but older adults failed more often overall. Failure was defined when the ball exceeded the escape angle. The bars show the mean percentage of failures for young (blue bars) and older (red bars) across the four blocks of practice. Error bars show standard error. Each block includes 60 trials. **(B)** Failure rate as a function of cup position for young and old subjects separately. By far the riskiest part of the ball and cup transit was stopping in the goal (at 0.4 m). Shown is the number of failed trials across all subjects as a function of the cup position at the time of failure.

ENERGY MARGIN

The safety margin was quantified in terms of an energy margin *EM*. An illustration of the *EM* and an exemplar early-practice *EM* time-history is shown for one older participant (**Figure 5**). The *EM* depends on the ball angle and angular velocity and cup acceleration, and therefore varied as these variables changed during a cup transit. When $EM > 0$ (light blue shading; **Figure 5A**), the ball will never escape from the cup, given the current cup acceleration. At the next instant in time the cup acceleration could change, which would update *EM*. An $EM \leq 0$ (light red shading; **Figure 5A**) signals that the ball will escape from the cup given the current cup acceleration. Therefore a corrective action is needed to keep the ball in the cup. For the latter case, the time-to-escape is shown (dashed red lines; **Figure 5A**). For $EM > 0$ the time-to-escape is infinite (the ball will just oscillate within the cup).

The critical energy threshold at $EM = 0$ is the escape energy E_{ESC}. This threshold can be visualized as a two-dimensional manifold in the three-dimensional task execution space (blue mesh; **Figure 5B**). Each cup transit forms a trajectory in this space; as long as the trajectory stays inside E_{ESC} manifold, the ball is not in danger of escaping from the cup. As shown in **Figure 6**, early in practice subjects typically had high trial-to-trial variability and frequently exceeded E_{ESC}. However, with practice the trajectories conformed to stay largely within the E_{ESC} manifold, except for the period of high deceleration at the end of the cup transit.

EM_{AVG} was higher in young subjects compared to older subjects [main effect $F_{(1, 15)} = 17.6$; $p < 0.001$; **Figure 7A**]. There was a significant effect of practice [main effect $F_{(3, 45)} = 7.0$; $p = 0.001$], but no interaction between age and practice ($p = 0.078$). For both the young and older subject groups, EM_{AVG} in blocks 2–4 was greater than in block 1 ($p < 0.018$), but blocks 2–4 were not different from each other ($p > 0.7$ for all comparisons). EM_{STD} was lower in young subjects compared to older subjects [main effect $F_{(1, 15)} = 18.3$; $p < 0.001$; **Figure 7B**], there was a significant effect of practice [main effect $F_{(1, 15)} = 18.5$; $p \leq 0.001$], but no interaction between age and practice ($p = 0.146$).

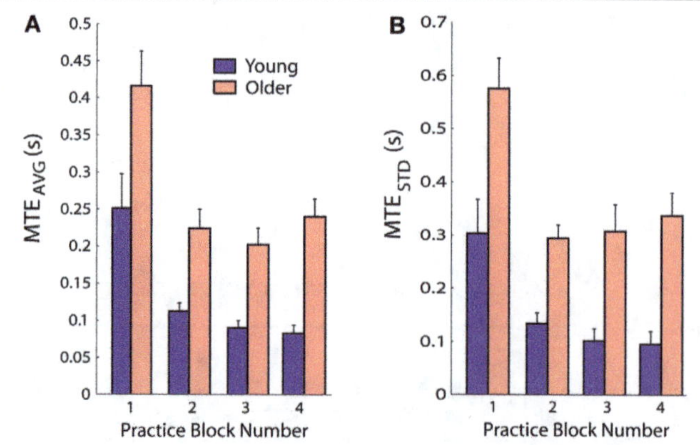

FIGURE 4 | (A) Average movement time error MTE_{AVG} improved with practice in both young and older subjects. **(B)** Trial-to-trial variability of movement time error MTE_{STD} decreased. Age-related differences in manipulation ability were reflected by main effects of age for MTE_{AVG} and MTE_{STD}. Error bars show standard errors; each block included 60 trials.

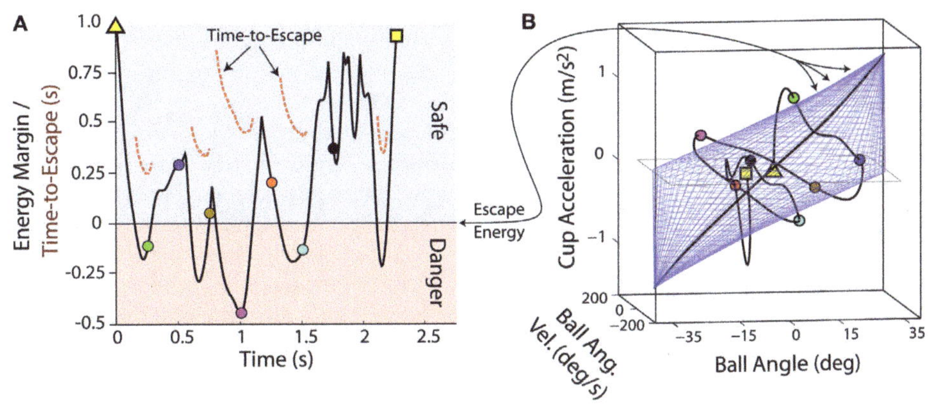

FIGURE 5 | (A) The energy margin *EM* as a function of time (black line) in one early practice trial for one older subject. If $EM > 0$, the ball will never escape from the cup, if the current cup acceleration is maintained. However, if $EM \leq 0$ the ball will escape from the cup, unless the cup acceleration is changed. For the latter case, the time-to-escape is shown (dashed red lines); for $EM > 0$ the time-to-escape is infinite (the ball will oscillate within the cup). **(B)** For the same trial, the three variables that determine *EM*, ball angle and angular velocity and cup acceleration, are shown in a three dimensional task execution space. The trial starts in the center (yellow triangle) and moves through the execution space as the trial progresses until the cup is stopped at the spatial target (yellow square). The blue mesh represents the critical *EM* level, i.e., where $EM = 0$. The colored circles provide timing landmarks every 0.25 s.

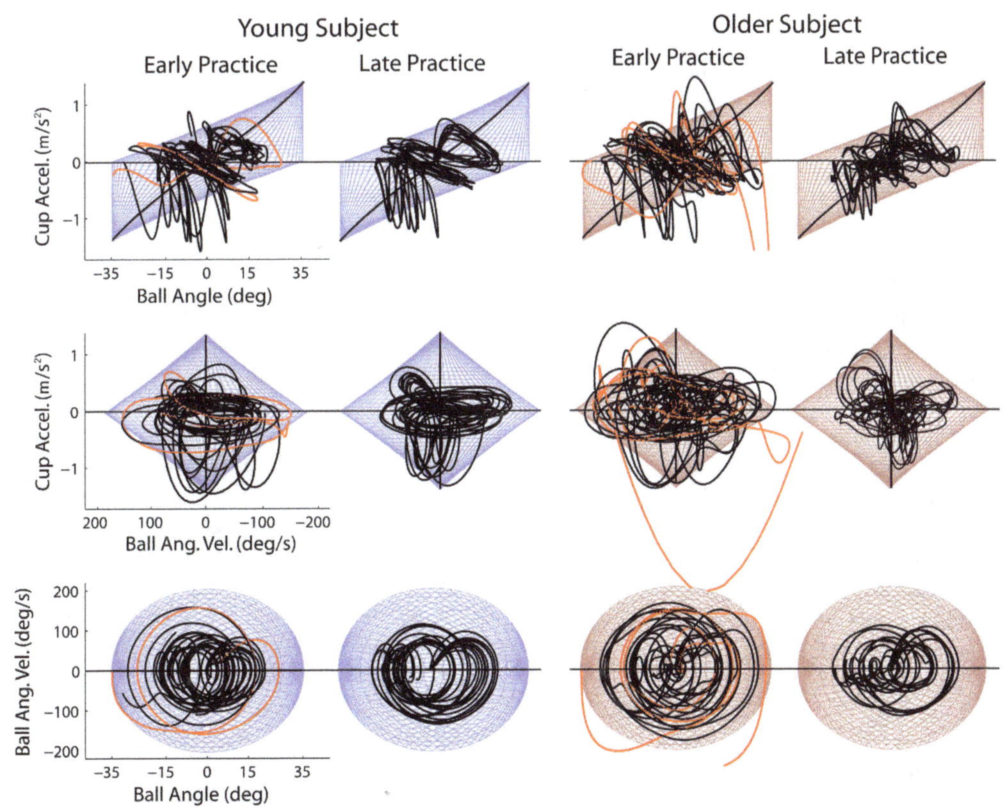

FIGURE 6 | Examples of early and late practice trials for a young and older subject. Trajectories are plotted in the execution space, defined by ball angle and velocity and cup acceleration. Three different views of the three-dimensional execution space are shown (three rows). Trials in which the ball escaped are shown in red.

DISCUSSION

Throughout practice of the virtual ball-and-cup transportation task the older adults employed a smaller safety margin, quantified in terms of an energy margin, than the younger adults, supporting hypothesis 1. Both the young and older adults increased their safety margins with practice, supporting hypothesis 2. This suggests that safety margins are learning-dependent, i.e., they were small when performance was low in

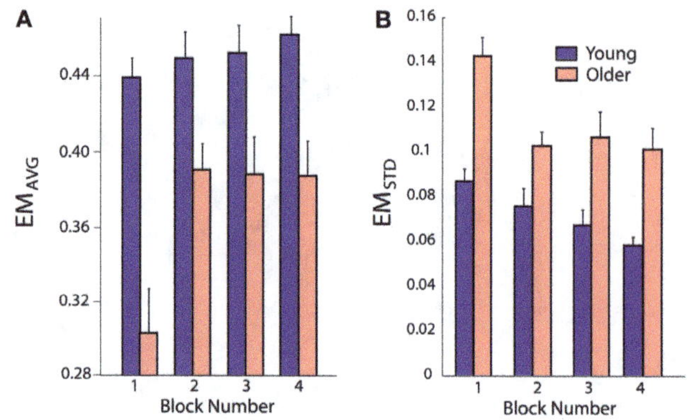

FIGURE 7 | (A) Both young and old subjects increased their mean energy margin EM_{AVG}. **(B)** Variability of EM_{STD} decreased from trial to trial. Overall the older subjects had smaller and more variable energy margins. Error bars show standard error; each block included 60 trials.

early skill acquisition, but increased in parallel to other performance measures.

SAFETY MARGINS AND AGE

The older adults used a movement strategy that was less safe than the young adults, placing them at a greater risk of failure, as shown by the greater number of ball escapes. This age-related reduction in safety margins is at odds with grip force studies that showed increased safety margins in older adults (Cole, 1991; Cole and Beck, 1994; Gilles and Wing, 2003). This could be explained by the dynamic challenges presented by the tasks. In the grip force studies (using older adults) the objects had rigid-body dynamics, i.e., the load was a linear function of the object's acceleration; the safety margins depended on only the ratio between the grip and load forces (Flanagan and Wing, 1990). In this case, the older adults may have been better able to predict the consequences of their manipulative actions, and therefore were able to maintain large safety margins. However, the increased dynamic challenge presented by the ball-and-cup object may have made it more difficult for the older adults to predict how the object would behave, reducing their ability to control the object and consequently maintain a sufficient safety margin. Note that the safety margin in the ball-and-cup task is a dynamic quantity that is a nonlinear function of three variables: the ball angle, the ball angular velocity, and the cup acceleration (Hasson et al., 2012b). The relatively smaller safety margins in the older adults is consistent with observations from whole-body tasks, such as posture and locomotion, in which older adults show reduced safety margins compared to younger adults (Slobounov et al., 1998; Begg and Sparrow, 2000; McFadyen and Prince, 2002; Van Wegen et al., 2002; Hamel et al., 2005). Together, the results of these studies suggest a link between the ability to control the dynamics of an object and the use of safety margins.

SAFETY MARGINS AND TASK PERFORMANCE

The connection between manipulation ability and safety margins is strengthened by the changes observed throughout practice. Despite having overall lower safety margins and performance (accuracy and precision), the older adults increased their safety margins by about 30% and improved performance by about 50%. These changes occurred almost entirely within the first half of task practice. In contrast, the young subjects showed much smaller increases (approximately 7%), and continued to improve their performance and increased safety margins throughout practice. The smaller relative increase in the younger adults could be due to a ceiling effect. Increases in the safety margin were paralleled by a decrease in the task failure rate, which over practice decreased by more than half in the older subjects. In young adults, it was reduced to almost zero. While changes in older subject task performance and safety margins leveled off with practice, the failure rate continued to decrease. This could be related to the binary nature of the failure rate, a large decrease in the failure rate could arise from a very small change in the safety margin if close to the safety margin threshold. Indeed, as shown in **Figure 2**, both young and older subjects came very close to the threshold as they brought the cup to the goal. This remained a "dangerous" point even after the practice period. Note that the safety margin does not necessarily increase with improvements in task performance, i.e., the safety margin could vary independently from the goal (accuracy and precision of the timing error) due to task redundancy afforded by the specification of a 2-s target time.

The reduced performance and lower safety margins of the older adults may be due to a combination of physiological limitations, such as less reliable sensory information (Light, 1990), slower sensory integration and cognitive processing (Myerson et al., 1990; Bashore et al., 1997), and increased neural noise and delays (Laidlaw et al., 2000; Pannese, 2011). Together, these changes may limit the ability of older subjects to make fast compensatory actions to keep the ball from escaping the cup, especially at the end of the movement, where the older adults had the lowest safety margin and lost the ball most frequently. Although the data are consistent with the hypothesis that safety margins are related to the ability of the older adults to control dynamics, a more nuanced view would suggest that additional factors might play a role in regulating safety margins. Maintaining large safety margins may incur an energy cost, i.e., lifting the foot high over an obstacle would require more effort than just clearing the obstacle (Chou et al., 1997). Large safety margins may also limit maneuverability, e.g., in posture keeping a large stability margin reduces the ability to make quick postural changes (Huang and Ahmed, 2011).

IMPLICATIONS AND APPLICATIONS

The task constraints imposed in the experiment raise the question of how these results may relate to the real world. The results show that, given a shallow cup and constrained movement time, older adults are less safe than younger adults. Instead of increasing their safety margins by improving their ability to control the dynamics of the ball and cup object, in real life older adults could take other steps to increase their safety margins. They could choose a very deep cup, place a lid on the cup, or move more slowly. The latter could reduce the cup accelerations, leading to less ball movement and therefore a greater safety margin. Along the same lines, older adults can increase the safety margins in activities like posture and locomotion by either walking more slowly and/or increasing the size of their base of support.

Experimentally, increasing the dynamic challenge presented to the subjects by adding movement time constraints had two key benefits. First, by stressing the neuromuscular system, limitations become clearer (Guadagnoli and Lee, 2004). If we had allowed subjects to slow down, it would have been unlikely that the age differences in safety margins would have been as large. In locomotor studies, if subjects walk on a level ground with no obstacles or cognitive challenges, there are no age differences in the safety margin (Winter et al., 1990). Second, there may be some instances in daily life, which preclude options, such as "slowing down." For example, while crossing the road one might need to quickly step up onto a curb due to errors in judging the speed of traffic. In this case, an inadequate safety margin may cause a fall leading to a serious injury or death.

LIMITATIONS

One of the challenges associated with the analysis of dynamically complex systems is the definition of the safety margin. For the ball-and-cup task we chose to define the safety margin in terms of the ball energy relative to escape. Clearly, there are other ways that the safety margin could be defined. For example, simpler versions could be just the angular distance of the ball from the cup rim, and/or the angular velocity of the ball as it approaches the rim. Our measure considers the ball angle, angular velocity, and cup acceleration, as all three variables determine the ball energy and thereby the risk of escape. More details about our rationale are provided in Hasson et al. (2012b).

CONCLUSIONS

This study demonstrated that in a constrained virtual ball-and-cup transportation task, older adults had less manipulation skill and utilized smaller safety margins compared to younger adults. However, with practice the older adults were able to improve their skill and increase their safety margins. These findings suggest that safety margins are related to the ability to control dynamics, and may explain why in tasks with simple dynamics older adults use adequate safety margins, but in more complex whole-body tasks safety margins are inadequate. Further, the results indicate that task-specific training may improve safety margins in older adults.

ACKNOWLEDGMENTS

This research was supported by a National Institutes of Health (NIH) Ruth L. Kirschstein National Research Service Award for Individual Postdoctoral Fellows (1F32AR061238) awarded to Christopher J. Hasson. Support was also provided by a National Institutes of Health grant (R01HD045639) and a National Science Foundation (NSF) grant (DMS-0928587) awarded to Dagmar Sternad. The contents of this manuscript are solely the responsibility of the authors and do not necessarily represent the official views of the NIH or NSF.

REFERENCES

Aoyagi, Y., and Shephard, R. J. (1992). Aging and muscle function. *Sports Med.* 14, 376–396. doi: 10.2165/00007256-199214060-00005

Bashore, T. R., Ridderinkhof, K. R., and Van Der Molen, M. W. (1997). The decline of cognitive processing speed in old age. *Curr. Dir. Psychol.* 6, 163–169. doi: 10.1111/1467-8721.ep10772944

Begg, R. K., and Sparrow, W. A. (2000). Gait characteristics of young and older individuals negotiating a raised surface: implications for the prevention of falls. *J. Gerontol A Biol. Sci. Med.* 55, M147–M154. doi: 10.1093/gerona/55.3.M147

Berg, W. P., Alessio, H. M., Mills, E. M., and Tong, C. (1997). Circumstances and consequences of falls in independent community-dwelling older adults. *Age Ageing* 26, 261–268. doi: 10.1093/ageing/26.4.261

Chou, L.-S., Draganich, L. F., and Song, S.-M. (1997). Minimum energy trajectories of the swing ankle when stepping over obstacles of different heights. *J. Biomech.* 30, 115–120. doi: 10.1016/S0021-9290(96)00111-X

Cole, K. J. (1991). Grasp force control in older adults. *J. Mot. Behav.* 23, 251–258. doi: 10.1080/00222895.1991.9942036

Cole, K. J., and Beck, C. L. (1994). The stability of precision grip force in older adults. *J. Mot. Behav.* 26, 171–177. doi: 10.1080/00222895.1994.9941671

Cole, K. J., Rotella, D. L., and Harper, J. G. (1999). Mechanisms for age-related changes of fingertip forces during precision gripping and lifting in adults. *J. Neurosci.* 19, 3238–3247.

Flanagan, J. R., and Wing, A. M. (1990). The stability of precision grip forces during cyclic arm movements with a hand-held load. *Exp. Brain Res.* 105, 455–464. doi: 10.1007/BF00233045

Flanagan, J. R., and Wing, A. M. (1993). Modulation of grip force with load force during point-to-point arm movements. *Exp. Brain Res.* 95, 131–143. doi: 10.1007/BF00229662

Folstein, M. F., Folstein, S. E., and McHugh, P. R. (1975). "Mini-mental state": a practical method for grading the cognitive state of patients for the clinician. *J. Psychiatr. Res.* 12, 189–198. doi: 10.1016/0022-3956(75)90026-6

Gilles, M. A., and Wing, A. M. (2003). Age-related changes in grip force and dynamics of hand movement. *J. Mot. Behav.* 35, 79–85. doi: 10.1080/00222890309602123

Goodpaster, B. H., Park, S. W., Harris, T. B., Kritchevsky, S. B., Nevitt, M., Schwartz, A. V., et al. (2006). The loss of skeletal muscle strength, mass, and quality in older adults: the health, aging and body composition study. *J. Gerontol A Biol. Sci. Med.* 61, 1059–1064. doi: 10.1093/gerona/61.10.1059

Guadagnoli, M. A., and Lee, T. D. (2004). Challenge point: a framework for conceptualizing the effects of various practice conditions in motor learning. *J. Mot. Behav.* 36, 212–224. doi: 10.3200/JMBR.36.2.212-224

Hamel, K. A., Okita, N., Higginson, J. S., and Cavanagh, P. R. (2005). Foot clearance during stair descent: effects of age and illumination. *Gait Posture* 21, 135–140. doi: 10.1016/j.gaitpost.2004.01.006

Hasson, C. J., Hogan, N., and Sternad, D. (2012a). "Human control of dynamically complex objects," in *4th International IEEE RAS & EMBS Conference on Biomedical Robotics and Biomechatronics* (Rome: BioRob), 1235–1240.

Hasson, C. J., Shen, T., and Sternad, D. (2012b). Energy margins in dynamic object manipulation. *J. Neurophysiol.* 108, 1349–1365. doi: 10.1152/jn.00019.2012

Huang, H. J., and Ahmed, A. A. (2011). Tradeoff between stability and maneuverability during whole-body movements. *PLoS ONE* 6:e21815. doi: 10.1371/journal.pone.0021815

Johansson, R. S., and Cole, K. J. (1992). Sensory-motor coordination during grasping and manipulative actions. *Cur. Opin. Neurobiol.* 2, 815–823. doi: 10.1007/BF00237997

Johansson, R., and Westling, G. (1984). Roles of glabrous skin receptors and sensorimotor memory in automatic control of precision grip when lifting rougher or more slippery objects. *Exp. Brain Res.* 56, 550–564. doi: 10.1016/0959-4388(92)90139-C

Laidlaw, D. H., Bilodeau, M., and Enoka, R. M. (2000). Steadiness is reduced and motor unit discharge is more variable in old adults. *Muscle Nerve* 23, 600–612. doi: 10.1002/(SICI)1097-4598(200004)23:4%3C600::AID-MUS20%3E3.0.CO;2-D

Light, K. E. (1990). Information processing for motor performance in aging adults. *Phys. Ther.* 70, 820–826.

McFadyen, B. J., and Prince, F. (2002). Avoidance and accommodation of surface height changes by healthy, community-dwelling, young, and elderly men. *J. Gerontol A Biol. Sci. Med.* 57, B166–B174. doi: 10.1093/gerona/57.4.B166

Myerson, J., Hale, S., Wagstaff, D., Poon, L. W., and Smith, G. A. (1990). The information-loss model: a mathematical theory of age-related cognitive slowing. *Psychol. Rev.* 97:475. doi: 10.1037/0033-295X.97.4.475

Onyshko, S., and Winter, D. (1980). A mathematical model for the dynamics of human locomotion. *J. Biomech.* 13, 361–368. doi: 10.1016/0021-9290(80)90016-0

Pannese, E. (2011). Morphological changes in nerve cells during normal aging. *Brain Struct. Func.* 216, 85–89. doi: 10.1007/s00429-011-0308-y

Salthouse, T. A. (1996). The processing-speed theory of adult age differences in cognition. *Psychol. Rev.* 103:403. doi: 10.1037/0033-295X.103.3.403

Slobounov, S. M., Moss, S. A., Slobounova, E. S., and Newell, K. M. (1998). Aging and time to instability in posture. *J. Gerontol. A Biol. Sci. Med.* 53, B71–B80. doi: 10.1093/gerona/53A.1.B71

Sternad, D., Huber, M. E., and Kuznetsov, N. (2014). "Acquisition of novel and complex motor skills: stable solutions where intrinsic noise matters less," in *Progress in Motor Control: Skill Learning, Performance, Health, and Injury, Chapter 8*, ed M. F. Levin (New York, NY: Springer).

Tombaugh, T. N., and McIntyre, N. J. (1992). The mini-mental state examination: a comprehensive review. *J. Am. Geriatr. Soc.* 40, 922–935.

Van der Linde, R., and Lammertse, P. (2003). HapticMaster–a generic force controlled robot for human interaction. *Ind. Robot.* 30, 515–524. doi: 10.1108/01439910310506783

Van Wegen, E., Van Emmerik, R., and Riccio, G. (2002). Postural orientation: age-related changes in variability and time-to-boundary. *Hum. Mov. Sci.* 21, 61–84. doi: 10.1016/S0167-9457(02)00077-5

Winter, D. A., Patla, A. E., Frank, J. S., and Walt, S. E. (1990). Biomechanical walking pattern changes in the fit and healthy elderly. *Phys. Ther.* 70, 340–347.

Ye, F., Nasseroleslami, B., and Sternad, D. (2014). "Predictability in human manipulation on nonlinear dynamic objects," in *IEEE Proceedings of the 40th Northeast Bioengineering Conference* (Boston, MA).

12

Using the zebrafish model for Alzheimer's disease research

Morgan Newman*, Esmaeil Ebrahimie and Michael Lardelli

School of Molecular and Biomedical Science, University of Adelaide, SA, Australia

Edited by:
Shin Murakami, Touro University California, USA

Reviewed by:
Fred Van Leeuwen, Maastricht University, Netherlands
Ruishan Wang, University of Tennessee Health Science Center, USA

****Correspondence:***
Morgan Newman, School of Molecular and Biomedical Science, University of Adelaide, SA 5005, Australia
e-mail: morgan.newman@adelaide.edu.au

Rodent models have been extensively used to investigate the cause and mechanisms behind Alzheimer's disease. Despite many years of intensive research using these models we still lack a detailed understanding of the molecular events that lead to neurodegeneration. Although zebrafish lack the complexity of advanced cognitive behaviors evident in rodent models they have proven to be a very informative model for the study of human diseases. In this review we give an overview of how the zebrafish has been used to study Alzheimer's disease. Zebrafish possess genes orthologous to those mutated in familial Alzheimer's disease and research using zebrafish has revealed unique characteristics of these genes that have been difficult to observe in rodent models. The zebrafish is becoming an increasingly popular model for the investigation of Alzheimer's disease and will complement studies using other models to help complete our understanding of this disease.

Keywords: zebrafish, Alzheimer disease, presenilins, gamma-secretase, amyloid beta-protein precursor, MAPT

ALZHEIMER'S DISEASE

Alzheimer's disease (AD) is the most prevalent form of dementia. It was estimated in 2010 that 36 million people were living with AD and this figure is predicted to increase to 66 million by 2030 (World Alzheimer report's, 2010). The main clinical feature of AD is progressive memory loss. However, AD can also be characterized by the impairment of speech and motor ability, depression, delusions, hallucinations, and aggressive behavior (Voisin and Vellas, 2009). Despite these recognizable behavioral differences it is actually difficult during the early stages of the disease to correctly diagnose someone as having AD (Blennow et al., 2006). There is significant neuronal loss in several brain regions in AD patients (Regeur et al., 1994; West et al., 1994). This is usually accompanied by extracellular aggregates of the amyloid-beta peptide and intracellular aggregates of the tau protein called neurofibrillary tangles (NFTs).

Alzheimer's disease can be classed as familial (FAD, usually with onset <65 years) or sporadic (SAD, onset >65 years). We have acquired most of our knowledge on the pathogenesis of AD through studies of FAD mutations. FAD is attributed to mutations in three genes, *PRESENILIN 1* (*PSEN1*), *PRESENILIN 2* (*PSEN2*), and the *AMYLOID BETA A4 PRECURSOR PROTEIN* (*APP*). The PSEN proteins are essential for γ-secretase activity that cleaves transmembrane domain proteins within lipid bilayers (reviewed in McCarthy et al., 2009). The PSEN proteins and four other proteins comprise γ-secretase complexes. PSEN (1 or 2), nicastrin (NCT), anterior pharynx defective 1 (APH1a or APH1b), and presenilin enhancer 2 (PSENEN) form active γ-secretase complexes in cellular membranes. These complexes are responsible for the cleavage of a number of single-pass transmembrane proteins such as APP and NOTCH. APP is initially cleaved by α- or β-secretases to release APPα or APPβ fragments, respectively. The subsequent cleavage of APP by γ-secretase after β-secretase cleavage liberates amyloid-β (Aβ) peptides of various lengths. The longer Aβ-42 peptide is prone to aggregation and is suggested to form toxic oligomers and fibrils that eventually deposit as amyloid plaques in the brain. Deposits of plaques and NFTs are common occurrences in the brains of those with FAD.

The common, late onset form of AD (accounting for >90% of cases) occurs sporadically (Blennow et al., 2006). Sporadic AD (SAD) has a complex etiology and is associated with many risk factors including old-age and possession of the ε4 allele of the *APOLIPOPROTEIN E* (*APOE*) gene. Human genome wide association studies have revealed a number of possible loci associated with risk for SAD [reviewed by Rademakers and Rovelet-Lecrux, 2009). There are numerous other risk factors associated with an individual's lifestyle that can also increase the likelihood of developing AD. These overlap considerably with the risk factors for cardiovascular disease (Kotze and van Rensburg, 2012) including hypertension, hypercholesterolemia and obesity (Martins et al., 2006). The molecular and cellular triggers for the onset of SAD are yet to be completely resolved, however, there have been many hypotheses suggested to explain how AD is initiated. Of the many hypotheses that have been postulated over the years, some that are gaining momentum attribute AD to vasculature dysfunction (Stone, 2008; Marchesi, 2011), oxidative stress (Nunomura et al., 2001), mitochondrial dysfunction (Selfridge et al., 2012) or hypoxia (Oresic et al., 2011).

The common observation of amyloid plaques in AD brains led to the formulation of the amyloid hypothesis in 1992 (Hardy and Higgins, 1992) that continues to dominate research thinking as a unifying hypothesis for FAD and SAD. The hypothesis suggests that toxic oligomerization of Aβ peptides is the initiating factor that triggers a cascade of subsequent cellular abnormalities such as inflammation and oxidative stress (Verdile et al., 2004). These secondary phenomena ultimately lead to neuronal dysfunction, degeneration and death. Although still widely accepted, doubts have arisen regarding its validity following several failed clinical trials of drugs intended to reduce Aβ levels (refer to www.alzforum.org regarding information on AD drugs in clinical trials).

Rodent models of AD have been exploited extensively and have given considerable insight into this disease. However, we still do not understand the events that trigger the neurodegeneration evident in AD. Research using the zebrafish model has revealed particular characteristics of the various genes implicated in AD that have been difficult to observe in other animal models (Liao et al., 2012; Newman et al., 2012). This review will focus on how the zebrafish has been used to study the genes and various cellular pathways implicated in FAD and SAD pathogenesis and will conclude by examining the limitations of the zebrafish and what the future may hold for use of this model in AD research.

THE ZEBRAFISH MODEL

The zebrafish are a small, hardy freshwater fish native to India and often kept in home aquaria. They were originally used as a model organism for the study of vertebrate development. However, over the last decade the zebrafish model has become increasingly employed for investigating a wide variety of human diseases (Lieschke and Currie, 2007). The zebrafish has a number of characteristics that make it a versatile animal model. Although they lack the advanced cognitive behaviors evident in rodent models, their transparent embryos, rapid development *ex utero* and large reproductive capacity (100+ embryos per spawning) provide obvious advantages over mammalian models. Furthermore, multiple genes can be manipulated simply and effectively in the zebrafish at physiologically relevant levels (Newman et al., 2012), which cannot be currently achieved in rodent models. While, in general, rodents more closely model human physiology than fish, zebrafish nevertheless are vertebrates and so are more relevant to understanding human biology than invertebrate models as *Drosophila melanogaster* and *Caenorhabditis elegans.* Zebrafish embryos are particularly manipulable due to their large size, ready availability and the ability to exploit changes in their development for assay of particular gene activities (Nornes et al., 2009). Thus, zebrafish embryos can often present a felicitous vertebrate system in which to examine the molecular and cellular functions of genes implicated in AD.

The zebrafish genome is extensively annotated. The zebrafish (teleost-bony fish) evolutionary lineage separated from the human (tetrapod) lineage approximately 450 million years ago (Kumar and Hedges, 1998). Teleosts appear to have undergone an additional round of genome duplication since their separation from the tetrapod lineage followed by loss of many of the duplicated genes (Catchen et al., 2011). However, in most cases, zebrafish genes can be identified that are clear orthologs of human genes. Zebrafish possess genes orthologous to the human genes that are thought to play essential roles in AD. The *psen1* (Leimer et al., 1999) and *psen2* (Groth et al., 2002) genes are orthologs of human *PSEN1* and *PSEN2*, respectively, while the *appa* and *appb* genes are "co-orthologs" of human *APP* (Musa et al., 2001). Zebrafish hold orthologous genes for the components of the gamma-secretase complex, *PSENEN* (*psenen*; Francis et al., 2002; Campbell et al., 2006), *NCTN* (*ncstn*; Strausberg et al., 2002) and *APH1b* (*aph1b*; Francis et al., 2002). While orthologs of β-secretase (*BACE1* and *BACE2*) have also recently been identified in zebrafish: *bace1* (Moussavi Nik et al., 2012) and *bace2* (van Bebber et al., 2013). The *microtubule-associated protein tau* (*MAPT*) gene in humans encodes the tau protein and our laboratory identified co-orthologs of this gene in zebrafish, *mapta*, and *maptb* (Chen et al., 2009). Zebrafish also possess co-orthologs of *APOE*: *apoea* and *apoeb* (Babin et al., 1997; Woods et al., 2005). Genes arising by duplication can have overlapping functions. This can be disadvantageous when analyzing gene function as particular loss-of-function phenotypes may be obscured unless the function of both duplicate genes is blocked. Alternatively, duplicate genes can have partially non-overlapping functions and this can facilitate functional analysis as loss-of-function phenotypes may be restricted to particular cells or tissues.

Zebrafish are an advantageous model for genetic and molecular studies. Zebrafish embryos are genetically malleable by injection of morpholino antisense oligonucleotides, mRNA, transgenes and more recently by genome engineering systems (reviewed in Hwang et al., 2013; Schmid and Haass, 2013; Hisano et al., 2014). These technologies can make both subtle and drastic changes in gene expression with the effects observed in the developing transparent embryos. Morpholinos are designed to bind to particular sites in transcripts from a gene of interest. Binding of a morpholino can either block mRNA translation (knockdown) or interfere with correct splicing of exons (e.g., Draper et al., 2001; Nornes et al., 2008; Berger et al., 2011). Injection of sense mRNA can allow overexpression of a particular gene of interest. The effects of morpholino and mRNA injection generally only persist during embryogenesis (2–3 days post-fertilization). Transgenic zebrafish can be generated using efficient vectors such as the Tol2 transposase system (Kawakami et al., 2000) to insert genes under the control of tissue specific promoters. Conditionally expressed transgenics can also be generated using the Cre/loxP (Hans et al., 2009) and GAL4-UAS (Halpern et al., 2008) systems for gene function analysis at particular time points. The absence of technology available to generate targeted mutations in the zebrafish genome was previously a disadvantage of the zebrafish model relative to rodents. In recent times however, zinc finger nucleases (ZFNs), transcription activator-like effector nucleases (TALENS) and the type II prokaryotic CRISPR (clustered regularly interspaced short palindromic repeats)/Cas systems have been developed for targeted modification of gene sequences in the zebrafish genome (Hwang et al., 2013; Schmid and Haass, 2013).

A search of the available scientific literature in the PubMed database using the term "zebrafish + alzheimer's disease" revealed 119 publications with 98 being original research papers (23rd May, 2014). **Figure 1** displays the research areas in which these papers have been published. There is an obvious concentration of research on Aβ and Presenilin function in zebrafish.

USING ZEBRAFISH TO INVESTIGATE GENES MUTATED IN FAD

THE PRESENILINS

The genes implicated in FAD have been extensively studied over the last 25 years, although our understanding of their normal functions is still far from complete. The *PSEN* genes

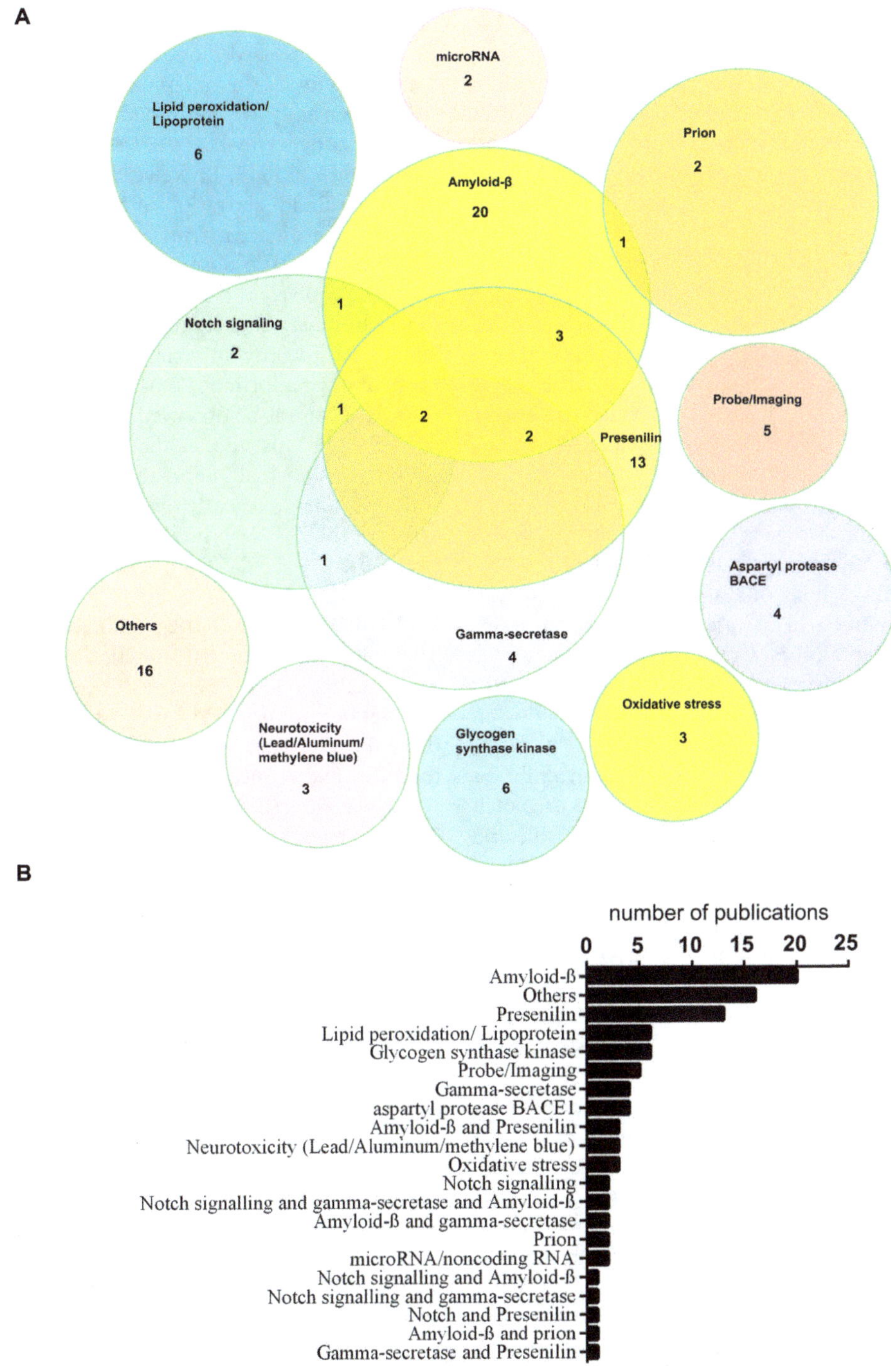

FIGURE 1 | Text mining analysis of the scientific literature to detect papers on the application of Zebrafish in Alzheimer's disease research. The PubMed database was mined for zebrafish and Alzheimer's disease using the search term, "zebrafish+alzheimer's disease," by the MedScan Reader 5 tool implemented in the Pathway Studio 9 Package (Nikitin et al., 2003b; Novichkova et al., 2003a). MedScan Reader 5 collects information and processes undertaken data using natural language processing (NLP). The language interprets these to logical concepts and extracts functional relationships between proteins, small molecules, and cellular processes (Nikitin et al., 2003b; Novichkova et al., 2003a). 119 publications were found. Abstracts of these publications were studied and review papers were removed such that 98 papers remained. **(A)** Venn diagram and **(B)** bar graph showing numbers of research papers in different areas. A concentration of research on Amyloidβ and Presenilin function is apparent.

play important roles in development. The zebrafish (as well-characterized model for studies of developmental biology) has been employed to investigate the normal functions of these genes. The *psen1* and *psen2* genes are ubiquitously expressed in zebrafish embryos (Leimer et al., 1999; Groth et al., 2002), implying a functional importance of these genes during development. Injection of morpholinos to knockdown *presenilin* gene expression revealed similar and dissimilar phenotypes compared to Presenilin knockout mice (*Psen1*$^{-/-}$). *Psen1*$^{-/-}$ mice die during development (Shen et al., 1997). To overcome this, conditional *Psen1* knockout mouse models have been developed (reviewed in van Tijn et al., 2011). Zebrafish embryos injected with a *psen1* translation-blocking morpholino are viable and have similar phenotypes (Nornes et al., 2003; Campbell et al., 2006; Nornes et al., 2008) to *Psen1*$^{-/-}$ mice such as aberrant somite formation and Notch signaling defects (Shen et al., 1997; Wong et al., 1997) Interestingly, a zebrafish mutant (discovered in a TILLING screen) lacking Psen1 activity is viable (Sundvik et al., 2013). These mutant fish have been used to study the brains histaminergic system (Sundvik et al., 2013). This system is essential in mediating cognitive functions affected in AD. Analysis of histamine neuron numbers in the *psen1*$^{-/-}$ zebrafish brains revealed that *psen1* in zebrafish is a regulator of histaminergic neuronal development (Sundvik et al., 2013). These mutant fish will be a valuable tool for further analysis of *psen1* function in zebrafish.

Blockage of Psen2 protein translation in zebrafish embryos (Nornes et al., 2008, 2009) appears to have major effects on Notch signaling in comparison to *Psen2*$^{-/-}$ mice which are viable and show only a minor phenotype (Herreman et al., 1999). Furthermore, loss of Psen2 expression affects the production of dorsal longitudinal ascending (DoLA) interneurons in the developing spinal cord of zebrafish larvae (Nornes et al., 2009). As loss of Psen1 does not affect DoLAs this observation provides an *in vivo* assay for Psen2 function. This assay was used to demonstrate a functional interaction between Psen1 and Psen2 in zebrafish (Nornes et al., 2009).

In the absence of technology available to analyze *PSEN* FAD missense mutations in zebrafish, our laboratory previously attempted to model *PSEN1* splicing mutations by injecting morpholinos that target splice acceptor sites of the orthologous *psen1* gene. We attempted to cause exon skipping to exclude exon 8 or 9 from zebrafish *psen1* transcripts to mimic the effects of the human *PSEN1 L271V* and Δ9 mutations, respectively,. However, instead of the (at that time) expected exon exclusion, injection of morpholinos blocking splice acceptor sites lead to the failure of introns 7 and 8 to be correctly spliced out of transcripts (Nornes et al., 2008). The inclusion of intron sequence lead to premature truncation of the open reading frame (ORF) after exons 6 and 7, respectively. It appeared that the aberrant transcripts induced by morpholino injection were able to evade nonsense-mediated decay and be translated into truncated protein molecules. Assays developed in our laboratory (discussed in the next section) demonstrated that truncation of the zebrafish *psen1* transcript ORF after exons 6 and 7 had potent dominant negative effects on Psen1 activity and could also suppress Psen2 activity (Nornes et al., 2008). These putative truncated proteins were subsequently expressed in embryos by injection of synthetic mRNAs. Injection of mRNAs coding for proteins truncated after exon 6- or 7-derived sequence had the same dominant effect on Psen1 activity as the morpholino-induced aberrant *psen1* transcripts. Recently we published results where we expanded the original study to analyze a series of *psen1* ORF truncations (i.e., after exon 4, 5, 6, 7, 8; Newman et al., 2014). We found differential, dominant activation of Notch signaling and APP cleavage amongst the different truncations of Psen1. Interestingly, similar effects were also observed after injection of synthetic mRNAs encoding equivalent truncations of human PSEN1. This supports the evolutionary conservation of function of these truncated proteins. A particularly important discovery from this study was that the activity of a form of Psen1 truncated after exon 4 sequence of the ORF) cannot be observed in the absence of normal endogenous Psen1. This implies that mutant forms of PSEN1 require endogenous normal PSEN1 to exert their effects. A similar observation was made recently by Heilig et al. for various FAD mutant forms of the PSEN1 protein in mouse embryo fibroblasts (Heilig et al., 2013).

OTHER COMPONENTS OF THE γ-SECRETASE COMPLEX

There has been limited functional analysis of the zebrafish genes orthlogous to the non-PRESENILIN components of the γ-secretase complex. Blockage of translation of Psenen or Aph1b proteins in zebrafish causes phenotypes including defective somitogenesis and reduced neuron formation as expected for loss of Notch signaling (that requires γ-secretase activity; Campbell et al., 2006). Furthermore, blockage of Psenen translation leads to destabilization of Psen1 protein and causes a much greater induction of apoptosis in developing embryos than blocking translation of Psen1, Psen2, or Aph1b (Campbell et al., 2006). Simultaneous inhibition of p53 translation was able to block the induction of apoptosis (Campbell et al., 2006).

THE AMYLOID-BETA PRECURSOR PROTEIN

The zebrafish *APP* "co-orthologs," *appa* and *appb* have widespread and overlapping expression from mid-gastrulation in the developing embryo (Musa et al., 2001). At 24hpf both genes are expressed in the developing forebrain and other tissues with only *appb* expressed in the spinal cord (Musa et al., 2001). In a zebrafish study by Lee and Cole a section of *appb* regulatory sequence was fused to GFP (Lee and Cole, 2007). Dissimilar to other expression studies, they observed expression of *appb* in the developing vasculature. More recently, Liao et al. (2012) isolated transposon gene trap integrations that contained RFP in the *appa* gene and in the closely related a*myloid beta precursor-like protein 2 gene (aplp2).* The gene traps caused fusions to RFP of the extracellular domains of both of the encoded proteins. The fusion proteins of these genes were accumulated in the vasculature. However, they could not detect the transcripts of these genes in the endothelial cells of the vasculature. Instead, transcripts were detected in neuronal cells. This suggests that these proteins are synthesized in neuronal cells and then accumulate in the vasculature.

Translation blocking morpholinos have also been employed to investigate the function of the Appa and Appb proteins (Joshi et al., 2009). Inhibition of Appa had little effect on the developing embryo while Appb translation inhibition resulted in defective convergent extension cellular movements and a reduced body length. These defects could be rescued by injecting Appb deficient embryos with mRNA coding for human APP. The rescue by human APP was more effective than injection of an mRNA encoding a human *APP* FAD mutant (the APP Swedish double mutation *K595N* and *M596L*). Loss of Appb activity has also been shown to cause defective neural development (Song and Pimplikar, 2012) including defective axonal out-growth patterning and synapse formation (Abramsson et al., 2013). In the study by Song and Pimplikar, only full-length human APP but not truncated forms could rescue the neuronal defects, revealing that both intracellular and extracellular domains of human APP are required for normal function (Song and Pimplikar, 2012). These studies demonstrate that zebrafish embryos can be exploited for the analysis of different mutant forms of human *APP*.

AMYLOID-BETA FUNCTION AND TOXICITY STUDIES IN ZEBRAFISH

Although Aβ was discovered over 25 years ago (Goate and Hardy, 2012) and many studies have examined its claimed toxicity, the non-pathological functions of the Aβ peptide are still poorly understood. A study by Cameron et al. (2012) demonstrated that high levels of Aβ can increase cerebrovascular branching in the developing zebrafish hindbrain. They then completed a follow up study to determine whether lowering Aβ levels would have the opposite effect (Luna et al., 2013). From 2 days post fertilization (dpf) APP-deficient (by morpholino injection) and Aβ deficient (endogenous Aβ production blocked using a β-secretase inhibitor) larvae presented with cerebrovascular defects. Interestingly, these defects could be rescued by treating the embryos with the human Aβ-42 peptide but not the shorter cleavage product of APP named p3 (that arises from cleavage of APP by α-secretase and γ-secretase). These results suggest that Aβ may play a role in maintaining normal cerebrovascular function. This interesting finding using the zebrafish model provided further evidence that caution should be taken when treating AD with drugs designed to inhibit Aβ production such as BSIs and γ-secretase inhibitors (GSIs).

As mentioned above the amyloid hypothesis of AD proposes that aggregations of Aβ peptides are toxic. Therefore, there has been a considerable effort put towards developing and discovering Aβ-lowering compounds to counter the toxicity. Inhibition of β-secretase, also known as beta-site APP cleaving enzyme (BACE1), is of prime interest for the development of amyloid-lowering drugs. BACE1 has become an attractive target for drug development as, in comparison to the lethality observed in *Psen1* null mice, *Bace1* knock-out mice are viable (Roberds et al., 2001; Luo et al., 2003) and have subtle phenotypes (Harrison et al., 2003; Willem et al., 2006). Furthermore no phenotypes have been reported for knockout of the *Bace1* homolog, *Bace2* and deletion of *Bace2* in mice did alter Aβ generation (Dominguez et al., 2005). Recently, *bace1* and *bace2* loss-of-function mutations have been introduced into the zebrafish genome by genome editing using ZFNs (van Bebber et al., 2013). *bace1* mutants had an increased number of mechanosensory neuromasts and, similar to observations in the mouse, *Bace1* knockout caused a decrease in myelination. *bace2* mutants had a distinct melanocyte migration phenotype that was not observed in the *bace1* mutants. There was no effect on myelination or neuromasts in the *bace2* mutants. The phenotypes observed in the single mutants were not enhanced further in the Bace1/2 double knockout. Together the data from this study suggests that, in zebrafish, Bace1 and Bace2, have distinct non-redundant physiological functions. These specific phenotypes observed in zebrafish *bace1* and *bace2* mutants have provided important information on BACE1 and BACE2 function and support that zebrafish can be a useful *in vivo* system for determining, e.g., whether BACE1 inhibitors also inhibit BACE2 function and vice versa. *In vivo* evaluation of BACE inhibitors is integral for establishing these drugs as a therapeutic option for AD.

The zebrafish is an excellent system for the screening of chemical libraries. Embryos and larvae placed into microtiter plates can be treated with various chemicals in their aqueous support medium. This strategy can be employed to reveal therapeutic compounds for various disease states modeled in the fish. The only published study that has generated a transgenic Aβ toxicity model in zebrafish involved fusing the human Aβ-42 sequence to the promoter of the *mitfa* (*nacre*) gene (Newman et al., 2010). This would drive expression of human Aβ-42 specifically in the melanin-containing pigment cells (melanocytes) of the zebrafish in the hope that it would produce an easily identifiable disrupted pigmentation pattern phenotype without being lethal to the zebrafish larvae. A disrupted pattern did become evident in the adult fish. However, unfortunately it only became apparent after 16 months which is too late for drug screening and was too late for breeding the old, infertile fish. Aβ toxicity can also be analyzed in zebrafish simply by exposing embryos to amyloid-beta in their supportive aqueous environment. Treatment of embryos with 2.5 μM Aβ-40 caused defective development including that of the vasculature and also accelerated cell senescence (Donnini et al., 2010). This system could be expanded to test Aβ-42 (more aggregative form) and also to find compounds that ameliorate these observed defects.

γ-secretase inhibitors (GSIs) have been investigated as a therapeutic option to inhibit the production of Aβ peptides. However, the use of GSIs comes with the potential side affects of also affecting Notch signaling. Testing the toxicity of GSIs on zebrafish has revealed important information on how Notch related pathways are adversely affected by GSIs (Yang et al., 2010).

ASSAYS FOR AD-RELEVANT CELLULAR PATHWAYS AND PROCESSES IN ZEBRAFISH

γ-SECRETASE ACTIVITY ASSAYS

There are a number of cellular pathways and processes that are aberrant in AD. The zebrafish are a useful system for investigating molecular events such as γ-secreatse activity and autophagy that have been implicated in AD pathogenesis.

There are over 70 proteins that are known to be substrates of γ-secreatse activity (Lleo and Saura, 2011). In zebrafish, γ-secretase activity was initially analyzed by observing changes in the expression of genes known to be downstream targets of Notch signaling such as *hairy-related 6* (Bernardos et al., 2005; Campbell et al., 2006; Arslanova et al., 2010) and *neurogenin* (Campbell et al.,

2006). However, gene expression can be under different transcriptional control in different regions of the embryo (Campbell et al., 2006; Arslanova et al., 2010). Therefore, using whole embryos in quantitative PCR analysis is not informative to assess changes in gene expression in response to various factors. To overcome this, changes in gene expression in a particular region of the embryos have been assessed by whole-mount *in situ* transcript hybridization (Campbell et al., 2006; Nornes et al., 2008; Arslanova et al., 2010). However, this is not normally used as a quantitative technique since many variables can influence the strength of the staining signal such as fixation conditions and incubation times. Consequently, use of this technique to assay relative differences in Notch signals under various treatments requires stringent controls.

Recently, the first assay to assess directly γ-secretase cleavage activity was developed by Wilson and Lardelli (2013). α- and β-secretase cleavage of Appa provide substrates for subsequent γ-secretase cleavage. Unfortunately these cleaved forms of Appa cannot be detected in zebrafish embryos prior to 48 hpf which currently makes monitoring endogenous Appa cleavage in manipulated zebrafish embryos difficult. Therefore, a fragment of Appa equivalent to the membrane-embedded remnant of APP following β-secretase cleavage was fused to GFP and expressed transiently in zebrafish embryos by the use of Tol2 vector transgenesis system. This construct is co-expressed with a set ratio of free GFP (for signal normalization). Western immunoblotting is then used to assess the ratio of the Appa:GFP substrate to free GFP (the γ-secretase cleavage product itself is too unstable to be observed). Once an Appa:GFP/ free GFP ratio is determined for a protein sample from a pool of manipulated embryos (e.g., drug treatment, morpholino or mRNA injection) it can then be compared to control embryos to determine how that particular manipulation is affecting γ-secretase cleavage activity.

ASSAYING PROTEIN DEGRADATION PATHWAYS IN ZEBRAFISH

Excess or aberrant cellular proteins can be degraded by the ubiquitin-proteasome system (UPS). Since protein aggregation is implicated in many neurodegenerative diseases (Ross and Poirier, 2004) it is unsurprising that problems with UPS function have been implicated in neurodegenerative disease such as AD (West et al., 1994; Nikitin et al., 2003a; Novichkova et al., 2003b) and Parkinson's disease (Olanow and McNaught, 2006). Zebrafish have been used to investigate UPS function in Parkinson's disease (Regeur et al., 1994); however, no analyses in zebrafish have yet examined the UPS with respect to AD.

Autophagy is an important mechanism required for the degradation of dysfunctional and unwanted cellular components (including incorrectly folded and aggregated proteins) through the actions of lysosomes. Indeed, autophagy has been identified as a pathway for the degradation of accumulated Aβ peptides (Nilsson et al., 2013). Recently, the Presenilin proteins were suggested to have a major role in autophagy with FAD mutations in human PSEN1 inhibiting this function (Lee et al., 2010). These authors presented evidence showing that PSEN1 acts as a chaperone in the ER for a transmembrane protein required for acidification of the lysosomes, the v-ATPase V0a1 subunit [Lee et al., 2010; however, other reports have disputed this finding (Coen et al., 2012; Zhang et al., 2012)]. They also demonstrated that this function of PSEN1 is dependent on the full-length PSEN1 holoprotein rather than the endoproteolysed form that is active in the γ-secretase complex. Furthermore, a γ-secretase inhibitor and loss of another γ-secretase complex component (NCT) had no effect on autophagy (Lee et al., 2010) suggesting that this function of PSEN1 is independent from its function in γ-secretase complexes.

Autophagy can be analyzed in zebrafish by observing induction of the LC3-II protein by western immunoblotting using a human antibody against LC3 that cross-reacts with zebrafish Lc3 (He et al., 2009; He and Klionsky, 2010). Transgenic zebrafish have also been developed that express GFP fused to Lc3 (He et al., 2009). As Presenilin protein expression can easily be manipulated in the zebrafish these autophagy assay are a useful tool for further investigation of the involvement of the Presenilins in autophagy.

USING THE ZEBRAFISH TO INVESTIGATE OTHER ASPECTS OF ALZHEIMER'S DISEASE ETIOLOGY

ANALYSIS OF HYPOXIA IN THE ZEBRAFISH

There is accumulating evidence suggesting that hypoxia is an important initiating factor in the pathogenesis of AD. Under hypoxic conditions the electron transport chain in the mitochondria increases free radical production that leads to increased oxidative stress (Bell et al., 2007). Biomarkers of hypoxia can differentiate between people with mild cognitive impairment that progress to AD and those who do not (Oresic et al., 2011). The risk factors for cardiovascular disease and AD are similar (Kotze and van Rensburg, 2012) and it is anticipated that vasculature problems would affect oxygenation of the brain. Interestingly, Aβ levels in serum have been shown to be elevated after cardiac arrest (Zetterberg et al., 2011).

Zebrafish are an advantageous system for analysis of the effects of hypoxia on various biological functions. Zebrafish embryos and adults can be exposed to real hypoxia by depleting their water environment of oxygen or to chemical mimicry of hypoxia through, e.g., sodium azide treatment (Moussavi Nik et al., 2011). Similarly to what is observed in humans (Lukiw et al., 2001; Pluta, 2005; De Gasperi et al., 2010; Zhang and Le, 2010), hypoxia upregulates *psen1*, *psen2*, *appa*, *appb*, and *bace1* in zebrafish adult brain and larvae (Moussavi Nik et al., 2012). This suggests that Aβ is produced as a protective response to hypoxia in both human and zebrafish cells – a response conserved over 450 Mya of evolutionary time. Note, however, that while all the enzymes required to cleave Aβ from Appa and/or Appb are present in zebrafish, the existence of Aβ itself has not yet been directly demonstrated (e.g., through immunoblotting or mass spectrometry). The study by Moussavi Nik et al. (2012) also demonstrated that, unlike in mammals, F2-isoprostanes are not a good marker of oxidative stress in zebrafish and that the upregulation of *catalase* gene expression can be a better alternative marker for demonstration of oxidative stress in zebrafish (Jin et al., 2011; Tseng et al., 2013).

APOE

The APOE ε4 allele has been identified has the main genetic risk factor for SAD. APOE is important for clearance of amyloid-beta from the brain (Huang and Mucke, 2012), while the AD risk-associated ε4 allele has been shown to impair the clearance of Aβ (Deane et al., 2008) and, more recently, to affect the integrity of the blood–brain barrier (Bell et al., 2012). There has been little research investigating APOE function in zebrafish. Expression studies of *apoea* (Raymond et al., 2006) and *apoeb* (Pujic et al., 2006) revealed expression in the developing retina and yolk syncytial layer. Furthermore, *apoeb* has also been observed in microglial cells (Veth et al., 2011), developing fins and epidermis (Monnot et al., 1999; Tingaud-Sequeira et al., 2006), regenerating fin tissue (Monnot et al., 1999), macrophages (Lien et al., 2006), liver, intestine, and ovary (Levi et al., 2012).

MAPT

The MAPT is the main component of the NFTs found in AD brains. Various dysfunctions of the tau protein are found in other neurodegenerative disorders such as frontotemporal dementia (FTD), corticobasal degeneration and progressive supranuclear palsy (Pittman et al., 2006). Diseases with tau-like pathology are collectively termed "tauopathies." A review by Bai and Burton (2011) discussed how the zebrafish has been used to investigate these diseases. A number of MAPT protein isoforms exist as a result of alternative splicing of *MAPT* transcripts. These isoforms can be classified into two groups, 3R or 4R, depending on the number of tubulin-binding motifs. It appears that an overall one-to-one ratio of 3R to 4R transcripts is required for normal functioning of the MAPT protein in the brain (Goedert and Spillantini, 2006). In most tauopathies this ratio is found to be changed (Goedert and Spillantini, 2006) and altered splicing of *MAPT* is also suggested to occur in AD brains (Conrad et al., 2007).

Transgenic zebrafish expressing human *MAPT* were generated and investigated prior to identification of the zebrafish ortholog(s) of *MAPT*. In these studies human *MAPT* was specifically expressed in zebrafish CNS neurons (Bai et al., 2007; Paquet et al., 2009). Bai et al. used the promoter of the *enolase 2* gene to drive the expression of MAPT 4R in zebrafish neurons at approximately eightfold higher levels than what is observed in human brain. This resulted in accumulations of tau protein (resembling NFTs) in the zebrafish brain. In the study by Paquet et al., the *HuC* promoter was employed to drive expression of a Gal4:VP16 fusion protein in neurons. This protein was then bound to UAS sites in a bidirectional promoter transcribing the DsRed fluorescent marker protein gene and a mutant form of human MAPT associated with FTD, *TAU-P301L*. The transgenic zebrafish larvae showed biochemical changes consistent with those observed in human tauopathies. However, it should be noted that no comparisons of phenotype were made between the non-mutant and mutant forms of human *MAPT* in the zebrafish. Furthermore, the expression levels of the transgenes relative to the endogenous zebrafish *mapt* genes were not assessed in these studies. Despite these limitations these transgenic zebrafish models provide a useful system to investigate whether chemical inhibitors can modulate the observed tauopathy-associated changes.

The zebrafish "co-orthologs" of the human *MAPT* gene, *mapta* and *maptb* have similar but not completely overlapping patterns of expression in developing embryos (Chen et al., 2009). They are both predominantly expressed in the developing CNS while only *maptb* has strong expression in the trigeminal ganglion and dorsal sensory neurons of the spinal cord. *Mapta* is spliced into 4R–6R isoforms while *maptb* is spliced mainly into 3R isoforms. This expression is in contrast to mouse *Mapt* which is mainly expressed as 3R in the brain (and hence may not be a good model of MAPT function for human pathologies). Manipulation of the expression of the zebrafish *mapt* isoforms may therefore be advantageous for understanding the function of 3R and 4R MAPT and the role(s) the 3R:4R ratio plays in pathogenesis.

THE FUTURE FOR MODELING ALZHEIMER'S DISEASE IN ZEBRAFISH

The zebrafish is rapidly emerging as an attractive model for AD research. They are an ideal model for drug testing prior to clinical testing in rodents. However, there are still aspects of this model that require better understanding. For the zebrafish system to be used to model aspects of AD pathobiology we need to better understand zebrafish brain structure and function and also gain a deeper understanding of adult zebrafish brain physiology. Work so far has revealed that the zebrafish brain does have a reasonable level of conservation of basic structure when compared to mammals as well as similar neuroanatomical and neurochemical pathways to those that play roles in human disease (reviewed in Santana et al., 2012). We have revealed various aspects of presenilin gene biology using the zebrafish that would otherwise be difficult to observe/analyze in other models. However, to analyze effectively future transgenic and mutant zebrafish models of AD we need to strengthen our understanding of the functions in zebrafish of some of the orthologs of the key genes implicated in human AD pathogenesis such as MAPT and APOE.

Whether the zebrafish can be employed to model a late-onset disease like AD is debatable since zebrafish have a profound capacity for regeneration and this must impact on the development of neurodegenerative phenotypes. Neurogenesis in the adult zebrafish brain is much more abundant than is observed in mammals (Kizil et al., 2012) consequently making analysis of neuronal loss difficult. Despite these limitations the recent availability and feasibility of using genome editing technologies presents an exciting opportunity to develop zebrafish genetic models of neurodegenerative diseases such as AD. ZFNs, TALENs and CRISP/Rs have been validated for use in the zebrafish [reviewed by Hwang et al., 2013; Schmid and Haass, 2013) and it is inevitable that FAD mutations will be introduced into zebrafish FAD gene orthologs.

Animal models are a useful tool in investigating the causes and pathologies of human diseases. Obviously such models can never reflect the complete pathology that is observed in human cases. The complexity of the human brain makes AD a particularly difficult disease to model in animals. However, by using a number of different models including the zebrafish, we can exploit the unique characteristics of each to unravel the molecular basis of this disease.

REFERENCES

Abramsson, A., Kettunen, P., Banote, R. K., Lott, E., Li, M., Arner, A., et al. (2013). The zebrafish amyloid precursor protein-b is required for motor neuron guidance and synapse formation. *Dev. Biol.* 381, 377–388. doi: 10.1016/j.ydbio.2013.06.026

Arslanova, D., Yang, T., Xu, X. Y., Wong, S. T., Augelli-Szafran, C. E., and Xia, W. M. (2010). Phenotypic analysis of images of zebrafish treated with Alzheimer's gamma-secretase inhibitors. *BMC Biotechnol.* 10:24. doi: 10.1186/1472-6750-10-24

Babin, P. J., Thisse, C., Durliat, M., Andre, M., Akimenko, M. A., and Thisse, B. (1997). Both apolipoprotein E and A-I genes are present in a nonmammalian vertebrate and are highly expressed during embryonic development. *Proc. Natl. Acad. Sci. U.S.A.* 94, 8622–8627. doi: 10.1073/pnas.94.16.8622

Bai, Q., and Burton, E. A. (2011). Zebrafish models of tauopathy. *Biochim. Biophys. Acta* 1812, 353–363. doi: 10.1016/j.bbadis.2010.09.004

Bai, Q., Garver, J. A., Hukriede, N. A., and Burton, E. A. (2007). Generation of a transgenic zebrafish model of Tauopathy using a novel promoter element derived from the zebrafish eno2 gene. *Nucleic Acids Res.* 35, 6501–6516. doi: 10.1093/nar/gkm608

Bell, E. L., Klimova, T. A., Eisenbart, J., Moraes, C. T., Murphy, M. P., Budinger, G. R. S., et al. (2007). The Q(o) site of the mitochondrial complex III is required for the transduction of hypoxic signaling via reactive oxygen species production. *J. Cell Biol.* 177, 1029–1036. doi: 10.1083/jcb.200609074

Bell, R. D., Winkler, E. A., Singh, I., Sagare, A. P., Deane, R., Wu, Z., et al. (2012). Apolipoprotein E controls cerebrovascular integrity via cyclophilin A. *Nature* 485, 512–516. doi: 10.1038/nature11087

Berger, J., Berger, S., Jacoby, A. S., Wilton, S. D., and Currie, P. D. (2011). Evaluation of exon-skipping strategies for Duchenne muscular dystrophy utilizing dystrophin-deficient zebrafish. *J. Cell Mol. Med.* 15, 2643–2651. doi: 10.1111/j.1582-4934.2011.01260.x

Bernardos, R. L., Lentz, S. I., Wolfe, M. S., and Raymond, P. A. (2005). Notch-Delta signaling is required for spatial patterning and Muller glia differentiation in the zebrafish retina. *Dev. Biol.* 278, 381–395. doi: 10.1016/j.ydbio.2004.11.018

Blennow, K., De Leon, M. J., and Zetterberg, H. (2006). Alzheimer's disease. *Lancet* 368, 387–403. doi: 10.1016/S0140-6736(06)69113-7

Cameron, D. J., Galvin, C., Alkam, T., Sidhu, H., Ellison, J., Luna, S., et al. (2012). Alzheimer's-related peptide amyloid-beta plays a conserved role in angiogenesis. *PLoS ONE* 7:e39598. doi: 10.1371/journal.pone.0039598

Campbell, W. A., Yang, H., Zetterberg, H., Baulac, S., Sears, J. A., Liu, T., et al. (2006). Zebrafish lacking Alzheimer presenilin enhancer 2 (Pen-2) demonstrate excessive p53-dependent apoptosis and neuronal loss. *J. Neurochem.* 96, 1423–1440. doi: 10.1111/j.1471-4159.2006.03648.x

Catchen, J. M., Braasch, I., and Postlethwait, J. H. (2011). Conserved synteny and the zebrafish genome. *Methods Cell Biol.* 104, 259–285. doi: 10.1016/B978-0-12-374814-0.00015-X

Chen, M., Martins, R. N., and Lardelli, M. (2009). Complex splicing and neural expression of duplicated tau genes in zebrafish embryos. *J. Alzheimers Dis.* 18, 305–317. doi: 10.3233/JAD-2009-1145

Coen, K., Flannagan, R. S., Baron, S., Carraro-Lacroix, L. R., Wang, D., Vermeire, W., et al. (2012). Lysosomal calcium homeostasis defects, not proton pump defects, cause endo-lysosomal dysfunction in PSEN-deficient cells. *J. Cell Biol.* 198, 23–35. doi: 10.1083/jcb.201201076

Conrad, C., Zhu, J., Conrad, C., Schoenfeld, D., Fang, Z., Ingelsson, M., et al. (2007). Single molecule profiling of tau gene expression in Alzheimer's disease. *J. Neurochem.* 103, 1228–1236. doi: 10.1111/j.1471-4159.2007.04857.x

De Gasperi, R., Sosa, M. A., Dracheva, S., and Elder, G. A. (2010). Presenilin-1 regulates induction of hypoxia inducible factor-1alpha: altered activation by a mutation associated with familial Alzheimer's disease. *Mol. Neurodegener.* 5:38. doi: 10.1186/1750-1326-5-38

Deane, R., Sagare, A., Hamm, K., Parisi, M., Lane, S., Finn, M. B., et al. (2008). apoE isoform-specific disruption of amyloid beta peptide clearance from mouse brain. *J. Clin. Invest.* 118, 4002–4013. doi: 10.1172/JCI36663 36663

Dominguez, D., Tournoy, J., Hartmann, D., Huth, T., Cryns, K., Deforce, S., et al. (2005). Phenotypic and biochemical analyses of BACE1- and BACE2-deficient mice. *J. Biol. Chem.* 280, 30797–30806. doi: 10.1074/jbc.M505249200

Donnini, S., Solito, R., Cetti, E., Corti, F., Giachetti, A., Carra, S., et al. (2010). A beta peptides accelerate the senescence of endothelial cells in vitro and in vivo, impairing angiogenesis. *FASEB J.* 24, 2385–2395. doi: 10.1096/Fj.09–146456

Draper, B. W., Morcos, P. A., and Kimmel, C. B. (2001). Inhibition of zebrafish fgf8 pre-mRNA splicing with morpholino oligos: a quantifiable method for gene knockdown. *Genesis* 30, 154–156. doi: 10.1002/gene.1053

Francis, R., Mcgrath, G., Zhang, J. H., Ruddy, D. A., Sym, M., Apfeld, J., et al. (2002). aph-1 and pen-2 are required for notch pathway signaling, gamma-secretase cleavage of beta APP, and presenilin protein accumulation. *Dev. Cell* 3, 85–97. doi: 10.1016/S1534-5807(02)00189-2

Goate, A., and Hardy, J. (2012). Twenty years of Alzheimer's disease-causing mutations. *J. Neurochem.* 120(Suppl. 1), 3–8. doi: 10.1111/j.1471-4159.2011.07575.x

Goedert, M., and Spillantini, M. G. (2006). A century of Alzheimer's disease. *Science* 314, 777–781. doi: 10.1126/science.1132814

Groth, C., Nornes, S., Mccarty, R., Tamme, R., and Lardelli, M. (2002). Identification of a second presenilin gene in zebrafish with similarity to the human Alzheimer's disease gene presenilin2. *Dev. Genes Evol.* 212, 486–490. doi: 10.1007/s00427-002-0269-5

Halpern, M. E., Rhee, J., Goll, M. G., Akitake, C. M., Parsons, M., and Leach, S. D. (2008). Gal4/UAS transgenic tools and their application to zebrafish. *Zebrafish* 5, 97–110. doi: 10.1089/zeb.2008.0530

Hans, S., Kaslin, J., Freudenreich, D., and Brand, M. (2009). Temporally-controlled site-specific recombination in zebrafish. *PLoS ONE* 4:e4640. doi: 10.1371/journal.pone.0004640

Hardy, J. A., and Higgins, G. A. (1992). Alzheimer's disease: the amyloid cascade hypothesis. *Science* 256, 184–185 doi: 10.1126/science.1566067

Harrison, S. M., Harper, A. J., Hawkins, J., Duddy, G., Grau, E., Pugh, P. L., et al. (2003). BACE1 (beta-secretase) transgenic and knockout mice: identification of neurochemical deficits and behavioral changes. *Mol. Cell. Neurosci.* 24, 646–655. doi: 10.1016/S1044-7431(03)00227-6

He, C., Bartholomew, C. R., Zhou, W., and Klionsky, D. J. (2009). Assaying autophagic activity in transgenic GFP-Lc3 and GFP-Gabarap zebrafish embryos. *Autophagy* 5, 520–526. doi: 10.4161/auto.5.4.7768

He, C., and Klionsky, D. J. (2010). Analyzing autophagy in zebrafish. *Autophagy* 6, 642–644. doi: 10.4161/auto.6.5.12092

Heilig, E. A., Gutti, U., Tai, T., Shen, J., and Kelleher, R. J. (2013). Trans-dominant negative effects of pathogenic PSEN1 mutations on gamma-secretase activity and Abeta production. *J. Neurosci.* 33, 11606–11617. doi: 10.1523/JNEUROSCI.0954-13.2013

Herreman, A., Hartmann, D., Annaert, W., Saftig, P., Craessaerts, K., Serneels, L., et al. (1999). Presenilin 2 deficiency causes a mild pulmonary phenotype and no changes in amyloid precursor protein processing but enhances the embryonic lethal phenotype of presenilin 1 deficiency. *Proc. Natl. Acad. Sci. U.S.A.* 96, 11872–11877. doi: 10.1073/pnas.96.21.11872

Hisano, Y., Ota, S., and Kawahara, A. (2014). Genome editing using artificial site-specific nucleases in zebrafish. *Dev. Growth Differ.* 56, 26–33. doi: 10.1111/dgd.12094

Huang, Y., and Mucke, L. (2012). Alzheimer mechanisms and therapeutic strategies. *Cell* 148, 1204–1222. doi: 10.1016/j.cell.2012.02.040

Hwang, W. Y., Fu, Y., Reyon, D., Maeder, M. L., Tsai, S. Q., Sander, J. D., et al. (2013). Efficient genome editing in zebrafish using a CRISPR-Cas system. *Nat. Biotechnol.* 31, 227–229. doi: 10.1038/nbt.2501

Jin, Y. X., Zheng, S. S., Pu, Y., Shu, L. J., Sun, L. W., Liu, W. P., et al. (2011). Cypermethrin has the potential to induce hepatic oxidative stress, DNA damage and apoptosis in adult zebrafish (*Danio rerio*). *Chemosphere* 82, 398–404. doi: 10.1016/j.chemosphere.2010.09.072

Joshi, P., Liang, J. O., Dimonte, K., Sullivan, J., and Pimplikar, S. W. (2009). Amyloid precursor protein is required for convergent–extension movements during zebrafish development. *Dev. Biol.* 335, 1–11. doi: 10.1016/j.ydbio.2009.07.041

Kawakami, K., Shima, A., and Kawakami, N. (2000). Identification of a functional transposase of the Tol2 element, an Ac-like element from the Japanese medaka fish, and its transposition in the zebrafish germ lineage. *Proc. Natl. Acad. Sci. U.S.A.* 97, 11403–11408. doi: 10.1073/pnas.97.21.11403

Kizil, C., Kaslin, J., Kroehne, V., and Brand, M. (2012). Adult neurogenesis and brain regeneration in zebrafish. *Dev. Neurobiol.* 72, 429–461. doi: 10.1002/dneu.20918

Kotze, M. J., and van Rensburg, S. J. (2012). Pathology supported genetic testing and treatment of cardiovascular disease in middle age for prevention of Alzheimer's disease. *Metab. Brain Dis.* 27, 255–266. doi: 10.1007/s11011-012-9296–9298

Kumar, S., and Hedges, S. B. (1998). A molecular timescale for vertebrate evolution. *Nature* 392, 917–920. doi: 10.1038/31927

Lee, J. A., and Cole, G. J. (2007). Generation of transgenic zebrafish expressing green fluorescent protein under control of zebrafish amyloid precursor protein gene regulatory elements. *Zebrafish* 4, 277–286. doi: 10.1089/zeb.2007.0516

Lee, J. H., Yu, W. H., Kumar, A., Lee, S., Mohan, P. S., Peterhoff, C. M., et al. (2010). Lysosomal proteolysis and autophagy require presenilin 1 and are disrupted by Alzheimer-related PS1 mutations. *Cell* 141, 1146–1158. doi: 10.1016/j.cell.2010.05.008

Leimer, U., Lun, K., Romig, H., Walter, J., Grunberg, J., Brand, M., et al. (1999). Zebrafish (*Danio rerio*) presenilin promotes aberrant amyloid beta-peptide production and requires a critical aspartate residue for its function in amyloidogenesis. *Biochemistry* 38, 13602–13609. doi: 10.1021/bi99 1453n

Levi, L., Ziv, T., Admon, A., Levavi-Sivan, B., and Lubzens, E. (2012). Insight into molecular pathways of retinal metabolism, associated with vitellogenesis in zebrafish. *Am. J. Physiol. Endocrinol. Metab.* 302, E626–E644. doi: 10.1152/ajpendo.00310.2011

Liao, H. K., Wang, Y., Watt, K. E. N., Wen, Q., Breitbach, J., Kemmet, C. K., et al. (2012). Tol2 gene trap integrations in the zebrafish amyloid precursor protein genes appa and aplp2 reveal accumulation of secreted APP at the embryonic veins. *Dev. Dyn.* 241, 415–425. doi: 10.1002/Dvdy.23725

Lien, C. L., Schebesta, M., Makino, S., Weber, G. J., and Keating, M. T. (2006). Gene expression analysis of zebrafish heart regeneration. *PLoS Biol.* 4:e260. doi: 10.1371/journal.pbio.0040260

Lieschke, G. J., and Currie, P. D. (2007). Animal models of human disease: zebrafish swim into view. *Nat. Rev. Genet.* 8, 353–367. doi: 10.1038/nrg2091

Lleo, A., and Saura, C. A. (2011). Gamma-secretase substrates and their implications for drug development in Alzheimer's disease. *Curr. Top. Med. Chem.* 11, 1513–1527. doi: 10.2174/156802611795861004

Lukiw, W. J., Gordon, W. C., Rogaev, E. I., Thompson, H., and Bazan, N. G. (2001). Presenilin-2 (PS2) expression up-regulation in a model of retinopathy of prematurity and pathoangiogenesis. *Neuroreport* 12, 53–57 doi: 10.1097/00001756-200101220-00019

Luna, S., Cameron, D. J., and Ethell, D. W. (2013). Amyloid-beta and APP deficiencies cause severe cerebrovascular defects: important work for an old villain. *PLoS ONE* 8:e75052. doi: 10.1371/journal.pone.0075052

Luo, Y., Bolon, B., Damore, M. A., Fitzpatrick, D., Liu, H., Zhang, J., et al. (2003). BACE1 (beta-secretase) knockout mice do not acquire compensatory gene expression changes or develop neural lesions over time. *Neurobiol. Dis.* 14, 81–88. doi: 10.1016/S0969-9961(03)00104-9

Marchesi, V. T. (2011). Alzheimer's dementia begins as a disease of small blood vessels, damaged by oxidative-induced inflammation and dysregulated amyloid metabolism: implications for early detection and therapy. *FASEB J.* 25, 5–13. doi: 10.1096/fj.11-0102ufm

Martins, I. J., Hone, E., Foster, J. K., Sunram-Lea, S. I., Gnjec, A., Fuller, S. J., et al. (2006). Apolipoprotein E, cholesterol metabolism, diabetes, and the convergence of risk factors for Alzheimer's disease and cardiovascular disease. *Mol. Psychiatry* 11, 721–736. doi: 10.1038/sj.mp.4001854

McCarthy, J. V., Twomey, C., and Wujek, P. (2009). Presenilin-dependent regulated intramembrane proteolysis and gamma-secretase activity. *Cell Mol. Life. Sci.* 66, 1534–1555. doi: 10.1007/s00018-009-8435-9

Monnot, M. J., Babin, P. J., Poleo, G., Andre, M., Laforest, L., Ballagny, C., et al. (1999). Epidermal expression of apolipoprotein E gene during fin and scale development and fin regeneration in zebrafish. *Dev. Dyn.* 214, 207–215. doi: 10.1002/(SICI)1097-0177(199903)214:3<207::AID-AJA4>3.0.CO;2-5

Moussavi Nik, S. H., Newman, M., and Lardelli, M. (2011). The response of HMGA1 to changes in oxygen availability is evolutionarily conserved. *Exp. Cell Res.* 317, 1503–1512. doi: 10.1016/j.yexcr.2011.04.004

Moussavi Nik, S. H., Wilson, L., Newman, M., Croft, K., Mori, T. A., Musgrave, I., et al. (2012). The BACE1-PSEN-AbetaPP regulatory axis has an ancient role in response to low oxygen/oxidative stress. *J. Alzheimers Dis.* 28, 515–530. doi: 10.3233/JAD-2011-110533

Musa, A., Lehrach, H., and Russo, V. A. (2001). Distinct expression patterns of two zebrafish homologues of the human APP gene during embryonic development. *Dev. Genes Evol.* 211, 563–567. doi: 10.1007/s00427-001-0189-9

Newman, M., Nornes, S., Martins, R. N., and Lardelli, M. T. (2012). Robust homeostasis of Presenilin1 protein levels by transcript regulation. *Neurosci. Lett.* 519, 14–19. doi: 10.1016/j.neulet.2012.04.064

Newman, M., Wilson, L., Camp, E., Verdile, G., Martins, R., and Lardelli, M. (2010). A zebrafish melanophore model of amyloid beta toxicity. *Zebrafish* 7, 155–159. doi: 10.1089/zeb.2009.0628

Newman, M., Wilson, L., Verdile, G., Lim, A., Khan, I., Moussavi Nik, S. H., et al. (2014). Differential, dominant activation and inhibition of Notch signalling and APP cleavage by truncations of PSEN1 in human disease. *Hum. Mol. Genet.* 23, 602–617. doi: 10.1093/hmg/ddt448

Nikitin, A., Egorov, S., Daraselia, N., and Mazo, I. (2003a). Pathway studio–the analysis and navigation of molecular networks. *Bioinformatics* 19, 2155–2157. doi: 10.1093/bioinformatics/btg290

Nikitin, A., Egorov, S., Daraselia, N., and Mazo, I. (2003b). Pathway studio–the analysis and navigation of molecular networks. *Bioinformatics* 19, 2155–2157. doi: 10.1093/bioinformatics/btg290

Nilsson, P., Loganathan, K., Sekiguchi, M., Matsuba, Y., Hui, K., Tsubuki, S., et al. (2013). Abeta secretion and plaque formation depend on autophagy. *Cell Rep.* 5, 61–69. doi: 10.1016/j.celrep.2013.08.042

Nornes, S., Groth, C., Camp, E., Ey, P., and Lardelli, M. (2003). Developmental control of Presenilin1 expression, endoproteolysis, and interaction in zebrafish embryos. *Exp. Cell Res.* 289, 124–132. doi: 10.1016/S0014-4827(03) 00257-X

Nornes, S., Newman, M., Verdile, G., Wells, S., Stoick-Cooper, C. L., Tucker, B., et al. (2008). Interference with splicing of Presenilin transcripts has potent dominant negative effects on Presenilin activity. *Hum. Mol. Genet.* 17, 402–412. doi: 10.1093/hmg/ddm317

Nornes, S., Newman, M., Wells, S., Verdile, G., Martins, R. N., and Lardelli, M. (2009). Independent and cooperative action of Psen2 with Psen1 in zebrafish embryos. *Exp. Cell Res.* 315, 2791–2801. doi: 10.1016/j.yexcr.2009.06.023

Novichkova, S., Egorov, S., and Daraselia, N. (2003a). MedScan, a natural language processing engine for MEDLINE abstracts. *Bioinformatics* 19, 1699–1706. doi: 10.1093/bioinformatics/btg207

Novichkova, S., Egorov, S., and Daraselia, N. (2003b). MedScan, a natural language processing engine for MEDLINE abstracts. *Bioinformatics* 19, 1699–1706. doi: 10.1093/bioinformatics/btg207

Nunomura, A., Perry, G., Aliev, G., Hirai, K., Takeda, A., Balraj, E. K., et al. (2001). Oxidative damage is the earliest event in Alzheimer disease. *J. Neuropathol. Exp. Neurol.* 60, 759–767.

Olanow, C. W., and McNaught, K. S. (2006). Ubiquitin-proteasome system and Parkinson's disease. *Mov. Disord.* 21, 1806–1823. doi: 10.1002/mds.21013

Oresic, M., Hyotylainen, T., Herukka, S.-K., Sysi-Aho, M., Mattila, I., Seppanan-Laakso, T., et al. (2011). Metabolome in progression to Alzheimer's disease. *Transl. Psychiatry* 1:e57. doi: 10.1038/tp.2011.55

Paquet, D., Bhat, R., Sydow, A., Mandelkow, E. M., Berg, S., Hellberg, S., et al. (2009). A zebrafish model of tauopathy allows in vivo imaging of neuronal cell death and drug evaluation. *J. Clin. Invest.* 119, 1382–1395. doi: 10.1172/JCI37537

Pittman, A. M., Fung, H. C., and De Silva, R. (2006). Untangling the tau gene association with neurodegenerative disorders. *Hum. Mol. Genet.* 15(Spec No. 2), R188–R195. doi: 10.1093/hmg/ddl190

Pluta, R. (2005). Pathological opening of the blood-brain barrier to horseradish peroxidase and amyloid precursor protein following ischemia-reperfusion brain injury. *Chemotherapy* 51, 223–226. doi: 10.1159/000086924

Pujic, Z., Omori, Y., Tsujikawa, M., Thisse, B., Thisse, C., and Malicki, J. (2006). Reverse genetic analysis of neurogenesis in the zebrafish retina. *Dev. Biol.* 293, 330–347. doi: 10.1016/j.ydbio.2005.12.056

Rademakers, R., and Rovelet-Lecrux, A. (2009). Recent insights into the molecular genetics of dementia. *Trends Neurosci.* 32, 451–461. doi: 10.1016/j.tins.2009.05.005

Raymond, P. A., Barthel, L. K., Bernardos, R. L., and Perkowski, J. J. (2006). Molecular characterization of retinal stem cells and their niches in adult zebrafish. *BMC Dev. Biol.* 6:36. doi: 10.1186/1471-213X-6-36

Regeur, L., Jensen, G. B., Pakkenberg, H., Evans, S. M., and Pakkenberg, B. (1994). No global neocortical nerve cell loss in brains from patients with senile dementia of Alzheimer's type. *Neurobiol. Aging* 15, 347–352. doi: 10.1016/0197-4580(94)90030-2

Roberds, S. L., Anderson, J., Basi, G., Bienkowski, M. J., Branstetter, D. G., Chen, K. S., et al. (2001). BACE knockout mice are healthy despite lacking the primary beta-secretase activity in brain: implications for Alzheimer's disease therapeutics. *Hum. Mol. Genet.* 10, 1317–1324. doi: 10.1093/hmg/10.12.1317

Ross, C. A., and Poirier, M. A. (2004). Protein aggregation and neurodegenerative disease. *Nat. Med.* 10(Suppl.), S10–S17. doi: 10.1038/nm1066

Santana, S., Rico, E. P., and Burgos, J. S. (2012). Can zebrafish be used as animal model to study Alzheimer's disease? *Am. J. Neurodegener. Dis.* 1, 32–48.

Schmid, B., and Haass, C. (2013). Genomic editing opens new avenues for zebrafish as a model for neurodegeneration. *J. Neurochem.* 127, 461–470. doi: 10.1111/jnc.12460

Selfridge, J. E., E, L., Lu, J., and Swerdlow, R. H. (2012). Role of mitochondrial homeostasis and dynamics in Alzheimer's disease. *Neurobiol. Dis.* 51, 3–12. doi: 10.1016/j.nbd.2011.12.057

Shen, J., Bronson, R. T., Chen, D. F., Xia, W., Selkoe, D. J., and Tonegawa, S. (1997). Skeletal and CNS defects in Presenilin-1-deficient mice. *Cell* 89, 629–639. doi: 10.1016/S0092-8674(00)80244-5

Song, P., and Pimplikar, S. W. (2012). Knockdown of amyloid precursor protein in zebrafish causes defects in motor axon outgrowth. *PLoS ONE* 7:e34209. doi: 10.1371/journal.pone.0034209

Stone, J. (2008). What initiates the formation of senile plaques? The origin of Alzheimer-like dementias in capillary haemorrhages. *Med. Hypotheses* 71, 347–359. doi: 10.1016/j.mehy.2008.04.007

Strausberg, R. L., Feingold, E. A., Grouse, L. H., Derge, J. G., Klausner, R. D., Collins, F. S., et al. (2002). Generation and initial analysis of more than 15,000 full-length human and mouse cDNA sequences. *Proc. Natl. Acad. Sci. U.S.A.* 99, 16899–16903. doi: 10.1073/pnas.242603899

Sundvik, M., Chen, Y. C., and Panula, P. (2013). Presenilin1 regulates histamine neuron development and behavior in zebrafish, danio rerio. *J. Neurosci.* 33, 1589–1597. doi: 10.1523/JNEUROSCI.1802-12.2013

Tingaud-Sequeira, A., Forgue, J., Andre, M., and Babin, P. J. (2006). Epidermal transient down-regulation of retinol-binding protein 4 and mirror expression of apolipoprotein Eb and estrogen receptor 2a during zebrafish fin and scale development. *Dev. Dyn.* 235, 3071–3079. doi: 10.1002/dvdy.20921

Tseng, W. E., Chen, C. M., Chen, Y. C., Yi, Z., Tan, E. K., and Wu, Y. R. (2013). Genetic Variations of GAK in two Chinese Parkinson's disease populations: a case–control study. *PLoS ONE* 8:e67506. doi: 10.1371/journal.pone.0067506

van Bebber, F., Hruscha, A., Willem, M., Schmid, B., and Haass, C. (2013). Loss of Bace2 in zebrafish affects melanocyte migration and is distinct from Bace1 knock out phenotypes. *J. Neurochem.* 127, 471–481. doi: 10.1111/jnc.12198

van Tijn, P., Kamphuis, W., Marlatt, M. W., Hol, E. M., and Lucassen, P. J. (2011). Presenilin mouse and zebrafish models for dementia: focus on neurogenesis. *Prog. Neurobiol.* 93, 149–164. doi: 10.1016/j.pneurobio.2010.10.008

Verdile, G., Fuller, S., Atwood, C. S., Laws, S. M., Gandy, S. E., and Martins, R. N. (2004). The role of beta amyloid in Alzheimer's disease: still a cause of everything or the only one who got caught? *Pharmacol. Res.* 50, 397–409. doi: 10.1016/j.phrs.2003.12.028

Veth, K. N., Willer, J. R., Collery, R. F., Gray, M. P., Willer, G. B., Wagner, D. S., et al. (2011). Mutations in zebrafish lrp2 result in adult-onset ocular pathogenesis that models myopia and other risk factors for glaucoma. *PLoS Genet.* 7:e1001310. doi: 10.1371/journal.pgen.1001310

Voisin, T., and Vellas, B. (2009). Diagnosis and treatment of patients with severe Alzheimer's disease. *Drugs Aging* 26, 135–144. doi: 10.2165/0002512-200926020-00005

West, M. J., Coleman, P. D., Flood, D. G., and Troncoso, J. C. (1994). Differences in the pattern of hippocampal neuronal loss in normal ageing and Alzheimer's disease. *Lancet* 344, 769–772. doi: 10.1016/S0140-6736(94)92338-8

Willem, M., Garratt, A. N., Novak, B., Citron, M., Kaufmann, S., Rittger, A., et al. (2006). Control of peripheral nerve myelination by the beta-secretase BACE1. *Science* 314, 664–666. doi: 10.1126/science.1132341

Wilson, L., and Lardelli, M. (2013). The development of an in vivo gamma-secretase assay using zebrafish embryos. *J. Alzheimers Dis.* 36, 521–534. doi: 10.3233/JAD-130332

Wong, P. C., Zheng, H., Chen, H., Becher, M. W., Sirinathsinghji, D. J., Trumbauer, M. E., et al. (1997). Presenilin 1 is required for Notch1 and DII1 expression in the paraxial mesoderm. *Nature* 387, 288–292. doi: 10.1038/387288a0

Woods, I. G., Wilson, C., Friedlander, B., Chang, P., Reyes, D. K., Nix, R., et al. (2005). The zebrafish gene map defines ancestral vertebrate chromosomes. *Genome Res.* 15, 1307–1314. doi: 10.1101/gr.4134305

World Alzheimer report. (2010). "Alzheimer's Disease International 2010," in *World Alzheimer Report 2010: The Global Impact of Dementia*, eds A. Wimo and M. Prince (London: Alzheimer's Disease International).

Yang, T., Arslanova, D., Xu, X., Li, Y. M., and Xia, W. (2010). In vivo manifestation of notch related phenotypes in zebrafish treated with Alzheimer's amyloid reducing gamma-secretase inhibitors. *J. Neurochem.* 113, 1200–1209. doi: 10.1111/j.1471-4159.2010.06681.x

Zetterberg, H., Mortberg, E., Song, L., Chang, L., Provuncher, G. K., Patel, P. P., et al. (2011). Hypoxia due to cardiac arrest induces a time-dependent increase in serum amyloid beta levels in humans. *PLoS ONE* 6:e28263. doi: 10.1371/journal.pone.0028263

Zhang, X., Garbett, K., Veeraraghavalu, K., Wilburn, B., Gilmore, R., Mirnics, K., et al. (2012). A role for presenilins in autophagy revisited: normal acidification of lysosomes in cells lacking PSEN1 and PSEN2. *J. Neurosci.* 32, 8633–8648. doi: 10.1523/JNEUROSCI.0556-12.2012

Zhang, X., and Le, W. (2010). Pathological role of hypoxia in Alzheimer's disease. *Exp. Neurol.* 223, 299–303. doi: 10.1016/j.expneurol.2009.07.033

13

Worming forward: amyotrophic lateral sclerosis toxicity mechanisms and genetic interactions in *Caenorhabditis elegans*

Martine Therrien[1] and J. Alex Parker[2]*

[1] Départment de Pathologie et Biologie Cellulaire, CRCHUM-Centre Hospitalier de l'Université de Montréal, Université de Montréal, Montréal, QC, Canada
[2] Départment de Pathologie et Biologie Cellulaire, Départment de Neurosciences, CRCHUM-Centre Hospitalier de l'Université de Montréal, Université de Montréal, Montréal, QC, Canada

Edited by:
Shin Murakami, Touro University-California, USA

Reviewed by:
Eirini Lionaki, Foundation for Research and Technology-Hellas, Greece
Maria Markaki, Foundation for Research and Technology -Hellas, Greece
Marta Artal Sanz, Pablo de Olavide University, Spain

***Correspondence:**
J. Alex Parker, CRCHUM- Centre Hospitalier de l'Université de Montréal, Université de Montréal, 900 St-Denis, Tour Viger, R09.440, Montréal, QC H2X 0A9, Canada
e-mail: ja.parker@umontreal.ca

Neurodegenerative diseases share pathogenic mechanisms at the cellular level including protein misfolding, excitotoxicity and altered RNA homeostasis among others. Recent advances have shown that the genetic causes underlying these pathologies overlap, hinting at the existence of a genetic network for neurodegeneration. This is perhaps best illustrated by the recent discoveries of causative mutations for amyotrophic lateral sclerosis (ALS) and frontotemporal degeneration (FTD). Once thought to be distinct entities, it is now recognized that these diseases exist along a genetic spectrum. With this wealth of discoveries comes the need to develop new genetic models of ALS and FTD to investigate not only pathogenic mechanisms linked to causative mutations, but to uncover potential genetic interactions that may point to new therapeutic targets. Given the conservation of many disease genes across evolution, *Caenorhabditis elegans* is an ideal system to investigate genetic interactions amongst these genes. Here we review the use of *C. elegans* to model ALS and investigate a putative genetic network for ALS/FTD that may extend to other neurological disorders.

Keywords: *C. elegans*, ALS (Amyotrophic lateral sclerosis), TDP-43, FUS, C9orf72, SOD1, genetic networks, motor neuron disease

INTRODUCTION

Amyotrophic lateral sclerosis (ALS) is a neurodegenerative disorder affecting 1–2/100,000 individuals. Most cases of ALS are sporadic, but 10% of cases are familial (Turner et al., 2013b). Mutations in the gene *superoxide dismutase 1 (SOD1)* were identified in 1993 (Rosen et al., 1993) as the first cause of familial ALS. Thanks to the recent advances in genetics, more than 20 genes are now linked to ALS (Chen et al., 2013) (**Table 1**). Genes recently shown to be mutated in ALS include the DNA/RNA binding proteins *TAR DNA binding protein 43 (TARDBP)* and *Fused-in-sarcoma (FUS)* (Kabashi et al., 2008; Sreedharan et al., 2008; Vance et al., 2009). More recently, mutations in *C9ORF72* have turned out to be a major cause of familial and sporadic ALS (DeJesus-Hernandez et al., 2011; Renton et al., 2011).

ALS is characterized by the selective loss of motor neurons in the motor cortex, the brainstem and the spinal cord, the loss of myelin in the spinal cord, and the presence of neuroinflammation (Robberecht and Philips, 2013). Onset of the disease usually begins in the lower limb and spreads toward the upper motor neurons leading to muscle weakness, fasciculation, and wasting. Death occurs 3–5 years after the beginning of the symptoms (Kiernan et al., 2011) and is caused by respiratory failure due to denervation of the respiratory muscles.

50% of ALS patients show cognitive impairment, of which 15% met the criteria of frontotemporal dementia (FTD) (Ringholz et al., 2005). FTD is a group of non-Alzheimer dementias characterized by atrophy of the frontal and/or temporal lobes causing mid-life behavioral changes or language impairment (Warren et al., 2013). Over the past few years, the identification of *TDP-43*, *C9ORF72* and *UBQLN2* as genes causing ALS and FTD has suggested a similarity for both diseases (Morris et al., 2012). Similar pathogenic mechanisms have been suggested for ALS and FTD (Van Langenhove et al., 2012; Ling et al., 2013) but so far it is unclear how patients with the same genetic mutations can have either ALS, FTD or both.

The genes involved in ALS have diverse functions and we still do not know how they interact to cause motor neuron degeneration. Most of the research over the past 20 years has focused on the toxicity caused by mutant SOD1. Among the proposed mechanisms of toxicity are mitochondrial dysfunction, axonal dysfunction, excitotoxicity and neuroinflammation (Turner et al., 2013b). However, TDP-43, FUS, and C9ORF72 proteins seem to point toward RNA toxicity (Ling et al., 2013). Most importantly, only one drug, riluzole, is used to slow disease progression and has only modest effects (Kiernan et al., 2011). Diagnosis is difficult and requires an experienced neurologist to differentiate between ALS and other neurological diseases (Turner et al., 2013a). It is thought that the clinical manifestations of ALS are downstream events that occur much later after the initial insult to the nervous system (Turner et al., 2013a). Therefore, the identification of biomarkers is essential for the rapid, early diagnosis of ALS, and the identification of new drugs limiting the degeneration of motor neuron is an essential unmet need for ALS patients.

Table 1 | ALS genes and their *C. elegans* orthologs.

Human gene	Function	*C. elegans* gene
MOST COMMON ALS GENES		
SOD1	Superoxide metabolism	*sod-1*
TARDBP	RNA metabolism	*tdp-1*
FUS	RNA metabolism	*fust-1*
OPTN	Vesicular transport	–
VCP	Vesicular transport	*cdc-48.1/2*
UBQLN2	Proteasome	*ubqnl-1*
C9ORF72	Unknown, DENN protein	*alfa-1*
SQSTM1	Autophagy	*sqst-2*
PFN1	Cytoskeleton dynamics	*pfn-1*
OTHER GENES INVOLVED IN ALS		
DCTN1	Cytoskeleton dynamics	*dnc-1*
ALS2	Endocytosis	–
CHMP2B	Vesicular transport	–
FIG4	Vesicular transport	*C34B7.2*
HNRNPA2B1	RNA metabolism	*hrp-1*
ELP3		–
SETX	RNA processing	–
HNRNPA1	RNA processing	*hrp-1*
ATXN2		*atx-2*
ANG	Blood vessels formation	–
SPG11	DNA damage	–
VAPB	Vesicular transport	*vpr-1*
NEFH	Cytoskeleton dynamics	*H39E23.3*
ARHGEF28	RNA metabolism	*rhgf-1*

To understand better the impact of the genetic mutations on the function of the different proteins involved in ALS, *in vivo* models have proved to be essential. Ever since the first SOD1 mouse was developed in 1994 (Gurney et al., 1994), several groups have tried to investigate ALS pathogenesis by expressing different ALS related mutations in mice, an approach that has recently been extended to other genes including TDP-43 and FUS for example. While the over expression of wild type SOD1 causes a mild denervation of neurons (Epstein et al., 1987), the over expression of $SOD1^{G93A}$ causes a loss of motor neurons, neuroinflammation, and reduces life span (Gurney et al., 1994; Guo et al., 2009). One model expressing mutant $TDP\text{-}43Q^{331K \text{ or } M337V}$ in the mouse central nervous system has shown selectivity for large caliber motor neuron neurodegeneration (Arnold et al., 2013), while others over expressing mutant $TDP\text{-}43^{G348C,\ A315T}$ and $FUS^{R512C,\ 14\Delta}$ have limited neuronal loss (Swarup et al., 2011; Verbeeck et al., 2012). Some rodent models display relevant ALS pathology, but given the time and expense to develop models for many of the recently discovered ALS genes, not to mention the difficulty of manipulating several genes at once, some laboratories have turned to simpler organisms to model ALS toxicity.

One model showing increasing popularity is the nematode *Caenorhabditis elegans*. This 1 mm long worm has a painstakingly characterized, invariant cell lineage that includes 302 neurons. The nervous system, its interconnections and its synapses are well studied which makes it an ideal model to study mechanisms of neuronal toxicity. The *C. elegans* genome was the first to be fully sequenced in 1998 and includes more than 19,000 genes on 6 chromosomes (*C. elegans* Sequencing Consortium, 1998). Since then, deletion mutants have been produced for many *C. elegans* genes and approximately 80% of *C. elegans* genes have a human homolog (Lai et al., 2000) (Shaye and Greenwald, 2011). *C. elegans* behavior is well studied and many experimental assays are available, including for worm locomotion. Worms initiate movement by bending their body to advance forward in a sinusoidal pattern, a process that is orchestrated by GABAergic and cholinergic neurons. Cholinergic neurons initiate the contraction along the dorsal or ventral body wall muscles while the GABAergic neurons send an inhibitory signal on the opposite side (Jorgensen, 2005).

C. elegans has been an important tool for the characterization of many neurodegenerative disorders (Li and Le, 2013). Many protein-misfolding disorders have been modeled in worms including Alzheimer's disease, Parkinson's disease, Huntington's disease and different spinocerebellar ataxias. Also, the toxicity of non-coding mutations in *C. elegans* resemble the toxicity in mammalian tissues (Wang et al., 2011b). Since many cellular stress and survival pathways are conserved in worms, our group and others have used *C. elegans* to model ALS. This review aims to summarize the work done modeling ALS in *C. elegans* and highlights the future possibilities and applications.

USE OF *C. elegans* TO MODEL SOD1 TOXICITY

SOD1 is an enzyme that catalyzes the conversion of O_2- into O_2 and H_2O_2. More than 160 mutations causative for ALS have been found in *SOD1* since 1993 (Al-Chalabi et al., 2012). Phenotypic heterogeneity is observed among *SOD1* mutation carriers where $SOD1^{A4V}$ seems to cause an aggressive form of ALS while $SOD1^{D90A}$ causes a milder, long duration ALS (Renton et al., 2014). It is hypothesized that *SOD1* mutations cause toxicity through a gain of function, even though a loss of enzyme activity have been observed in patients and some models (Saccon et al., 2013). Many pathogenic mechanisms have been hypothesized but no consensus has been reached, although it is thought that the misfolding of mutant SOD1, and sometimes wild type SOD1, may be an important first step of the pathogenesis observed in patients (Pickles and Vande Velde, 2012). Based on pathological evidence, it is now acknowledged that ALS caused by mutations in SOD1 is a distinctive form of ALS (Mackenzie et al., 2007).

Several groups have used *C. elegans* to model SOD1 toxicity (**Table 2**) starting with Oeda and colleagues who showed that the ubiquitous expression of human mutant SOD1 impairs the worm's response to oxidative stress and causes protein aggregates (Oeda et al., 2001). It was later shown that expression of mutant SOD1 throughout the worm's entire nervous system resulted in locomotion defects and impaired neuronal transmission (Wang et al., 2009). Interestingly, the formation of aggregates seemed to be restricted to certain mechanosensory neurons despite the pan neuronal expression of SOD1. Other models are non-neuronal in nature and have relied on the expression of SOD1 proteins in the body wall muscles where it was observed that distinct SOD1 mutations have varying propensities to aggregate (Gidalevitz et al., 2009). More recently a *C. elegans* model was generated

Table 2 | Summary of transgenic SOD1 models.

Study	Promoter	Gene	Motor phenotype	Aggregation	Neuro-degeneration	Synaptic dysfunction
Oeda et al., 2001	*hsp-16.2:* all tissues except the germline	$SOD1^{A4V}$	n.d	n.d.	n.d	n.d
		$SOD1^{G37R}$	n.d	n.d	n.d	n.d
		$SOD1^{G93R}$	n.d	n.d	n.d	n.d
	myo-3: muscle cells	$SOD1^{A4V}$	n.d	yes	n.a	n.a
Wang et al., 2009	*snb-1:* entire nervous system	$SOD1^{WT}$	No	No	n.d	Normal
		$SOD1^{G83R}$	Yes	Yes	n.d	Impaired
Gidalevitz et al., 2009	*unc-54:* muscle cells	$SOD1^{WT}$	No	No	n.a.	n.a
		$SOD1^{G85R}$	Yes	Yes	n.a.	n.a.
		$SOD1^{G93A}$	Yes	Yes	n.a.	n.a.
		$SOD1^{127X}$	Yes	Yes	n.a.	n.a.
Li et al., 2013a	*unc-25:* GABAergic motor neurons	$SOD1^{WT}$	Yes	Yes	Yes	n.d.
		$SOD1^{G93A}$	Yes	Yes	Yes	n.d.

n.d., not determined; n.a., not applicable.

based on the expression of SOD1 in the worm's motor neurons showing neurodegeneration in the absence of caspases (Li et al., 2013a), an intriguing finding since the motor neuron loss observed in mouse models is associated with caspase activation (Pasinelli et al., 2000). Whether this reflects a difference between invertebrate and vertebrate systems, or reflects a novel mechanism of neurodegeneration remains to be determined.

The *C. elegans sod-1* gene has a similar function to human *SOD1*. *sod-1* loss of function mutants have increased O_2- levels, shorter lifespan and are sensitive to some environmental stresses (Yanase et al., 2009). Inversely, overexpression of the worm *sod-1* increases lifespan and increases the level of H_20_2, the by-product of the catalase reaction of SOD1. However, the increased lifespan seems to be independent of SOD-1 catalase activity, but may be due to altered endoplasmic reticulum (ER) stress signaling (Cabreiro et al., 2011). Interestingly, Van Raamsdonk et al. have generated a *sod* null worm, where all five *C. elegans sod* genes have been mutated and these worms have a normal lifespan and response to oxidative damage but are sensitive to many acute environmental stresses (Van Raamsdonk and Hekimi, 2012).

In summary, many aspects of SOD1 function and toxicity are conserved in worms, but some questions remain. It is known that mutant SOD1 is found in association with the mitochondria in SOD1 mouse model and ALS patients (Pickles and Vande Velde, 2012). To our knowledge, no group has yet investigated the effects of human mutant SOD1 in worm mitochondria. However, it was recently shown that a cleavage product of *vpr-1,* the ortholog of VAPB also involved in ALS, affects mitochondrial organization in muscle cells (Han et al., 2013). A similar analysis of the different SOD1 transgenic models would be interesting and could help identify pathways and drugs that act specifically on this important aspect of ALS pathogenesis.

USE OF *C. elegans* TO MODEL TDP-43 TOXICITY

TDP-43 is a protein encoded by the *TARDBP* gene on chromosome 1. The protein contains two RNA binding domains, a glycine rich domain and nuclear export and import signals. TDP-43 is similar to the members of the ribonucleoprotein family. TDP-43 was identified in 2006 as the main constituents of sporadic and familial ALS/FTD aggregates (Neumann et al., 2006). In patients, the ubiquitinated aggregates are present in the most affected regions of the brain and spinal cord. These aggregates contain a hyperphosphorylated form of TDP-43 and the C terminus cleaved fragment (Neumann et al., 2006). In 2008, mutations in the *TARDBP* gene were linked to familial and sporadic ALS/FTD cases (Kabashi et al., 2008; Sreedharan et al., 2008; Sreedharan and Brown, 2013). So far, more than 40 mutations in *TARDBP* have been linked to ALS/FTD and most of them are found in the C terminus region of the protein, a region involved in protein-protein interactions (Al-Chalabi et al., 2012).

Under normal cellular conditions, TDP-43 protein shuttles from the nucleus to the cytoplasm. The normal function of TDP-43 is still unclear but the protein participates in transcription, miRNA processing, mRNA splicing, RNA transport and stress granule formation (Ling et al., 2013). The pathogenic effect of the mutant proteins is not well understood and it is still unclear if the toxicity is a gain of function, a loss of function, or both (Ling et al., 2013; Vanden Broeck et al., 2014). An important aspect of TDP-43 toxicity was discovered when characterizing TDP-43 wild type mice. Mice with elevated expression of wild type TDP-43 also have characteristics of TDP-43 mutant proteins (Xu et al., 2010). Therefore, expression level is important and should be considered when generating different transgenic models.

To clarify the toxicity caused by the expression of mutant TDP-43, several groups have developed *C. elegans* models (**Table 3**). In 2010, Ash and colleagues developed the first TDP-43 overexpression model in *C. elegans.* The pan neuronal expression of human TDP-43 and *C. elegans* TDP-1 resulted in worms with uncoordinated, slow movements and defasciculation of the GABAergic motor neurons (Ash et al., 2010). The results regarding the expression of human TDP-43 were confirmed by Liachko and colleagues who also observed motility defects and degeneration phenotypes from the expression of mutant TDP-43 proteins throughout the worms nervous system (Liachko et al., 2010).

Table 3 | Summary of transgenic TDP-43 models.

Study	Promoter	Gene	Motor phenotype	Aggregation	Neuro-degeneration	Synaptic dysfunction
Ash et al., 2010	*snb-1:* entire nervous system	TDP-1	Yes	n.d.	n.d.	n.d.
		TDP-43^{WT}	Yes	n.d.	GABAergic	n.d.
		TDP-43$^{\Delta RRM1}$	No	n.d.	n.d.	n.d.
		TDP-43$^{\Delta RRM2}$	No	n.d.	n.d.	n.d.
		TDP-43$^{\Delta C\ terminus}$	No	n.d.	n.d.	n.d.
		TDP-43$^{no\ caspase}$	Yes	n.d.	n.d.	n.d.
		TDP-43$^{no\ NLS}$	No	n.d.	n.d.	n.d.
Liachko et al., 2010	*snb-1:* entire nervous system	TDP-43^{WT}	Yes	Yes	No	n.d.
		TDP-43^{G290A}	Yes	Yes	GABAergic and dopaminergic	n.d.
		TDP-43^{A315T}	Yes	Yes	GABAergic and dopaminergic	n.d.
		TDP-43^{M337V}	Yes	Yes	GABAergic and dopaminergic	n.d.
Zhang et al., 2012b	*snb-1:* entire nervous system	TDP-43^{WT}	Yes	Yes	No	Impaired
		TDP-43^{G331K}	Yes	n.d.	No	Impaired
		TDP-43^{M337V}	Yes	n.d.	No	Impaired
		TDP-43$^{C\ terminus}$	Yes	Yes	No	Impaired
Vaccaro et al., 2012c	*unc-47*: GABAergic neurons	TDP-43^{WT}	No	No	No	No
		TDP-43^{A315T}	Yes	Yes	GABAergic	Impaired

n.d., not determined; NLS, nuclear localization signal; ΔRRM, deletion of RNA recognition motif; ΔC terminus, deletion of C terminus; no caspase, mutations in TDP-43 that block caspase cleavage.

These phenotypes also highly correlated with protein phosphorylation levels where hyperphosphorylation increased the toxicity of mutant TDP-43 proteins similarly to what is observed in ALS patients (Liachko et al., 2010). The TDP-43 C terminus fragment shows another similarity with patients. Zhang and colleagues showed that the pan neuronal expression of human TDP-43 C′ fragment caused a phenotype similar to the expression of wild type or mutant TDP-43 (Zhang et al., 2011). Even though no neuronal loss was observed in the latter model, all strains displayed synaptic transmission abnormalities. In worms, GABAergic neurons seem to be particularly sensitive to the expression of TDP-43 (Liachko et al., 2010). To evaluate if the effect of TDP-43 expression in these neurons could cause locomotor defects, our group developed models in which human wild type or mutant TDP-43 were expressed specifically in GABAergic motor neurons as directed by an *unc-47* promoter (McIntire et al., 1997). Interestingly, the overexpression of mutant TDP-43, but not wild type TDP-43, caused an adult-onset, progressive paralysis phenotype accompanied by GABAergic neurodegeneration and synaptic transmission impairment (Vaccaro et al., 2012b). Finally, some of these models showed aggravation of the phenotypes during aging recapitulating an important feature of ALS and neurodegeneration (Liachko et al., 2010; Vaccaro et al., 2012b).

It is still unclear if the toxicity of mutant TDP-43 proteins in ALS patients arises from a gain of function, a loss of function or if both mechanisms are employed. The transgenic *C. elegans* models of TDP-43 are based on the overexpression of TDP-43 in worms and likely represent a gain of function rather than a loss of function. However, the *C. elegans* genome has an ortholog of TDP-43 called TDP-1. TDP-1 is a primarily nuclear protein expressed in most tissues including body wall muscles, pharynx and neurons (Vaccaro et al., 2012c; Zhang et al., 2012b). TDP-1 contains two RNA binding motifs, a nuclear localization signal and an export signal but lacks the glycine rich domain found in human TDP-43. TDP-1 seems to be functionally conserved because the expression of human TDP-43 can rescue the toxicity of a loss of function of a *tdp-1* mutant (Zhang et al., 2012b).

Mutant *tdp-1* animals show numerous phenotypes including slow development, and locomotion defects (Liachko et al., 2010; Zhang et al., 2012b). TDP-1 was also shown to be involved in lifespan and the cellular stress response. Somewhat paradoxically, worms lacking *tdp-1* have a longer lifespan but are more sensitive to oxidative and osmotic stresses (Vaccaro et al., 2012c; Zhang et al., 2012b). The expression of *tdp-1* can be induced by oxidative stress, either chemically or from activation of the ER stress response, and it is thought that chronic induction of *tdp-1* by stress is ultimately cytotoxic and reduces the worms lifespan (Vaccaro et al., 2012c). Furthermore, several studies have shown that wild type TDP-1 protein may contribute to the neurodegeneration elicited by mutant protein in *C. elegans*. Neurodegeneration was suppressed by deleting *tdp-1* from worms in several ALS models (Vaccaro et al., 2012c; Zhang et al., 2012b) as well as in a *C. elegans* model of Huntington's disease (Tauffenberger et al., 2013a) suggesting there may be genetic interactions amongst genes linked to neurodegeneration. Interestingly, a transcriptome analysis of *tdp-1(ok803)* showed that one of the biological process that was highly affected in the mutant worms was the ER unfolded protein response (Zhang et al., 2012b). ER stress and proteostasis have been a recurrent theme in ALS research (Matus et al., 2013; Musarò, 2013) which is of interest since sporadic and familial cases of ALS are known to have an abnormal ER stress response (Ilieva et al., 2007; Atkin et al., 2008; Hetz et al., 2009; Ito et al., 2009).

USE OF *C. elegans* TO MODEL FUS TOXICITY

After the identification of TDP-43, several groups examined related RNA-binding proteins for their potential contributions to ALS. In 2009, a protein with a similar function, FUS, was identified as causative of ALS (Kwiatkowski et al., 2009; Vance et al., 2009). Similar to TDP-43, FUS contains a RNA binding domain and a glycine rich domain but also has a two arginine glycine rich regions and one large glutamine, glycine, serine, tyrosine domain in N terminus. Because of their high degree of structural similarity, it was hypothesized that FUS and TDP-43 share common functions. It is known that FUS can bind DNA and RNA and is involved in many of the same RNA processing activities of TDP-43 (Ling et al., 2013). FUS transgenic models are relatively recent additions to the research field and much remains to be learned about the function of FUS and the implication of the mutant protein in neurodegeneration.

Two transgenic models have been developed in *C. elegans* for FUS (**Table 4**). Murakami et al. (2012) expressed several *FUS* mutations and two truncated FUS proteins throughout the worm's nervous system. Interestingly, only the mutations that caused aggregation resulted in motor phenotypes in worms. The motor phenotype could not be rescued by the expression of wild type *FUS* suggesting a gain of function mechanism. Our group confirmed a similar toxicity mechanism in models expressing *FUS* in the worm motor neurons. Expression of *FUS* wild type did not cause aggregation but expression of mutant *FUS* caused aggregation accompanied by paralysis, neuronal synaptic impairment and neurodegeneration (Vaccaro et al., 2012b).

FUS is well conserved and the *C. elegans* ortholog is named *fust-1*. In contrast to *tdp-1*, a *fust-1* deletion mutant could not alleviate the toxicity induced by the expression of C′ TDP-43 fragment (Zhang et al., 2012b), suggesting a different role in proteotoxicity. In *Drosophila*, *Cabeza* (*Caz*), the *Drosophila* ortholog of *FUS*, is expressed in motor neurons and a decreased expression of *Caz* causes a motor phenotype and motor neuron degeneration (Wang et al., 2011a; Sasayama et al., 2012). These results suggest a link between the expression and function of FUS, and the specificity of ALS neurodegeneration and we await further investigations of *fust-1* in *C. elegans*.

USE OF *C. elegans* TO MODEL C9ORF72 TOXICITY

A region of chromosome 9 had been linked to ALS for several years (Morita et al., 2006; Vance et al., 2006; van Es et al., 2009; Shatunov et al., 2010) but the gene was only identified in 2011 (DeJesus-Hernandez et al., 2011; Renton et al., 2011) and has since been shown to be a major cause of sporadic and familial ALS (Turner et al., 2013b). The basis of the mutation is a GGGGCC repeat expansion within the first intron of *C9ORF72*. Many questions remain to be answered about the role of *C9ORF72* in the pathogenesis of ALS. It is still not clear whether the GGGGCC repeat expansion results in a loss of function, a gain of function or both, or if the size of the repeat has differential effects on these potential mechanisms. Recent reports have observed decreased expression of *C9ORF72* when the GGGGCC repeat reaches pathogenic length (DeJesus-Hernandez et al., 2011; Ciura et al., 2013; Xi et al., 2013). Whether decreased expression contributes to ALS pathogenesis is unknown since very little is known about the biological role of C9ORF72 other than its sequence similarity to the GDP/GTP exchange factor "Differentially Expressed in Normal and Neoplasia" (DENN) (Zhang et al., 2012a; Levine et al., 2013). DENN proteins are involved in the regulation of Rab-GTPases and endocytosis. Recently, C9ORF72 was shown to be implicated in endosomal trafficking (Farg et al., 2014), confirming its role as a DENN protein. In *C. elegans*, work has been previously done regarding some Rab proteins using deletion mutants and GFP reporters (Sato et al., 2008) to investigate endocytosis (Fares and Grant, 2002). *C. elegans* would be an ideal model to confirm the involvement of *C9ORF72* in this pathway. The *C. elegans* homolog of *C9ORF72* is named *alfa-1* (**ALS**/**FTD** **a**ssociated gene homolog). Our group characterized the loss of function mutant *alfa-1(ok3062)* where we observed that decreased expression of *alfa-1* causes a motility defect, neurodegeneration specifically of the motor neurons and sensitivity to osmotic stress (Therrien et al., 2013). Further characterization still remains to be done but it is interesting that loss of *alfa-1* is linked

Table 4 | Summary of transgenic FUS models.

Study	Promoter	Gene	Motor phenotype	Aggregation	Neuro-degeneration	Synaptic dysfunction
Murakami et al., 2012	*rgef-1*: entire nervous system	FUS^{WT}	No	No	n.d.	n.d.
		FUS^{R514G}	No	No	n.d.	n.d.
		FUS^{R521G}	No	No	n.d.	n.d.
		FUS^{R522G}	Yes	Yes	n.d.	n.d.
		FUS^{P525L}	Yes	Yes	n.d.	n.d.
		$FUS^{501trunc}$	Yes	Yes	n.d.	n.d.
		$FUS^{513trunc}$	Yes	Yes	n.d.	n.d.
Vaccaro et al., 2012c	*unc-47*: GABAergic neurons	FUS^{WT}	No	No	No	Normal
		$FUS^{S57\Delta}$	Yes	Yes	GABAergic neurons	Impaired

n.d., not determined; trunc, truncation.

to neuronal integrity specifically for GABAergic motor neurons in worm.

GGGGCC repeat expansions are found in the first intron of *C9ORF72* and the presence of such long non-coding repeats is suggestive of a toxic gain of function mechanism driving neurodegeneration as seen in many of the trinucleotide repeat expansion diseases. In patients, the repeat was shown to induce abnormal translation (non-ATG translation of the repeat, also called RAN translation) leading to the production of different dipeptides(Ash et al., 2013; Mori et al., 2013b). Also of interest were the presence of RNA foci containing the expanded GGGGCC repeat in patients (DeJesus-Hernandez et al., 2011). It is unknown whether a toxic gain of function is caused by the presence of toxic RNA or the presence of toxic protein, or both. So far, no groups have generated transgenic worms to model this aspect of the toxicity however the expression of the non-coding GGGGCC repeat in *Drosophila* causes neurodegeneration (Xu et al., 2013). *C. elegans* may be useful to model non-coding repeats based on previous efforts studying the expression of non-coding CUG repeats that were toxic to worms (Chen et al., 2007) and recapitulated aspects of RNA foci toxicity (Wang et al., 2011b).

STRESS RESPONSE AND AGE-DEPENDENT NEURODEGENERATION IN *C. elegans*

With the identification of TDP-43 in most ALS aggregates and later the identification of mutations affecting *TARDBP* and *FUS* genes, RNA metabolism has become an important area of investigation in ALS research. Under normal conditions, both proteins are mainly observed in the nucleus but the mutant proteins are also found in the cytoplasm. FUS and TDP-43 contain a low-complexity prion-like domain and a RNA binding domain suggesting a role in RNA metabolism (Li et al., 2013b). High throughput RNA-sequencing experiments have been used to identify targets of TDP-43 and FUS in normal or disease states. In worms, the transcriptome of the *tdp-1(ok803)* mutant has been studied (Zhang et al., 2012b) and showed the involvement of TDP-1 in various aspects of development.

Under cellular stress, wild type and mutant TDP-43 and FUS proteins form RNA granules (Bosco et al., 2010; Dormann et al., 2010; Liu-Yesucevitz et al., 2010; Gal et al., 2011; McDonald et al., 2011). These granules are usually formed in order to protect RNA from degradation under stress conditions. In worms, a variety of different RNA granules exist: P granules, P bodies and stress granules. P granules are the most characterized RNA granules in worms and are highly involved in cellular development (Updike and Strome, 2010). However, human proteins found in P bodies and stress granules, such as TIA1, the decapping enzymes and polyA binding proteins, have *C. elegans* ortholog and their role seem conserved regarding RNA granules (Jud et al., 2008; Sun et al., 2011). An active area of research concerns whether mutant TDP-43 and/or FUS proteins interfere with stress granule homeostasis. In a transgenic model of FUS, wild type and mutant FUS were shown to colocalize to stress granules after a heat shock but only the recruitment of mutant FUS to the stress granules caused persistent motility defects in the worms (Murakami et al., 2012). Most work done in *C. elegans* to study stress granules have used thermal stress as an inducer of the granule (Sun et al., 2011). In cells, formation of granules containing FUS is also initiated by other environmental stresses such as osmotic stress (Baron et al., 2013) and oxidative stress (Vance et al., 2013), thus the effect of these other stresses would be interesting to evaluate. Since most of the components of the granules are conserved in worms, *C. elegans* could be a powerful system to investigate stress biology in the context of aging, an aspect not easily studied in cellular systems.

Since TDP-43 and FUS are components of stress granules, this has led to the hypothesis that both proteins may be involved in the cellular stress response. The genetic pathways governing cellular stress signaling have been studied to great success in *C. elegans*. The different stress response pathways are highly characterized in worms with the insulin/IGF-1 pathway being a major, conserved signaling axis (Lau and Chalasani, 2014). In worms, the insulin/IGF-1 pathway has a sole insulin/IGF-1 receptor, DAF-2, that acts through the kinases AGE-1, PDK and AKT to phosphorylate the FOXO transcription factor DAF-16, and regulate stress resistance and longevity (Lapierre and Hansen, 2012). The most common stresses applied to worms in laboratory settings include exposure to thermal, oxidative, osmotic or hypoxic stresses (Rodriguez et al., 2013). While each is a damaging stress, they can elicit distinct genetic signaling pathways with diverse outcomes. An open question in the field of late-onset neurodegeneration is whether environmental components exist to account for the range in disease onset and progression for what are many highly penetrant, monogenic, dominantly acting disorders. A stress intrinsic to ALS and many neurodegenerative diseases is proteotoxicity. Here mutant proteins misfold leading to a diverse range of proteotoxic consequences. Thus, cells maintain an extensive network of mechanisms, including the insulin/IGF-1 pathway, to maintain protein homeostasis in the face of environmentally derived damage or genetically encoded misfolded proteins.

Work from *C. elegans* directly linked *tdp-1* to the insulin/IGF-1 pathway and proteotoxicity. In *C. elegans tdp-1* is required for the stress resistance of *daf-2* mutants and the stress-induced expression of *tdp-1* was dependent on *daf-16*. These data suggest a role for TDP-1/TDP-43 in the insulin/IGF-1 pathway and it remains to see if insulin/IGF-1 signaling is altered by disease-associated TDP-43 mutations.

Interestingly, in Vaccaro et al., mutant TDP-43 and mutant FUS proteins were only expressed in the 26 GABAergic motor neurons but activated the ER unfolded protein response chaperone HSP-4 in intestinal tissue (Vaccaro et al., 2012c). This observation suggests that proteotoxic insults can induce stress-signaling pathways in other tissues. It is not known if this is due to a diffusible signaling molecule, or if the mutant proteins make their way from the nervous system to adjacent tissue. TDP-43, FUS, HNRNPA1, HNRNAP2B and TAF15 all contain a prion-like domain (Couthouis et al., 2011; Polymenidou and Cleveland, 2011; Kim et al., 2013) and misfolded SOD1 protein may be able to self propagate (Grad and Cashman, 2014). Thus, these proteins could share properties with toxic prion protein (PrPsc) that misfolds, become infectious, and spreads from cell to cell (Kabir and Safar, 2014). The development of ALS symptoms, starting usually in the lower limb and spreading upward, also suggests a propagation mechanism. Little is known about the propagation potential of the ALS associated misfolded proteins in *C. elegans* transgenic models. Mutant TDP-43 and FUS proteins in the worm's motor neurons were shown to induce the expression of HSP-4 in the intestine, but the proteins were not visualized outside of the neurons where they were expressed (Vaccaro et al., 2012c). A prion model was however characterized expressing Sup35NM, a yeast prion protein, in the body wall muscle of the worm. The most toxic form of the protein was shown between muscle cells, in the intestine and the coelomocytes, and the toxic fibrils were able to induce protein misfolding (Nussbaum-Krammer et al., 2013). Also, proteostasis, ER stress resistance and longevity, all major ALS research topics, have been recently shown to have important cell-non-autonomous components (Taylor and Dillin, 2013; van Oosten-Hawle et al., 2013). Since *C. elegans* is transparent, direct visualization of tagged proteins during development and aging is possible. The development of additional tools should help establish if a propagation mechanism exists for mutant TDP-43, FUS and SOD1 proteins.

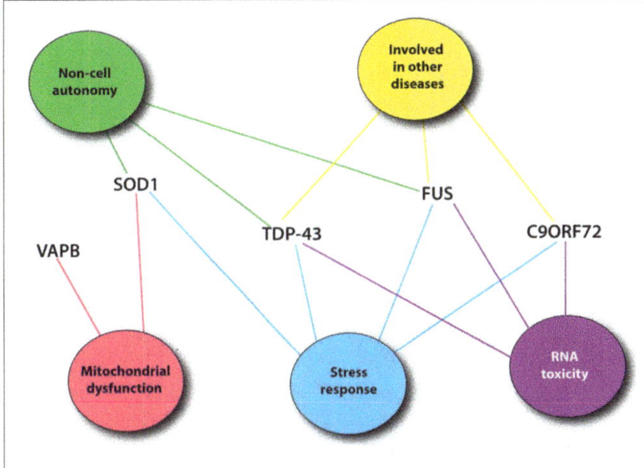

FIGURE 1 | Most common ALS genes and pathogenic pathways. Shown are mutant proteins associated with ALS and putative, shared toxicity mechanisms including RNA toxicity, the cellular stress response, mitochondrial impairment and cell autonomy/non-autonomy. Many of these pathways can be easily investigated using *C. elegans*.

IDENTIFICATION OF GENETIC INTERACTIONS

Recent genetic advances have identified many new causative genes for familial cases of ALS (**Table 1**). Moreover, genome-wide association studies (GWAS) have also been done in sporadic ALS cohorts to identify potential genes (Renton et al., 2014). With the increasing number of genes linked to ALS along with the diverse functions of these genes, it is essential to identify common pathological pathways relevant to ALS. Genetic interactions amongst genes can refer to functional relationships amongst a group of genes (Boucher and Jenna, 2013). However, genetic interactions are not always easy to interpret and do not necessarily point toward genes that function in the same pathway but rather identify functional similarity between genes that could be in the same pathway or in compensatory pathways (Boucher and Jenna, 2013). Therefore, identification of genetic interactions between ALS genes could point toward potential therapeutic avenues for ALS patients (**Figure 1**).

Among the proteins identified, TDP-43, SOD1, FUS, OPTN, UBQLN2, and NEFH proteins are found in familial and sporadic ALS inclusions (Al-Chalabi et al., 2012). In zebrafish and *Drosophila*, FUS, and TDP-43 were shown to interact genetically together but independently of SOD1 (Kabashi et al., 2011; Lanson et al., 2011; Wang et al., 2011a). The rapid development of phenotypes and the availability of multiple mutants or RNAi clones make *C. elegans* an expedient model to study genetic interactions. In worms, TDP-1 was shown to participate in the neurotoxicity observed in motor neuron caused by human TDP-43 and human FUS (Vaccaro et al., 2012c). However, FUS and TDP-43 seem to interact differently with PGRN, a gene involved in FTD, and C9ORF72/ALFA-1 (Tauffenberger et al., 2013a; Therrien et al., 2013). Those results provide an interesting start to the identification of common pathological pathways in ALS. Finally, the characterization of the loss of function mutant of *pgrn-1*, the *C. elegans* ortholog of progranulin, showed that PGRN-1 is involved in apoptotic cell clearance (Kao et al., 2011). Understanding how *pgrn-1* interacts with the different genes involved in ALS/FTD could help to better understand the variation observed along ALS/FTD continuum (Mackenzie et al., 2011).

At a broader level, screening for potential genetic modifiers using RNAi has brought a new understanding of the pathogenesis. For example, SOD1 aggregation was linked to motor dysfunction in worms, but upon decreasing the expression of chaperone proteins, the worms exhibited larger aggregates and increased locomotion deficits (Wang et al., 2009). A non-biased screening approach has recently demonstrated that targeting proteins that affect the phosphorylation levels of TDP-43 greatly affects its neuronal toxicity, setting the stage for novel therapeutic approaches (Liachko et al., 2013). Thus far, only a handful of genetic screens have been described for *C. elegans* ALS models but future studies may help uncover pathogenic mechanisms and therapeutic strategies.

TDP-43 aggregates were shown to be the main protein found in non-SOD1 ALS cases (Neumann et al., 2006). However, the presence of TDP-43 aggregates is not exclusive to ALS. TDP-43 aggregates are observed in other neurodegenerative diseases such as Huntington's disease, Parkinson's disease, Alzheimer's disease, and FTD (Mackenzie et al., 2010). FUS is also found in the aggregates of polyglutamine disorders (Woulfe et al., 2010) and mutations in *FUS* were linked to essential tremor (Merner et al., 2012). Recently, FIG4 and VCP were also identified in different neurodegenerative aggregates (Mori et al., 2013a; Kon et al., 2014). Uncovering specific genetic interactions that involve these proteins could also help our understanding of their recruitment to the aggregates of so many neurodegenerative disorders. Using other models, groups have shown that intermediate polyglutamine repeat of *ATXN2* gene and EPHA4 are potent modulators of ALS toxicity (Elden et al., 2010; Van Hoecke et al., 2012). Therefore, a genetic interaction map may extend the role of these genes beyond ALS and perhaps into other neurodegenerative disorders.

USING *C. elegans* MODEL FOR ALS DRUG DISCOVERY

The small size of *C. elegans*, its rapid life cycle, its ease of cultivation and ability to obtain large numbers of animals makes it an attractive model for drug discovery. Furthermore, worms can be grown on solid media or in liquid culture, the latter being relatively easy to adapt for drug screening purposes often through use of multiwell plates and/or automated screening methods (O'Reilly et al., 2013). The transparency of *C. elegans* makes it an ideal model for neurodegeneration applications since protein aggregation and neuronal morphology can be easily assayed as a complement to behavioral phenotypes.

Boyd and colleagues have shown that drugs identified from cell based systems often have relevance in *C. elegans* (Boyd et al., 2013). A screen to identify compounds that decrease TDP-43 aggregation was performed in cell lines and many of the molecules identified were able to suppress the impaired motility phenotype of worms expressing mutant human TDP-43 (Boyd et al., 2013).

Our group has also developed a high-throughput drug-screening assay. We observed that the paralysis phenotype that typically manifests over 5–12 days on solid media can be observed after just hours when the worms are placed in liquid culture (Vaccaro et al., 2012b; Therrien et al., 2013). Using this technique, more than 4000 FDA approved compounds were screened in our laboratory. From this screen, we identified a number of molecules including methylene blue and others acting on the ER stress response that decrease the toxicity of TDP-43 (Vaccaro et al., 2012a, 2013). Interestingly, these drugs were also confirmed in zebrafish ALS models confirming that these compounds can be effective across species. These compounds are therefore promising leads for testing in mammalian models.

Even though in the disease state, aging and neurodegeneration seem to go hand in hand, we have shown that the drugs that act on neurodegeneration can be separated from those that broadly affect lifespan (Tauffenberger et al., 2013b) suggesting that lifespan extension is not a strong predictor of neuroprotection.

OTHER MOTOR NEURON DISEASES

ALS is part of the neurological group of disorders called motor neuron diseases. This group also includes spinal muscular atrophy (SMA), primary lateral sclerosis (PLS), hereditary spastic paraplegia (HSP) and many others affecting the upper and/or lower motor neurons. The causative genes of these diseases are involved in many cellular functions, however they all share a common toxic pathways since they mainly affect motor neurons. Finding similarities and differences among those diseases could highly increase our understanding of motor neuron toxicity. *C. elegans* has been used to study two of these, SMA and HSP.

HSP is a group of disorders affecting mainly the lower motor neurons. More than 40 loci have been linked to HSP and the genes identify are involved in axon pathfinding and myelination, mitochondrial maintenance and membrane trafficking (Blackstone, 2012). Recently, a large network including many of these genes have been identify and this network is highly similar to Parkinson's, ALS and Alzheimer's diseases (Novarino et al., 2014). Using *C. elegans*, the function and toxicity of two HSP genes have been investigated. First, *spas-1*, the *C. elegans* ortholog of *spastin*, also called *SPG4*, was shown to be involved in the development of microtubules. SPAS-1 is expressed in the cytoskeleton and is involved specifically in the disassembly of microtubules (Matsushita-Ishiodori et al., 2007). Then, the pan neuronal expression of *NIPA-1* associated mutations led to motor deficits and shortened the lifespan of transgenic worms probably through the activation of caspases and increased ER toxicity (Zhao et al., 2008). With the rapid discovery of new HSP genes, more models are surely to come and will help unravel similarities between these diseases.

SMA is a rare autosomal recessive disorder and a leading genetic cause of infant death. All genetic causes of SMA lead to a decreased expression of the proteins survival of motor neuron (SMN) 1 and 2 (Arnold and Burghes, 2013). It mainly affects the lower motor neurons, but recent evidences suggest that it can be a systemic disease affecting the vascular, cardiac and hepatic functions as well as affecting bone formation (Hamilton and Gillingwater, 2013). *C. elegans* possesses one ortholog of the *SMN* gene, *smn-1*. In 1999, Miguel-Aliaga and colleagues showed that decreased expression of *smn-1* in worms resulted in severe locomotion defects and sterility (Miguel-Aliaga et al., 1999). Then SMN-1 was shown to interact with SMI-1, a known interactor of SMN in humans (Burt et al., 2006). Briese and colleagues characterized the first *smn-1* deletion mutant observing that the mutants displayed early developmental arrest, which could be rescued by reintroducing expression of *smn-1* in the nervous system, while expression in muscle cells was ineffective (Briese et al., 2009). Little is known about any downstream targets of SMN and no drugs are available. Thus, several groups have used *C. elegans* to identify modifiers of the *smn-1* phenotypes. In a cross-species study, it was shown that proteins involved in endocytosis and mRNA regulation could modify the toxicity (Dimitriadi et al., 2010). Also, knowing that the ubiquitin-proteasome pathway degrades SMN, decreased expression of *Mibl*, an E3 ligase, was shown to ameliorate *smn-1* phenotypes (Kwon et al., 2013). Since the *smn-1* deletion allele o*k355* is an early larval lethal phenotype, to aid the development of drug screening Sleigh and colleagues identified a less severe mutant allele that more closely resembles the severity of SMA (Sleigh et al., 2011). Using this mutant, they identified several small molecules that alleviate *smn-1* phenotypes of the worms, therefore, being highly promising compounds for SMA drug development (Sleigh et al., 2011).

PERSPECTIVES

With the discovery of many new ALS genes comes the need to better understand their functions, expression patterns and their modes of toxicity. *C. elegans* has proven to be an informative model to study neurodegeneration mechanisms arising from multiple ALS related proteins. We envision that the introduction of new transgenic and genetic models will help unravel important questions about the normal and pathogenic roles of these proteins.

Most models explained here recapitulate some if not many, important features of ALS, however, phenotypic variations are seen amongst the different models, for a number of reasons. First, the models do not all use the same mutations, thus the resulting mutant proteins may not all be equally toxic, or display the same interactions with other proteins. Also, the level of expression is important to consider as for example, there is considerable evidence that TDP-43 levels are tightly regulated (Budini and Buratti, 2011), and elevated expression is toxic in nearly every system studied (Ash et al., 2010; Xu et al., 2010; Estes et al., 2011). The most common method to generate transgenic worms is by microinjection to create stable lines followed by radiation to integrate the transgene in the genome. This procedure typically produces transgenics with multiple copies of the gene inserted in the genome, thus some of the toxicity observed may be due to overexpression. Aware of this issue, a new generation of ALS transgenic worms should be constructed based on single copy integration (Frøkjaer-Jensen et al., 2008) or with the CRISPR-Cas9 method (Friedland et al., 2013) instead to ensure that transgenic lines have a similar level of expression from the same genomic location. Finally, the phenotypic variance may also be due to the promoter used. Some models have used pan neuronal expression constructs, while others have targeted transgenic expression to specific neuronal populations. In humans, most of these proteins are expressed ubiquitously but only specific neuronal populations are sensitive to degeneration. Thus, worm models based on motor neuron transgenics could be ideal model to uncover conserved mechanisms of motor neuron degeneration. To confirm the specificity of each phenotype, mutant and wild type proteins should be carefully compared and similar changes should be confirmed in higher eukaryotes. For example, mutant TDP-43 and FUS proteins induce an ER stress response in worms which is not observed when the wild type proteins are expressed (Vaccaro et al., 2012b). Also, the ER stress response was shown to be activated in other ALS models and in patients (see section above).

These models are setting the stage for novel toxicity hypothesis. The immune system seems to play an important role in the neurodegeneration observed in ALS. Protein aggregation could activate the immune response and neuroinflammation actively contributes to disease progression (McCombe and Henderson, 2011). *C. elegans* relies on an evolutionary conserved, innate immune response (Engelmann and Pujol, 2010) that coordinates its activity with the insulin/IGF-1 pathway (Singh and Aballay, 2009) suggesting these may be pathways worth investigating. Also, in the past year, a convergence of data has suggested a role for glial cells in ALS neurodegeneration (Parisi et al., 2013; Valori et al., 2013; Chiu et al., 2014). The worm has 56 glial cells and some are found at the neuromuscular junction (Oikonomou and Shaham, 2011). Characterization of the cross talk between the neurons and the glial cells would also be an interesting area of investigation.

An important topic related to ALS and to other neurodegenerative disorders is aging. The risk of ALS increases with age, peaking between 70 and 80 years old (Gordon, 2013). Aging pathways are well characterized in worms and among others, include the insulin/IGF-1, the target of rapamycin (TOR) and germline signaling pathways. There is a strong overlap between protetotoxicity and aging where autophagy and lipid metabolism are major targets (Lapierre and Hansen, 2012). Evaluating the toxic impact of mutant proteins during aging is not feasible in many models, but is easily accomplished using *C. elegans*. The development of models with age-related toxicity is essential and could help understand the link between the proteotoxicity and aging.

When using *C. elegans* or other animal models, most studies have focused on the toxicity of known ALS genes. It is important to note that almost 90% of ALS cases are sporadic ALS with no link to known genetic abnormalities. Therefore, we still do not know how most patients develop ALS. However, it is important to know that sporadic and familial cases of ALS are clinically indistinguishable (Al-Chalabi and Hardiman, 2013). Given that ALS patients can live between 6 months and 6 years after diagnosis, it has been hypothesized that environmental factors may influence disease onset and progression (Al-Chalabi and Hardiman, 2013). Many environmental factors have been examined in relation to ALS but there is no consensus for their contribution to the disease (Al-Chalabi and Hardiman, 2013). *C. elegans* could be useful to study some of the environmental risks hypothesized. In fact, several groups have identified compounds that could cause specific degeneration of motor neurons (Du and Wang, 2009; Negga et al., 2012; Estevez et al., 2014) opening the door to identifying environmental modifiers of degeneration in ALS models.

However, how relevant are any of these findings to humans? Will any of the drugs identified in *C. elegans* translate to mammalian models let alone ALS patients? So far, many drugs identified using rodent models focusing mainly on protein aggregation and cell death mechanisms have failed in subsequent clinical trials. Using *C. elegans* to identify drugs acting on early neuronal dysfunction mechanisms could be an effective way to prevent ensuing cellular decline and death. From a liquid culture screen, our group has identified a compound with this property (unpublished results). The compound is effective in vertebrate ALS animal models and is now being tested in ALS patients. Therefore, large screens using *C. elegans* targeting specific early aspects of neurodegeneration seem promising and show relevance in higher organisms.

ACKNOWLEDGMENTS

Funding from ALS Canada, the Canadian Institutes of Health Research, the Congressionally Directed Medical Research Program (CDMRP) Amyotrophic Lateral Sclerosis Research Program (USA), and the Muscular Dystrophy Association (USA) supported this work.

REFERENCES

Al-Chalabi, A., and Hardiman, O. (2013). The epidemiology of ALS: a conspiracy of genes, environment and time. *Nat. Rev. Neurol.* 9, 617–628. doi: 10.1038/nrneurol.2013.203

Al-Chalabi, A., Jones, A., Troakes, C., King, A., Al-Sarraj, S., and van den Berg, L. H., (2012). The genetics and neuropathology of amyotrophic lateral sclerosis. *Acta Neuropathol.* 124, 339–352. doi: 10.1007/s00401-012-1022-4

Arnold, E. S., Ling, S.-C., Huelga, S. C., Lagier-Tourenne, C., Polymenidou, M., Ditsworth, D., et al. (2013). ALS-linked TDP-43 mutations produce aberrant RNA splicing and adult-onset motor neuron disease without aggregation or loss of nuclear TDP-43. *Proc. Natl. Acad. Sci. U.S.A.* 110, E736–E745. doi: 10.1073/pnas.1222809110

Arnold, W. D., and Burghes, A. H. M. (2013). Spinal muscular atrophy: development and implementation of potential treatments. *Ann. Neurol.* 74, 348–362. doi: 10.1002/ana.23995

Ash, P. E. A., Bieniek, K. F., Gendron, T. F., Caulfield, T., Lin, W.-L., DeJesus-Hernandez, M., et al. (2013). Unconventional translation of C9ORF72 GGGGCC expansion generates insoluble polypeptides specific to c9FTD/ALS. *Neuron* 77, 639–646. doi: 10.1016/j.neuron.2013.02.004

Ash, P. E. A., Zhang, Y. J., Roberts, C. M., Saldi, T., Hutter, H., Buratti, E., et al. (2010). Neurotoxic effects of TDP-43 overexpression in *C. elegans*. *Hum. Mol. Genet.* 19, 3206–3218. doi: 10.1093/hmg/ddq230

Atkin, J. D., Farg, M. A., Walker, A. K., McLean, C., Tomas, D., and Horne, M. K. (2008). Endoplasmic reticulum stress and induction of the unfolded protein response in human sporadic amyotrophic lateral sclerosis. *Neurobiol. Dis.* 30, 400–407. doi: 10.1016/j.nbd.2008.02.009

Baron, D. M., Kaushansky, L. J., Ward, C. L., Sama, R. R. K., Chian, R.-J., Boggio, K. J., et al. (2013). Amyotrophic lateral sclerosis-linked FUS/TLS alters stress granule assembly and dynamics. *Mol. Neurodegener.* 8:30. doi: 10.1186/1750-1326-8-30

Blackstone, C. (2012). Cellular pathways of hereditary spastic paraplegia. *Annu. Rev. Neurosci.* 35, 25–47. doi: 10.1146/annurev-neuro-062111-150400

Bosco, D. A., Lemay, N., Ko, H. K., Zhou, H., Burke, C., Kwiatkowski, T. J., et al. (2010). Mutant FUS proteins that cause amyotrophic lateral sclerosis incorporate into stress granules. *Hum. Mol. Genet.* 19, 4160–4175. doi: 10.1093/hmg/ddq335

Boucher, B., and Jenna, S. (2013). Genetic interaction networks: better understand to better predict. *Front. Genet.* 4:290. doi: 10.3389/fgene.2013.00290

Boyd, J. D., Lee-Armandt, J. P., Feiler, M. S., Zauur, N., Liu, M., Kraemer, B., et al. (2013). A high-content screen identifies novel compounds that inhibit stress-induced TDP-43 cellular aggregation and associated cytotoxicity. *J. Biomol. Screen.* 19, 44–56. doi: 10.1177/1087057113501553

Briese, M., Esmaeili, B., Fraboulet, S., Burt, E. C., Christodoulou, S., Towers, P. R., et al. (2009). Deletion of smn-1, the *Caenorhabditis elegans* ortholog of the spinal muscular atrophy gene, results in locomotor dysfunction and reduced lifespan. *Hum. Mol. Genet.* 18, 97–104. doi: 10.1093/hmg/ddn320

Budini, M., and Buratti, E. (2011). TDP-43 autoregulation: implications for disease. *J. Mol. Neurosci.* 45, 473–479. doi: 10.1007/s12031-011-9573-8

Burt, E. C., Towers, P. R., and Sattelle, D. B. (2006). *Caenorhabditis elegans* in the study of SMN-interacting proteins: a role for SMI-1, an orthologue of human Gemin2 and the identification of novel components of the SMN complex. *Invert. Neurosci.* 6, 145–159. doi: 10.1007/s10158-006-0027-x

C. elegans Sequencing Consortium. (1998). Genome sequence of the nematode *C. elegans*: a platform for investigating biology. *Science* 282, 2012–2018. doi: 10.1126/science.282.5396.2012

Cabreiro, F., Ackerman, D., Doonan, R., Araiz, C., Back, P., Papp, D., et al. (2011). Increased life span from overexpression of superoxide dismutase in *Caenorhabditis elegans* is not caused by decreased oxidative damage. *Free Radic. Biol. Med.* 51, 1575–1582. doi: 10.1016/j.freeradbiomed.2011.07.020

Chen, K.-Y., Pan, H., Lin, M.-J., Li, Y.-Y., Wang, L.-C., Wu, Y.-C., et al. (2007). Length-dependent toxicity of untranslated CUG repeats on *Caenorhabditis elegans*. *Biochem. Biophys. Res. Commun.* 352, 774–779. doi: 10.1016/j.bbrc.2006.11.102

Chen, S., Sayana, P., Zhang, X., and Le, W. (2013). Genetics of amyotrophic lateral sclerosis: an update. *Mol. Neurodegener.* 8:28. doi: 10.1186/1750-1326-8-28

Chiu, H., Alqadah, A., and Chang, C. (2014). The role of microRNAs in regulating neuronal connectivity. *Front. Cell. Neurosci.* 7:283. doi: 10.3389/fncel.2013.00283

Ciura, S., Lattante, S., Le Ber, I., Latouche, M., Tostivint, H., Brice, A., et al. (2013). Loss of function of C9orf72 causes motor deficits in a zebrafish model of Amyotrophic Lateral Sclerosis. *Ann Neurol.* 74, 180–187. doi: 10.1002/ana.23946

Couthouis, J., Hart, M. P., Shorter, J., DeJesus-Hernandez, M., Erion, R., Oristano, R., et al. (2011). A yeast functional screen predicts new candidate ALS disease genes. *Proc. Natl. Acad. Sci.U.S.A.* 108, 20881–20890. doi: 10.1073/pnas.1109434108

DeJesus-Hernandez, M., Mackenzie, I. R., Boeve, B. F., Boxer, A. L., Baker, M., Rutherford, N. J., et al. (2011). Expanded GGGGCC hexanucleotide repeat in noncoding region of C9ORF72 causes chromosome 9p-linked FTD and ALS. *Neuron* 72, 245–256. doi: 10.1016/j.neuron.2011.09.011

Dimitriadi, M., Sleigh, J. N., Walker, A., Chang, H. C., Sen, A., Kalloo, G., et al. (2010). Conserved genes act as modifiers of invertebrate SMN loss of function defects. *PLoS Genet.* 6:e1001172. doi: 10.1371/journal.pgen.1001172

Dormann, D., Rodde, R., Edbauer, D., Bentmann, E., Fischer, I., Hruscha, A., et al. (2010). ALS-associated fused in sarcoma (FUS) mutations disrupt Transportin-mediated nuclear import. *EMBO J.* 29, 2841–2857. doi: 10.1038/emboj.2010.143

Du, M., and Wang, D. (2009). The neurotoxic effects of heavy metal exposure on GABAergic nervous system in nematode *Caenorhabditis elegans*. *Environ. Toxicol. Pharmacol.* 27, 314–320. doi: 10.1016/j.etap.2008.11.011

Elden, A. C., Kim, H.-J., Hart, M. P., Chen-Plotkin, A. S., Johnson, B. S., Fang, X., et al. (2010). Ataxin-2 intermediate-length polyglutamine expansions are associated with increased risk for ALS. *Nature* 466, 1069–1075. doi: 10.1038/nature09320

Engelmann, I., and Pujol, N. (2010). Innate immunity in *C. elegans*. *Adv. Exp. Med. Biol.* 708, 105–121. doi: 10.1007/978-1-4419-8059-5_6

Epstein, C. J., Avraham, K. B., Lovett, M., Smith, S., Elroy-Stein, O., Rotman, G., et al. (1987). Transgenic mice with increased Cu/Zn-superoxide dismutase activity: animal model of dosage effects in Down syndrome. *Proc. Natl. Acad. Sci. U.S.A.* 84, 8044–8048. doi: 10.1073/pnas.84.22.8044

Estes, P. S., Boehringer, A., Zwick, R., Tang, J. E., Grigsby, B., and Zarnescu, D. C. (2011). Wild-type and A315T mutant TDP-43 exert differential neurotoxicity in a Drosophila model of ALS. *Hum. Mol. Genet.* 20, 2308–2321. doi: 10.1093/hmg/ddr124

Estevez, A. O., Morgan, K. L., Szewczyk, N. J., Gems, D., and Estevez, M. (2014). The neurodegenerative effects of selenium are inhibited by FOXO and PINK1/PTEN regulation of insulin/insulin-like growth factor signaling in *Caenorhabditis elegans*. *Neurotoxicology* 41, 28–43. doi: 10.1016/j.neuro.2013.12.012

Fares, H., and Grant, B. (2002). Deciphering endocytosis in *Caenorhabditis elegans*. *Traffic* 3, 11–19. doi: 10.1034/j.1600-0854.2002.30103.x

Farg, M. A., Sundaramoorthy, V., Sultana, J. M., Yang, S., Atkinson, R. A. K., Levina, V., et al. (2014). C9ORF72, implicated in amytrophic lateral sclerosis and frontotemporal dementia, regulates endosomal trafficking. *Hum. Mol. Genet.* doi: 10.1093/hmg/ddu068. [Epub ahead of print].

Friedland, A. E., Tzur, Y. B., Esvelt, K. M., Colaiácovo, M. P., Church, G. M., and Calarco, J. A. (2013). Heritable genome editing in *C. elegans* via a CRISPR-Cas9 system. *Nat. Meth.* 10, 741–743. doi: 10.1038/nmeth.2532

Frøkjaer-Jensen, C., Davis, M. W., Hopkins, C. E., Newman, B. J., Thummel, J. M., Olesen, S.-P., et al. (2008). Single-copy insertion of transgenes in *Caenorhabditis elegans*. *Nat. Genet.* 40, 1375–1383. doi: 10.1038/ng.248

Gal, J., Zhang, J., Kwinter, D. M., Zhai, J., Jia, H., Jia, J., et al. (2011). Nuclear localization sequence of FUS and induction of stress granules by ALS mutants. *Neurobiol. Aging* 32, 2323.e27–e40. doi: 10.1016/j.neurobiolaging.2010.06.010

Gidalevitz, T., Krupinski, T., Garcia, S., and Morimoto, R. I. (2009). Destabilizing protein polymorphisms in the genetic background direct phenotypic expression of mutant SOD1 toxicity. *PLoS Genet.* 5:e1000399. doi: 10.1371/journal.pgen.1000399

Gordon, P. H. (2013). Amyotrophic lateral sclerosis: an update for 2013 clinical features, pathophysiology, management and therapeutic trials. *Aging Dis.* 4, 295–310. doi: 10.14336/AD.2013.0400295

Grad, L. I., and Cashman, N. R. (2014). Prion-like activity of Cu/Zn superoxide dismutase: implications for amyotrophic lateral sclerosis. *Prion* 8, 35–43. doi: 10.4161/pri.27602

Guo, Y.-S., Wu, D.-X., Wu, H.-R., Wu, S.-Y., Yang, C., Li, B., et al. (2009). Sensory involvement in the SOD1-G93A mouse model of amyotrophic lateral sclerosis. *Exp. Mol. Med.* 41, 140–150. doi: 10.3858/emm.2009.41.3.017

Gurney, M. E., Pu, H., Chiu, A. Y., Dal Canto, M. C., Polchow, C. Y., Alexander, D. D., et al. (1994). Motor neuron degeneration in mice that express a human Cu,Zn superoxide dismutase mutation. *Science* 264, 1772–1775. doi: 10.1126/science.8209258

Hamilton, G., and Gillingwater, T. H. (2013). Spinal muscular atrophy: going beyond the motor neuron. *Trends Mol. Med.* 19, 40–50. doi: 10.1016/j.molmed.2012.11.002

Han, S. M., Oussini, E. L. H., Scekic-Zahirovic, J., Vibbert, J., Cottee, P., and Miller, M. A. (2013). VAPB/ALS8 MSP ligands regulate striated muscle energy metabolism critical for adult survival in *Caenorhabditis elegans*. *PLoS Genet.* 9:e1003738. doi: 10.1371/journal.pgen.1003738

Hetz, C., Thielen, P., Matus, S., Nassif, M., Court, F., Kiffin, R., et al. (2009). XBP-1 deficiency in the nervous system protects against amyotrophic lateral sclerosis by increasing autophagy. *Genes Dev.* 23, 2294–2306. doi: 10.1101/gad.1830709

Ilieva, E. V., Ayala, V., Jové, M., Dalfó, E., Cacabelos, D., Povedano, M., et al. (2007). Oxidative and endoplasmic reticulum stress interplay in sporadic amyotrophic lateral sclerosis. *Brain* 130, 3111–3123. doi: 10.1093/brain/awm190

Ito, Y., Yamada, M., Tanaka, H., Aida, K., Tsuruma, K., Shimazawa, M., et al. (2009). Involvement of CHOP, an ER-stress apoptotic mediator, in both human sporadic ALS and ALS model mice. *Neurobiol. Dis.* 36, 470–476. doi: 10.1016/j.nbd.2009.08.013

Jorgensen, E. M. (2005). GABA. *WormBook* 1–13. doi: 10.1895/wormbook.1.14.1

Jud, M. C., Czerwinski, M. J., Wood, M. P., Young, R. A., Gallo, C. M., Bickel, J. S., et al. (2008). Large P body-like RNPs form in *C. elegans* oocytes in response to arrested ovulation, heat shock, osmotic stress, and anoxia and are regulated by the major sperm protein pathway. *Dev. Biol.* 318, 38–51. doi: 10.1016/j.ydbio.2008.02.059

Kabashi, E., Bercier, V., Lissouba, A., Liao, M., Brustein, E., Rouleau, G. A., et al. (2011). FUS and TARDBP but not SOD1 interact in genetic models of amyotrophic lateral sclerosis. *PLoS Genet.* 7:e1002214. doi: 10.1371/journal.pgen.1002214

Kabashi, E., Valdmanis, P. N., Dion, P., Spiegelman, D., McConkey, B. J., Vande Velde, C., et al. (2008). TARDBP mutations in individuals with sporadic and familial amyotrophic lateral sclerosis. *Nat. Genet.* 40, 572–574. doi: 10.1038/ng.132

Kabir, M. E., and Safar, J. G. (2014). Implications of prion adaptation and evolution paradigm for human neurodegenerative diseases. *Prion* 8, 113–118. doi: 10.4161/pri.27661

Kao, A. W., Eisenhut, R. J., Martens, L. H., Nakamura, A., Huang, A., Bagley, J. A., et al. (2011). A neurodegenerative disease mutation that accelerates the clearance of apoptotic cells. *Proc. Natl. Acad. Sci.* 108, 4441–4446. doi: 10.1073/pnas.1100650108

Kiernan, M. C., Vucic, S., Cheah, B. C., Turner, M. R., Eisen, A., Hardiman, O., et al. (2011). Amyotrophic lateral sclerosis. *Lancet* 377, 942–955. doi: 10.1016/S0140-6736(10)61156-7

Kim, H. J., Kim, N. C., Wang, Y.-D., Scarborough, E. A., Moore, J., Diaz, Z., et al. (2013). Mutations in prion-like domains in hnRNPA2B1 and hnRNPA1 cause multisystem proteinopathy and ALS. *Nature* 495, 467–473. doi: 10.1038/nature11922

Kon, T., Mori, F., Tanji, K., Miki, Y., Toyoshima, Y., Yoshida, M., et al. (2014). ALS-associated protein FIG4 is localized in Pick and Lewy bodies, and also neuronal nuclear inclusions, in polyglutamine and intranuclear inclusion body diseases. *Neuropathology* 34, 19–26. doi: 10.1111/neup.12056

Kwiatkowski, T. J., Bosco, D. A., LeClerc, A. L., Tamrazian, E., Vanderburg, C. R., Russ, C., et al. (2009). Mutations in the FUS/TLS gene on chromosome 16 cause familial amyotrophic lateral sclerosis. *Science* 323, 1205–1208. doi: 10.1126/science.1166066

Kwon, D. Y., Dimitriadi, M., Terzic, B., Cable, C., Hart, A. C., Chitnis, A., et al. (2013). The E3 ubiquitin ligase mind bomb 1 ubiquitinates and promotes the degradation of survival of motor neuron protein. *Mol. Biol. Cell* 24, 1863–1871. doi: 10.1091/mbc.E13-01-0042

Lai, C. H., Chou, C. Y., Ch'ang, L. Y., Liu, C. S., and Lin, W. (2000). Identification of novel human genes evolutionarily conserved in *Caenorhabditis elegans* by comparative proteomics. *Genome Res.* 10, 703–713. doi: 10.1101/gr.10.5.703

Lanson, N. A., Maltare, A., King, H., Smith, R., Kim, J. H., Taylor, J. P., et al. (2011). A Drosophila model of FUS-related neurodegeneration reveals genetic interaction between FUS and TDP-43. *Hum. Mol. Genet.* 20, 2510–2523. doi: 10.1093/hmg/ddr150

Lapierre, L. R., and Hansen, M. (2012). Lessons from *C. elegans*: signaling pathways for longevity. *Trends Endocrinol. Metab.* 23, 637–644. doi: 10.1016/j.tem.2012.07.007

Lau, H. E., and Chalasani, S. H. (2014). Divergent and convergent roles for insulin-like peptides in the worm, fly and mammalian nervous systems. *Invert. Neurosci.* doi: 10.1007/s10158-013-0166-9. [Epub ahead of print].

Levine, T. P., Daniels, R. D., Gatta, A. T., Wong, L. H., and Hayes, M. J. (2013). The product of C9orf72, a gene strongly implicated in neurodegeneration, is structurally related to DENN Rab-GEFs. *Bioinformatics* 29, 499–503. doi: 10.1093/bioinformatics/bts725

Li, J., and Le, W. (2013). Modeling neurodegenerative diseases in *Caenorhabditis elegans*. *Exp. Neurol.* 250, 94–103. doi: 10.1016/j.expneurol.2013.09.024

Li, J., Li, T., Zhang, X., Tang, Y., Yang, J., and Le, W. (2013a). Human superoxide dismutase 1 overexpression in motor neurons of *Caenorhabditis elegans* causes axon guidance defect and neurodegeneration. *Neurobiol. Aging* 35, 837–846. doi: 10.1016/j.neurobiolaging.2013.09.003

Li, Y. R., King, O. D., Shorter, J., and Gitler, A. D. (2013b). Stress granules as crucibles of ALS pathogenesis. *J. Cell Biol.* 201, 361–372. doi: 10.1083/jcb.201302044

Liachko, N. F., Guthrie, C. R., and Kraemer, B. C. (2010). Phosphorylation promotes neurotoxicity in a *Caenorhabditis elegans* Model of TDP-43 proteinopathy. *J. Neurosci.* 30, 16208–16219. doi: 10.1523/JNEUROSCI.2911-10.2010

Liachko, N. F., McMillan, P. J., Guthrie, C. R., Bird, T. D., Leverenz, J. B., and Kraemer, B. C. (2013). CDC7 inhibition blocks pathological TDP-43 phosphorylation and neurodegeneration. *Ann Neurol.* 74, 39–52. doi: 10.1002/ana.23870

Ling, S.-C., Polymenidou, M., and Cleveland, D. W. (2013). Converging mechanisms in ALS and FTD: disrupted RNA and protein homeostasis. *Neuron* 79, 416–438. doi: 10.1016/j.neuron.2013.07.033

Liu-Yesucevitz, L., Bilgutay, A., Zhang, Y.-J., Vanderweyde, T., Vanderwyde, T., Citro, A., et al. (2010). Tar DNA binding protein-43 (TDP-43) associates with stress granules: analysis of cultured cells and pathological brain tissue. *PLoS ONE* 5:e13250. doi: 10.1371/journal.pone.0013250

Mackenzie, I. R. A., Ansorge, O., Strong, M., Bilbao, J., Zinman, L., Ang, L. C., et al. (2011). Pathological heterogeneity in amyotrophic lateral sclerosis with FUS mutations: two distinct patterns correlating with disease severity and mutation. *Acta Neuropathol.* 122, 87–98. doi: 10.1007/s00401-011-0838-7

Mackenzie, I. R. A., Bigio, E. H., Ince, P. G., Geser, F., Neumann, M., Cairns, N. J., et al. (2007). Pathological TDP-43 distinguishes sporadic amyotrophic lateral sclerosis from amyotrophic lateral sclerosis with SOD1 mutations. *Ann. Neurol.* 61, 427–434. doi: 10.1002/ana.21147

Mackenzie, I. R., Rademakers, R., and Neumann, M. (2010). TDP-43 and FUS in amyotrophic lateral sclerosis and frontotemporal dementia. *Lancet Neurol* 9, 995–1007. doi: 10.1016/S1474-4422(10)70195-2

Matsushita-Ishiodori, Y., Yamanaka, K., and Ogura, T. (2007). The *C. elegans* homologue of the spastic paraplegia protein, spastin, disassembles microtubules. *Biochem. Biophys. Res. Commun.* 359, 157–162. doi: 10.1016/j.bbrc.2007.05.086

Matus, S., Valenzuela, V., Medinas, D. B., and Hetz, C. (2013). ER dysfunction and protein folding stress in ALS. *Int. J. Cell Biol.* 2013, 674751. doi: 10.1155/2013/674751

McCombe, P. A., and Henderson, R. D. (2011). The role of immune and inflammatory mechanisms in ALS. *Curr. Mol. Med.* 11, 246–254. doi: 10.2174/156652411795243450

McDonald, K. K., Aulas, A., Destroismaisons, L., Pickles, S., Beleac, E., Camu, W., et al. (2011). TAR DNA-binding protein 43 (TDP-43) regulates stress granule dynamics via differential regulation of G3BP and TIA-1. *Hum. Mol. Genet.* 20, 1400–1410. doi: 10.1093/hmg/ddr021

McIntire, S. L., Reimer, R. J., Schuske, K., Edwards, R. H., and Jorgensen, E. M. (1997). Identification and characterization of the vesicular GABA transporter. *Nature* 389, 870–876. doi: 10.1038/39908

Merner, N. D., Girard, S. L., Catoire, H., Bourassa, C. V., Belzil, V. V., Rivière, J.-B., et al. (2012). Exome sequencing identifies FUS mutations as a cause of essential tremor. *Am. J. Hum. Genet.* 91, 313–319. doi: 10.1016/j.ajhg.2012.07.002

Miguel-Aliaga, I., Culetto, E., Walker, D. S., Baylis, H. A., Sattelle, D. B., and Davies, K. E. (1999). The *Caenorhabditis elegans* orthologue of the human gene responsible for spinal muscular atrophy is a maternal product critical for germline maturation and embryonic viability. *Hum. Mol. Genet.* 8, 2133–2143. doi: 10.1093/hmg/8.12.2133

Mori, F., Tanji, K., Toyoshima, Y., Sasaki, H., Yoshida, M., Kakita, A., et al. (2013a). Valosin-containing protein immunoreactivity in tauopathies, synucleinopathies, polyglutamine diseases and intranuclear inclusion body disease. *Neuropathology* 33, 637–644. doi: 10.1111/neup.12050

Mori, K., Weng, S.-M., Arzberger, T., May, S., Rentzsch, K., Kremmer, E., et al. (2013b). The C9orf72 GGGGCC repeat is translated into aggregating dipeptide-repeat proteins in FTLD/ALS. *Science* 339, 1335–1338. doi: 10.1126/science.1232927

Morita, M., Al-Chalabi, A., Andersen, P. M., Hosler, B., Sapp, P., Englund, E., et al. (2006). A locus on chromosome 9p confers susceptibility to ALS and frontotemporal dementia. *Neurology* 66, 839–844. doi: 10.1212/01.wnl.0000200048.53766.b4

Morris, H. R., Waite, A. J., Williams, N. M., Neal, J. W., and Blake, D. J. (2012). Recent advances in the genetics of the ALS-FTLD complex. *Curr. Neurol. Neurosci. Rep.* 12, 243–250. doi: 10.1007/s11910-012-0268-5

Murakami, T., Yang, S.-P., Xie, L., Kawano, T., Fu, D., Mukai, A., et al. (2012). ALS mutations in FUS cause neuronal dysfunction and death in *Caenorhabditis elegans* by a dominant gain-of-function mechanism. *Hum. Mol. Genet.* 21, 1–9. doi: 10.1093/hmg/ddr417

Musarò, A. (2013). Understanding ALS: new therapeutic approaches. *FEBS J.* 280, 4315–4322. doi: 10.1111/febs.12087

Negga, R., Stuart, J. A., Machen, M. L., Salva, J., Lizek, A. J., Richardson, S. J., et al. (2012). Exposure to glyphosate- and/or Mn/Zn-ethylene-bis-dithiocarbamate-containing pesticides leads to degeneration of γ-aminobutyric acid and dopamine neurons in *Caenorhabditis elegans*. *Neurotox. Res.* 21, 281–290. doi: 10.1007/s12640-011-9274-7

Neumann, M., Sampathu, D. M., Kwong, L. K., Truax, A. C., Micsenyi, M. C., Chou, T. T., et al. (2006). Ubiquitinated TDP-43 in frontotemporal lobar degeneration and amyotrophic lateral sclerosis. *Science* 314, 130–133. doi: 10.1126/science.1134108

Novarino, G., Fenstermaker, A. G., Zaki, M. S., Hofree, M., Silhavy, J. L., Heiberg, A. D., et al. (2014). Exome sequencing links corticospinal motor neuron disease to common neurodegenerative disorders. *Science* 343, 506–511. doi: 10.1126/science.1247363

Nussbaum-Krammer, C. I., Park, K.-W., Li, L., Melki, R., and Morimoto, R. I. (2013). Spreading of a prion domain from cell-to-cell by vesicular transport in *Caenorhabditis elegans*. *PLoS Genet.* 9:e1003351. doi: 10.1371/journal.pgen.1003351

Oeda, T., Shimohama, S., Kitagawa, N., Kohno, R., Imura, T., Shibasaki, H., et al. (2001). Oxidative stress causes abnormal accumulation of familial amyotrophic lateral sclerosis-related mutant SOD1 in transgenic *Caenorhabditis elegans*. *Hum. Mol. Genet.* 10, 2013–2023. doi: 10.1093/hmg/10.19.2013

Oikonomou, G., and Shaham, S. (2011). The glia of *Caenorhabditis elegans*. *Glia* 59, 1253–1263. doi: 10.1002/glia.21084

O'Reilly, L. P., Luke, C. J., Perlmutter, D. H., Silverman, G. A., and Pak, S. C. (2013). *C. elegans* in high-throughput drug discovery. *Adv. Drug Deliv. Rev.* doi: 10.1016/j.addr.2013.12.001. [Epub ahead of print].

Parisi, C., Arisi, I., D'Ambrosi, N., Storti, A. E., Brandi, R., D'Onofrio, M., et al. (2013). Dysregulated microRNAs in amyotrophic lateral sclerosis microglia modulate genes linked to neuroinflammation. *Cell Death Dis.* 4, e959. doi: 10.1038/cddis.2013.491

Pasinelli, P., Houseweart, M. K., Brown, R. H., and Cleveland, D. W. (2000). Caspase-1 and -3 are sequentially activated in motor neuron death in Cu,Zn superoxide dismutase-mediated familial amyotrophic lateral sclerosis. *Proc. Natl. Acad. Sci. U.S.A.* 97, 13901–13906. doi: 10.1073/pnas.240305897

Pickles, S., and Vande Velde, C. (2012). Misfolded SOD1 and ALS: zeroing in on mitochondria. *Amyotroph Lateral Scler* 13, 333–340. doi: 10.3109/17482968.2012.648645

Polymenidou, M., and Cleveland, D. W. (2011). The seeds of neurodegeneration: prion-like spreading in ALS. *Cell* 147, 498–508. doi: 10.1016/j.cell.2011.10.011

Renton, A. E., Chiò, A., and Traynor, B. J. (2014). State of play in amyotrophic lateral sclerosis genetics. *Nat. Neurosci.* 17, 17–23. doi: 10.1038/nn.3584

Renton, A. E., Majounie, E., Waite, A., Simón-Sánchez, J., Rollinson, S., Gibbs, J. R., et al. (2011). A hexanucleotide repeat expansion in C9ORF72 is the cause of chromosome 9p21-linked ALS-FTD. *Neuron* 72, 257–268. doi: 10.1016/j.neuron.2011.09.010

Ringholz, G. M., Appel, S. H., Bradshaw, M., Cooke, N. A., Mosnik, D. M., and Schulz, P. E. (2005). Prevalence and patterns of cognitive impairment in sporadic ALS. *Neurology* 65, 586–590. doi: 10.1212/01.wnl.0000172911.39167.b6

Robberecht, W., and Philips, T. (2013). The changing scene of amyotrophic lateral sclerosis. *Nat. Rev. Neurosci.* 14, 248–264. doi: 10.1038/nrn3430

Rodriguez, M., Snoek, L. B., De Bono, M., and Kammenga, J. E. (2013). Worms under stress: *C. elegans* stress response and its relevance to complex human disease and aging. *Trends Genet.* 29, 367–374. doi: 10.1016/j.tig.2013.01.010

Rosen, D. R., Siddique, T., Patterson, D., Figlewicz, D. A., Sapp, P., Hentati, A., et al. (1993). Mutations in Cu/Zn superoxide dismutase gene are associated with familial amyotrophic lateral sclerosis. *Nature* 362, 59–62. doi: 10.1038/362059a0

Saccon, R. A., Bunton-Stasyshyn, R. K. A., Fisher, E. M. C., and Fratta, P. (2013). Is SOD1 loss of function involved in amyotrophic lateral sclerosis? *Brain* 136, 2342–2358. doi: 10.1093/brain/awt097

Sasayama, H., Shimamura, M., Tokuda, T., Azuma, Y., Yoshida, T., Mizuno, T., et al. (2012). Knockdown of the Drosophila fused in sarcoma (FUS) homologue causes deficient locomotive behavior and shortening of motoneuron terminal branches. *PLoS ONE* 7:e39483. doi: 10.1371/journal.pone.0039483

Sato, M., Sato, K., Liou, W., Pant, S., Harada, A., and Grant, B. D. (2008). Regulation of endocytic recycling by *C. elegans* Rab35 and its regulator RME-4, a coated-pit protein. *EMBO J.* 27, 1183–1196. doi: 10.1038/emboj.2008.54

Shatunov, A., Mok, K., Newhouse, S., Weale, M. E., Smith, B., Vance, C., et al. (2010). Chromosome 9p21 in sporadic amyotrophic lateral sclerosis in the UK and seven other countries: a genome-wide association study. *Lancet Neurol.* 9, 986–994. doi: 10.1016/S1474-4422(10)70197-6

Shaye, D. D., and Greenwald, I. (2011). OrthoList: a compendium of *C. elegans* genes with human orthologs. *PLoS ONE* 6:e20085. doi: 10.1371/journal.pone.0020085

Singh, V., and Aballay, A. (2009). Regulation of DAF-16-mediated innate immunity in *Caenorhabditis elegans*. *J. Biol. Chem.* 284, 35580–35587. doi: 10.1074/jbc.M109.060905

Sleigh, J. N., Buckingham, S. D., Esmaeili, B., Viswanathan, M., Cuppen, E., Westlund, B. M., et al. (2011). A novel *Caenorhabditis elegans* allele, smn-1(cb131), mimicking a mild form of spinal muscular atrophy, provides a convenient drug screening platform highlighting new and pre-approved compounds. *Hum. Mol. Genet.* 20, 245–260. doi: 10.1093/hmg/ddq459

Sreedharan, J., Blair, I. P., Tripathi, V. B., Hu, X., Vance, C., Rogelj, B., et al. (2008). TDP-43 mutations in familial and sporadic amyotrophic lateral sclerosis. *Science* 319, 1668–1672. doi: 10.1126/science.1154584

Sreedharan, J., and Brown, R. H. (2013). Amyotrophic lateral sclerosis: problems and prospects. *Ann. Neurol.* 74, 309–316. doi: 10.1002/ana.2401

Sun, Y., Yang, P., Zhang, Y., Bao, X., Li, J., Hou, W., et al. (2011). A genome-wide RNAi screen identifies genes regulating the formation of P bodies in *C. elegans* and their functions in NMD and RNAi. *Protein Cell* 2, 918–939. doi: 10.1007/s13238-011-1119-x

Swarup, V., Phaneuf, D., Bareil, C., Robertson, J., Rouleau, G. A., Kriz, J., et al. (2011). Pathological hallmarks of amyotrophic lateral sclerosis/frontotemporal lobar degeneration in transgenic mice produced with TDP-43 genomic fragments. *Brain* 134, 2610–2626. doi: 10.1093/brain/awr159

Tauffenberger, A., Chitramuthu, B. P., Bateman, A., Bennett, H. P. J., and Parker, J. A. (2013a). Reduction of polyglutamine toxicity by TDP-43, FUS and progranulin in Huntington's disease models. *Hum. Mol. Genet.* 22, 782–794. doi: 10.1093/hmg/dds485

Tauffenberger, A., Julien, C., and Parker, J. A. (2013b). Evaluation of longevity enhancing compounds against transactive response DNA-binding protein-43 neuronal toxicity. *Neurobiol. Aging* 34, 2175–2182. doi: 10.1016/j.neurobiolaging.2013.03.014

Taylor, R. C., and Dillin, A. (2013). XBP-1 is a cell-nonautonomous regulator of stress resistance and longevity. *Cell* 153, 1435–1447. doi: 10.1016/j.cell.2013.05.042

Therrien, M., Rouleau, G. A., Dion, P. A., and Parker, J. A. (2013). Deletion of C9ORF72 results in motor neuron degeneration and stress sensitivity in *C. elegans*. *PLoS ONE* 8:e83450. doi: 10.1371/journal.pone.0083450

Turner, M. R., Bowser, R., Bruijn, L., Dupuis, L., Ludolph, A., McGrath, M., et al. (2013a). Mechanisms, models and biomarkers in amyotrophic lateral sclerosis. *Amyotroph. Lateral Scler. Frontotemporal Degener.* 14(Suppl. 1), 19–32. doi: 10.3109/21678421.2013.778554

Turner, M. R., Hardiman, O., Benatar, M., Brooks, B. R., Chiò, A., de Carvalho, M., et al. (2013b). Controversies and priorities in amyotrophic lateral sclerosis. *Lancet Neurol.* 12, 310–322. doi: 10.1016/S1474-4422(13)70036-X

Updike, D., and Strome, S. (2010). P granule assembly and function in *Caenorhabditis elegans* germ cells. *J. Androl.* 31, 53–60. doi: 10.2164/jandrol.109.008292

Vaccaro, A., Patten, S. A., Aggad, D., Julien, C., Maios, C., Kabashi, E., et al. (2013). Pharmacological reduction of ER stress protects against TDP-43 neuronal toxicity *in vivo*. *Neurobiol. Dis.* 55, 64–75. doi: 10.1016/j.nbd.2013.03.015

Vaccaro, A., Patten, S. A., Ciura, S., Maios, C., Therrien, M., Drapeau, P., et al. (2012a). Methylene blue protects against TDP-43 and FUS neuronal toxicity in *C. elegans* and *D. rerio*. *PLoS ONE* 7:e42117. doi: 10.1371/journal.pone.0042117

Vaccaro, A., Tauffenberger, A., Aggad, D., Rouleau, G., Drapeau, P., and Parker, J. A. (2012b). Mutant TDP-43 and FUS cause age-dependent paralysis and neurodegeneration in *C. elegans*. *PLoS ONE* 7:e31321. doi: 10.1371/journal.pone.0031321

Vaccaro, A., Tauffenberger, A., Ash, P. E. A., Carlomagno, Y., Petrucelli, L., and Parker, J. A. (2012c). TDP-1/TDP-43 regulates stress signaling and age-dependent proteotoxicity in *Caenorhabditis elegans*. *PLoS Genet.* 8:e1002806. doi: 10.1371/journal.pgen.1002806

Valori, C. F., Brambilla, L., Martorana, F., and Rossi, D. (2013). The multifaceted role of glial cells in amyotrophic lateral sclerosis. *Cell. Mol. Life Sci.* 71, 287–297. doi: 10.1007/s00018-013-1429-7

Vance, C., Al-Chalabi, A., Ruddy, D., Smith, B. N., Hu, X., Sreedharan, J., et al. (2006). Familial amyotrophic lateral sclerosis with frontotemporal dementia is linked to a locus on chromosome 9p13.2-21.3. *Brain* 129, 868–876. doi: 10.1093/brain/awl030

Vance, C., Rogelj, B., Hortobágyi, T., De Vos, K. J., Nishimura, A. L., Sreedharan, J., et al. (2009). Mutations in FUS, an RNA processing protein, cause familial amyotrophic lateral sclerosis type 6. *Science* 323, 1208–1211. doi: 10.1126/science.1165942

Vance, C., Scotter, E. L., Nishimura, A. L., Troakes, C., Mitchell, J. C., Kathe, C., et al. (2013). ALS mutant FUS disrupts nuclear localization and sequesters wild-type FUS within cytoplasmic stress granules. *Hum. Mol. Genet.* 22, 2676–2688. doi: 10.1093/hmg/ddt117

Vanden Broeck, L., Callaerts, P., and Dermaut, B. (2014). TDP-43-mediated neurodegeneration: towards a loss-of-function hypothesis? *Trends Mol. Med.* 20, 66–71. doi: 10.1016/j.molmed.2013.11.003

van Es, M. A., Veldink, J. H., Saris, C. G. J., Blauw, H. M., van Vught, P. W. J., Birve, A., et al. (2009). Genome-wide association study identifies 19p13.3 (UNC13A) and 9p21.2 as susceptibility loci for sporadic amyotrophic lateral sclerosis. *Nat. Genet.* 41, 1083–1087. doi: 10.1038/ng.442

Van Hoecke, A., Schoonaert, L., Lemmens, R., Timmers, M., Staats, K. A., Laird, A. S., et al. (2012). EPHA4 is a disease modifier of amyotrophic lateral sclerosis in animal models and in humans. *Nat. Med.* 18, 1418–1422. doi: 10.1038/nm.2901

Van Langenhove, T., van der Zee, J., and Van Broeckhoven, C. (2012). The molecular basis of the frontotemporal lobar degeneration-amyotrophic lateral sclerosis spectrum. *Ann. Med.* 44, 817–828. doi: 10.3109/07853890.2012.665471

van Oosten-Hawle, P., Porter, R. S., and Morimoto, R. I. (2013). Regulation of organismal proteostasis by transcellular chaperone signaling. *Cell* 153, 1366–1378. doi: 10.1016/j.cell.2013.05.015

Van Raamsdonk, J. M., and Hekimi, S. (2012). Superoxide dismutase is dispensable for normal animal lifespan. *Proc. Natl. Acad. Sci. U.S.A.* 109, 5785–5790. doi: 10.1073/pnas.1116158109

Verbeeck, C., Deng, Q., DeJesus-Hernandez, M., Taylor, G., Ceballos-Diaz, C., Kocerha, J., et al. (2012). Expression of Fused in sarcoma mutations in mice recapitulates the neuropathology of FUS proteinopathies and provides insight into disease pathogenesis. *Mol. Neurodegener.* 7:53. doi: 10.1186/1750-1326-7-53

Wang, J., Farr, G. W., Hall, D. H., Li, F., Furtak, K., Dreier, L., et al. (2009). An ALS-linked mutant SOD1 produces a locomotor defect associated with aggregation and synaptic dysfunction when expressed in neurons of *Caenorhabditis elegans*. *PLoS Genet* 5:e1000350. doi: 10.1371/journal.pgen.1000350

Wang, J.-W., Brent, J. R., Tomlinson, A., Shneider, N. A., and McCabe, B. D. (2011a). The ALS-associated proteins FUS and TDP-43 function together to affect Drosophila locomotion and life span. *J. Clin. Invest.* 121, 4118–4126. doi: 10.1172/JCI57883

Wang, L.-C., Chen, K.-Y., Pan, H., Wu, C.-C., Chen, P.-H., Liao, Y.-T., et al. (2011b). Muscleblind participates in RNA toxicity of expanded CAG and CUG repeats in *Caenorhabditis elegans*. *Cell. Mol. Life Sci.* 68, 1255–1267. doi: 10.1007/s00018-010-0522-4

Warren, J. D., Rohrer, J. D., and Rossor, M. N. (2013). Clinical review. Frontotemporal dementia. *BMJ* 347, f4827. doi: 10.1136/bmj.f4827

Woulfe, J., Gray, D. A., and Mackenzie, I. R. A. (2010). FUS-immunoreactive intranuclear inclusions in neurodegenerative disease. *Brain Pathol.* 20, 589–597. doi: 10.1111/j.1750-3639.2009.00337.x

Xi, Z., Zinman, L., Moreno, D., Schymick, J., Liang, Y., Sato, C., et al. (2013). Hypermethylation of the CpG island near the G4C2 repeat in ALS with a C9orf72 expansion. *Am. J. Hum. Genet.* 92, 981–989. doi: 10.1016/j.ajhg.2013.04.017

Xu, Y.-F., Gendron, T. F., Zhang, Y.-J., Lin, W.-L., D'Alton, S., Sheng, H., et al. (2010). Wild-type human TDP-43 expression causes TDP-43 phosphorylation, mitochondrial aggregation, motor deficits, and early mortality in transgenic mice. *J. Neurosci.* 30, 10851–10859. doi: 10.1523/JNEUROSCI.1630-10.2010

Xu, Z., Poidevin, M., Li, X., Li, Y., Shu, L., Nelson, D. L., et al. (2013). Expanded GGGGCC repeat RNA associated with amyotrophic lateral sclerosis and frontotemporal dementia causes neurodegeneration. *Proc. Natl. Acad. Sci. U.S.A.* 110, 7778–7783. doi: 10.1073/pnas.1219643110

Yanase, S., Onodera, A., Tedesco, P., Johnson, T. E., and Ishii, N. (2009). SOD-1 deletions in *Caenorhabditis elegans* alter the localization of intracellular reactive oxygen species and show molecular compensation. *J. Gerontol. A Bio. Sci. Med. Sci.* 64, 530–539. doi: 10.1093/gerona/glp020

Zhang, D., Iyer, L. M., He, F., and Aravind, L. (2012a). Discovery of Novel DENN Proteins: implications for the evolution of eukaryotic intracellular membrane structures and human disease. *Front. Genet.* 3:283. doi: 10.3389/fgene.2012.00283

Zhang, T., Hwang, H. Y., Hao, H., Talbot, C., and Wang, J. (2012b). *Caenorhabditis elegans* RNA-processing protein TDP-1 regulates protein homeostasis and life span. *J. Biol. Chem.* 287, 8371–8382. doi: 10.1074/jbc.M111.311977

Zhang, T., Mullane, P. C., Periz, G., and Wang, J. (2011). TDP-43 neurotoxicity and protein aggregation modulated by heat shock factor and insulin/IGF-1 signaling. *Hum. Mol. Genet.* 20, 1952–1965. doi: 10.1093/hmg/ddr076

Zhao, J., Matthies, D. S., Botzolakis, E. J., Macdonald, R. L., Blakely, R. D., and Hedera, P. (2008). Hereditary spastic paraplegia-associated mutations in the NIPA1 gene and its *Caenorhabditis elegans* homolog trigger neural degeneration *in vitro* and *in vivo* through a gain-of-function mechanism. *J. Neurosci.* 28, 13938–13951. doi: 10.1523/JNEUROSCI.4668-08.2008

14

A semi-automated motion-tracking analysis of locomotion speed in the *C. elegans* transgenics overexpressing beta-amyloid in neurons

Kevin Machino[1], Christopher D. Link[2], Susan Wang[1], Hana Murakami[1] and Shin Murakami[1]*

[1] Department of Basic Sciences, College of Osteopathic Medicine, Touro University California, Vallejo, CA, USA
[2] Institute of Behavioral Genetics, University of Colorado, Boulder, Boulder, CO, USA

Edited by:
Nektarios Tavernarakis, University of Crete, Foundation for Research and Technology-Hellas, Greece

Reviewed by:
Eirini Lionaki, Foundation for Research and Technology-Hellas, Greece
Vassiliki Nikoletopoulou, Institute of Molecular Biology and Biotechnology, Greece
Maria Markaki, Foundation for Research and Technology-Hellas, Greece

***Correspondence:**
Shin Murakami, College of Osteopathic Medicine, Touro University California, 1310 Club Drive, Mare Island, Vallejo, CA 94594, USA
e-mail: shin.murakami@tu.edu

Multi-Worm Tracker (MWT) is a real-time computer vision system that can simultaneously quantify motional patterns of multiple worms. MWT provides several behavioral parameters, including analysis of accurate real-time locomotion speed in the nematode, *Caenorhabditis elegans*. Here, we determined locomotion speed of the Alzheimer's disease (AD) transgenic strain that over-expresses human beta-amyloid1-42 (Aβ) in the neurons. The MWT analysis showed that the AD strain logged a slower average speed than the wild type (WT) worms. The results may be consistent with the observation that the AD patients with dementia tend to show deficits in physical activities, including frequent falls. The AD strain showed reduced ability of the eggs to hatch and slowed hatching of the eggs. Thus, over-expression of Aβ in neurons causes negative effects on locomotion and hatchability. This study sheds light on new examples of detrimental effects that Aβ deposits can exhibit using *C. elegans* as a model system. The information gathered from this study indicates that the motion tracking analysis is a cost-effective, efficient way to assess the deficits of Aβ over-expression in the *C. elegans* system.

Keywords: Alzheimer's disease, beta amyloid, age-related memory impairment (AMI), frailty, behavioral aging, motion tracking, automated system, Alzheimer's disease in children

INTRODUCTION

Alzheimer's disease (AD) is a type of amyloidosis and is the major neurodegenerative disorder that causes dementia. Amyloidosis is characterized by fibril deposits that contain at least 30 fibril proteins in humans and 10 fibril proteins in animals, according to the 2012 the Nomenclature Committee of the International Society of Amyloidosis (Sipe et al., 2012). Of them, accumulation of Aβ has been observed in the AD and congophilic cerebral angiopathy (CAA) (Selkoe, 2001; Revesz et al., 2003). AD leads to cognitive deficits due to abnormal deposits of β-amyloid (Aβ) peptides in the brain, while CAA is characterized by vascular deposits in the central nervous system, in which hemorrhage is a major clinical feature (Samarasekera et al., 2012). CAA is often observed in AD patients, in which case it has been diagnosed as AD (Wright, 2013).

In AD, deposits of the Aβ peptides arise from the proteolytic processing of amyloid precursor proteins (APP), commonly observed in patients with AD (Nicholson et al., 2012). Aβ deposits and tau tangles are well known hallmarks for AD, which may trigger inflammation worsening the disease (Nicholson et al., 2012; Jack and Holtzman, 2013). Aβ toxicity may be linked to tau hyperphysphorylation observed in tau tangles (Lloret et al., 2011; Ermak and Davies, 2013). Although it is believed that Aβ is involved in initiation of AD in the presence of tau pathologies and that tau is correlated with severity of AD (reviewed in LaFerla, 2010; Castillo-Carranza et al., 2014), molecular mechanisms of AD remain unclear. Details of clinical pathogenesis and biomarkers have been reviewed elsewhere (Jack and Holtzman, 2013).

This study aimed to assess the effects of Aβ toxicity on a behavioral parameter, average speed of movement. A transgenic strain overexpressing the signal peptide::$A\beta^{1-42}$ in the neurons (Dosanjh et al., 2010; Lublin and Link, 2013) was used for this study. Over-expression of Aβ in the neurons may affect the serotonin system (Dosanjh et al., 2010). Previously, locomotion has been assessed in a manual assay that measures the rate of body bend, which is an indirect measure with relatively high variability (Dosanjh et al., 2010; Lublin and Link, 2013); the manual assay may have been missed early signs of motility defect. In addition, another neural Aβ strain is tagged by a behavioral marker (i.e., roller phenotype) (McColl et al., 2012), which is difficult to assess locomotion speed. We used behavioral tracking software, Multi Worm Tracker (MWT) (Swierczek et al., 2010), to record and collect data on the speed. MWT is a program designed to quantify the behavior of multiple worms on a petri plate with minimal human effort. The main advantage is that it allows for a more accurate and detailed assessment of locomotion speed compared to the traditional method that measures body bends. Thus, our hypothesis is that the strain overexpressing Aβ in the neurons show defects in locomotion speed. We reason that motion tracking analysis, including MWT analysis, should contribute to understanding the harmful effects of Aβ toxicity in *C. elegans*.

MATERIALS AND METHODS

STRAINS, MEDIA, AND STAINING

Wild-type strain, N2, was used (referred to as WT strain). As a control, we also used the *smg-1*^{ts} strain [*smg-1*^{ts}*(cc546)*], which generated similar results as N2 in the assays (i.e., locomotion and hatchability) used in this study (data not shown). The strain CL2355 [*smg-1*^{ts}*(cc546)*; *snb-1*::Aβ_{1-42}::long 3′-UTR] that utilizes the *C. elegans* promotor of the synaptobrevin (*snb-1*) gene to cause a pan-neuronal overexpression of the signal peptide::Aβ^{1-42} (Dosanjh et al., 2010; Lublin and Link, 2013) was used (referred to as AD strain). For simplicity, the transgenic strain CL2355 is referred to as the AD strain for the duration of the paper. All strains were maintained at 15°C in a nematode growth media (NGM) spotted with *Escherichia coli*, OP50, as a food source (Murakami et al., 2005). The following procedure adopted from Stiernagle (2006) was used to prepare NGM plates. Before autoclaving, 17 g agar, 2.5 g peptone, 3 g NaCl, and 975 mL distilled H_2O was added to a flask and covered with aluminum foil. Then the flask was autoclaved for 50 min. After autoclaving the mixture, 1 mL of 1 M $CaCl_2$, 1 mL of 5 mg/mL cholesterol in ethanol, 1 mL of 1 M $MgSO_4$, and 25 mL of 1 M KPO_4 (pH 6.0) was added to the flask. Then petri plates were filled 2/3 with agar. Plates were left at room temperature for 2–3 days to allow excess moisture to evaporate. For immunofluorescence staining, we used the procedure described in Link (1995). Transgenic worms were fixed, permeabilized, and stained with the anti-Aβ monoclonal antibody 4G8 and anti-TOR-2 polyclonal sera as a counterstain. DNA was visualized using 4′,6-diamidino-2-phenylindole (DAPI).

GROWTH CONDITIONS

Strains were grown on NGM agar plates at 15°C. To assess hatchability, eggs were layed on NGM plates at 15°C and incubated at the temperature indicated in the text (15 or 25°C). Unhatched eggs were counted after 24 h or the time specified in the text. Hatched eggs (larvae) were also counted to confirm the result. To prepare adult worms, eggs were layed and grown into adults for 4 days. Adults at the age of day 5 (i.e., 1 day after they start to lay eggs) was defined as "younger adults." Adults at the age of day 7 was defined as "middle-aged adults." Adults at the age of day 13–14 was defined as "older adults."

MULTI WORM TRACKER (MWT) ANALYSIS

Videos of the worms were recorded under a stereomicroscope using ToupView, a video capturing software (Amscope.com, Irvine, CA). The parameters of 3 min for duration and 6 s for bin size was set when capturing the video, which created a video file that was 35 s in length. To analyze the speed of the worms, the video file was uploaded into MWT, a behavioral tracking software (Swierczek et al., 2010). In a typical assay, about five worms in a microscopic field was computed and average speed of the worms were calculated. A measure for speed (in pixels/s) was made at a series of ages indicated in the text. We used the conversion rate in the system: 1 pixel/s = 0.035 cm/s at the images of 72 PPI (pixels per inch). Death was determined by observing no movement of the worms. Statistical analysis has been performed by ANOVA using NCSS 2007 statistics software (NCSS, LLC, Kaysville, Utah, USA).

RESULTS

We sought to assay the locomotion of the transgenic *C. elegans* strain CL2355 (Dosanjh et al., 2010), which expresses a human Aβ_{42} minigene under the control of the pan-neuronal synaptobrevin (*snb-1*) promoter. Expression of Aβ using this promoter leads to intraneuronal deposition of Aβ, particularly detectable in the nerve ring area (**Figure 1**).

Video images of the worms on NGM agar were captured for 3 min and the speed of the worms was determined using MWT. We compared the results of the WT (wild type) and AD strains (over-expressing amyloid beta) (Materials and Methods). As described in the Method, adults that had grown for 5 days were defined as "younger adults." Adults that had grown for 7 days were defined as "middle-aged adults." Adults that had grown for 13 days were defined as "older adults."

THE AD TRANSGENIC STRAIN SHOWING SLOWER MOVEMENT

Table 1 summarizes the results. For the younger adults (day 5), WT had a mean speed of 0.18 ± 0.15 cm/s whereas the AD had a mean speed of 0.05 ± 0.06 cm/s ($p > 0.0001$; **Figure 2A**;

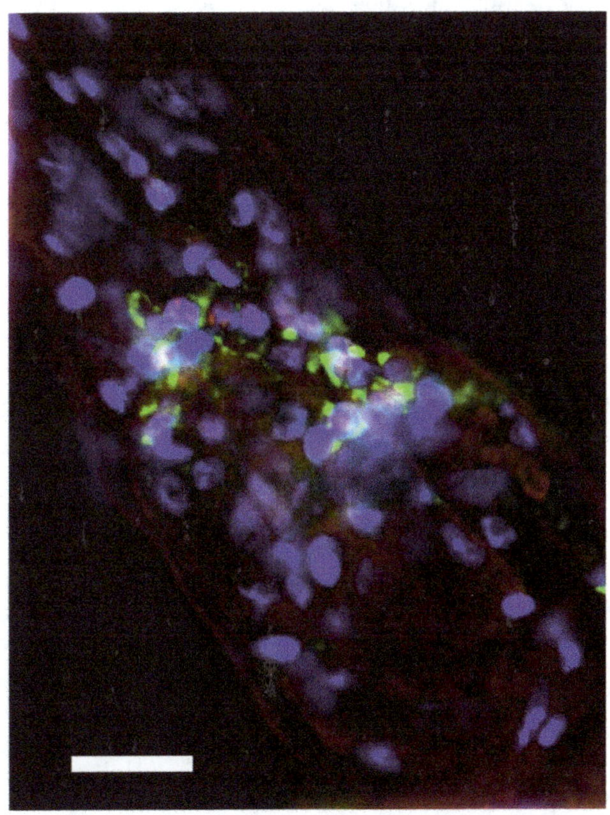

FIGURE 1 | Intraneuronal deposition of Aβ in transgenic *C. elegans*. Anterior region of transgenic *C. elegans* is shown. The strain was immune-stained by anti-Aβ monoclonal antibody 4G8 (green), anti-TOR-2 polyclonal sera (red), and DAPI (blue). Note cytoplasmic accumulation of Aβ in nerve ring neurons. Size bar = 10 μM.

Table 1 | Locomotion speed (mean ± standard deviation) as assessed by MWT analysis for various stages in the life cycle (* $p < 0.0001$).

Life stage (day #)	Type of strain	Average speed (cm/s)
Younger adult (day 5)	WT	0.18 ± 0.15
	AD	0.05 ± 0.06*
(day 6)	WT	0.52 ± 0.25
	AD	0.21 ± 0.17*
Middle-aged (day 7)	WT	0.43 ± 0.19
	AD	0.05 ± 0.05*
(day 10)	WT	0.10 ± 0.11
	AD	0.08 ± 0.12
Older adult (day 13)	WT	0.11 ± 0.07
	AD	0.12 ± 0.07

Table 1). Slow locomotion speed in the AD strain compared to WT was observed from day 5 (younger adults) to day 7 (middle age) ($p > 0.0001$; **Figures 2A,B**; **Table 1**). Interestingly, there was a peak of locomotion speed at the age of day 5 (**Figure 2E**), which was consistent with previous study as assessed in a classical assay that measured body bends, an indicator of locomotion speed (Murakami et al., 2008).

Slow locomotion speed in the AD strain was also evident in the still images (**Figure 3**) and **Supplementary Video** (Supplementary Figure). In the sill images taken every 7 s (**Figure 2**), the WT worms were located in different positions (**Figure 3A**), while the AD worms were nearly stagnant from 0 to 35 s (**Figure 3B**). Thus, a difference in the worm movements was clearly visible.

Older worms at day 10 and 13 showed similar results for the WT and AD strains. Day 10 WT worms had an average speed of 0.10 ± 0.11 cm/s whereas Day 10 AD worms moved at an average speed of 0.08 ± 0.12 cm/s for four worms (**Figure 2C**; **Table 1**). Finally, in the older adult at the age of Day 13, WT worms logged an average speed of 0.11 ± 0.07 cm/s and Day 13 AD worms showed similar locomotion speed (0.12 ± 0.07 cm/s) (**Figure 2D**; **Table 1**). Overall, worms with overexpressed Aβ resulted in slower movement up to middle-aged (**Figure 2**).

Aβ TOXICITY IN THE EMBRYONIC STAGE

Hatching of the eggs from the WT (N2) and AD (CL2355) strains were compared. We measured total number of unhatched eggs 24 h at restrictive temperature (25°C) after egg lay. We also counted hatched larvae to confirm the results. In the WT strain, there were 16.3% (37/227) eggs that remained unhatched and 83.7% (190/227) hatched (**Figure 4A**). For the AD strain, 89.2% (182/204) eggs remained unhatched and 10.8% (22/204) hatched. The rate of hatching in the control strain (*smg-1^ts^*), was similar to WT (data now shown), excluding the possibility that the background mutation lowered the rate of hatching. Thus, the AD strain showed an approximately 7.8 folds lower hatching after 24 h of egg lay. We also investigated the time course of hatchability at permissive temperature, 15°C. Most of the eggs in the WT strain hatched 1 day after egg lay (Day 2; **Figure 4B**). In contrast, the AD strain hatched much slower than the WT strain, taking 2 days after egg lay (Day 3; **Figure 4B**). Thus, the AD strain shows reduced hatching and a delayed timing of egg hatching. We also observed a low rate of fecundity (Blood size: WT, 248 ± 22, $n = 10$; AD, 50 ± 12, $n = 20$; $p < 0.001$).

DISCUSSION

In this study, we used MWT analysis to measure locomotion speed. Compared to a manual assay to measure the number of body bends, MWT analysis provides a more accurate measure of multiple worms for a longer time (MWT for 3 min; Manual assay for 1 min). Young wild-type worm (locomotion speed: 0.18 ± 0.15 cm/s) was within the range of previously reported results (lower range of 0.13 cm/s, Ramot et al., 2008; upper range of 0.22 cm/s, Ryu and Samuel, 2002). They have also reported locomotion speed, ranging from 0.14 to 0.33 cm/s at the temperatures ranging from 17 to 27°C. The groups used other worm tracking systems, which suggests that MWT analysis results are consistent with those from the other worm tracking systems. It is worth noting that our MWT system is one of the most cost effective systems. The total cost was estimated to be up to US$200 for a routine USB-camera (as of April, 2014; our cost was zero since we recycled the camera, excluding the cost of software, computer, and microscope), which is much less than the cost estimated for MWT elsewhere (US$7,000) (Husson et al., 2012).

The AD strain showed an approximately 7.8-fold decrease in hatching compared to the WT strain. Likewise, the AD strain showed reduced hatching even at the permissive temperature, where Aβ is expressed, but at a lower level. The reduced level of hatching seen in the AD strain could be attributed to Aβ overexpression, suggesting the negative effect of Aβ on embryogenesis due to its toxicity. It is worth noting that some CL2355 worms are completely sterile (no eggs laid). This is a surprising observation if the defects in the CL2355 strain are restricted to neurons, as fertility in *C. elegans* is not strongly neuronally regulated. The fertility/sterility phenotypes of CL2355 were observed in the precursor extrachromosomal line, suggesting that these defects are not due to gene disruption caused by chromosomal integration of the transgene. We also observed that worms show larval arrest and death, suggesting defects in development caused by Aβ (data not shown).

The findings also suggest that Aβ accumulation has detrimental effects on locomotion speed in the adult life cycle, except for late-life in which all worms move poorly. In younger adults and middle-aged adults (corresponding to Day 5 and 7, respectively), the AD worms exhibited a slower speed than the WT worms (**Figure 1**). The middle-aged AD worms showed the greatest amount of difference from that of the WT worms; the approximate 8.3-fold difference in speed indicates that the presence of Aβ is correlated with the slower movement in the worms. This may be consistent with frailty seen in the Alzheimer's patients (Koch et al., 2013; Kulmala et al., 2014) and gait problems in the mouse models of AD (APP and APP/PS1 mice) (Lalonde et al., 2012; Wang et al., 2012a), though some other mice models [APP23, J20, APP + PDAPP, PS1 [Tg2576 + PS1 (M146L)], TgCRND8, TG2576, and 3 × Tg-AD mice] show increased locomotion due to

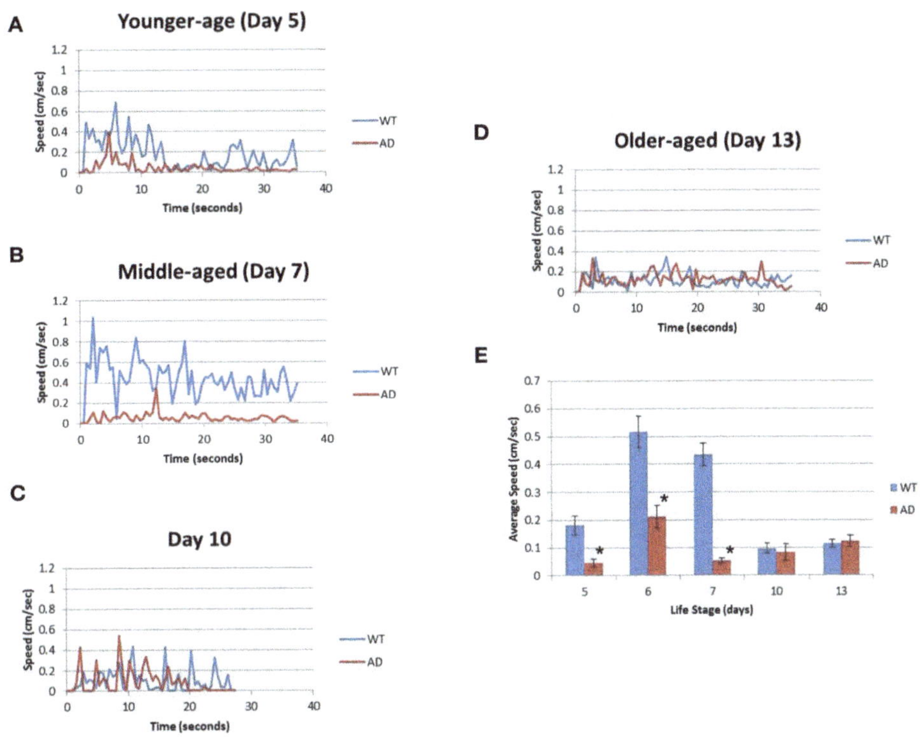

FIGURE 2 | The AD strain exhibits slower speeds than WT in the life cycle. (A) The graph represents the locomotion speed of adult worms measured at the age of day 5 (younger age). **(B)** The graph represents the speed for worms measured at the age of day 7 (middle age). **(C)** The graph represents the speed for middle-aged worms measured at the age of day 10. **(D)** The graph represents the speed for older adult worms measured at the age of day 13 (older age). **(E)** Comparison of the average speeds for WT (blue) and AD (red) worms at various ages over the course of their life span. Error bars indicate standard error of the mean. $^{*}p > 0.0001$. WT worms (blue); and AD worms (red). See also **Table 1**.

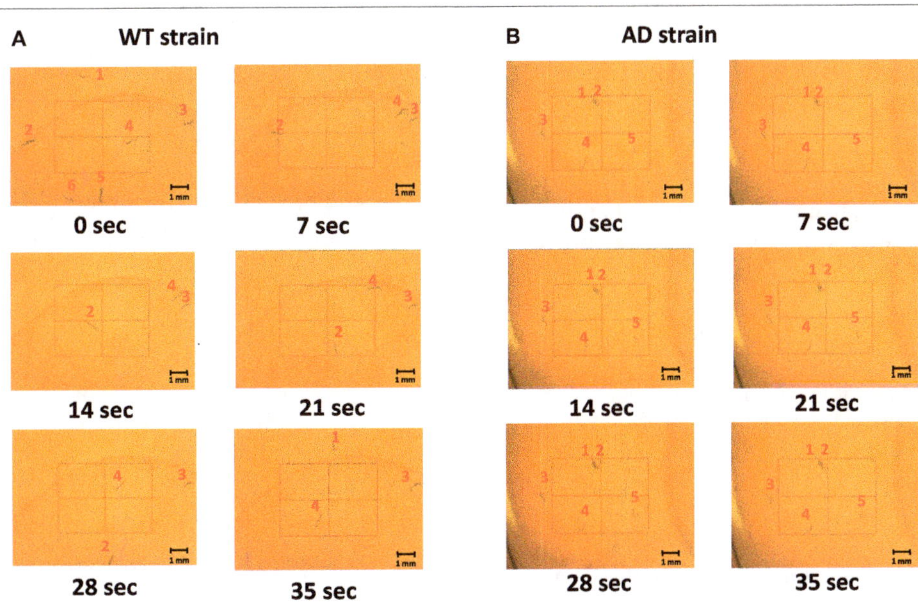

FIGURE 3 | Images of middle-aged (day 7) worms on the NGM plates at various time points. The images captured were taken every 7 s from 0 to 35 s. The worms were labeled 1–6 for the WT and 1–5 for the AD strain so that the difference in movement could be seen between and amongst frames. **(A)** An example of the WT worms. They moved throughout the plate as time progressed. **(B)** An example of the AD worms. They hardly moved as time elapsed.

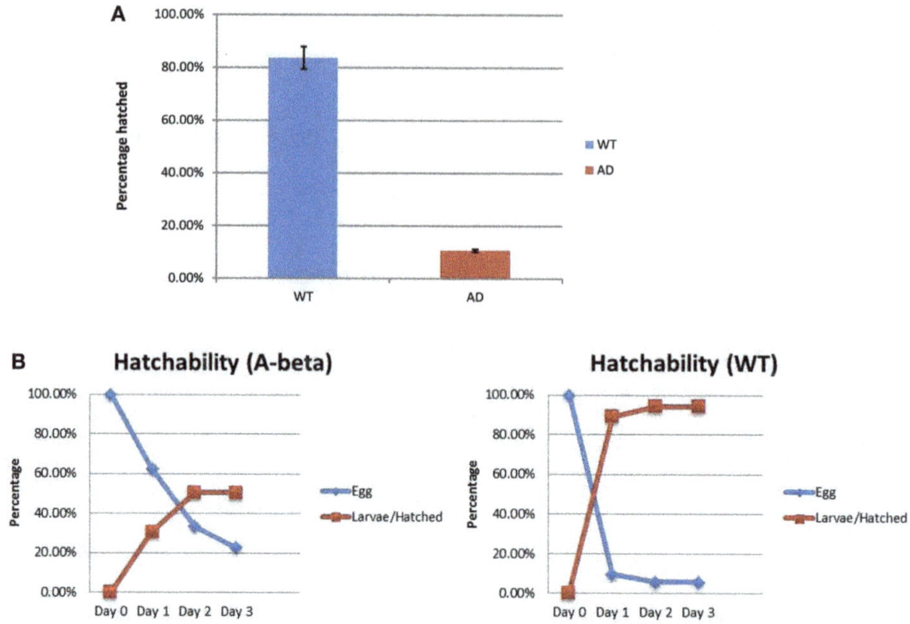

FIGURE 4 | Rate of egg hatching (hatchability) in the WT and AD strains. (A) Percentage of eggs unhatched after 24 h. There were more AD eggs (red) that remained unhatched compared to the WT eggs (blue). **(B)** Time course of the percentage of eggs that hatched from day 0 (the day of egg lay) to day 3 for both strains. Error bars indicate standard error of the mean.

aggression and other behavioral problems (Webster et al., 2014). Thus, locomotion is not always defective in AD patients and in AD models but rather altered. It is critical to assess locomotion in each AD system. In addition to our finding, locomotion defects have been observed in the fruit fly model of Aβ toxicity, while paralysis has been observed in the other strains over-expressing Aβ in the muscles and in the neurons (McColl et al., 2012; Wang et al., 2012b; Lublin and Link, 2013; Prüßing et al., 2013; Carrillo-Mora et al., 2014). Technical difficulties in the previous studies have been discussed above.

This study provides evidence that Aβ toxicity affects the embryonic stage as well as the adult phases. Since the AD transgenic strain used in this study has Aβ overexpression, the data can be used to assess the effects of Aβ toxicity on embryonic and behavioral parameters. Assessing the hatchability and speed of the worms allows for the analysis of the strains and the impact Aβ toxicity has on embryonic health and movement. The research will be beneficial as AD is one of the most common causes of dementia, and the number of Americans aged 65 and older affected by AD is predicted to triple by 2050 (Hebert et al., 2013). Currently, there are drugs there are drugs that can treat memory impairment in AD patients, but there are no cure for the disease itself. It is worth noting that a chaperone, HSP-16, is strongly associated with the Aβ deposits in the neuronal expression lines (reviewed in Lublin and Link, 2013). The future direction of this study aims to explore the relationship between AD drugs and potential Aβ clearance. The hope is that future studies will demonstrate the effectiveness of current FDA-approved AD treatment interventions to help alleviate the Aβ buildup seen in AD patients and enhance future treatments by potentially slowing or stopping the disease.

ACKNOWLEDGMENTS

We thank Dr. Rex Kirr (Janeila Farm Research Campus, Ashburn, VA) for technical assistance of MWT analysis and Mr. Chris Koebler for editing the manuscript. The work was supported by research support from the Tour University California (Shin Murakami) and NIH grant R01 AG012423 (Christopher D. Link).

SUPPLEMENTARY MATERIAL

Supplementary Video | Video images of day 7 worms shown in Figure 2. (Video 1). Video shows the WT strain (File name: Machino et al. WT strain Day 7.mwv). **(Video 2)** Video shows the AD strain (File name: Machino et al. AD strain Day 7.mwv). As described in Materials and Methods, 3 min-long videos were shortened into 35 s in length. Due to the conversion from AVI to MP4 format to reduce the size of the files, the video have lower quality compared to the originals.

REFERENCES

Carrillo-Mora, P., Luna, R., and Colín-Barenque, L. (2014). Amyloid beta: multiple mechanisms of toxicity and only some protective effects? *Oxid. Med. Cell. Longev.* 2014:795375. doi: 10.1155/2014/795375

Castillo-Carranza, D. L., Guerrero-Muñoz, M. J., and Kayed, R. (2014). Immunotherapy for the treatment of Alzheimer's disease: amyloid-β or tau, which is the right target? *ImmunoTargets and Therapy* 3, 19–28. doi: 10.2147/ITT.S40131

Dosanjh, L. E., Brown, M. K., Rao, G., Link, C. D., and Luo, Y. (2010). Behavioral phenotyping of a transgenic *Caenorhabditis elegans* expressing neuronal amyloid-beta. *J. Alzheimers. Dis.* 19, 681–690. doi: 10.3233/JAD-2010-1267

Ermak, G., and Davies, K. J. (2013). Chronic high levels of the RCAN1-1 protein may promote neurodegeneration and Alzheimer disease. *Free Radic. Biol. Med.* 62, 47–51. doi: 10.1016/j.freeradbiomed.2013.01.016

Hebert, L. E., Weuve, J., Scherr, P. A., and Evans, D. A. (2013). Alzheimer disease in the United States (2010-2050) estimated using the 2010 census. *Neurology* 80, 1778–1783. doi: 10.1212/WNL.0b013e31828726f5

Husson, S. J., Costa, W. S., Schmitt, C., and Gottschalk, A. (2012). *Keeping Track of Worm Trackers. WormBook, the C. elegans Research Community*. Availbale online at: http://www.wormbook.org

Jack, C. R. Jr., and Holtzman, D. M. (2013). Biomarker modeling of Alzheimer's disease. *Neuron.* 80, 1347–1358. doi: 10.1016/j.neuron.2013.12.003

Koch, G., Belli, L., Giudice, T. L., Lorenzo, F. D., Sancesario, G. M., Sorge, R., et al. (2013). Frailty among Alzheimer's disease patients. *CNS Neurol. Disord. Drug Targets.* 12, 507–511. doi: 10.2174/1871527311312040010

Kulmala, J., Nykänen, I., Mänty, M., and Hartikainen, S. (2014). Association between Frailty and Dementia: a population-based study. *Gerontology.* 60, 16–21. doi: 10.1159/000353859

LaFerla, F. M. (2010). Pathways linking Abeta and tau pathologies. *Biochem. Soc. Trans.* 38, 993–995. doi: 10.1042/BST0380993

Lalonde, R., Fukuchi, K., and Strazielle, C. (2012). Neurologic and motor dysfunctions in APP transgenic mice. *Rev. Neurosci.* 23, 363–379. doi: 10.1515/revneuro-2012-0041

Link, C. D. (1995). Expression of human beta-amyloid peptide in transgenic *Caenorhabditis elegans. Proc. Natl. Acad. Sci. U.S.A.* 92, 9368–9372.

Lloret, A., Badia, M. C., Giraldo, E., Ermak, G., Alonso, M. D., Pallardó, F. V., et al. (2011). Amyloid-β toxicity and tau hyperphosphorylation are linked via RCAN1 in Alzheimer's disease. *J. Alzheimers. Dis.* 27, 701–709. doi: 10.3233/JAD-2011-110890

Lublin, A. L., and Link, C. D. (2013). Alzheimer's disease drug discovery: *in vivo* screening using *Caenorhabditis elegans* as a model for β-amyloid peptide-induced toxicity. *Drug Discov. Today Technol.* 10, e115–e119. doi: 10.1016/j.ddtec.2012.02.002

McColl, G., Roberts, B. R., Pukala, T. L., Kenche, V. B., Roberts, C. M., Link, C. D., et al. (2012). Utility of an improved model of amyloid-beta ($A\beta_{1-42}$) toxicity in *Caenorhabditis elegans* for drug screening for Alzheimer's disease. *Mol. Neurodegener.* 7:57. doi: 10.1186/1750-1326-7-57

Murakami, H., Bessinger, K., Hellmann, J., Luerman, G. C., and Murakami, S. (2008). Manipulation of serotonin signal suppresses early phase of behavioral aging in *Caenorhabditis elegans. Neurobiol. Aging* 29, 1093–100. doi: 10.1016/j.neurobiolaging.2007.01.013

Murakami, H., Bessinger, K., Hellmann, J., and Murakami, S. (2005). Aging-dependent and independent regulation of learning by insulin/IGF-1 signal in *C. elegans. J. Neurosci.* 25, 10894–10904. doi: 10.1523/JNEUROSCI.3600-04.2005

Nicholson, A. M., Wold, L. A., Walsh, D. M., and Ferreira, A. (2012). β-Amyloid carrying the dutch mutation has diverse effects on calpain-mediated toxicity in hippocampal neurons. *Mol. Med.* 18, 178–185. doi: 10.2119/molmed.2011.00366

Prüßing, K., Voigt, A., and Schulz, J. B. (2013). Drosophila melanogaster as a model organism for Alzheimer's disease. *Mol. Neurodegener.* 8:35 doi: 10.1186/1750-1326-8-35

Ramot, D., MacInnis, B. L., Lee, H. C., and Goodman, M. B. (2008). Thermotaxis is a robust mechanism for thermoregulation in *Caenorhabditis elegans* nematodes. *J. Neurosci.* 1928, 12546–12557. doi: 10.1523/JNEUROSCI.2857-08.2008

Revesz, T., Ghiso, J., Lashley, T., Plant, G., Rostagno, A., Frangione, B., et al. (2003). Cerebral amyloid angiopathies: a pathologic, biochemical, and genetic view. *J. Neuropathol. Exp. Neurol.* 62, 885–898.

Ryu, W. S., and Samuel, A. D. (2002). Thermotaxis in *Caenorhabditis elegans* analyzed by measuring responses to defined Thermal stimuli. *J. Neurosci.* 22, 5727–5733.

Samarasekera, N., Smith, C., and Al-Shahi Salman, R. (2012). The association between cerebral amyloid angiopathy and intracerebral haemorrhage: systematic review and meta-analysis. *J. Neurol. Neurosurg. Psychiatry* 83, 275–281. doi: 10.1136/jnnp-2011-300371

Selkoe, D. J. (2001). Alzheimer's disease: genes, proteins, and therapy. *Physiol. Rev.* 81, 741–766.

Sipe, J. D., Benson, M. D., Buxbaum, J. N., Ikeda, S., Merlini, G., Saraiva, M. J., et al. (2012). Nomenclature Committee of the International Society of Amyloidosis. Amyloid fibril protein nomenclature: 2012 recommendations from the Nomenclature Committee of the International Society of Amyloidosis. *Amyloid* 19, 167–170. doi: 10.3109/13506129.2012.734345

Stiernagle, T. (2006). "Maintenance of *C. elegans*," in *WormBook*, Vol. 11, 1–11. doi: 10.1895/wormbook.1.101.1

Swierczek, N. A., Giles, A. C., Rankin, C. H., and Kerr, R. A. (2010). High-throughput behavioral analysis in *C. elegans. Nat Methods* 8, 592–598. doi: 10.1038/nmeth.1625

Wang, H., He, J., Zhang, R., Zhu, S., Wang, J., Kong, L., et al. (2012a). Sensorimotor gating and memory deficits in an APP/PS1 double transgenic mouse model of Alzheimer's disease. *Behav. Brain Res.* 233, 237–243. doi: 10.1016/j.bbr.2012.05.007

Wang, L., Chiang, H.-C., Wu, W., Liang, B., Xie, Z., Yao, X., et al. (2012b). Epidermal growth factor receptor is a preferred target for treating Amyloid-β-induced memory loss *Proc. Natl. Acad. Sci. U.S.A.* 109, 16743–16748. doi: 10.1073/pnas.1208011109

Webster, S. J., Bachstetter, A. D., Nelson, P. T., Schmitt, F. A., and Van Eldik, L. J. (2014). Using mice to model Alzheimer's dementia: an overview of the clinical disease and the preclinical behavioral changes in 10 mouse models. *Front. Genet.* 5:88. doi: 10.3389/fgene.2014.00088

Wright, C. B. (2013). "Etiology, clinical manifestations, and diagnosis of vascular dementia," in *UpToDate,* eds S. T. DeKosky and A. F. Eichler (Waltham, MA: UpToDate).

15

Using mice to model Alzheimer's dementia: an overview of the clinical disease and the preclinical behavioral changes in 10 mouse models

Scott J. Webster[1], **Adam D. Bachstetter**[1], **Peter T. Nelson**[1,2], **Frederick A. Schmitt**[1,3] **and Linda J. Van Eldik**[1,4]*

[1] *Sanders-Brown Center on Aging, University of Kentucky, Lexington, KY, USA*
[2] *Division of Neuropathology, Department of Pathology and Laboratory Medicine, University of Kentucky, Lexington, KY, USA*
[3] *Department of Neurology, University of Kentucky, Lexington, KY, USA*
[4] *Department of Anatomy and Neurobiology, University of Kentucky, Lexington, KY, USA*

Edited by:
Shin Murakami, Touro University-California, USA

Reviewed by:
James C. Vickers, University of Tasmania, Australia
Danna Zimmer, University of Maryland Medical School, USA

***Correspondence:**
Linda J. Van Eldik, Sanders-Brown Center on Aging, 800 S. Limestone, Lexington, KY 40536-0230, USA
e-mail: linda.vaneldik@uky.edu

The goal of this review is to discuss how behavioral tests in mice relate to the pathological and neuropsychological features seen in human Alzheimer's disease (AD), and present a comprehensive analysis of the temporal progression of behavioral impairments in commonly used AD mouse models that contain mutations in amyloid precursor protein (APP). We begin with a brief overview of the neuropathological changes seen in the AD brain and an outline of some of the clinical neuropsychological assessments used to measure cognitive deficits associated with the disease. This is followed by a critical assessment of behavioral tasks that are used in AD mice to model the cognitive changes seen in the human disease. Behavioral tests discussed include spatial memory tests [Morris water maze (MWM), radial arm water maze (RAWM), Barnes maze], associative learning tasks (passive avoidance, fear conditioning), alternation tasks (Y-Maze/T-Maze), recognition memory tasks (Novel Object Recognition), attentional tasks (3 and 5 choice serial reaction time), set-shifting tasks, and reversal learning tasks. We discuss the strengths and weaknesses of each of these behavioral tasks, and how they may correlate with clinical assessments in humans. Finally, the temporal progression of both cognitive and non-cognitive deficits in 10 AD mouse models (PDAPP, TG2576, APP23, TgCRND8, J20, APP/PS1, TG2576 + PS1 (M146L), APP/PS1 KI, 5×FAD, and 3×Tg-AD) are discussed in detail. Mouse models of AD and the behavioral tasks used in conjunction with those models are immensely important in contributing to our knowledge of disease progression and are a useful tool to study AD pathophysiology and the resulting cognitive deficits. However, investigators need to be aware of the potential weaknesses of the available preclinical models in terms of their ability to model cognitive changes observed in human AD. It is our hope that this review will assist investigators in selecting an appropriate mouse model, and accompanying behavioral paradigms to investigate different aspects of AD pathology and disease progression.

Keywords: Alzheimer's disease, mouse models, neuropsychological assessment, behavior, cognition, APP mice, APP/PS1 mice, 3×TG-AD mice

INTRODUCTION

Alzheimer's disease (AD) is characterized by a progressive decline in cognitive function, usually starting with memory complaints and eventually progressing to involve multiple cognitive, neuropsychological and behavioral domains. The definitive diagnosis of AD comes from postmortem analysis of the neuropathological changes in the brain. Analyses of both clinical and pathological features, i.e., clinicopathological correlation studies, have provided important insights into how the pathology correlates with cognitive status. Complementing these studies in humans has been the development of preclinical model systems of AD pathology. These preclinical animal models, especially mouse models, have been extremely useful to test mechanistic hypotheses about AD pathophysiology and to predict outcomes from pharmacological interventions. However, no animal model recapitulates the entirety of AD in humans, and therefore it is important to understand both the utility and limitations of particular animal models. With this in mind, we will present an overview of the neuropathological changes seen in the AD patient population as individuals transition from normal cognitive aging to dementia, review the clinical neuropsychological assessments used in the AD field, review the mouse behavioral tasks commonly used in preclinical testing and discuss how they relate to these clinical neuropsychological assessments, and outline the temporal progression of cognitive and non-cognitive deficits seen in the commonly used mouse models of AD.

OVERVIEW OF NEUROPATHOLOGICAL CHANGES IN AD

In 2012, new consensus guidelines for neuropathologic evaluation of AD were adopted (Hyman et al., 2012; Montine et al., 2012). The AD neuropathologic change is now ranked on three parameters (Amyloid, Braak, CERAD) to obtain an "ABC" score: histopathologic assessments of beta-amyloid (Aβ)-containing amyloid plaques (A), Braak staging of neurofibrillary tangles (B), and scoring of neuritic amyloid plaques (C). Standard approaches for the workup of cases, preferred staining methods, reporting of results and clinicopathological correlations are also recommended. Unlike the prior AD neuropathologic criteria (Hyman and Trojanowski, 1997) that required a history of dementia, the current guidelines recognize that AD neuropathologic changes can be present in the brain in the apparent absence of cognitive impairment. The updated guidelines thus emphasize the continuum of neuropathologic changes that underlie AD. For a disease process that is known to occur over a decade or more (Blennow and Zetterberg, 2013; Rosen and Zetterberg, 2013; Rosen et al., 2013), and encompasses the age range where people are likely to die of other causes, it is inevitable that many people will die in a prodromal or "preclinical" stage of AD. This consideration points to the complexity that clinicopathological studies face when examining AD pathological contributions to cognitive deficits (Nelson et al., 2009b).

There have been numerous clinicopathological studies attempting to correlate amyloid plaques with the cognitive deficits seen in AD (Blessed et al., 1968; Tomlinson et al., 1970; Duyckaerts et al., 1990, 1998; Berg et al., 1998; Gold et al., 2000; Mungas et al., 2001; Tiraboschi et al., 2002, 2004; Guillozet et al., 2003; Kraybill et al., 2005; Holtzer et al., 2006; Markesbery et al., 2006; Nelson et al., 2007a, 2009a; Beach et al., 2009; Sabbagh et al., 2010; Robinson et al., 2011). Apparent inconsistencies in the conclusions of these studies are due to differences in study cohorts, methodology used to classify plaque subcategories, plaque-counting techniques, and metrics used to assess cognitive deficits. Nevertheless, several important concepts have emerged pertaining to plaque pathology and cognition. First, the strongest correlation between amyloid plaques and cognition is in the early stages of the disease and this association weakens as NFTs and gross neocortical neurodegeneration become more widespread (Thal et al., 2002; Nelson et al., 2009b, 2012). As the disease progresses into the later stages, there is little evidence to support a continued contribution by amyloid plaques to the late-stage AD cognitive decline (Nelson et al., 2009b, 2012). Second, it appears that density of neuritic plaques correlates more strongly with the cognitive deficits than do "diffuse" amyloid plaques (Mckee et al., 1991; Crystal et al., 1993; Tiraboschi et al., 2004; Nelson et al., 2007a; Braak et al., 2011).

In contrast to the literature concerning amyloid plaques, a large number of studies have arrived at a common finding, namely, there is a strong link between neocortical NFTs and cognitive decline (Tomlinson et al., 1970; Duyckaerts et al., 1990, 1997, 1998; Mckee et al., 1991; Arriagada et al., 1992; Bierer et al., 1995; Davis et al., 1995; Dickson et al., 1995; Nagy et al., 1995, 1999; Cummings et al., 1996; Berg et al., 1998; Grober et al., 1999; Sabbagh et al., 1999; Gold et al., 2000; Mungas et al., 2001; Riley et al., 2002; Silver et al., 2002; Tiraboschi et al., 2002; Guillozet et al., 2003; Bennett et al., 2004; Kraybill et al., 2005; Holtzer et al., 2006; Markesbery et al., 2006; Koepsell et al., 2008; Whitwell et al., 2008; Beach et al., 2009; Brayne et al., 2009; Giannakopoulos et al., 2009; Sabbagh et al., 2010; Robinson et al., 2011). It should be noted that outside of frontotemporal lobar degeneration (FTLD), one does not see widespread cortical NFTs without abundant plaque pathology. In the earliest stages of AD (Braak stage I-II), NFTs are restricted to the entorhinal cortex (Braak and Del Tredici, 2011; Braak et al., 2011). NFTs spread to the limbic and medial temporal lobe (Braak stage III-IV), and this stage correlates with early AD symptoms related to memory (Schmitt et al., 2000; Riley et al., 2011). During the late stages (Braak stage V–VI), NFTs increase in number and manifest in neocortical areas responsible for higher cognitive domains such as executive function, visuospatial capacities, and speech in synchrony with observed AD-related cognitive deficits in these respective cognitive domains. Not all AD cases fall within the standard NFT distribution described by the Braak staging (Hof et al., 1997; Abner et al., 2011; Murray et al., 2011). Some cases classified as "high level" of AD neuropathological changes may show subtle or undetectable cognitive impairment, yet all cases with quantifiably "end stage" neocortical NFT pathology show cognitive impairment (Dickson et al., 1995; Berlau et al., 2007; Nelson et al., 2009a, 2012; Abner et al., 2011; Santacruz et al., 2011; Jicha et al., 2012). In sum, the correlations noted in human material support the hypothesis that plaques and tangles correlate with cognitive status. The data also support the "Amyloid Cascade Hypothesis"(Karran et al., 2011), a deceptively complex hypothesis which posits that beta-amyloid/plaque pathology kindles widespread tau/NFT pathology, with the tau/NFT pathology constituting the more direct cause of the cell loss and synapse elimination underlying clinical disease (Nelson et al., 2009b, 2012).

COGNITIVE NEUROPSYCHOLOGICAL ASSESSMENTS USED IN THE AD FIELD

Neuropsychological assessment is the most reliable means to clinically evaluate the cognitive deficits seen in humans. Many neuropsychological tests have been developed which are highly sensitive to the cognitive behavioral symptoms seen in AD, and these tests are extensively used as clinical diagnostic tools (Schmitt, 1994) as well as to track the progression of the disease (Flicker et al., 1984; Morris et al., 1989; Storandt and Hill, 1989; Storandt, 1991; Welsh et al., 1991, 1992; Locascio et al., 1995; Albert, 1996; Storandt et al., 1998; Schmitt et al., 2000; Salmon and Bondi, 2009). Current neuropsychological assessments (from the National Institute on Aging workgroups on diagnostic guidelines for AD) aim to detect disruptions in cognitive domains such as episodic memory, semantic memory, working memory, and attention, as well as dysfunction in language, praxis, and executive functioning (Flicker et al., 1984; Baddeley et al., 1986, 1991, 2001; Huff et al., 1987; Knopman and Ryberg, 1989; Hodges et al., 1992; Parasuraman and Nestor, 1993; Hodges and Patterson, 1995; Perry and Hodges, 1999; Salmon et al., 1999; Perry et al., 2000; Backman et al., 2001; Lambon Ralph et al., 2003). In the following section, we will cover several of the most common neuropsychological tests used clinically to assess the mental status and memory disruptions in AD (for more in depth reviews see Perry and Hodges, 1999; Budson and Price, 2005; Bondi et al., 2008; Weintraub et al., 2012). **Table 1** provides an overview of four mental status examinations and two brief memory tests commonly used clinically.

MENTAL STATUS EXAMS

Mental status examinations assess multiple mental functions and cognitive abilities across multiple domains (see **Table 1**), and are generally more encompassing than specific verbal and visual memory tests (examples also seen in **Table 1**). Both categories of tests are clinically useful in assessing the cognitive progression of AD. Most mental status examinations assess mental functions and cognitive ability across a wide range of areas such as: language skills, arithmetic ability, visuospatial ability, attention, memory, and orientation to time and place.

The Mini-Mental Status Examination (MMSE) is one of the most commonly used neuropsychological screening tools for cognitive impairments seen in AD (Simard and Van Reekum, 1999; Snyderman and Rovner, 2009). The MMSE is a brief questionnaire that can both diagnose cognitive impairment and track the severity of this cognitive impairment throughout the pathogenesis of the disease. The MMSE covers multiple areas such as: attention, memory (semantic and episodic), orientation to time and place, and working memory. The scoring system ranges from 0 to 30 points. In general, a score of 27 or greater reflects normal cognition, a score of 19–24 represents mild impairment, a score of 10–18 represents moderate impairment, and a score below 9 indicates severe cognitive impairment. The MMSE has excellent reproducibility that lends itself well to longitudinal use in tracking the progression of the cognitive impairments associated with AD (Jacqmin-Gadda et al., 1997; Aevarsson and Skoog, 2000; Chatfield et al., 2007).

The Montreal Cognitive Assessment (MoCA) is a more recent mental status examination used for cognitive dysfunction seen in AD. This test battery takes approximately 10 min to administer and covers many similar cognitive domains to that of the MMSE. The total possible score is 30 points, with a score of 26 or above considered within the normal range. An example of a task included in the MoCA is the forward and backward digit span test. In the forward digit span test, a sequence of five numbers is read at a rate of one number per second and the test taker is required to repeat a set of numbers in exactly the same sequence as they were presented. In the backward digit span task, the test taker is required to repeat a three number sequence in the reverse order in which it was presented. One point is awarded for each of the digit span tests in which the test taker made no errors. The MoCA also includes a delayed recall memory test. Relatively near the beginning of the test, the examiner presents a short word list for the patient to remember. At the end of the test, the patient is again prompted to recall the word list and for each of the words correctly remembered one point is awarded.

Another commonly used test battery is that of the Short Blessed Test (SBT) which consists of a six-item test designed to identify the cognitive dysfunction seen in AD (Katzman et al., 1983). An appealing advantage of the SBT is the ease and speed with which it can be administered (often taking only a few minutes). In the SBT, errors are scored for incorrect answers and the scoring range falls between 0 and 28, with a score of 0–4 representing normal cognition, a score of 5–9 representing early impairment, and a score of 10 or more representing impaired cognition. Despite the simplicity and brevity of the SBT, the results that it produces have demonstrated excellent reliability (Fuld, 1978). Similarly, the SBT was the first mental status examination to be correlated with amyloid plaque burden at autopsy (Carpenter et al., 2011).

The Alzheimer's Disease Assessment Scale (ADAS) was specifically developed to measure the severity of symptoms commonly seen in AD (Rosen et al., 1984). Initially, it was developed in two parts (sub-scales): one for cognitive symptoms and one for non-cognitive symptoms. The cognitive sub-scale of the ADAS is commonly referred to as the ADAS-cog, and has become one of the most common neuropsychological tests used to assess AD progression. The scoring for the ADAS-cog ranges from 0 to 70, with a low score representing a cognitively intact person and a high score representing someone with cognitive impairment. Because the ADAS-cog has an excellent test-retest reliability and is considered to be one of the most sensitive scales for assessing cognitive changes related to AD (Emilien et al., 2004), this test is extensively used in AD clinical trials as an outcome measure of cognitive change (Schmitt and Wichems, 2006; Connor and Sabbagh, 2008).

MEMORY TESTS

Individual memory tests are generally shorter than mental status examinations and focus solely on assessing memory deficits. Both verbal and visual memory tests are commonly used clinically as stand alone tests or incorporated into a more comprehensive mental status examination. Examples of such memory tests are the Logical Memory Test I and II (LM-I and LM-II) and the Benton Visual Retention Test (BVRT) (Benton, 1992; Wechsler, 1997).

The LM-I and LM-II were originally developed as subtests to the Wechsler memory scale, but are commonly used as standalone memory tests. Both are verbal based memory tests that involve a short story read to the patient. In the LM-I, the patient answers immediate questions related to the narrative, whereas in the LM-II there is a delay between the presentation of the story and the questions. Thus, these memory tests are used to assess immediate recall (LM-I) and delayed recall (LM-II).

In the BVRT, the patient is shown 10 different visual designs, one at a time, and is then asked to reproduce each one from memory exactly as it appeared. While scoring the BVRT, errors of omissions, distortions, perseverations, rotations, misplacements, and size are all looked for and can give some insight into the progression of the disease. For example, if the patient has a high number of perseveration errors it is likely that the AD pathology has manifest itself in neocortical areas responsible for higher cognitive domains such as executive function, and visuospatial capacities (Braak Stage V–VI).

COGNITIVE NEUROPSYCHOLOGICAL ASSESSMENT SUMMARY

Each of the tests described above is aimed at assessing deficits in different cognitive domains. Each of these domains has been

Table 1 | Common neuropsychological assessment tasks seen clinically.

Task	Description	Cognitive domains	References
MENTAL STATUS EXAMS			
Mini-Mental State Examination (MMSE)	Nineteen item (30 points) test of general cognitive status	Working memory, attention, memory (semantic), praxis, etc.	Folstein et al., 1975
Montreal Cognitive Assessment (MoCA)	A rapid screening method to assess mild cognitive dysfunction	Working memory, memory (semantic and episodic), attention, visuospatial memory, etc.	Nasreddine et al., 2005
Short Blessed Test (SBT)	A short six item test measuring general cognitive status	Memory (semantic and episodic), working memory, and attention, etc.	Blessed et al., 1968
Alzheimer's Disease Assessment Scale (ADAS)	An 11 part test that measures cognitive dysfunction	Memory (semantic and episodic), and attention, etc.	Rosen et al., 1984
MEMORY TESTS			
Logical memory test I and II	A short story is presented to the patient and used to test immediate memory (test I) and delayed memory (test II)	Memory (episodic), verbal recall, etc.	Wechsler, 1997
Benton Visual Retention Test (BRVT)	Visual based test of general memory	Memory (episodic), and working memory etc.	Benton, 1992

shown to be impaired at some point in the spectrum of human AD. However, they are not uniformly affected throughout the course of the disease. Deficits in some domains occur relatively early, while deficits in others occur much later in the progression of the disease. **Figure 1A** depicts an overview of the time course of affected cognitive domains in human AD. It has become increasingly clear that identifying and targeting the cognitive deficits that occur early in the course of the disease is critical to producing the maximum impact of treatment on cognitive function and quality of life (Salmon et al., 2002). Thus, great efforts have been made to better understand the profile of cognitive deficits associated with early AD, and have resulted in earlier and more reliable clinical diagnosis (Bondi et al., 1995, 1999; Jacobson et al., 2002; Lange et al., 2002; Mickes et al., 2007).

Some of the earliest neuropathological changes in AD are in the hippocampus and entorhinal cortex, followed by changes in the medial temporal lobe. Consistent with this progression of pathology, the earliest detectable deficits in cognition are seen in medial temporal lobe-dependent episodic memory (Bondi et al., 1999; Collie and Maruff, 2000; Schmitt et al., 2000; Smith et al., 2007). These early deficits in episodic memory are followed closely by deficits in semantic memory, and both are developed before other deficits in cognitive domains such as attention, visuospatial memory, or executive function (Bondi et al., 2008). This suggests that cognitive functions such as episodic and semantic memory that depend heavily on the neural circuitry of the medial and lateral temporal lobes may be impaired earlier than cognitive abilities that depend on the circuitry of other brain regions. Further support for this idea comes from the time course of the frontal lobe dependent executive function deficits observed in patients. Slight deficits in executive functioning are first detectable near the end of the preclinical phase of AD but after the observed deficits in episodic and semantic memory (Storandt et al., 2006; Twamley et al., 2006). As the patient moves from the preclinical phase of AD into MCI, more cognitive domains begin to be affected. Most studies of MCI patients show consistent impairments in verbal recall (Larrieu et al., 2002; Tuokko et al., 2005; Kryscio et al., 2006) and a decline in general memory functioning (Tuokko et al., 2005; Bondi et al., 2008). Once the AD patient progresses past MCI and into dementia, general cognition continues to decline with deficits appearing in all respective cognitive domains (Huff et al., 1987; Locascio et al., 1995; Lambon Ralph et al., 2003; Mckhann et al., 2011).

The importance of neuropsychological testing cannot be overstated, as it is the only measure that provides information about a patient's current cognitive status and remains the most reliable means to clinically diagnose probable AD. Neuropsychological testing provides information on both general cognitive status and specific information on different cognitive domains affected in AD. Composite scores encompassing multiple neuropsychological tests are often used and can provide some of the most reliable assessments of global cognitive status relating to AD as well as serving as efficacy outcome measures in clinical trials (Bernick et al., 2012).

HOW COMMONLY USED PRECLINICAL MOUSE BEHAVIORAL TASKS RELATE TO THE CLINICAL NEUROPSYCHOLOGICAL ASSESSMENT TESTS IN HUMAN AD?

Ideally, preclinical rodent cognitive testing would assess identical cognitive domains to those examined through neuropsychological testing in human AD. Indeed, many rodent behavioral tasks have been specifically designed with this in mind, and while each task varies with respect to face, construct, and predictive validity, they all attempt to model different aspects of the cognition disrupted in AD and targeted by the human neuropsychological assessments listed in the previous section. Some cognitive domains disrupted in AD have been extensively modeled (reference memory, working memory and executive function), some less so (attention), and some nearly not at all (episodic memory). Reference memory, while not used clinically to describe human cognition, refers to learned knowledge for an aspect of a task that remains constant throughout the behavioral task and most closely correlates to human semantic memory. Working memory refers to a mental processing system used to hold transitory information for a limited time where it can be manipulated and operated on and used to guide behavior. Recognition

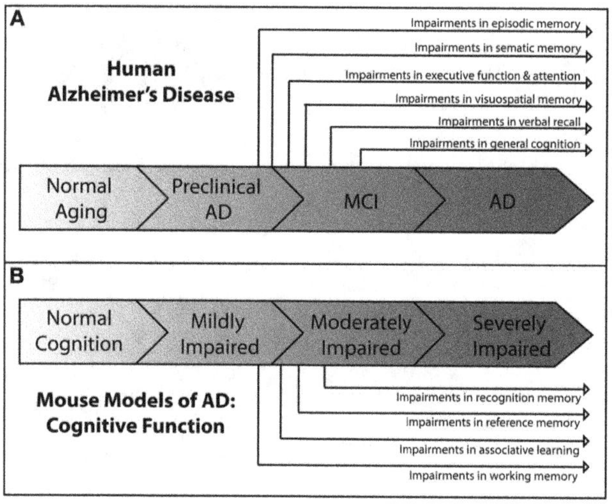

FIGURE 1 | Overview of the progression of cognitive deficits in human AD and in mouse models of AD. (A) In the human disease, the earliest AD-related cognitive deficits present themselves as episodic memory impairment during the late preclinical phase of the disease (Backman et al., 2005; Twamley et al., 2006; Bondi et al., 2008). Semantic memory deficits are the next to develop (Tuokko et al., 2005; Storandt et al., 2006), followed by impairments in executive functioning (Bondi et al., 2008), attention (Bondi et al., 2008), and visuospatial memory (Twamley et al., 2006) near the beginning of the MCI phase of the disease. As MCI progresses, deficits in verbal recall (Kryscio et al., 2006; Bondi et al., 2008) develop and impairments in general cognition (Bondi et al., 2008) become apparent. As the patient transitions into AD, all cognitive domains become affected. **(B)** The development of cognitive deficits in APP mouse models of AD shows similar patterns of progression. Consistently, the earliest observable impairments are in spatial working memory (Webster et al., 2013), as assessed through the use of water maze based tasks. These impairments are generally followed temporally by impairments in associative learning and reference memory, as assessed by maze alternation (Lalonde et al., 2012) and fear conditioning tasks (Kobayashi and Chen, 2005). Deficits in recognition memory usually present later in the spectrum of cognitive impairment than deficits in other domains (Eriksen and Janus, 2007; Hall and Roberson, 2012; Webster et al., 2013).

memory refers to the ability to recognize previously encountered events, objects, or individuals and is classified as part of long-term declarative memory. Other cognitive domains impaired in human AD such as those involving language (i.e., verbal acuity tasks and verbal recall tasks) simply cannot be modeled in rodent models. **Table 2** provides a short description of various behavioral tasks used to assess AD-like cognitive deficits in mice, and summarizes the respective cognitive domains measured by each task.

MODELING WORKING MEMORY

Working memory is perhaps one of the most well modeled aspects of the memory deficits in AD. Clinically, many of the neuropsychological tests that assess working memory rely heavily on the use of verbal tasks (Kaplan et al., 1978; Benedict et al., 1998; Spreen and Strauss, 1998; Delis et al., 2000), employing language as a core construct and thus are not feasible to model using mice. Instead, spatial based working memory tasks are heavily employed in murine working memory testing and likely are more depictive of the visuospatial working memory tasks used clinically (Benton, 1992; Benedict and Groninger, 1994).

The most widely used paradigms for working memory in mice are maze type tasks which require spatial working memory to solve. The earliest variants of these are the T-maze and Y-maze alternation tasks, which are relatively simple tests consisting of three arms with a single intersection. These tasks rely on the natural exploratory behavior (tendency to choose an alternative arm over an arm which has been previously explored) of rodents and are considered the most rudimentary tasks to assess spatial working memory (Dudchenko, 2004). A more complex maze type task used to test murine spatial working memory is that of the Radial Arm Maze (RAM), consisting of several arms (usually 6–8) radiating outwards from a central platform (Olton and Samuelson, 1976; Olton et al., 1979). In the RAM, the animal is started in the center area and then some of the arms or all of the arms can be baited with a food reward. Depending on the baiting paradigm, unimpaired rats and mice will quickly learn where the food reward is and which arms have previously been visited, and will avoid re-entering a previously entered arm. Perhaps the most widely employed spatial working memory task is that of the Morris Water Maze (MWM) (Morris et al., 1982). The MWM consists of a large open pool with a hidden (submerged) escape platform located somewhere within the pool. Animals must learn where the platform is, remember the platform's location, and then use spatial cues on subsequent trials to navigate back to the hidden platform. Large numbers of AD mouse models have been tested in the MWM and most show AD related cognitive deficits (Webster et al., 2013). Other common tasks of murine spatial working memory are the Radial Arm Water Maze (RAWM) and the Barnes Maze (Barnes, 1979; Diamond et al., 1999; Alamed et al., 2006).

It is important to note that while many of the previously described behavioral tasks are considered tasks of working memory they can also be modified to test reference memory depending on the testing protocol used. Similarly, not all models of murine working memory are spatial working memory tasks. For example, there exist versions of both the RAM and RAWM that are considered non-spatial working memory tasks (Olton and Feustle, 1981; Crusio et al., 1993; Hyde et al., 2000). Other examples of non-spatial working memory tasks are operant tasks such as the Delayed Match to Sample (DMTS), Delayed Non-Match to Sample (DNMTS), and Delayed Stimulus Discrimination Task (DSDT) (Dudchenko, 2004; Buccafusco et al., 2008). In these non-spatial working memory tasks the animal is required to remember a stimulus (over a delay period) that is paired with a particular type of response (generally a lever press or a nose poke) and a correct response is rewarded. In many of the non-spatial operant working memory tasks each animal can perform many trials per day and thus can serve as its own control. This lends itself nicely to pharmacological based studies assessing potential therapeutic compounds for the treatment of the cognitive deficits seen in AD (Buccafusco et al., 2008).

MODELING EXECUTIVE FUNCTION

Executive function refers to a broad range of higher cognitive processes such as: reasoning, planning, cognitive flexibility,

Table 2 | Commonly used mouse behavioral tasks.

Task	Description	Cognitive domains	References
Morris Water Maze (MWM)	Widely used behavioral task where mice are placed in a circular pool and must find a hidden escape platform	Reference memory and working memory	Morris et al., 1982
Radial Arm Maze (RAM)	The maze usually consists of 6–8 arms radiating from a round central space. Various arms are baited with a food reward.	Reference memory and working memory	Olton and Samuelson, 1976
Radial Arm Water Maze (RAWM)	A submerged version of the RAM where the food reward is replaced by an escape platform.	Reference memory and working memory	Diamond et al., 1999
Barnes maze	Consists of a circular platform with holes around the circumference and an escape box	Reference memory and working memory	Barnes, 1979
T-Maze/Y-Maze alternation	A three arm maze which forces the animal to choose between two arms	Reference memory and working memory	Blodgett and Mccutchan, 1947; Glickman and Jensen, 1961
Novel Object Recognition (NOR)	A two trial memory task which uses the animal's innate exploratory behavior to assess memory	Recognition memory	Ennaceur and Delacour, 1988
Contextual and cued fear conditioning	The animal learns to predict an aversive stimulus based on an associated context/cue	Reference memory (associative learning/memory)	Fanselow, 1980; Curzon et al., 2009
Passive avoidance	An avoidance task where the animal must refrain from entering a chamber where an aversive stimulus was previously administered	Reference memory (associative learning/memory)	Van Der Poel, 1967
Active avoidance	A fear-motivated associative avoidance test where an animal must actively avoid an aversive stimulus	Reference memory and working memory (associative learning/memory)	Vanderwolf, 1964
Delayed Matching (non-matching) to Position/Sample (DMTP/DMTS)	The animal receives a sample stimulus and then after a short delay is required to choose the correct corresponding response	Working memory	Dunnett, 1993; Robinson and Crawley, 1993
Multiple-Choice Serial Reaction Time Task (CSRTT)	The animal must attend to several spatial locations (usually 3–5), observe a corresponding stimulus, and then correctly respond	Attention, impulsivity, and executive function	Carli et al., 1983
Attentional set-shifting tasks	The animal must shift back and forth between changing rules to successfully obtain a reward	Executive function and cognitive flexibility	Birrell and Brown, 2000
Reversal learning	Adjustment to changes in reward contingency	Executive function and working memory	Butter, 1969; Bussey et al., 1997
What-Where-Which Task (WWWhich)	The animal must associate an object (What) with its location (Where) in a specific visuospatial context (Which) to form an integrated memory	Recognition memory and episodic-like memory	Davis et al., 2013a,b

sequencing, response inhibition, and abstract concept formation. The current mouse models of executive function most closely replicate the human aspects of cognitive flexibility and response inhibition in executive function. Attentional set-shifting tasks are one of the main behavioral tasks used to assess executive function in the mouse. In many ways, set-shifting tasks are similar to the Wisconsin Card Sorting Task in that they form the gold standard for assessing executive function (Drewe, 1974; Robinson et al., 1980; Arnett et al., 1994). In both the Wisconsin Card Sorting Task in humans and set-shifting tasks in mice, the dorsolateral and orbital prefrontal cortex is critical for successful performance (Weinberger et al., 1986; Berman et al., 1995; Brigman et al., 2005; Bissonette et al., 2008). In the most common version of the murine set-shifting task, mice are required to select a bowl in which to dig for a food reward. Bowls can be discriminated from each other according to different stimulus dimensions such as texture and odor. Successful completion of the task requires the animal to shift between stimuli dimensions to successfully retrieve the food reward. The ability to extract knowledge from different stimuli dimensions suggests that the mouse is capable of using at least some aspects of higher-order cognitive functions seen in human executive functioning (Chudasama, 2011). Numerous different transgenic mouse models of AD have shown deficits in set-shifting tasks (Zhuo et al., 2007, 2008; Marchese et al., 2013).

Reversal learning is another way that aspects of executive function are modeled in the mouse. While less complex than attentional set shifting, reversal learning does require both cognitive flexibility and impulse control, thus tapping into components of human executive function (Chudasama, 2011; Stopford et al.,

2012). There are many different variations of reversal learning tasks in mouse behavior, but they all work on the same principle. The animal first learns that a particular response to a stimulus will be rewarded, while a response to a different stimulus will be unrewarded. Then the stimulus-reward is switched so that the previously unrewarded stimulus becomes the rewarded stimulus. The animal must learn to reverse responses in order to receive the reward. Wild type control mice are able to quickly adjust their response in order to obtain the reward. However, animals with prefrontal cortex lesions display profound deficits in reversal learning (Chudasama, 2011; Izquierdo and Jentsch, 2012). Similarly, many different AD mouse models have shown impairment in reversal learning (Angelo et al., 2003; Dong et al., 2005; Filali et al., 2012; Cheng et al., 2013; Musilli et al., 2013; Papadopoulos et al., 2013).

Another aspect of executive function that is modeled in mice is response inhibition. Response inhibition is required for the appropriate control of an individual's behavioral actions in response to a stimulus (Robbins, 1996; Humby et al., 1999; Perry and Hodges, 1999; Romberg et al., 2013a). The five choice serial reaction time task (5-CSRTT) is a behavioral task that measures the response inhibition component of executive function (5-CSRTT is also used to model aspects of attention, see below section) in mice (Robbins, 2002; Bari et al., 2008; Chudasama, 2011; Romberg et al., 2013a). The 5-CSRTT can test two different aspects of response inhibition: (1) a failure to withhold the impulsive urge to respond while anticipating correct response (premature responses) and (2) a failure to disengage from repeating past correct responses (perseveration responses) (Chudasama, 2011). Several mouse models of AD have shown deficits in response inhibition using the 5-CSRTT (Romberg et al., 2011, 2013b).

MODELING ATTENTION

Several behavioral tasks have been developed for modeling attention in mice that provide reliable measures comparable to the neuropsychological assessments used in AD. The most widely used of these tasks is the 5-CSRTT (Muir, 1996; Humby et al., 1999; Robbins, 2002; De Bruin et al., 2006; Gibson et al., 2006; Lambourne et al., 2007; Pattij et al., 2007). This task employs an operant box with nose poke holes on the front wall of the chamber. Animals are trained to respond to brief flashes of light corresponding to five different spatial locations on this front side of the chamber and correct responses are rewarded with a food pellet released to a feeder box at the rear of the chamber. Touchscreen versions of this task are also available in which the nose poke holes and stimulus lights are replaced with an LCD screen (Romberg et al., 2011; Bussey et al., 2012). For both standard and touchscreen versions of the task, multiple trials are run each day and both the duration of the stimulus itself or the interval between the stimulus and response can be manipulated to increase the attention demands placed on the animal. Sustained attention is measured by examining when the animal responds to a different (incorrect) hole than where the stimulus light appeared (called errors of commission), fails to respond within the allotted time to the stimulus (errors of omission), and the speed with which the animal responds (reaction time). Aspects of selective attention can also be modeled with the 5-CSRTT by introducing brief bursts of white noise that the animal must ignore while still detecting the visual stimulus as it is presented (Robbins, 2002; Bari et al., 2008). The rodent 5-CSRTT is analogous to Leonard's 5-CSRTT used in humans (Wilkinson, 1963). Both tasks require subjects (mouse and human respectively) to utilize sustained attention divided among multiple spatial locations across which a large number of trials and errors of commission, omission, and reaction time are scored. Another task that can be considered somewhat analogous to the 5-CSRTT is the human Continuous Performance Tests (CPT) of sustained attention (Beck et al., 1956). In this task, the subjects are asked to respond to signal and non-signal events across numerous trials, and scores of hits, misses, rejections, and false alarms are recorded. Errors of commission in the 5-CSRTT are thought to be analogous to CPT false alarms rates. Similarly, errors of omission in the 5-CSRTT are thought to be analogous to CPT misses. AD mice such as the 3×Tg-AD mice have been shown to have deficits in sustained attention using the 5-CSRTT (Romberg et al., 2011). However, the homology between mouse and human versions of these tasks is far from perfect, and caution should be used when drawing conclusions from the rodent 5-CSRTT and applying them to human attention (Young et al., 2009).

MODELING EPISODIC MEMORY

Episodic memory refers to the ability to encode and recall personal past events and experiences. Episodic memory has also been referred to as the "what, when, and where" aspect of a particular experience. Modeling AD-related deficits in episodic memory in mice is a less well-explored area than that of other aspects of working memory, executive function, or attention. Historically, episodic memory was thought to be unique to humans (Tulving and Markowitsch, 1998). However, work over the past few decades on episodic-like memory across a number of animal species has suggested otherwise, and several mouse behavioral tasks designed at assessing episodic-like memory have been developed (Clayton and Dickinson, 1998; Clayton et al., 2001; Griffiths and Clayton, 2001; Morris, 2001; Davis et al., 2013a,b). One such task is the What-Where-Which Task (WWWhich). This task is an adaptation of the NOR task. While the NOR task itself is too simplistic a task to be considered a true episodic memory task (rather it is considered a task of recognition memory), the WWWhich task is able to model episodic-like memory. In the WWWhich task, the animal must integrate the location of a particular object with specific contextual cues to form an episodic-like memory (Davis et al., 2013a,b). Several studies employing the WWWhich task have observed performance deficits related to the aging process and to AD disease state in several transgenic mouse lines (Davis et al., 2013a,b). While the WWWhich task models episodic memory in the mouse, it is not very comparable to any of the episodic memory tasks commonly used in neuropsychological testing for AD. This is largely because the human tasks rely on language as a foundational construct for assessment. Obviously, there exists no such component in the WWWhich task for mice. Therefore, caution should be used when attempting to correlate any preclinical finding concerning episodic memory in mice to that of human cognition.

SUMMARY OF MOUSE BEHAVIORAL TESTS

All of the rodent behavioral tasks discussed in this section have been specifically developed to assess deficits in cognitive domains related to what is seen in human AD. Just as multiple neuropsychological tests assessing different cognitive domains are often used clinically to provide a global cognitive profile, so multiple behavioral tasks assessing different cognitive domains should ideally be used when characterizing the profile of AD-related cognitive impairment in a particular mouse model of AD.

TEMPORAL PROGRESSION OF THE COGNITIVE DEFICITS SEEN IN THE COMMONLY USED AD MOUSE MODELS

Cognitive decline is a defining feature of AD, and many mouse models have been developed that recapitulate aspects of the cognitive impairments seen in AD (Elder et al., 2010; Hochgrafe et al., 2013; Platt et al., 2013). Although no one animal model fully replicates the progression of cognitive impairments seen in the human disease, AD mouse models have been invaluable in advancing our knowledge of the disease. It should be noted that most of the AD mouse models are representative of the familial form of AD (FAD) which accounts for only a small percentage of the total AD cases each year (Campion et al., 1999). In addition, the contributions of both background strain and likely overexpression of mutant human APP genes on brain development and function must always be considered with regard to observed cognitive deficits in the various AD mouse models. Each transgenic mouse model of AD provides different insights into aspects of AD pathogenesis and the cognitive deficits associated with the disease. A generalized time course of the development of cognitive deficits across the various mouse models is depicted in **Figure 1B**. For each specific mouse model the temporal time course and progression of cognitive deficits in each cognitive domain can be different. In addition, in some models, cognitive deficits can be detected prior to the appearance of significant neuropathology. Careful forethought is therefore required in the selection of an optimal model displaying the AD related cognitive deficits desired based on the specific research interests of the investigator. An overview of the progressive cognitive deficits and the time of appearance of amyloid pathology is presented in **Table 3** for five mouse models that contain amyloid precursor protein (APP) mutations and in **Table 4** for five other common mouse models that contain APP and presenilin (PS1) mutations, or APP/PS1/Tau mutations. These tables are by no means an all-encompassing list of mouse models; rather they are simply meant to be examples of some of the commonly used mouse models of AD that are characterized by APP mutations. For recent reviews of additional AD mouse strains not included here, see (Ashe and Zahs, 2010; Elder et al., 2010; Epis et al., 2010; Hall and Roberson, 2012; Platt et al., 2013).

PDAPP

(Promoter: Platelet-Derived (PDGF) Promoter, Symbol: Tg (APPV717F) 109Ili, MGI ID: 2151935)

The PDAPP mouse was first described by Games in 1995 and is considered one of the earliest mouse models of AD (Chartier-Harlin et al., 1991; Games et al., 1995). In this model, the cognitive deficits first present themselves in spatial working memory at 4 months of age when assessed by MWM testing (Hartman et al., 2005). These deficits in working memory in the MWM are present throughout the rest of the life span for this model (Chen et al., 2000; Daumas et al., 2008). Deficits in recognition memory appear to develop after the working memory deficits in this model, as the first reported deficits in the NOR task are at 6 months old (Dodart et al., 1999). The cognitive deficits in recognition memory do not appear as robust as those in working memory in this model as there are inconsistent reports in the literature (Dodart et al., 1999, 2002; Chen et al., 2000). The cognitive defects in this model appear to present themselves before the appearance of plaque deposition (first appear at approximately 6 months) or other gross amyloid pathologies (Games et al., 1995; Hsiao et al., 1996; Schenk et al., 1999; Chen et al., 2000; Morgan, 2003).

TG2576

(Promoter: Hamster PrP Promoter, Symbol: Tg (APPSWE) 2576Kha, MGI ID: 2385631)

In the Tg2576 mouse (Hsiao et al., 1996), the first presentation of cognitive deficits is seen at 5 months of age in spatial working memory (Arendash et al., 2004). These spatial working memory deficits are generally accepted to be present across the rest of the life span for this model (Hsiao et al., 1996; Westerman et al., 2002; Arendash et al., 2004). However, methodology used to assess spatial memory appears to be very important, as several different reports have failed to observe these same deficits at various ages (Hsiao et al., 1996; Arendash et al., 2001a; King and Arendash, 2002). Non-spatial working memory tasks show a similar time course progression, first appearing at 3–5 months of age and persisting across the lifespan (Hsiao et al., 1996; Chapman et al., 1999; King and Arendash, 2002; Lalonde et al., 2003; Ohno et al., 2004). Deficits in recognition memory do not appear until much later, first appearing at 12 months of age in the NOR task (Oules et al., 2012; Yassine et al., 2013).

APP23

(Promoter: Thy-1, Symbol: Tg (Thy1-APP) 3Somm, MGI ID: 2447146)

The APP23 mouse model was reported in 1997 (Sturchler-Pierrat et al., 1997). In this model, the cognitive deficits begin to first appear in both recognition memory and spatial working memory at 3 months of age. The deficits appear to be progressive with age, and at 12 months old the animals also show cognitive deficits in a reference memory version of the Barnes maze (Prut et al., 2007). This model develops non-spatial working memory deficits very late in the progression of the disease (only after 19 months of age) (Lalonde et al., 2002; Dumont et al., 2004). Interestingly, cognitive performance in passive avoidance memory tasks follows the same progression as non-spatial working memory deficits in this model, unimpaired at 15 months of age and then developing deficits between 19 and 20 months of age (Kelly et al., 2003).

TgCRND8

(Promoter: PrP, Symbol: Tg (PRNP-APPSweInd) 8Dwst, MGI ID: 3589475)

The TgCRND8 model, described by Chishti et al. (2001), exhibits early cognitive impairment that spans across multiple cognitive domains (Chishti et al., 2001). TgCRND8 are impaired on spatial

Table 3 | Progression of cognitive deficits in APP mouse models of AD.

Strain	Passive avoidance	Fear Conditioning	Y/T-Maze Alternation	NOR	RAWM	MWM	Barnes Maze	Age in Months
PDAPP: [1]					[2]	[2]		1-2m
				[3]		[4]		3-5m
				[3] [5]	[6]			6-8m*
				[3]		[4]		9-11m
				[6]		[6]		12-14m
					[2]	[4]		15-18m
				[6]		[6]		≥19m
Tg2576: [7]		[8]	[9]					1-2m
	[10]	[8]	[10] [7]		[11]	[12]		3-5m
			[13] [11]	[14]	[12] [11]	[15] [11]	[14]	6-8m
	[10]	[8]	[7, 9]			[7] [10]		9-11m*
	[10]	[16]		[17]		[15] [10]		12-14m
		[18]	[16] [11]	[17] [14]	[19]	[15]	[14]	15-18m
	[10]		[10]			[15] [10]		≥19m
APP23: [20]	[21]					[21]		1-2m
	[21]			[22]		[21]		3-5m
	[21]			[23]		[21]		6-8m*
								9-11m
							[24]	12-14m
	[25]		[26]			[26]		15-18m
	[25]		[27]			[25]		≥19m
TgCRND8: [28]			[29]					1-2m
		[30]		[31-33]		[28]	[32]	3-5m*
		[30]	[29]		[34]	[35]		6-8m
			[29]			[36]		9-11m
		[30]				[36]		12-14m
								15-18m
								≥19m
J20: [37]				[38]				1-2m
		[39]		[38] [40]	[41]	[42]		3-5m
		[39]		[43]	[44]	[45]		6-8m*
			[46]	[47]	[48]	[46]		9-11m
		[49]	[49]	[49]	[44]	[50]		12-14m
								15-18m
					[44]			≥19m

Data not found | Same as control | Increased from control | Decreased from control

The strain is presented in the left column and age is presented in the right column. Black cells represent impairment, light gray cells represent no impairment compared to controls, dark gray cells represent increases from control (very few such cases), and white cells represent time points where no data are available for the respective behavior. The asterisk appearing in the age column represents when diffuse amyloid plaques are first observable in the brain for that particular mouse model of AD. The numbers within each cell correspond to the following references: 1: (Games et al., 1995), 2: (Nilsson et al., 2004), 3: (Dodart et al., 1999), 4: (Hartman et al., 2005), 5: (Dodart et al., 2002), 6: (Chen et al., 2000), 7: (Hsiao et al., 1996), 8: (Dineley et al., 2002), 9: (Chapman et al., 1999), 10: (King et al., 1999), 11: (Arendash et al., 2001a), 12: (Arendash et al., 2004), 13: (Ohno et al., 2004), 14: (Yassine et al., 2013), 15: (Westerman et al., 2002), 16: (Corcoran et al., 2002), 17: (Oules et al., 2012), 18: (Lassalle et al., 2008), 19: (Morgan et al., 2000), 20: (Sturchler-Pierrat et al., 1997), 21: (Van Dam et al., 2003), 22: (Huang et al., 2006), 23: (Heneka et al., 2006), 24: (Prut et al., 2007), 25: (Kelly et al., 2003), 26: (Lalonde et al., 2002), 27: (Dumont et al., 2004), 28: (Chishti et al., 2001), 29: (Hyde et al., 2005), 30: (Hanna et al., 2012), 31:(Ambree et al., 2009), 32: (Gortz et al., 2008), 33:(Richter et al., 2008), 34: (Lovasic et al., 2005), 35: (Janus, 2004), 36: (Hanna et al., 2009), 37: (Mucke et al., 2000), 38: (Harris et al., 2010), 39: (Saura et al., 2005), 40: (Simon et al., 2009), 41: (Lustbader et al., 2004), 42: (Cheng et al., 2007), 43: (Cisse et al., 2011), 44: (Du et al., 2011), 45: (Palop et al., 2003), 46: (Murakami et al., 2011), 47: (Escribano et al., 2009), 48: (Fang et al., 2012), 49: (Karl et al., 2012), 50: (Galvan et al., 2006).

Table 4 | Progression of memory deficits in other mouse models of AD (APP + PS1/Tau).

Strain	Passive avoidance	Fear Conditioning	Y/T -Maze Alternation	Novel Object Recognition	RAWM	MWM	Barn es Maze	Age in Months
APP/PS1: [1]								1-2m
					[2]			3-5m*
		[3] [4]	[5, 6]		[7]	[6]	[4]	6-8m
		[3]			[8]	[3]		9-11m
	[9]	[10]			[2]	[11]		12-14m
						[11]	[12]	15-18m
								≥19m
APP + PS1: [13]		[14]				[15]		1-2m
		[14]	[13, 16]		[17]	[16]		3-5m
					[15] [16]	[15] [13]		6-8m*
		[14]				[13]		9-11m
				[18]				12-14m
			[16, 17]		[19]	[17]		15-18m
					[20]	[21]		≥19m
APP/PS1KI: [22]								1-2m
								3-5m
				[23]	[23]			6-8m*
				[23]	[23]			9-11m
								12-14m
				[23]	[23]			15-18m
				[23]	[23]			≥19m
5xFAD: [24]			[24]					1-2m*
		[25]	[24] [26]	[26]		[25]		3-5m
		[27]	[26, 28]	[18]		[25]		6-8m
		[27]	[26]			[29]		9-11m
		[27]	[26, 28]					12-14m
								15-18m
								≥19m
3xTgAD: [30]				[31]		[31]		1-2m
	[31]		[32]			[31] [33]		3-5m*
		[34]	[35]	[31]		[34]		6-8m
	[35]		[32]	[31]		[36]		9-11m
	[37]		[32]	[37, 38]		[33]	[39]	12-14m
				[40]		[36]		15-18m
								≥19m

Data not found	Same as control	Increased from control	Decreased from control

The strain is presented in the left column and age is presented in the right column. Black cells represent impairment, light gray cells represent no impairment compared to controls, dark gray cells represent increases from control (very few such cases), and white cells represent time points where no data are available for the respective behavior. The asterisk appearing in the age column represents when diffuse amyloid plaques are first observable in the brain for that particular mouse model of AD. The numbers within each cell correspond to the following references: 1: (Jankowsky et al., 2001), 2: (Park et al., 2006), 3: (Cramer et al., 2012), 4: (Reiserer et al., 2007), 5:(Cao et al., 2007) 6:(Lalonde et al., 2004), 7: (Volianskis et al., 2010), 8: (Sood et al., 2007), 9: (Zhang et al., 2011), 10: (Knafo et al., 2009), 11: (Lalonde et al., 2005), 12: (O'leary and Brown, 2009), 13: (Holcomb et al., 1999), 14: (Dineley et al., 2002), 15: (Trinchese et al., 2004), 16: (Arendash et al., 2001a), 17: (Arendash et al., 2001b), 18: (Tohda et al., 2012), 19: (Morgan et al., 2000), 20: (Wilcock et al., 2004), 21: (Sadowski et al., 2004), 22: (Flood et al., 2002), 23: (Webster et al., 2013), 24: (Oakley et al., 2006), 25: (Ohno et al., 2006), 26: (Shukla et al., 2013), 27: (Devi and Ohno, 2010), 28:(Devi and Ohno, 2012), 29: (Urano and Tohda, 2010), 30: (Oddo et al., 2003), 31: (Clinton et al., 2007), 32: (Carroll et al., 2007), 33: (Gimenez-Llort et al., 2007), 34: (Billings et al., 2005), 35: (Nelson et al., 2007b), 36: (Pietropaolo et al., 2008), 37: (Filali et al., 2012), 38: (Arsenault et al., 2011), 39: (Stewart et al., 2011), 40: (Halagappa et al., 2007).

working memory tasks starting at 3 months of age. These deficits are seen in the MWM and progress with age of the animal (Janus et al., 2000; Chishti et al., 2001; Gortz et al., 2008; Richter et al., 2008; Ambree et al., 2009). Reference memory deficits via Barnes maze testing are also present at 3 months of age (Gortz et al., 2008; Richter et al., 2008; Ambree et al., 2009). Similar to this observed temporal time course of spatial working memory and reference memory deficits are the development of deficits in both recognition memory and fear conditioning (Gortz et al., 2008; Richter et al., 2008; Ambree et al., 2009; Hanna et al., 2012). Deficits in alternation tasks develop by 6 and 9 months in Y-maze and T-maze alternation tasks, respectively (Hyde et al., 2005).

J20

(Promoter: Platelet-Derived (PDGF), Symbol: Tg (PDGFB-APPSwInd) 20Lms, MGI ID: 3057148)

The J20 mouse model was developed by (Mucke et al., 2000).This model is unique in that the first presented cognitive deficits are observed very early (at 1–2 months of age) in recognition memory (Harris et al., 2010). These deficits in recognition memory are present when assessed at several other time points (Escribano et al., 2009; Simon et al., 2009; Cisse et al., 2011). However, they do not appear to progress with the age of the animal and there has even been a report of no recognition memory deficits in old animals in advanced stages of the disease (Karl et al., 2012). Early memory deficits can also be observed in spatial working memory at 3 months of age when assessed by the MWM and the RAWM tasks (Lustbader et al., 2004; Cheng et al., 2007; Meilandt et al., 2008). These spatial working memory deficits are present across the rest of this model's lifespan (Palop et al., 2003; Galvan et al., 2006; Cisse et al., 2011; Du et al., 2011; Murakami et al., 2011; Fang et al., 2012). Fear conditioning deficits appear consistent with the presentation of spatial working memory and recognition memory deficits in this model (Saura et al., 2005). Interestingly, this model does not appear to display working memory deficits on tasks of alternation such as the Y-maze (Murakami et al., 2011; Karl et al., 2012).

APP/PS1

(Promoter: PrP, Symbol: Tg (APPswe, PSEN1de9) 85Dbo, MGI ID: 3524957)

The cognitive deficits in the APP/PS1 mouse model, first described by Jankowsky et al. (2001), have been well characterized. Cognitive deficits are first seen at 3 months of age in the RAWM spatial working memory task and are also reported by 6 months of age in the MWM (Cao et al., 2007; Ding et al., 2008). Further, these deficits have been well characterized across the lifespan of this mouse model in water based spatial working memory tasks (Lalonde et al., 2005; Park et al., 2006; Cao et al., 2007; Sood et al., 2007; Ding et al., 2008; Volianskis et al., 2010; Zhang et al., 2011; Cramer et al., 2012; Ma et al., 2012). Impairments in reference memory develop by 6 months and persist through the rest of the life of this model (Reiserer et al., 2007; Bernardo et al., 2009; O'leary and Brown, 2009). Deficits in associative learning have also been described in fear conditioning tasks starting at 6–8 months of age (Knafo et al., 2009; Cramer et al., 2012). Similarly, passive avoidance deficits have also been described at 12 months of age (Zhang et al., 2011). No deficits were seen in alternation tasks of working memory for this model (Lalonde et al., 2004; Cao et al., 2007).

APP + PS1

(Promoter: Hamster PrP Promoter, Symbol: Tg (APPSWE) 2576kha, MGI ID: 2385631) × (Platelet-Derived (PDGF), Symbol: Tg (PDGFB-PSEN1M146L) 2Jhd, MGI ID: 2447326)

Holcomb described a mouse model in 1998 that has been widely used to study cognitive deficits related to AD (Holcomb et al., 1998). The first observable deficits in this model are shown in associative learning and present themselves between 4 and 5 months of age (Dineley et al., 2002). The progression of the spatial working memory impairment in this model is relatively slow compared to most other models. The first reported impairment in spatial working memory was observed using 6-month-old animals (Trinchese et al., 2004). However, these cognitive deficits are not robust at this age, as others have observed no such deficit (Holcomb et al., 1999; Arendash et al., 2001a). By 15 months of age the spatial working memory is consistently impaired throughout the rest of the life span (Morgan et al., 2000; Arendash et al., 2001b; Gordon et al., 2001; Sadowski et al., 2004; Wilcock et al., 2004). Similarly, deficits in recognition memory occur later in this model, first observed at 12 months of age (Mori et al., 2013). No deficits were observed in alternation tasks of working memory (Holcomb et al., 1998; Arendash et al., 2001a).

APP/PS1 KI

(Promoter: Endogenous, Symbol: Apptm1.1Cep, MGI ID: 2652346) × (Promoter: Endogenous, Symbol: Psen1tm1Dgf, MGI ID: 3608968)

The APP/PS1 knock-in mouse model (first described in Flood et al., 2002) uses endogenous promoters to drive the expression of humanized amyloid beta sequence, and AD-like pathology and cognitive deficits develop in the absence of APP or PS1 overexpression (Flood et al., 2002). The earliest reports of cognitive deficits are reported at 7 months in this model (Bruce-Keller et al., 2011). However, the majority of cognitive deficits appear later. We have shown previously that the cognitive deficits in spatial working memory (assessed by RAWM testing) first appear at 9 months of age (Webster et al., 2013). These deficits are followed by impairments in associative memory (appearing by 14 months of age Thibault et al., 2012) and in recognition memory (not developing until 15 months of age Webster et al., 2013).

5×FAD

(Promoter: Thy-1, Symbol: Tg (APPSwFlLon, PSEN1*M146L*L286V) 6799Vas, MGI ID: 3693208)

The 5×FAD model, first described by Oakley et al. (2006), develops progressive cognitive deficits with age. This model develops cognitive deficits by 3 months of age in spatial working memory (Ohno et al., 2006; Urano and Tohda, 2010). These working memory deficits are followed temporally with the development of associative learning impairment in fear conditioning (Ohno et al., 2006; Devi and Ohno, 2010) as well as the development of deficits in a working memory version of the Y-maze (Oakley et al., 2006; Devi and Ohno, 2012; Shukla et al., 2013). As with several of the other models (PDAPP, Tg2576, APP/PS1, and APP/PS1 KI) this model develops deficits in recognition memory later than the observed deficits in spatial working memory (Tohda et al., 2012).

3×Tg-AD

(Promoter: Thy-1, Symbol: Tg (APPSwe,tauP301L) 1Lfa, MGI ID: 2672831) × (Promoter: Endogenous, Symbol: Psen1tm1Mpm, MGI ID: 1930937)

The 3×Tg-AD mouse model, developed by Oddo et al. (2003), shows progressive cognitive impairments starting at a young age. The first deficits observed in this model are those of associative learning deficits, which begin between 3 and 5 months of age. These are then followed by deficits in spatial working memory at 6 months of age in the MWM task. Both Y-maze alternation and contextual fear conditioning impairment follow a similar temporal time course. Then deficits in recognition memory present themselves between 9 and 11 months of age. Finally, reference memory impairment in the Barnes maze task is observed at 12 months of age.

TEMPORAL PROGRESSION OF AD-LIKE NON-COGNITIVE BEHAVIORAL ABNORMALITIES SEEN IN THE COMMONLY USED MOUSE MODELS

While most AD research has focused on the neurobiological mechanisms underlying the cognitive deficits seen in AD pathogenesis, there is a wide range of non-cognitive neuropsychiatric symptoms also associated with the disease. Indeed, these non-cognitive symptoms are seen as a very important concern among the family members of the patients and caregivers alike (Tan et al., 2005). These non-cognitive symptoms are often more difficult to deal with, as they compose important sources of distress and psychological burden on the family members/caregivers and can drastically affect the quality of life of patients by leading to institutionalization (Hope et al., 1998; Shin et al., 2005). Non-cognitive neuropsychological symptoms associated with AD include activity disturbances, affective disturbances, aggression, stereotypic behavior, circadian rhythm disturbances, and anxiety (Ancoli-Israel et al., 1989; Okawa et al., 1991; Vitiello et al., 1992; Bliwise, 1994; Satlin et al., 1995; Van Someren et al., 1996; Hope et al., 1998; Harper et al., 2004; Shin et al., 2005; Tan et al., 2005). While there has been less emphasis placed on the modeling of these non-cognitive neuropsychological disturbances in murine models of AD, several of the commonly used mouse models of AD do show a number of these disruptions. Non-cognitive symptoms associated with AD shown in the mouse include increased locomotor activity (Dodart et al., 1999; King et al., 1999; Arendash et al., 2001b; Dumont et al., 2004; Hyde et al., 2005; Cheng et al., 2007; Gil-Bea et al., 2007; Pietropaolo et al., 2008; Sanchez-Mejia et al., 2008; Ambree et al., 2009; Cisse et al., 2011; Mori et al., 2013), anxiety (Moechars et al., 1996, 1999; Lalonde et al., 2003, 2004; Gil-Bea et al., 2007; Reiserer et al., 2007; Lassalle et al., 2008; Espana et al., 2010; Bedrosian et al., 2011; Cisse et al., 2011; Murakami et al., 2011; Filali et al., 2012), circadian disturbances (Huitron-Resendiz et al., 2002; Vloeberghs et al., 2004; Wisor et al., 2005; Ambree et al., 2006; Sterniczuk et al., 2010; Bedrosian et al., 2011), and increased aggression (Moechars et al., 1996, 1998; Van Dorpe et al., 2000; Ambree et al., 2006; Vloeberghs et al., 2006; Pugh et al., 2007; Alexander et al., 2011).

LOCOMOTOR ACTIVITY

Most of the commonly used AD mouse models exhibit increased locomotor activity (Dodart et al., 1999; King et al., 1999; Arendash et al., 2001b; Dumont et al., 2004; Hyde et al., 2005; Cheng et al., 2007; Gil-Bea et al., 2007; Pietropaolo et al., 2008; Sanchez-Mejia et al., 2008; Ambree et al., 2009; Cisse et al., 2011; Mori et al., 2013). These disturbances include hyperactivity, stereotypic behaviors, and home cage activity disturbances (Dodart et al., 1999; Janus and Westaway, 2001; Auld et al., 2002; Dumont et al., 2004; Hyde et al., 2005; Cheng et al., 2007; Gil-Bea et al., 2007; Gimenez-Llort et al., 2007; Pietropaolo et al., 2008; Cisse et al., 2011) and have been linked to altered APP metabolism, amyloid levels, and disease progression (Van Someren et al., 1996; Harper et al., 2004). These activity disturbances do not seem to be constant, but rather present themselves with more severity at different times of the day. For example, in the TgCRND8 mice, the deficits seem most severe near the end of their wake cycle and less severe at other times of the day (Ambree et al., 2006). Further, these disturbances increase with the age of the animals and with the severity of the disease. Likewise, in the APP23 mice there have been reports of increased activity in the second half of the nocturnal phase (end of the active phase of the wake cycle) (Vloeberghs et al., 2004). These increased activity disturbances at the end of the activity cycle have been suggested to be similar to the exacerbation of activity behavioral symptoms observed in human AD patients late in the afternoon and evening time termed sundowning syndrome (Vitiello et al., 1992; Bliwise, 1994). Other AD mouse models that show activity disturbances are the PDAPP, TG2576, J20, APP + PS1 [Tg2576 + PS1 (M146L)], and 3×Tg-AD mouse models of AD. The onset of the disturbances is different for each model, with the J20 and the TgCRND8 mice developing disruptions earliest (approximately 1 month of age), followed by PDAPP and TG2576 (approximately 3 months of age), and the PS1 [Tg2576 + PS1 (M146L)], 3×TgAD, and APP23 mice developing last (approximately 6–9 months of age) (Dodart et al., 1999; King et al., 1999; Arendash et al., 2001b; Dumont et al., 2004; Hyde et al., 2005; Cheng et al., 2007; Gil-Bea et al., 2007; Gimenez-Llort et al., 2007; Pietropaolo et al., 2008; Sanchez-Mejia et al., 2008; Ambree et al., 2009; Harris et al., 2010; Cisse et al., 2011; Mori et al., 2013).

CIRCADIAN RHYTHM AND SLEEP DISRUPTIONS

Similar to the reported activity disturbances, circadian rhythm disruptions are also observed in many of the AD mouse models (Huitron-Resendiz et al., 2002; Vloeberghs et al., 2004; Wisor et al., 2005; Ambree et al., 2006; Sterniczuk et al., 2010; Bedrosian et al., 2011). Circadian rhythm disturbances have also been well described in human AD patients (Ancoli-Israel et al., 1989; Okawa et al., 1991; Vitiello et al., 1992; Van Someren et al., 1996; Auld et al., 2002; Harper et al., 2004). These disturbances are characterized by the AD patient's propensity to frequently awaken during the nighttime and to increase the amount of time slept during the day (Ancoli-Israel et al., 1989; Okawa et al., 1991). While this behavior is in itself a non-cognitive behavior, it has been reported to possibly have important effects on patient cognition (Smith, 1985; Graves et al., 2001). Several mouse models of AD also display sleep disruption. Other similarities between the sleep disturbances seen clinically and those seen in the AD mouse models are: (1) as the severity of the disease progresses, the worse the sleep disturbances become (Smith, 1985; Graves et al., 2001; Huitron-Resendiz et al., 2002, 2005) and (2) the greater the sleep disruptions are, the more severe the cognitive decline seems to be (Huitron-Resendiz et al., 2002, 2005).

ANXIETY DISTURBANCES

Anxiety disturbances have been reported in many of the AD mouse models (Moechars et al., 1996, 1999; Lalonde et al., 2003, 2004; Gil-Bea et al., 2007; Reiserer et al., 2007; Lassalle et al., 2008; Espana et al., 2010; Bedrosian et al., 2011; Cisse et al., 2011; Murakami et al., 2011; Filali et al., 2012). The prevailing thought is that these anxiolytic-like behaviors stem from disinhibitory tendencies resulting from the underlying AD pathology (Lalonde et al., 2003; Ognibene et al., 2005). Both APP function (as these anxiolytic behaviors are more common in APP transgenic mice) (Moechars et al., 1996, 1999; Lalonde et al., 2003, 2004; Lassalle et al., 2008; Murakami et al., 2011; Filali et al., 2012) and disruption of the cholinergic system (Apelt et al., 2002; Klingner et al., 2003; Luth et al., 2003) because of its well-known role in behavioral inhibition (and disruption in several of the AD mouse lines) have been proposed as underlying causes of this behavioral abnormality. The temporal time course of these anxiety-like disturbances can vary depending on the mouse model. For example, in some models the behavioral disturbances start early at 1–2 months of age or 3–6 months of age for the J20 and the APP/PS1 models, respectively (Lalonde et al., 2004; Reiserer et al., 2007; Harris et al., 2010). Other models such as the TG2576 develop the anxiety-like disturbances later at the age of 9–11 months of age (Gil-Bea et al., 2007). It is also important to note that not all murine AD models exhibit anxiety disturbances (Arendash et al., 2001b; Lalonde et al., 2002; Webster et al., 2013). Still, the majority of models do display these disturbances and the prevailing thought is that this behavioral phenotype of disinhibition may be akin to the disinhibition seen in AD patients (exemplified by unacceptable behavior and inappropriate euphoria) (Daffner et al., 1992; Chung and Cummings, 2000).

AGGRESSIVE BEHAVIORS

Increased aggressive behaviors are another common behavioral symptom of AD and present themselves in as much as 65% of AD patients (Burns et al., 1990b). As with other non-cognitive behavioral symptoms of AD, increased aggression can be emotionally stressful to both the patient and caregivers (Murman et al., 2002a,b). The exact mechanism that underlies these increased aggressive behaviors is not known but proposed mechanisms deal with dysregulation of different neurotransmitter systems such as serotonin, norepinephrine, dopamine, and GABA (Arsland, 1995; Meltzer et al., 1998). Many AD mouse models also display increased aggressive behavior (Moechars et al., 1996, 1998; Van Dorpe et al., 2000; Ambree et al., 2006; Vloeberghs et al., 2006; Pugh et al., 2007; Alexander et al., 2011). For example, in the TG2576 mouse increased aggressive behaviors display themselves in both the frequency of attacks on other home cage mice as well as on the latency to first attack when interacting with a novel mouse (Alexander et al., 2011). The APP23 mouse model of AD also shows increased aggressive behaviors (Vloeberghs et al., 2006). These aggressive disruptions appear to develop later than the onset of cognitive deficits in this model (Kelly et al., 2003; Van Dam et al., 2003; Vloeberghs et al., 2006). The aggression alterations in the APP23 model appear by 6 months of age (after amyloid pathology and behavioral deficits) and seem to remain relatively constant throughout the rest of the course of disease (Vloeberghs et al., 2006). This suggests that perhaps aggressive deficits correlate best with moderate to severe stages of the disease, which is also what is observed clinically in human AD (Senanarong et al., 2004).

DEPRESSIVE SYMPTOMS

Depressive symptoms/behaviors are a very common comorbidity with AD. The exact prevalence of this comorbidity is not known but is believed to range from as low as 2% to as high as 85% (variability likely due to methods of assessment, diagnostic criteria, stage of AD participants, and other factors) (Mendez et al., 1990; Burns et al., 1990a; Migliorelli et al., 1995a,b; Devanand et al., 1996; Cummings, 2000; Apostolova and Cummings, 2008). Numerous meta-analysis studies have linked depression and AD (Chen et al., 1999; Charlson and Peterson, 2002; Ownby et al., 2006; Lenoir et al., 2011; Diniz et al., 2013), and several even consider late-life depression a significant risk factor for future development of AD (Butters et al., 2000, 2008; Diniz et al., 2013). Generally, depressive symptoms precede the onset of AD (Devanand et al., 1996) and usually worsen with the progression of the disease (Mega et al., 1996). Similarly, patients with a history of depression prior to a diagnosis of AD are much more likely to experience depressive episodes in the course of AD (Pearlson et al., 1990; Strauss and Ogrocki, 1996). Despite this well documented connection between depression and AD and having a wide range of potentially applicable tools to study depression in animal models (Seligman et al., 1975; Jolly et al., 1999; Song and Leonard, 2005; Flint and Shifman, 2008; Nestler and Hyman, 2010), very little work has been devoted to determining the range of depressive behavioral symptoms in the commonly used mouse models of AD. Depressive-like behaviors have been reported in at least one mouse model of AD (Filali et al., 2009), and likely exist in many of the other commonly used models.

CONCLUSIONS

No one animal model fully replicates the pathogenesis of AD, but rather only model different aspects of the disease. Consequently, no one model recapitulates all of the cognitive deficits observed in human AD. Further, the anatomical makeup and cognitive ability of mice make it difficult to model all of the intricacies of higher-order cognitive function exclusive to humans. Instead, each mouse model allows us insight into different aspects of cognition related to AD. Several important points should be taken away from the preceding discussion of the temporal development of cognitive deficits in the various mouse models of AD. First, the temporal time course and progression of cognitive deficits in a specific cognitive domain/behavioral task can be quite different among the different mouse models. Investigators should use careful forethought in selection of an optimal model and planning experiments based on the progression of that model's specific deficits. Secondly, most models display deficits in spatial working memory earlier than the deficits in other cognitive domains. Similarly, most of the studies using mouse models of AD have focused on understanding/correcting the cognitive deficits associated with the disease. However, AD is not just a memory disorder, rather it is a complex disease with many different non-cognitive neuropsychiatric symptoms which are an important source of distress and a psychological burden on family members and caregivers alike. These non-cognitive symptoms are present across many of the different mouse models of AD and more emphasis should be placed on understanding/correcting these deficits, as well as the cognitive aspects of the disease. It is our hope that this comprehensive review of the spectrum of behavioral deficits present in commonly used AD mouse models and how well they model human cognitive and non-cognitive symptoms will assist investigators in selecting an appropriate mouse model to investigate different aspects of AD pathology and disease progression.

ACKNOWLEDGMENTS

Research in our laboratories is supported by funds from the National Institutes of Health (National Institute on Aging, National Institute of Neurological Disorders and Stroke, National Institute of Child Health and Human Development, and National Institute of Nursing Research).

REFERENCES

Abner, E. L., Kryscio, R. J., Schmitt, F. A., Santacruz, K. S., Jicha, G. A., Lin, Y., et al. (2011). "End-stage" neurofibrillary tangle pathology in preclinical Alzheimer's disease: fact or fiction? *J. Alzheimers Dis.* 25, 445–453. doi: 10.3233/JAD-2011-101980

Aevarsson, O., and Skoog, I. (2000). A longitudinal population study of the mini-mental state examination in the very old: relation to dementia and education. *Dement. Geriatr. Cogn. Disord.* 11, 166–175. doi: 10.1159/000017231

Alamed, J., Wilcock, D. M., Diamond, D. M., Gordon, M. N., and Morgan, D. (2006). Two-day radial-arm water maze learning and memory task; robust resolution of amyloid-related memory deficits in transgenic mice. *Nat. Protoc.* 1, 1671–1679. doi: 10.1038/nprot.2006.275

Albert, M. S. (1996). Cognitive and neurobiologic markers of early Alzheimer disease. *Proc. Natl. Acad. Sci. U.S.A.* 93, 13547–13551. doi: 10.1073/pnas.93.24.13547

Alexander, G., Hanna, A., Serna, V., Younkin, L., Younkin, S., and Janus, C. (2011). Increased aggression in males in transgenic Tg2576 mouse model of Alzheimer's disease. *Behav. Brain Res.* 216, 77–83. doi: 10.1016/j.bbr.2010.07.016

Ambree, O., Richter, H., Sachser, N., Lewejohann, L., Dere, E., De Souza Silva, M. A., et al. (2009). Levodopa ameliorates learning and memory deficits in a murine model of Alzheimer's disease. *Neurobiol. Aging* 30, 1192–1204. doi: 10.1016/j.neurobiolaging.2007.11.010

Ambree, O., Touma, C., Gortz, N., Keyvani, K., Paulus, W., Palme, R., et al. (2006). Activity changes and marked stereotypic behavior precede Abeta pathology in TgCRND8 Alzheimer mice. *Neurobiol. Aging* 27, 955–964. doi: 10.1016/j.neurobiolaging.2005.05.009

Ancoli-Israel, S., Parker, L., Sinaee, R., Fell, R. L., and Kripke, D. F. (1989). Sleep fragmentation in patients from a nursing home. *J. Gerontol.* 44, M18–M21. doi: 10.1093/geronj/44.1.M18

Angelo, M., Plattner, F., Irvine, E. E., and Giese, K. P. (2003). Improved reversal learning and altered fear conditioning in transgenic mice with regionally restricted p25 expression. *Eur. J. Neurosci.* 18, 423–431. doi: 10.1046/j.1460-9568.2003.02746.x

Apelt, J., Kumar, A., and Schliebs, R. (2002). Impairment of cholinergic neurotransmission in adult and aged transgenic Tg2576 mouse brain expressing the Swedish mutation of human beta-amyloid precursor protein. *Brain Res.* 953, 17–30. doi: 10.1016/S0006-8993(02)03262-6

Apostolova, L. G., and Cummings, J. L. (2008). Neuropsychiatric manifestations in mild cognitive impairment: a systematic review of the literature. *Dement. Geriatr. Cogn. Disord.* 25, 115–126. doi: 10.1159/000112509

Arendash, G. W., Gordon, M. N., Diamond, D. M., Austin, L. A., Hatcher, J. M., Jantzen, P., et al. (2001a). Behavioral assessment of Alzheimer's transgenic mice following long-term Abeta vaccination: task specificity and correlations between Abeta deposition and spatial memory. *DNA Cell Biol.* 20, 737–744. doi: 10.1089/10445490152717604

Arendash, G. W., King, D. L., Gordon, M. N., Morgan, D., Hatcher, J. M., Hope, C. E., et al. (2001b). Progressive, age-related behavioral impairments in transgenic mice carrying both mutant amyloid precursor protein and presenilin-1 transgenes. *Brain Res.* 891, 42–53. doi: 10.1016/S0006-8993(00)03186-3

Arendash, G. W., Lewis, J., Leighty, R. E., Mcgowan, E., Cracchiolo, J. R., Hutton, M., et al. (2004). Multi-metric behavioral comparison of APPsw and P301L models for Alzheimer's disease: linkage of poorer cognitive performance to tau pathology in forebrain. *Brain Res.* 1012, 29–41. doi: 10.1016/j.brainres.2004.02.081

Arnett, P. A., Rao, S. M., Bernardin, L., Grafman, J., Yetkin, F. Z., and Lobeck, L. (1994). Relationship between frontal lobe lesions and Wisconsin Card Sorting Test performance in patients with multiple sclerosis. *Neurology* 44, 420–425. doi: 10.1212/WNL.44.3_Part_1.420

Arriagada, P. V., Growdon, J. H., Hedley-Whyte, E. T., and Hyman, B. T. (1992). Neurofibrillary tangles but not senile plaques parallel duration and severity of Alzheimer's disease. *Neurology* 42, 631–639. doi: 10.1212/WNL.42.3.631

Arsenault, D., Julien, C., Tremblay, C., and Calon, F. (2011). DHA improves cognition and prevents dysfunction of entorhinal cortex neurons in 3xTg-AD mice. *PLoS ONE* 6:e17397. doi: 10.1371/journal.pone.0017397

Arsland, D. (1995). Aggressive-behavior in dementia and its pharmacological treatment - a review. *Nord. J. Psychiatry* 49, 111–118. doi: 10.3109/08039489509011892

Ashe, K. H., and Zahs, K. R. (2010). Probing the biology of Alzheimer's disease in mice. *Neuron* 66, 631–645. doi: 10.1016/j.neuron.2010.04.031

Auld, D. S., Kornecook, T. J., Bastianetto, S., and Quirion, R. (2002). Alzheimer's disease and the basal forebrain cholinergic system: relations to beta-amyloid peptides, cognition, and treatment strategies. *Prog. Neurobiol.* 68, 209–245. doi: 10.1016/S0301-0082(02)00079-5

Backman, L., Jones, S., Berger, A. K., Laukka, E. J., and Small, B. J. (2005). Cognitive impairment in preclinical Alzheimer's disease: a meta-analysis. *Neuropsychology* 19, 520–531. doi: 10.1037/0894-4105.19.4.520

Backman, L., Small, B. J., and Fratiglioni, L. (2001). Stability of the preclinical episodic memory deficit in Alzheimer's disease. *Brain* 124, 96–102. doi: 10.1093/brain/124.1.96

Baddeley, A., Logie, R., Bressi, S., Della Sala, S., and Spinnler, H. (1986). Dementia and working memory. *Q. J. Exp. Psychol. A* 38, 603–618. doi: 10.1080/14640748608401616

Baddeley, A. D., Baddeley, H. A., Bucks, R. S., and Wilcock, G. K. (2001). Attentional control in Alzheimer's disease. *Brain* 124, 1492–1508. doi: 10.1093/brain/124.8.1492

Baddeley, A. D., Bressi, S., Della Sala, S., Logie, R., and Spinnler, H. (1991). The decline of working memory in Alzheimer's disease. A longitudinal study. *Brain* 114(Pt 6), 2521–2542. doi: 10.1093/brain/114.6.2521

Bari, A., Dalley, J. W., and Robbins, T. W. (2008). The application of the 5-choice serial reaction time task for the assessment of visual attentional processes and impulse control in rats. *Nat. Protoc.* 3, 759–767. doi: 10.1038/nprot.2008.41

Barnes, C. A. (1979). Memory deficits associated with senescence: a neurophysiological and behavioral study in the rat. *J. Comp. Physiol. Psychol.* 93, 74–104. doi: 10.1037/h0077579

Beach, T. G., Adler, C. H., Lue, L., Sue, L. I., Bachalakuri, J., Henry-Watson, J., et al. (2009). Unified staging system for Lewy body disorders: correlation with nigrostriatal degeneration, cognitive impairment and motor dysfunction. *Acta Neuropathol.* 117, 613–634. doi: 10.1007/s00401-009-0538-8

Beck, L. H., Bransome, E. D. Jr., Mirsky, A. F., Rosvold, H. E., and Sarason, I. (1956). A continuous performance test of brain damage. *J. Consult. Psychol.* 20, 343–350. doi: 10.1037/h0043220

Bedrosian, T. A., Herring, K. L., Weil, Z. M., and Nelson, R. J. (2011). Altered temporal patterns of anxiety in aged and amyloid precursor protein (APP) transgenic mice. *Proc. Natl. Acad. Sci. USA.* 108, 11686–11691. doi: 10.1073/pnas.1103098108

Benedict, R. H. B., and Groninger, L. (1994). Preliminary standardization and validation of a multiple-form test for the assessment of visuospatial memory. *Arch. Clin. Neuropsychol.* 9, 109–110.

Benedict, R. H. B., Schretlen, D., Groninger, L., and Brandt, J. (1998). Hopkins verbal learning test revised: normative data and analysis of inter-form and test-retest reliability. *Clin. Neuropsychol.* 12, 43–55. doi: 10.1076/clin.12.1.43.1726

Bennett, D. A., Schneider, J. A., Wilson, R. S., Bienias, J. L., and Arnold, S. E. (2004). Neurofibrillary tangles mediate the association of amyloid load with clinical Alzheimer disease and level of cognitive function. *Arch. Neurol.* 61, 378–384. doi: 10.1001/archneur.61.3.378

Benton, A. L. (1992). *Benton Visual Retention Test, 5th Edn.* San Antonio, TX: The Psychological Corporation.

Berg, L., Mckeel, D. W. Jr., Miller, J. P., Storandt, M., Rubin, E. H., Morris, J. C., et al. (1998). Clinicopathologic studies in cognitively healthy aging and Alzheimer's disease: relation of histologic markers to dementia severity, age, sex, and apolipoprotein E genotype. *Arch. Neurol.* 55, 326–335. doi: 10.1001/archneur.55.3.326

Berlau, D. J., Kahle-Wrobleski, K., Head, E., Goodus, M., Kim, R., and Kawas, C. (2007). Dissociation of neuropathologic findings and cognition: case report of an apolipoprotein E epsilon2/epsilon2 genotype. *Arch. Neurol.* 64, 1193–1196. doi: 10.1001/archneur.64.8.1193

Berman, K. F., Ostrem, J. L., Randolph, C., Gold, J., Goldberg, T. E., Coppola, R., et al. (1995). Physiological activation of a cortical network during performance of the Wisconsin Card Sorting Test: a positron emission tomography study. *Neuropsychologia* 33, 1027–1046. doi: 10.1016/0028-3932(95)00035-2

Bernardo, A., Harrison, F. E., Mccord, M., Zhao, J., Bruchey, A., Davies, S. S., et al. (2009). Elimination of GD3 synthase improves memory and reduces amyloid-beta plaque load in transgenic mice. *Neurobiol. Aging* 30, 1777–1791. doi: 10.1016/j.neurobiolaging.2007.12.022

Bernick, C., Cummings, J., Raman, R., Sun, X., and Aisen, P. (2012). Age and rate of cognitive decline in Alzheimer disease: implications for clinical trials. *Arch. Neurol.* 69, 901–905. doi: 10.1001/archneurol.2011.3758

Bierer, L. M., Hof, P. R., Purohit, D. P., Carlin, L., Schmeidler, J., Davis, K. L., et al. (1995). Neocortical neurofibrillary tangles correlate with dementia severity in Alzheimer's disease. *Arch. Neurol.* 52, 81–88. doi: 10.1001/archneur.1995.00540250089017

Billings, L. M., Oddo, S., Green, K. N., Mcgaugh, J. L., and Laferla, F. M. (2005). Intraneuronal Abeta causes the onset of early Alzheimer's disease-related cognitive deficits in transgenic mice. *Neuron* 45, 675–688. doi: 10.1016/j.neuron.2005.01.040

Birrell, J. M., and Brown, V. J. (2000). Medial frontal cortex mediates perceptual attentional set shifting in the rat. *J. Neurosci.* 20, 4320–4324. Available online at: http://www.jneurosci.org/content/20/11/4320.long

Bissonette, G. B., Martins, G. J., Franz, T. M., Harper, E. S., Schoenbaum, G., and Powell, E. M. (2008). Double dissociation of the effects of medial and orbital prefrontal cortical lesions on attentional and affective shifts in mice. *J. Neurosci.* 28, 11124–11130. doi: 10.1523/JNEUROSCI.2820-08.2008

Blennow, K., and Zetterberg, H. (2013). The application of cerebrospinal fluid biomarkers in early diagnosis of Alzheimer disease. *Med. Clin. North Am.* 97, 369–376. doi: 10.1016/j.mcna.2012.12.012

Blessed, G., Tomlinson, B. E., and Roth, M. (1968). The association between quantitative measures of dementia and of senile change in the cerebral grey matter of elderly subjects. *Br. J. Psychiatry* 114, 797–811. doi: 10.1192/bjp.114.512.797

Bliwise, D. L. (1994). What is sundowning? *J. Am. Geriatr. Soc.* 42, 1009–1011.

Blodgett, H. C., and Mccutchan, K. (1947). Place versus response learning in the simple T-maze. *J. Exp. Psychol.* 37, 412–422. doi: 10.1037/h0059305

Bondi, M. W., Jak, A. J., Delano-Wood, L., Jacobson, M. W., Delis, D. C., and Salmon, D. P. (2008). Neuropsychological contributions to the early identification of Alzheimer's disease. *Neuropsychol. Rev.* 18, 73–90. doi: 10.1007/s11065-008-9054-1

Bondi, M. W., Salmon, D. P., Galasko, D., Thomas, R. G., and Thal, L. J. (1999). Neuropsychological function and apolipoprotein E genotype in the preclinical detection of Alzheimer's disease. *Psychol. Aging* 14, 295–303. doi: 10.1037/0882-7974.14.2.295

Bondi, M. W., Salmon, D. P., Monsch, A. U., Galasko, D., Butters, N., Klauber, M. R., et al. (1995). Episodic memory changes are associated with the APOE-epsilon 4 allele in nondemented older adults. *Neurology* 45, 2203–2206. doi: 10.1212/WNL.45.12.2203

Braak, H., and Del Tredici, K. (2011). The pathological process underlying Alzheimer's disease in individuals under thirty. *Acta Neuropathol.* 121, 171–181. doi: 10.1007/s00401-010-0789-4

Braak, H., Thal, D. R., Ghebremedhin, E., and Del Tredici, K. (2011). Stages of the pathologic process in Alzheimer disease: age categories from 1 to 100 years. *J. Neuropathol. Exp. Neurol.* 70, 960–969. doi: 10.1097/NEN.0b013e318232a379

Brayne, C., Richardson, K., Matthews, F. E., Fleming, J., Hunter, S., Xuereb, J. H., et al. (2009). Neuropathological correlates of dementia in over-80-year-old brain donors from the population-based Cambridge city over-75s cohort (CC75C) study. *J. Alzheimers Dis.* 18, 645–658. doi: 10.3233/JAD-2009-1182

Brigman, J. L., Bussey, T. J., Saksida, L. M., and Rothblat, L. A. (2005). Discrimination of multidimensional visual stimuli by mice: intra- and extradimensional shifts. *Behav. Neurosci.* 119, 839–842. doi: 10.1037/0735-7044.119.3.839

Bruce-Keller, A. J., Gupta, S., Knight, A. G., Beckett, T. L., Mcmullen, J. M., Davis, P. R., et al. (2011). Cognitive impairment in humanized APPxPS1 mice is linked to Abeta (1-42) and NOX activation. *Neurobiol. Dis.* 44, 317–326. doi: 10.1016/j.nbd.2011.07.012

Buccafusco, J. J., Terry, A. V. Jr., Webster, S. J., Martin, D., Hohnadel, E. J., Bouchard, K. A., et al. (2008). The scopolamine-reversal paradigm in rats and monkeys: the importance of computer-assisted operant-conditioning memory tasks for screening drug candidates. *Psychopharmacology (Berl.)* 199, 481–494. doi: 10.1007/s00213-007-0887-8

Budson, A. E., and Price, B. H. (2005). Memory dysfunction. *N. Engl. J. Med.* 352, 692–699. doi: 10.1056/NEJMra041071

Burns, A., Jacoby, R., and Levy, R. (1990a). Psychiatric phenomena in Alzheimer's disease. II: Disorders of perception. *Br. J. Psychiatry* 157, 76–81, 92–74.

Burns, A., Jacoby, R., and Levy, R. (1990b). Psychiatric phenomena in Alzheimer's disease. IV: Disorders of behaviour. *Br. J. Psychiatry* 157, 86–94. doi: 10.1192/bjp.157.1.86

Bussey, T. J., Holmes, A., Lyon, L., Mar, A. C., Mcallister, K. A., Nithianantharajah, J., et al. (2012). New translational assays for preclinical modelling of cognition in schizophrenia: the touchscreen testing method for mice and rats. *Neuropharmacology* 62, 1191–1203. doi: 10.1016/j.neuropharm.2011.04.011

Bussey, T. J., Muir, J. L., Everitt, B. J., and Robbins, T. W. (1997). Triple dissociation of anterior cingulate, posterior cingulate, and medial frontal cortices on visual discrimination tasks using a touchscreen testing procedure for the rat. *Behav. Neurosci.* 111, 920–936. doi: 10.1037/0735-7044.111.5.920

Butter, C. M. (1969). Perseveration in extinction and in discrimination reversal tasks following selective frontal ablations in *Macaca mulatta*. *Physiol. Behav.* 4, 163–171. doi: 10.1016/0031-9384(69)90075-4

Butters, M. A., Becker, J. T., Nebes, R. D., Zmuda, M. D., Mulsant, B. H., Pollock, B. G. 3rd., et al. (2000). Changes in cognitive functioning following treatment of late-life depression. *Am. J. Psychiatry* 157, 1949–1954. doi: 10.1176/appi.ajp.157.12.1949

Butters, M. A., Young, J. B., Lopez, O., Aizenstein, H. J., Mulsant, B. H., Reynolds, C. F., et al. (2008). Pathways linking late-life depression to persistent cognitive impairment and dementia. *Dialogues Clin. Neurosci.* 10, 345–357.

Campion, D., Dumanchin, C., Hannequin, D., Dubois, B., Belliard, S., Puel, M., et al. (1999). Early-onset autosomal dominant Alzheimer disease: prevalence, genetic heterogeneity, and mutation spectrum. *Am. J. Hum. Genet.* 65, 664–670. doi: 10.1086/302553

Cao, D., Lu, H., Lewis, T. L., and Li, L. (2007). Intake of sucrose-sweetened water induces insulin resistance and exacerbates memory deficits and amyloidosis in a transgenic mouse model of Alzheimer disease. *J. Biol. Chem.* 282, 36275–36282. doi: 10.1074/jbc.M703561200

Carli, M., Robbins, T. W., Evenden, J. L., and Everitt, B. J. (1983). Effects of lesions to ascending noradrenergic neurones on performance of a 5-choice serial reaction task in rats; implications for theories of dorsal noradrenergic bundle function based on selective attention and arousal. *Behav. Brain Res.* 9, 361–380. doi: 10.1016/0166-4328(83)90138-9

Carpenter, C. R., Bassett, E. R., Fischer, G. M., Shirshekan, J., Galvin, J. E., and Morris, J. C. (2011). Four sensitive screening tools to detect cognitive dysfunction in geriatric emergency department patients: brief Alzheimer's Screen, Short Blessed Test, Ottawa 3DY, and the caregiver-completed AD8. *Acad. Emerg. Med.* 18, 374–384. doi: 10.1111/j.1553-2712.2011.01040.x

Carroll, J. C., Rosario, E. R., Chang, L., Stanczyk, F. Z., Oddo, S., Laferla, F. M., et al. (2007). Progesterone and estrogen regulate Alzheimer-like neuropathology in female 3xTg-AD mice. *J. Neurosci.* 27, 13357–13365. doi: 10.1523/JNEUROSCI.2718-07.2007

Chapman, P. F., White, G. L., Jones, M. W., Cooper-Blacketer, D., Marshall, V. J., Irizarry, M., et al. (1999). Impaired synaptic plasticity and learning in aged amyloid precursor protein transgenic mice. *Nat. Neurosci.* 2, 271–276. doi: 10.1038/6374

Charlson, M., and Peterson, J. C. (2002). Medical comorbidity and late life depression: what is known and what are the unmet needs? *Biol. Psychiatry* 52, 226–235. doi: 10.1016/S0006-3223(02)01422-1

Chartier-Harlin, M. C., Crawford, F., Houlden, H., Warren, A., Hughes, D., Fidani, L., et al. (1991). Early-onset Alzheimer's disease caused by mutations at codon 717 of the beta-amyloid precursor protein gene. *Nature* 353, 844–846. doi: 10.1038/353844a0

Chatfield, M., Matthews, F. E., Brayne, C., Medical Research Council Cognitive, F., and Ageing, S. (2007). Using the Mini-Mental State Examination for tracking cognition in the older population based on longitudinal data. *J. Am. Geriatr. Soc.* 55, 1066–1071. doi: 10.1111/j.1532-5415.2007.01216.x

Chen, G., Chen, K. S., Knox, J., Inglis, J., Bernard, A., Martin, S. J., et al. (2000). A learning deficit related to age and beta-amyloid plaques in a mouse model of Alzheimer's disease. *Nature* 408, 975–979. doi: 10.1038/35046031

Chen, P., Ganguli, M., Mulsant, B. H., and Dekosky, S. T. (1999). The temporal relationship between depressive symptoms and dementia: a community-based prospective study. *Arch. Gen. Psychiatry* 56, 261–266. doi: 10.1001/archpsyc.56.3.261

Cheng, D., Low, J. K., Logge, W., Garner, B., and Karl, T. (2013). Novel behavioural characteristics of female APP/PS1DeltaE9 double transgenic mice. *Behav. Brain Res.* 260, 111–118. doi: 10.1016/j.bbr.2013.11.046

Cheng, I. H., Scearce-Levie, K., Legleiter, J., Palop, J. J., Gerstein, H., Bien-Ly, N., et al. (2007). Accelerating amyloid-beta fibrillization reduces oligomer levels and functional deficits in Alzheimer disease mouse models. *J. Biol. Chem.* 282, 23818–23828. doi: 10.1074/jbc.M701078200

Chishti, M. A., Yang, D. S., Janus, C., Phinney, A. L., Horne, P., Pearson, J., et al. (2001). Early-onset amyloid deposition and cognitive deficits in transgenic mice expressing a double mutant form of amyloid precursor protein 695. *J. Biol. Chem.* 276, 21562–21570. doi: 10.1074/jbc.M100710200

Chudasama, Y. (2011). Animal models of prefrontal-executive function. *Behav. Neurosci.* 125, 327–343. doi: 10.1037/a0023766

Chung, J. A., and Cummings, J. L. (2000). Neurobehavioral and neuropsychiatric symptoms in Alzheimer's disease: characteristics and treatment. *Neurol. Clin.* 18, 829–846. doi: 10.1016/S0733-8619(05)70228-0

Cisse, M., Sanchez, P. E., Kim, D. H., Ho, K., Yu, G. Q., and Mucke, L. (2011). Ablation of cellular prion protein does not ameliorate abnormal neural network activity or cognitive dysfunction in the J20 line of human amyloid precursor protein transgenic mice. *J. Neurosci.* 31, 10427–10431. doi: 10.1523/JNEUROSCI.1459-11.2011

Clayton, N. S., and Dickinson, A. (1998). Episodic-like memory during cache recovery by scrub jays. *Nature* 395, 272–274. doi: 10.1038/26216

Clayton, N. S., Griffiths, D. P., Emery, N. J., and Dickinson, A. (2001). Elements of episodic-like memory in animals. *Philos. Trans. R. Soc. Lond. B Biol. Sci.* 356, 1483–1491. doi: 10.1098/rstb.2001.0947

Clinton, L. K., Billings, L. M., Green, K. N., Caccamo, A., Ngo, J., Oddo, S., et al. (2007). Age-dependent sexual dimorphism in cognition and stress response in the 3xTg-AD mice. *Neurobiol. Dis.* 28, 76–82. doi: 10.1016/j.nbd.2007.06.013

Collie, A., and Maruff, P. (2000). The neuropsychology of preclinical Alzheimer's disease and mild cognitive impairment. *Neurosci. Biobehav. Rev.* 24, 365–374. doi: 10.1016/S0149-7634(00)00012-9

Connor, D. J., and Sabbagh, M. N. (2008). Administration and scoring variance on the ADAS-Cog. *J. Alzheimers Dis.* 15, 461–464.

Corcoran, K. A., Lu, Y., Turner, R. S., and Maren, S. (2002). Overexpression of hAPPswe impairs rewarded alternation and contextual fear conditioning in a transgenic mouse model of Alzheimer's disease. *Learn. Mem.* 9, 243–252. doi: 10.1101/lm.51002

Cramer, P. E., Cirrito, J. R., Wesson, D. W., Lee, C. Y., Karlo, J. C., Zinn, A. E., et al. (2012). ApoE-directed therapeutics rapidly clear beta-amyloid and reverse deficits in AD mouse models. *Science* 335, 1503–1506. doi: 10.1126/science.1217697

Crusio, W. E., Schwegler, H., and Brust, I. (1993). Covariations between hippocampal mossy fibres and working and reference memory in spatial and non-spatial radial maze tasks in mice. *Eur. J. Neurosci.* 5, 1413–1420. doi: 10.1111/j.1460-9568.1993.tb00927.x

Crystal, H. A., Dickson, D. W., Sliwinski, M. J., Lipton, R. B., Grober, E., Marks-Nelson, H., et al. (1993). Pathological markers associated with normal aging and dementia in the elderly. *Ann. Neurol.* 34, 566–573. doi: 10.1002/ana.410340410

Cummings, B. J., Pike, C. J., Shankle, R., and Cotman, C. W. (1996). Beta-amyloid deposition and other measures of neuropathology predict cognitive status in Alzheimer's disease. *Neurobiol. Aging* 17, 921–933. doi: 10.1016/S0197-4580(96)00170-4

Cummings, J. L. (2000). Cognitive and behavioral heterogeneity in Alzheimer's disease: seeking the neurobiological basis. *Neurobiol. Aging* 21, 845–861. doi: 10.1016/S0197-4580(00)00183-4

Curzon, P., Rustay, N. R., and Browman, K. E. (2009). "Cued and Contextual Fear Conditioning for Rodents," in *Methods of Behavior Analysis in Neuroscience, Chapter 2, 2nd Edn.* ed J. J. Buccafusco (Boca Raton, FL: CRC Press), 26–49.

Daffner, K. R., Scinto, L. F., Weintraub, S., Guinessey, J. E., and Mesulam, M. M. (1992). Diminished curiosity in patients with probable Alzheimer's disease as measured by exploratory eye movements. *Neurology* 42, 320–328. doi: 10.1212/WNL.42.2.320

Daumas, S., Sandin, J., Chen, K. S., Kobayashi, D., Tulloch, J., Martin, S. J., et al. (2008). Faster forgetting contributes to impaired spatial memory in the PDAPP mouse: deficit in memory retrieval associated with increased sensitivity to interference? *Learn. Mem.* 15, 625–632. doi: 10.1101/lm.990208

Davis, K. E., Eacott, M. J., Easton, A., and Gigg, J. (2013a). Episodic-like memory is sensitive to both Alzheimer's-like pathological accumulation and normal ageing processes in mice. *Behav. Brain Res.* 254, 73–82. doi: 10.1016/j.bbr.2013.03.009

Davis, K. E., Easton, A., Eacott, M. J., and Gigg, J. (2013b). Episodic-like memory for what-where-which occasion is selectively impaired in the 3xTgAD mouse model of Alzheimer's disease. *J. Alzheimers Dis.* 33, 681–698. doi: 10.3233/JAD-2012-121543

Davis, P. C., Gearing, M., Gray, L., Mirra, S. S., Morris, J. C., Edland, S. D., et al. (1995). The CERAD experience, Part VIII: neuroimaging-neuropathology correlates of temporal lobe changes in Alzheimer's disease. *Neurology* 45, 178–179. doi: 10.1212/WNL.45.1.178

De Bruin, N. M., Fransen, F., Duytschaever, H., Grantham, C., and Megens, A. A. (2006). Attentional performance of (C57BL/6Jx129Sv) F2 mice in the five-choice serial reaction time task. *Physiol. Behav.* 89, 692–703. doi: 10.1016/j.physbeh.2006.08.009

Delis, D. C., Kaplan, E., Kramer, J. H., and Ober, B. A. (2000). *California Verbal Learning Test - Second Edition (CVLT - II) Manual.* San Antonio, TX: Psychological Corperation.

Devanand, D. P., Sano, M., Tang, M. X., Taylor, S., Gurland, B. J., Wilder, D., et al. (1996). Depressed mood and the incidence of Alzheimer's disease in the elderly living in the community. *Arch. Gen. Psychiatry* 53, 175–182. doi: 10.1001/archpsyc.1996.01830020093011

Devi, L., and Ohno, M. (2010). Genetic reductions of beta-site amyloid precursor protein-cleaving enzyme 1 and amyloid-beta ameliorate impairment of conditioned taste aversion memory in 5XFAD Alzheimer's disease model mice. *Eur. J. Neurosci.* 31, 110–118. doi: 10.1111/j.1460-9568.2009.07031.x

Devi, L., and Ohno, M. (2012). Mitochondrial dysfunction and accumulation of the beta-secretase-cleaved C-terminal fragment of APP in Alzheimer's disease transgenic mice. *Neurobiol. Dis.* 45, 417–424. doi: 10.1016/j.nbd.2011.09.001

Diamond, D. M., Park, C. R., Heman, K. L., and Rose, G. M. (1999). Exposing rats to a predator impairs spatial working memory in the radial arm water maze. *Hippocampus* 9, 542–552.

Dickson, D. W., Crystal, H. A., Bevona, C., Honer, W., Vincent, I., and Davies, P. (1995). Correlations of synaptic and pathological markers with cognition of the elderly. *Neurobiol. Aging* 16, 285–298. discussion: 298–304. doi: 10.1016/0197-4580(95)00013-5

Dineley, K. T., Xia, X., Bui, D., Sweatt, J. D., and Zheng, H. (2002). Accelerated plaque accumulation, associative learning deficits, and up-regulation of alpha 7 nicotinic receptor protein in transgenic mice co-expressing mutant human presenilin 1 and amyloid precursor proteins. *J. Biol. Chem.* 277, 22768–22780. doi: 10.1074/jbc.M200164200

Ding, Y., Qiao, A., Wang, Z., Goodwin, J. S., Lee, E. S., Block, M. L., et al. (2008). Retinoic acid attenuates beta-amyloid deposition and rescues memory deficits in an Alzheimer's disease transgenic mouse model. *J. Neurosci.* 28, 11622–11634. doi: 10.1523/JNEUROSCI.3153-08.2008

Diniz, B. S., Butters, M. A., Albert, S. M., Dew, M. A., and Reynolds, C. F. 3rd. (2013). Late-life depression and risk of vascular dementia and Alzheimer's disease: systematic review and meta-analysis of community-based cohort studies. *Br. J. Psychiatry* 202, 329–335. doi: 10.1192/bjp.bp.112.118307

Dodart, J. C., Bales, K. R., Gannon, K. S., Greene, S. J., Demattos, R. B., Mathis, C., et al. (2002). Immunization reverses memory deficits without reducing brain Abeta burden in Alzheimer's disease model. *Nat. Neurosci.* 5, 452–457. doi: 10.1038/nn842

Dodart, J. C., Meziane, H., Mathis, C., Bales, K. R., Paul, S. M., and Ungerer, A. (1999). Behavioral disturbances in transgenic mice overexpressing the V717F beta-amyloid precursor protein. *Behav. Neurosci.* 113, 982–990. doi: 10.1037/0735-7044.113.5.982

Dong, H., Csernansky, C. A., Martin, M. V., Bertchume, A., Vallera, D., and Csernansky, J. G. (2005). Acetylcholinesterase inhibitors ameliorate behavioral deficits in the Tg2576 mouse model of Alzheimer's disease. *Psychopharmacology (Berl.)* 181, 145–152. doi: 10.1007/s00213-005-2230-6

Drewe, E. A. (1974). The effect of type and area of brain lesion on Wisconsin card sorting test performance. *Cortex* 10, 159–170. doi: 10.1016/S0010-9452(74)80006-7

Du, H., Guo, L., Zhang, W., Rydzewska, M., and Yan, S. (2011). Cyclophilin D deficiency improves mitochondrial function and learning/memory in aging Alzheimer disease mouse model. *Neurobiol. Aging* 32, 398–406. doi: 10.1016/j.neurobiolaging.2009.03.003

Dudchenko, P. A. (2004). An overview of the tasks used to test working memory in rodents. *Neurosci. Biobehav. Rev.* 28, 699–709. doi: 10.1016/j.neubiorev.2004.09.002

Dumont, M., Strazielle, C., Staufenbiel, M., and Lalonde, R. (2004). Spatial learning and exploration of environmental stimuli in 24-month-old female APP23 transgenic mice with the Swedish mutation. *Brain Res.* 1024, 113–121. doi: 10.1016/j.brainres.2004.07.052

Dunnett, S. B. (1993). The role and repair of forebrain cholinergic systems in short-term memory. Studies using the delayed matching-to-position task in rats. *Adv. Neurol.* 59, 53–65.

Duyckaerts, C., Bennecib, M., Grignon, Y., Uchihara, T., He, Y., Piette, F., et al. (1997). Modeling the relation between neurofibrillary tangles and intellectual status. *Neurobiol. Aging* 18, 267–273. doi: 10.1016/S0197-4580(97)80306-5

Duyckaerts, C., Colle, M. A., Dessi, F., Piette, F., and Hauw, J. J. (1998). Progression of Alzheimer histopathological changes. *Acta Neurol. Belg.* 98, 180–185.

Duyckaerts, C., Delaere, P., Hauw, J. J., Abbamondi-Pinto, A. L., Sorbi, S., Allen, I., et al. (1990). Rating of the lesions in senile dementia of the Alzheimer type: concordance between laboratories. A European multicenter study under the auspices of EURAGE. *J. Neurol. Sci.* 97, 295–323. doi: 10.1016/0022-510X(90)90226-D

Elder, G. A., Gama Sosa, M. A., and De Gasperi, R. (2010). Transgenic mouse models of Alzheimer's disease. *Mt. Sinai J. Med.* 77, 69–81. doi: 10.1002/msj.20159

Emilien, G., Durlach, C., Minaker, K. L., Winblad, B., Gauthier, S., and Maloteaux, J.-M. (2004). *Alzheimer Disease: Neuropsychology and Pharmacology.* Basel: Birkhauser Verlag.

Ennaceur, A., and Delacour, J. (1988). A new one-trial test for neurobiological studies of memory in rats. 1: Behavioral data. *Behav. Brain Res.* 31, 47–59. doi: 10.1016/0166-4328(88)90157-X

Epis, R., Gardoni, F., Marcello, E., Genazzani, A., Canonico, P. L., and Di Luca, M. (2010). Searching for new animal models of Alzheimer's disease. *Eur. J. Pharmacol.* 626, 57–63. doi: 10.1016/j.ejphar.2009.10.020

Eriksen, J. L., and Janus, C. G. (2007). Plaques, tangles, and memory loss in mouse models of neurodegeneration. *Behav. Genet.* 37, 79–100. doi: 10.1007/s10519-006-9118-z

Escribano, L., Simon, A. M., Perez-Mediavilla, A., Salazar-Colocho, P., Del Rio, J., and Frechilla, D. (2009). Rosiglitazone reverses memory decline and hippocampal glucocorticoid receptor down-regulation in an Alzheimer's disease mouse model. *Biochem. Biophys. Res. Commun.* 379, 406–410. doi: 10.1016/j.bbrc.2008.12.071

Espana, J., Gimenez-Llort, L., Valero, J., Minano, A., Rabano, A., Rodriguez-Alvarez, J., et al. (2010). Intraneuronal beta-amyloid accumulation in the amygdala enhances fear and anxiety in Alzheimer's disease transgenic mice. *Biol. Psychiatry* 67, 513–521. doi: 10.1016/j.biopsych.2009.06.015

Fang, F., Chen, X., Huang, T., Lue, L. F., Luddy, J. S., and Yan, S. S. (2012). Multi-faced neuroprotective effects of Ginsenoside Rgl in an Alzheimer mouse model. *Biochim. Biophys. Acta* 1822, 286–292. doi: 10.1016/j.bbadis.2011.10.004

Fanselow, M. S. (1980). Conditioned and unconditional components of post-shock freezing. *Pavlov. J. Biol. Sci.* 15, 177–182.

Filali, M., Lalonde, R., and Rivest, S. (2009). Cognitive and non-cognitive behaviors in an APPswe/PS1 bigenic model of Alzheimer's disease. *Genes Brain Behav.* 8, 143–148. doi: 10.1111/j.1601-183X.2008.00453.x

Filali, M., Lalonde, R., Theriault, P., Julien, C., Calon, F., and Planel, E. (2012). Cognitive and non-cognitive behaviors in the triple transgenic mouse model of Alzheimer's disease expressing mutated APP, PS1, and Mapt (3xTg-AD). *Behav. Brain Res.* 234, 334–342. doi: 10.1016/j.bbr.2012.07.004

Flicker, C., Bartus, R. T., Crook, T. H., and Ferris, S. H. (1984). Effects of aging and dementia upon recent visuospatial memory. *Neurobiol. Aging* 5, 275–283. doi: 10.1016/0197-4580(84)90003-4

Flint, J., and Shifman, S. (2008). Animal models of psychiatric disease. *Curr. Opin. Genet. Dev.* 18, 235–240. doi: 10.1016/j.gde.2008.07.002

Flood, D. G., Reaume, A. G., Dorfman, K. S., Lin, Y. G., Lang, D. M., Trusko, S. P., et al. (2002). FAD mutant PS-1 gene-targeted mice: increased A beta 42 and A beta deposition without APP overproduction. *Neurobiol. Aging* 23, 335–348. doi: 10.1016/S0197-4580(01)00330-X

Folstein, M. F., Folstein, S. E., and Mchugh, P. R. (1975). "Mini-mental state." A practical method for grading the cognitive state of patients for the clinician. *J. Psychiatr. Res.* 12, 189–198. doi: 10.1016/0022-3956(75)90026-6

Fuld, P. (1978). *Psychological Testing in the Differential Diagnosis of the Dementias.* New York, NY: Raven Press.

Galvan, V., Gorostiza, O. F., Banwait, S., Ataie, M., Logvinova, A. V., Sitaraman, S., et al. (2006). Reversal of Alzheimer's-like pathology and behavior in human APP transgenic mice by mutation of Asp664. *Proc. Natl. Acad. Sci. U.S.A.* 103, 7130–7135. doi: 10.1073/pnas.0509695103

Games, D., Adams, D., Alessandrini, R., Barbour, R., Berthelette, P., Blackwell, C., et al. (1995). Alzheimer-type neuropathology in transgenic mice overexpressing V717F beta-amyloid precursor protein. *Nature* 373, 523–527. doi: 10.1038/373523a0

Giannakopoulos, P., Kovari, E., Gold, G., Von Gunten, A., Hof, P. R., and Bouras, C. (2009). Pathological substrates of cognitive decline in Alzheimer's disease. *Front. Neurol. Neurosci.* 24, 20–29. doi: 10.1159/000197881

Gibson, A. P., Bettinger, T. L., Patel, N. C., and Crismon, M. L. (2006). Atomoxetine versus stimulants for treatment of attention deficit/hyperactivity disorder. *Ann. Pharmacother.* 40, 1134–1142. doi: 10.1345/aph.1G582

Gil-Bea, F. J., Aisa, B., Schliebs, R., and Ramirez, M. J. (2007). Increase of locomotor activity underlying the behavioral disinhibition in tg2576 mice. *Behav. Neurosci.* 121, 340–344. doi: 10.1037/0735-7044.121.2.340

Gimenez-Llort, L., Blazquez, G., Canete, T., Johansson, B., Oddo, S., Tobena, A., et al. (2007). Modeling behavioral and neuronal symptoms of Alzheimer's disease in mice: a role for intraneuronal amyloid. *Neurosci. Biobehav. Rev.* 31, 125–147. doi: 10.1016/j.neubiorev.2006.07.007

Glickman, S. E., and Jensen, G. D. (1961). The effects of hunger and thirst on Y-maze exploration. *J. Comp. Physiol. Psychol.* 54, 83–85. doi: 10.1037/h0049301

Gold, G., Bouras, C., Kovari, E., Canuto, A., Glaria, B. G., Malky, A., et al. (2000). Clinical validity of Braak neuropathological staging in the oldest-old. *Acta Neuropathol.* 99, 579–582. discussion: 583–574. doi: 10.1007/s004010051163

Gordon, M. N., King, D. L., Diamond, D. M., Jantzen, P. T., Boyett, K. V., Hope, C. E., et al. (2001). Correlation between cognitive deficits and Abeta deposits in transgenic APP+PS1 mice. *Neurobiol. Aging* 22, 377–385. doi: 10.1016/S0197-4580(00)00249-9

Gortz, N., Lewejohann, L., Tomm, M., Ambree, O., Keyvani, K., Paulus, W., et al. (2008). Effects of environmental enrichment on exploration, anxiety, and memory in female TgCRND8 Alzheimer mice. *Behav. Brain Res.* 191, 43–48. doi: 10.1016/j.bbr.2008.03.006

Graves, L., Pack, A., and Abel, T. (2001). Sleep and memory: a molecular perspective. *Trends Neurosci.* 24, 237–243. doi: 10.1016/S0166-2236(00)01744-6

Griffiths, D. P., and Clayton, N. S. (2001). Testing episodic memory in animals: a new approach. *Physiol. Behav.* 73, 755–762. doi: 10.1016/S0031-9384(01)00532-7

Grober, E., Dickson, D., Sliwinski, M. J., Buschke, H., Katz, M., Crystal, H., et al. (1999). Memory and mental status correlates of modified Braak staging. *Neurobiol. Aging* 20, 573–579. doi: 10.1016/S0197-4580(99)00063-9

Guillozet, A. L., Weintraub, S., Mash, D. C., and Mesulam, M. M. (2003). Neurofibrillary tangles, amyloid, and memory in aging and mild cognitive impairment. *Arch. Neurol.* 60, 729–736. doi: 10.1001/archneur.60.5.729

Halagappa, V. K., Guo, Z., Pearson, M., Matsuoka, Y., Cutler, R. G., Laferla, F. M., et al. (2007). Intermittent fasting and caloric restriction ameliorate age-related behavioral deficits in the triple-transgenic mouse model of Alzheimer's disease. *Neurobiol. Dis.* 26, 212–220. doi: 10.1016/j.nbd.2006.12.019

Hall, A. M., and Roberson, E. D. (2012). Mouse models of Alzheimer's disease. *Brain Res. Bull.* 88, 3–12. doi: 10.1016/j.brainresbull.2011.11.017

Hanna, A., Horne, P., Yager, D., Eckman, C., Eckman, E., and Janus, C. (2009). Amyloid beta and impairment in multiple memory systems in older transgenic APP TgCRND8 mice. *Genes Brain Behav.* 8, 676–684. doi: 10.1111/j.1601-183X.2009.00510.x

Hanna, A., Iremonger, K., Das, P., Dickson, D., Golde, T., and Janus, C. (2012). Age-related increase in amyloid plaque burden is associated with impairment in conditioned fear memory in CRND8 mouse model of amyloidosis. *Alzheimers Res. Ther.* 4, 21. doi: 10.1186/alzrt124

Harper, D. G., Stopa, E. G., Mckee, A. C., Satlin, A., Fish, D., and Volicer, L. (2004). Dementia severity and Lewy bodies affect circadian rhythms in Alzheimer disease. *Neurobiol. Aging* 25, 771–781. doi: 10.1016/j.neurobiolaging.2003.04.009

Harris, J. A., Devidze, N., Halabisky, B., Lo, I., Thwin, M. T., Yu, G. Q., et al. (2010). Many neuronal and behavioral impairments in transgenic mouse models of Alzheimer's disease are independent of caspase cleavage of the amyloid precursor protein. *J. Neurosci.* 30, 372–381. doi: 10.1523/JNEUROSCI.5341-09.2010

Hartman, R. E., Izumi, Y., Bales, K. R., Paul, S. M., Wozniak, D. F., and Holtzman, D. M. (2005). Treatment with an amyloid-beta antibody ameliorates plaque load, learning deficits, and hippocampal long-term potentiation in a mouse model of Alzheimer's disease. *J. Neurosci.* 25, 6213–6220. doi: 10.1523/JNEUROSCI.0664-05.2005

Heneka, M. T., Ramanathan, M., Jacobs, A. H., Dumitrescu-Ozimek, L., Bilkei-Gorzo, A., Debeir, T., et al. (2006). Locus ceruleus degeneration promotes Alzheimer pathogenesis in amyloid precursor protein 23 transgenic mice. *J. Neurosci.* 26, 1343–1354. doi: 10.1523/JNEUROSCI.4236-05.2006

Hochgrafe, K., Sydow, A., and Mandelkow, E. M. (2013). Regulatable transgenic mouse models of Alzheimer disease: onset, reversibility and spreading of Tau pathology. *FEBS J.* 280, 4371–4381. doi: 10.1111/febs.12250

Hodges, J. R., and Patterson, K. (1995). Is semantic memory consistently impaired early in the course of Alzheimer's disease? Neuroanatomical and diagnostic implications. *Neuropsychologia* 33, 441–459. doi: 10.1016/0028-3932(94)00127-B

Hodges, J. R., Salmon, D. P., and Butters, N. (1992). Semantic memory impairment in Alzheimer's disease: failure of access or degraded knowledge? *Neuropsychologia* 30, 301–314. doi: 10.1016/0028-3932(92)90104-T

Hof, P. R., Vogt, B. A., Bouras, C., and Morrison, J. H. (1997). Atypical form of Alzheimer's disease with prominent posterior cortical atrophy: a review of lesion distribution and circuit disconnection in cortical visual pathways. *Vision Res.* 37, 3609–3625. doi: 10.1016/S0042-6989(96)00240-4

Holcomb, L., Gordon, M. N., Mcgowan, E., Yu, X., Benkovic, S., Jantzen, P., et al. (1998). Accelerated Alzheimer-type phenotype in transgenic mice carrying both mutant amyloid precursor protein and presenilin 1 transgenes. *Nat. Med.* 4, 97–100. doi: 10.1038/nm0198-097

Holcomb, L. A., Gordon, M. N., Jantzen, P., Hsiao, K., Duff, K., and Morgan, D. (1999). Behavioral changes in transgenic mice expressing both amyloid precursor protein and presenilin-1 mutations: lack of association with amyloid deposits. *Behav. Genet.* 29, 177–185. doi: 10.1023/A:1021691918517

Holtzer, R., Irizarry, M. C., Sanders, J., Hyman, B. T., Wegesin, D. J., Riba, A., et al. (2006). Relation of quantitative indexes of concurrent alpha-synuclein abnormalities to clinical outcome in autopsy-proven Alzheimer disease. *Arch. Neurol.* 63, 226–230. doi: 10.1001/archneur.63.2.226

Hope, T., Keene, J., Gedling, K., Fairburn, C. G., and Jacoby, R. (1998). Predictors of institutionalization for people with dementia living at home with a carer. *Int. J. Geriatr. Psychiatry* 13, 682–690.

Hsiao, K., Chapman, P., Nilsen, S., Eckman, C., Harigaya, Y., Younkin, S., et al. (1996). Correlative memory deficits, Abeta elevation, and amyloid plaques in transgenic mice. *Science* 274, 99–102. doi: 10.1126/science.274.5284.99

Huang, S. M., Mouri, A., Kokubo, H., Nakajima, R., Suemoto, T., Higuchi, M., et al. (2006). Neprilysin-sensitive synapse-associated amyloid-beta peptide oligomers impair neuronal plasticity and cognitive function. *J. Biol. Chem.* 281, 17941–17951. doi: 10.1074/jbc.M601372200

Huff, F. J., Becker, J. T., Belle, S. H., Nebes, R. D., Holland, A. L., and Boller, F. (1987). Cognitive deficits and clinical diagnosis of Alzheimer's disease. *Neurology* 37, 1119–1124. doi: 10.1212/WNL.37.7.1119

Huitron-Resendiz, S., Sanchez-Alavez, M., and Criado, J. R. (2005). Sleep-wake states in transgenic mouse models overexpressing the human beta-amyloid precursor protein. *Am. J. Alzheimers Dis. Other Demen.* 20, 87–90. doi: 10.1177/153331750502000204

Huitron-Resendiz, S., Sanchez-Alavez, M., Gallegos, R., Berg, G., Crawford, E., Giacchino, J. L., et al. (2002). Age-independent and age-related deficits in visuospatial learning, sleep-wake states, thermoregulation and motor activity in PDAPP mice. *Brain Res.* 928, 126–137. doi: 10.1016/S0006-8993(01)03373-X

Humby, T., Laird, F. M., Davies, W., and Wilkinson, L. S. (1999). Visuospatial attentional functioning in mice: interactions between cholinergic manipulations and genotype. *Eur. J. Neurosci.* 11, 2813–2823. doi: 10.1046/j.1460-9568.1999.00701.x

Hyde, L. A., Kazdoba, T. M., Grilli, M., Lozza, G., Brusa, R., Zhang, Q., et al. (2005). Age-progressing cognitive impairments and neuropathology in transgenic CRND8 mice. *Behav. Brain Res.* 160, 344–355. doi: 10.1016/j.bbr.2004.12.017

Hyde, L. A., Sherman, G. F., and Denenberg, V. H. (2000). Non-spatial water radial-arm maze learning in mice. *Brain Res.* 863, 151–159. doi: 10.1016/S0006-8993(00)02113-2

Hyman, B. T., Phelps, C. H., Beach, T. G., Bigio, E. H., Cairns, N. J., Carrillo, M. C., et al. (2012). National Institute on Aging-Alzheimer's Association guidelines for the neuropathologic assessment of Alzheimer's disease. *Alzheimers Dement.* 8, 1–13. doi: 10.1016/j.jalz.2011.10.007

Hyman, B. T., and Trojanowski, J. Q. (1997). Consensus recommendations for the postmortem diagnosis of Alzheimer disease from the National Institute on Aging and the Reagan Institute Working Group on diagnostic criteria for the neuropathological assessment of Alzheimer disease. *J. Neuropathol. Exp. Neurol.* 56, 1095–1097. doi: 10.1097/00005072-199710000-00002

Izquierdo, A., and Jentsch, J. D. (2012). Reversal learning as a measure of impulsive and compulsive behavior in addictions. *Psychopharmacology (Berl.)* 219, 607–620. doi: 10.1007/s00213-011-2579-7

Jacobson, M. W., Delis, D. C., Bondi, M. W., and Salmon, D. P. (2002). Do neuropsychological tests detect preclinical Alzheimer's disease: individual-test versus cognitive-discrepancy score analyses. *Neuropsychology* 16, 132–139. doi: 10.1037/0894-4105.16.2.132

Jacqmin-Gadda, H., Fabrigoule, C., Commenges, D., and Dartigues, J. F. (1997). A 5-year longitudinal study of the Mini-Mental State Examination in normal aging. *Am. J. Epidemiol.* 145, 498–506. doi: 10.1093/oxfordjournals.aje.a009137

Jankowsky, J. L., Slunt, H. H., Ratovitski, T., Jenkins, N. A., Copeland, N. G., and Borchelt, D. R. (2001). Co-expression of multiple transgenes in mouse CNS: a comparison of strategies. *Biomol. Eng.* 17, 157–165. doi: 10.1016/S1389-0344(01)00067-3

Janus, C. (2004). Search strategies used by APP transgenic mice during navigation in the Morris water maze. *Learn. Mem.* 11, 337–346. doi: 10.1101/lm.70104

Janus, C., Pearson, J., Mclaurin, J., Mathews, P. M., Jiang, Y., Schmidt, S. D., et al. (2000). A beta peptide immunization reduces behavioural impairment and plaques in a model of Alzheimer's disease. *Nature* 408, 979–982. doi: 10.1038/35050110

Janus, C., and Westaway, D. (2001). Transgenic mouse models of Alzheimer's disease. *Physiol. Behav.* 73, 873–886. doi: 10.1016/S0031-9384(01)00524-8

Jicha, G. A., Abner, E. L., Schmitt, F. A., Kryscio, R. J., Riley, K. P., Cooper, G. E., et al. (2012). Preclinical AD Workgroup staging: pathological correlates and potential challenges. *Neurobiol. Aging* 33, 622.e621–622.e616. doi: 10.1016/j.neurobiolaging.2011.02.018

Jolly, D. C., Richards, J. B., and Seiden, L. S. (1999). Serotonergic mediation of DRL 72s behavior: receptor subtype involvement in a behavioral screen for antidepressant drugs. *Biol. Psychiatry* 45, 1151–1162. doi: 10.1016/S0006-3223(98)00014-6

Kaplan, E. F., Goodglass, H., and Weintraub, S., (1978). *The Boston Naming Test.* Philadelphia, PA: Lea & Febiger.

Karl, T., Bhatia, S., Cheng, D., Kim, W. S., and Garner, B. (2012). Cognitive phenotyping of amyloid precursor protein transgenic J20 mice. *Behav. Brain Res.* 228, 392–397. doi: 10.1016/j.bbr.2011.12.021

Karran, E., Mercken, M., and De Strooper, B. (2011). The amyloid cascade hypothesis for Alzheimer's disease: an appraisal for the development of therapeutics. *Nat. Rev. Drug Discov.* 10, 698–712. doi: 10.1038/nrd3505

Katzman, R., Brown, T., Fuld, P., Peck, A., Schechter, R., and Schimmel, H. (1983). Validation of a short Orientation-Memory-Concentration Test of cognitive impairment. *Am. J. Psychiatry* 140, 734–739.

Kelly, P. H., Bondolfi, L., Hunziker, D., Schlecht, H. P., Carver, K., Maguire, E., et al. (2003). Progressive age-related impairment of cognitive behavior in

APP23 transgenic mice. *Neurobiol. Aging* 24, 365–378. doi: 10.1016/S0197-4580(02)00098-2

King, D. L., and Arendash, G. W. (2002). Behavioral characterization of the Tg2576 transgenic model of Alzheimer's disease through 19 months. *Physiol. Behav.* 75, 627–642. doi: 10.1016/S0031-9384(02)00639-X

King, D. L., Arendash, G. W., Crawford, F., Sterk, T., Menendez, J., and Mullan, M. J. (1999). Progressive and gender-dependent cognitive impairment in the APP(SW) transgenic mouse model for Alzheimer's disease. *Behav. Brain Res.* 103, 145–162. doi: 10.1016/S0166-4328(99)00037-6

Klingner, M., Apelt, J., Kumar, A., Sorger, D., Sabri, O., Steinbach, J., et al. (2003). Alterations in cholinergic and non-cholinergic neurotransmitter receptor densities in transgenic Tg2576 mouse brain with beta-amyloid plaque pathology. *Int. J. Dev. Neurosci.* 21, 357–369. doi: 10.1016/j.ijdevneu.2003.08.001

Knafo, S., Venero, C., Merino-Serrais, P., Fernaud-Espinosa, I., Gonzalez-Soriano, J., Ferrer, I., et al. (2009). Morphological alterations to neurons of the amygdala and impaired fear conditioning in a transgenic mouse model of Alzheimer's disease. *J. Pathol.* 219, 41–51. doi: 10.1002/path.2565

Knopman, D. S., and Ryberg, S. (1989). A verbal memory test with high predictive accuracy for dementia of the Alzheimer type. *Arch. Neurol.* 46, 141–145. doi: 10.1001/archneur.1989.00520380041011

Kobayashi, D. T., and Chen, K. S. (2005). Behavioral phenotypes of amyloid-based genetically modified mouse models of Alzheimer's disease. *Genes Brain Behav.* 4, 173–196. doi: 10.1111/j.1601-183X.2005.00124.x

Koepsell, T. D., Kurland, B. F., Harel, O., Johnson, E. A., Zhou, X. H., and Kukull, W. A. (2008). Education, cognitive function, and severity of neuropathology in Alzheimer disease. *Neurology* 70, 1732–1739. doi: 10.1212/01.wnl.0000284603.85621.aa

Kraybill, M. L., Larson, E. B., Tsuang, D. W., Teri, L., Mccormick, W. C., Bowen, J. D., et al. (2005). Cognitive differences in dementia patients with autopsy-verified AD, Lewy body pathology, or both. *Neurology* 64, 2069–2073. doi: 10.1212/01.WNL.0000165987.89198.65

Kryscio, R. J., Schmitt, F. A., Salazar, J. C., Mendiondo, M. S., and Markesbery, W. R. (2006). Risk factors for transitions from normal to mild cognitive impairment and dementia. *Neurology* 66, 828–832. doi: 10.1212/01.wnl.0000203264.71880.45

Lalonde, R., Dumont, M., Staufenbiel, M., Sturchler-Pierrat, C., and Strazielle, C. (2002). Spatial learning, exploration, anxiety, and motor coordination in female APP23 transgenic mice with the Swedish mutation. *Brain Res.* 956, 36–44. doi: 10.1016/S0006-8993(02)03476-5

Lalonde, R., Fukuchi, K., and Strazielle, C. (2012). Neurologic and motor dysfunctions in APP transgenic mice. *Rev. Neurosci.* 23, 363–379. doi: 10.1515/revneuro-2012-0041

Lalonde, R., Kim, H. D., and Fukuchi, K. (2004). Exploratory activity, anxiety, and motor coordination in bigenic APPswe + PS1/DeltaE9 mice. *Neurosci. Lett.* 369, 156–161. doi: 10.1016/j.neulet.2004.07.069

Lalonde, R., Kim, H. D., Maxwell, J. A., and Fukuchi, K. (2005). Exploratory activity and spatial learning in 12-month-old APP(695) SWE/co+PS1/DeltaE9 mice with amyloid plaques. *Neurosci. Lett.* 390, 87–92. doi: 10.1016/j.neulet.2005.08.028

Lalonde, R., Lewis, T. L., Strazielle, C., Kim, H., and Fukuchi, K. (2003). Transgenic mice expressing the betaAPP695SWE mutation: effects on exploratory activity, anxiety, and motor coordination. *Brain Res.* 977, 38–45. doi: 10.1016/S0006-8993(03)02694-5

Lambon Ralph, M. A., Patterson, K., Graham, N., Dawson, K., and Hodges, J. R. (2003). Homogeneity and heterogeneity in mild cognitive impairment and Alzheimer's disease: a cross-sectional and longitudinal study of 55 cases. *Brain* 126, 2350–2362. doi: 10.1093/brain/awg236

Lambourne, S. L., Humby, T., Isles, A. R., Emson, P. C., Spillantini, M. G., and Wilkinson, L. S. (2007). Impairments in impulse control in mice transgenic for the human FTDP-17 tauV337M mutation are exacerbated by age. *Hum. Mol. Genet.* 16, 1708–1719. doi: 10.1093/hmg/ddm119

Lange, K. L., Bondi, M. W., Salmon, D. P., Galasko, D., Delis, D. C., Thomas, R. G., et al. (2002). Decline in verbal memory during preclinical Alzheimer's disease: examination of the effect of APOE genotype. *J. Int. Neuropsychol. Soc.* 8, 943–955. doi: 10.1017/S1355617702870096

Larrieu, S., Letenneur, L., Orgogozo, J. M., Fabrigoule, C., Amieva, H., Le Carret, N., et al. (2002). Incidence and outcome of mild cognitive impairment in a population-based prospective cohort. *Neurology* 59, 1594–1599. doi: 10.1212/01.WNL.0000034176.07159.F8

Lassalle, J. M., Halley, H., Daumas, S., Verret, L., and Frances, B. (2008). Effects of the genetic background on cognitive performances of TG2576 mice. *Behav. Brain Res.* 191, 104–110. doi: 10.1016/j.bbr.2008.03.017

Lenoir, H., Dufouil, C., Auriacombe, S., Lacombe, J. M., Dartigues, J. F., Ritchie, K., et al. (2011). Depression history, depressive symptoms, and incident dementia: the 3C Study. *J. Alzheimers Dis.* 26, 27–38. doi: 10.3233/JAD-2011-101614

Locascio, J. J., Growdon, J. H., and Corkin, S. (1995). Cognitive test performance in detecting, staging, and tracking Alzheimer's disease. *Arch. Neurol.* 52, 1087–1099. doi: 10.1001/archneur.1995.00540350081020

Lovasic, L., Bauschke, H., and Janus, C. (2005). Working memory impairment in a transgenic amyloid precursor protein TgCRND8 mouse model of Alzheimer's disease. *Genes Brain Behav.* 4, 197–208. doi: 10.1111/j.1601-183X.2004.00104.x

Lustbader, J. W., Cirilli, M., Lin, C., Xu, H. W., Takuma, K., Wang, N., et al. (2004). ABAD directly links Abeta to mitochondrial toxicity in Alzheimer's disease. *Science* 304, 448–452. doi: 10.1126/science.1091230

Luth, H. J., Apelt, J., Ihunwo, A. O., Arendt, T., and Schliebs, R. (2003). Degeneration of beta-amyloid-associated cholinergic structures in transgenic APP SW mice. *Brain Res.* 977, 16–22. doi: 10.1016/S0006-8993(03)02658-1

Ma, T., Du, X., Pick, J. E., Sui, G., Brownlee, M., and Klann, E. (2012). Glucagon-like peptide-1 cleavage product GLP-1(9-36) amide rescues synaptic plasticity and memory deficits in Alzheimer's disease model mice. *J. Neurosci.* 32, 13701–13708. doi: 10.1523/JNEUROSCI.2107-12.2012

Marchese, M., Cowan, D., Head, E., Ma, D., Karimi, K., Ashthorpe, V., et al. (2013). Autoimmune Manifestations in the 3xTg-AD Model of Alzheimer's Disease. *J. Alzheimers Dis.* 39, 191–210. doi: 10.3233/JAD-131490

Markesbery, W. R., Schmitt, F. A., Kryscio, R. J., Davis, D. G., Smith, C. D., and Wekstein, D. R. (2006). Neuropathologic substrate of mild cognitive impairment. *Arch. Neurol.* 63, 38–46. doi: 10.1001/archneur.63.1.38

Mckee, A. C., Kosik, K. S., and Kowall, N. W. (1991). Neuritic pathology and dementia in Alzheimer's disease. *Ann. Neurol.* 30, 156–165. doi: 10.1002/ana.410300206

Mckhann, G. M., Knopman, D. S., Chertkow, H., Hyman, B. T., Jack, C. R. Jr., Kawas, C. H., et al. (2011). The diagnosis of dementia due to Alzheimer's disease: recommendations from the National Institute on Aging-Alzheimer's Association workgroups on diagnostic guidelines for Alzheimer's disease. *Alzheimers Dement.* 7, 263–269. doi: 10.1016/j.jalz.2011.03.005

Mega, M. S., Cummings, J. L., Fiorello, T., and Gornbein, J. (1996). The spectrum of behavioral changes in Alzheimer's disease. *Neurology* 46, 130–135. doi: 10.1212/WNL.46.1.130

Meilandt, W. J., Yu, G. Q., Chin, J., Roberson, E. D., Palop, J. J., Wu, T., et al. (2008). Enkephalin elevations contribute to neuronal and behavioral impairments in a transgenic mouse model of Alzheimer's disease. *J. Neurosci.* 28, 5007–5017. doi: 10.1523/JNEUROSCI.0590-08.2008

Meltzer, C. C., Smith, G., Dekosky, S. T., Pollock, B. G., Mathis, C. A., Moore, R. Y., et al. (1998). Serotonin in aging, late-life depression, and Alzheimer's disease: the emerging role of functional imaging. *Neuropsychopharmacology* 18, 407–430. doi: 10.1016/S0893-133X(97)00194-2

Mendez, M. F., Martin, R. J., Smyth, K. A., and Whitehouse, P. J. (1990). Psychiatric symptoms associated with Alzheimer's disease. *J. Neuropsychiatry Clin. Neurosci.* 2, 28–33.

Mickes, L., Wixted, J. T., Fennema-Notestine, C., Galasko, D., Bondi, M. W., Thal, L. J., et al. (2007). Progressive impairment on neuropsychological tasks in a longitudinal study of preclinical Alzheimer's disease. *Neuropsychology* 21, 696–705. doi: 10.1037/0894-4105.21.6.696

Migliorelli, R., Petracca, G., Teson, A., Sabe, L., Leiguarda, R., and Starkstein, S. E. (1995a). Neuropsychiatric and neuropsychological correlates of delusions in Alzheimer's disease. *Psychol. Med.* 25, 505–513. doi: 10.1017/S0033291700033420

Migliorelli, R., Teson, A., Sabe, L., Petracchi, M., Leiguarda, R., and Starkstein, S. E. (1995b). Prevalence and correlates of dysthymia and major depression among patients with Alzheimer's disease. *Am. J. Psychiatry* 152, 37–44.

Moechars, D., Dewachter, I., Lorent, K., Reverse, D., Baekelandt, V., Naidu, A., et al. (1999). Early phenotypic changes in transgenic mice that overexpress different mutants of amyloid precursor protein in brain. *J. Biol. Chem.* 274, 6483–6492. doi: 10.1074/jbc.274.10.6483

Moechars, D., Gilis, M., Kuiperi, C., Laenen, I., and Van Leuven, F. (1998). Aggressive behaviour in transgenic mice expressing APP is alleviated by serotonergic drugs. *Neuroreport* 9, 3561–3564. doi: 10.1097/00001756-199811160-00004

Moechars, D., Lorent, K., De Strooper, B., Dewachter, I., and Van Leuven, F. (1996). Expression in brain of amyloid precursor protein mutated in the alpha-secretase site causes disturbed behavior, neuronal degeneration and premature death in transgenic mice. *EMBO J.* 15, 1265–1274.

Montine, T. J., Phelps, C. H., Beach, T. G., Bigio, E. H., Cairns, N. J., Dickson, D. W., et al. (2012). National Institute on Aging-Alzheimer's Association guidelines for the neuropathologic assessment of Alzheimer's disease: a practical approach. *Acta Neuropathol.* 123, 1–11. doi: 10.1007/s00401-011-0910-3

Morgan, D. (2003). Learning and memory deficits in APP transgenic mouse models of amyloid deposition. *Neurochem. Res.* 28, 1029–1034. doi: 10.1023/A:1023255106106

Morgan, D., Diamond, D. M., Gottschall, P. E., Ugen, K. E., Dickey, C., Hardy, J., et al. (2000). A beta peptide vaccination prevents memory loss in an animal model of Alzheimer's disease. *Nature* 408, 982–985. doi: 10.1038/35050116

Mori, T., Koyama, N., Guillot-Sestier, M. V., Tan, J., and Town, T. (2013). Ferulic acid is a nutraceutical beta-secretase modulator that improves behavioral impairment and alzheimer-like pathology in transgenic mice. *PLoS ONE* 8:e55774. doi: 10.1371/journal.pone.0055774

Morris, J. C., Heyman, A., Mohs, R. C., Hughes, J. P., Van Belle, G., Fillenbaum, G., et al. (1989). The Consortium to Establish a Registry for Alzheimer's Disease (CERAD). Part I. Clinical and neuropsychological assessment of Alzheimer's disease. *Neurology* 39, 1159–1165. doi: 10.1212/WNL.39.9.1159

Morris, R. G. (2001). Episodic-like memory in animals: psychological criteria, neural mechanisms and the value of episodic-like tasks to investigate animal models of neurodegenerative disease. *Philos. Trans. R. Soc. Lond. B Biol. Sci.* 356, 1453–1465. doi: 10.1098/rstb.2001.0945

Morris, R. G., Garrud, P., Rawlins, J. N., and O'keefe, J. (1982). Place navigation impaired in rats with hippocampal lesions. *Nature* 297, 681–683. doi: 10.1038/297681a0

Mucke, L., Masliah, E., Yu, G. Q., Mallory, M., Rockenstein, E. M., Tatsuno, G., et al. (2000). High-level neuronal expression of abeta 1-42 in wild-type human amyloid protein precursor transgenic mice: synaptotoxicity without plaque formation. *J. Neurosci.* 20, 4050–4058. Available online at: http://www.jneurosci.org/content/20/11/4050.long

Muir, J. L. (1996). Attention and stimulus processing in the rat. *Brain Res. Cogn. Brain Res.* 3, 215–225. doi: 10.1016/0926-6410(96)00008-0

Mungas, D., Reed, B. R., Ellis, W. G., and Jagust, W. J. (2001). The effects of age on rate of progression of Alzheimer disease and dementia with associated cerebrovascular disease. *Arch. Neurol.* 58, 1243–1247. doi: 10.1001/archneur.58.8.1243

Murakami, K., Yokoyama, S., Murata, N., Ozawa, Y., Irie, K., Shirasawa, T., et al. (2011). Insulin receptor mutation results in insulin resistance and hyperinsulinemia but does not exacerbate Alzheimer's-like phenotypes in mice. *Biochem. Biophys. Res. Commun.* 409, 34–39. doi: 10.1016/j.bbrc.2011.04.101

Murman, D. L., Chen, Q., Colucci, P. M., Colenda, C. C., Gelb, D. J., and Liang, J. (2002a). Comparison of healthcare utilization and direct costs in three degenerative dementias. *Am. J. Geriatr. Psychiatry* 10, 328–336. doi: 10.1097/00019442-200205000-00013

Murman, D. L., Chen, Q., Powell, M. C., Kuo, S. B., Bradley, C. J., and Colenda, C. C. (2002b). The incremental direct costs associated with behavioral symptoms in AD. *Neurology* 59, 1721–1729. doi: 10.1212/01.WNL.0000036904.73393.E4

Murray, M. E., Graff-Radford, N. R., Ross, O. A., Petersen, R. C., Duara, R., and Dickson, D. W. (2011). Neuropathologically defined subtypes of Alzheimer's disease with distinct clinical characteristics: a retrospective study. *Lancet Neurol.* 10, 785–796. doi: 10.1016/S1474-4422(11)70156-9

Musilli, M., Nicolia, V., Borrelli, S., Scarpa, S., and Diana, G. (2013). Behavioral effects of Rho GTPase modulation in a model of Alzheimer's disease. *Behav. Brain Res.* 237, 223–229. doi: 10.1016/j.bbr.2012.09.043

Nagy, Z., Esiri, M. M., Jobst, K. A., Morris, J. H., King, E. M., Mcdonald, B., et al. (1995). Relative roles of plaques and tangles in the dementia of Alzheimer's disease: correlations using three sets of neuropathological criteria. *Dementia* 6, 21–31.

Nagy, Z., Hindley, N. J., Braak, H., Braak, E., Yilmazer-Hanke, D. M., Schultz, C., et al. (1999). The progression of Alzheimer's disease from limbic regions to the neocortex: clinical, radiological and pathological relationships. *Dement. Geriatr. Cogn. Disord.* 10, 115–120. doi: 10.1159/000017111

Nasreddine, Z. S., Phillips, N. A., Bédirian, V., Charbonneau, S., Whitehead, V., Collin, I., et al. (2005). The Montreal Cognitive Assessment (MoCA): a brief screening tool for mild cognitive impairment. *J. Am. Geriatr. Soc.* 53, 695–699. doi: 10.1111/j.1532-5415.2005.53221.x

Nelson, P. T., Abner, E. L., Scheff, S. W., Schmitt, F. A., Kryscio, R. J., Jicha, G. A., et al. (2009a). Alzheimer's-type neuropathology in the precuneus is not increased relative to other areas of neocortex across a range of cognitive impairment. *Neurosci. Lett.* 450, 336–339. doi: 10.1016/j.neulet.2008.11.006

Nelson, P. T., Alafuzoff, I., Bigio, E. H., Bouras, C., Braak, H., Cairns, N. J., et al. (2012). Correlation of Alzheimer disease neuropathologic changes with cognitive status: a review of the literature. *J. Neuropathol. Exp. Neurol.* 71, 362–381. doi: 10.1097/NEN.0b013e31825018f7

Nelson, P. T., Braak, H., and Markesbery, W. R. (2009b). Neuropathology and cognitive impairment in Alzheimer disease: a complex but coherent relationship. *J. Neuropathol. Exp. Neurol.* 68, 1–14. doi: 10.1097/NEN.0b013e3181919a48

Nelson, P. T., Jicha, G. A., Schmitt, F. A., Liu, H., Davis, D. G., Mendiondo, M. S., et al. (2007a). Clinicopathologic correlations in a large Alzheimer disease center autopsy cohort: neuritic plaques and neurofibrillary tangles "do count" when staging disease severity. *J. Neuropathol. Exp. Neurol.* 66, 1136–1146. doi: 10.1097/nen.0b013e31815c5efb

Nelson, R. L., Guo, Z., Halagappa, V. M., Pearson, M., Gray, A. J., Matsuoka, Y., et al. (2007b). Prophylactic treatment with paroxetine ameliorates behavioral deficits and retards the development of amyloid and tau pathologies in 3xTgAD mice. *Exp. Neurol.* 205, 166–176. doi: 10.1016/j.expneurol.2007.01.037

Nestler, E. J., and Hyman, S. E. (2010). Animal models of neuropsychiatric disorders. *Nat. Neurosci.* 13, 1161–1169. doi: 10.1038/nn.2647

Nilsson, L. N., Arendash, G. W., Leighty, R. E., Costa, D. A., Low, M. A., Garcia, M. F., et al. (2004). Cognitive impairment in PDAPP mice depends on ApoE and ACT-catalyzed amyloid formation. *Neurobiol. Aging* 25, 1153–1167. doi: 10.1016/j.neurobiolaging.2003.12.011

O'leary, T. P., and Brown, R. E. (2009). Visuo-spatial learning and memory deficits on the Barnes maze in the 16-month-old APPswe/PS1dE9 mouse model of Alzheimer's disease. *Behav. Brain Res.* 201, 120–127. doi: 10.1016/j.bbr.2009.01.039

Oakley, H., Cole, S. L., Logan, S., Maus, E., Shao, P., Craft, J., et al. (2006). Intraneuronal beta-amyloid aggregates, neurodegeneration, and neuron loss in transgenic mice with five familial Alzheimer's disease mutations: potential factors in amyloid plaque formation. *J. Neurosci.* 26, 10129–10140. doi: 10.1523/JNEUROSCI.1202-06.2006

Oddo, S., Caccamo, A., Shepherd, J. D., Murphy, M. P., Golde, T. E., Kayed, R., et al. (2003). Triple-transgenic model of Alzheimer's disease with plaques and tangles: intracellular Abeta and synaptic dysfunction. *Neuron* 39, 409–421. doi: 10.1016/S0896-6273(03)00434-3

Ognibene, E., Middei, S., Daniele, S., Adriani, W., Ghirardi, O., Caprioli, A., et al. (2005). Aspects of spatial memory and behavioral disinhibition in Tg2576 transgenic mice as a model of Alzheimer's disease. *Behav. Brain Res.* 156, 225–232. doi: 10.1016/j.bbr.2004.05.028

Ohno, M., Chang, L., Tseng, W., Oakley, H., Citron, M., Klein, W. L., et al. (2006). Temporal memory deficits in Alzheimer's mouse models: rescue by genetic deletion of BACE1. *Eur. J. Neurosci.* 23, 251–260. doi: 10.1111/j.1460-9568.2005.04551.x

Ohno, M., Sametsky, E. A., Younkin, L. H., Oakley, H., Younkin, S. G., Citron, M., et al. (2004). BACE1 deficiency rescues memory deficits and cholinergic dysfunction in a mouse model of Alzheimer's disease. *Neuron* 41, 27–33. doi: 10.1016/S0896-6273(03)00810-9

Okawa, M., Mishima, K., Hishikawa, Y., Hozumi, S., Hori, H., and Takahashi, K. (1991). Circadian rhythm disorders in sleep-waking and body temperature in elderly patients with dementia and their treatment. *Sleep* 14, 478–485.

Olton, D. S., Becker, J. T., and Handelmann, G. E. (1979). Hippocampus, Space, and Memory. *Behav. Brain Sci.* 2, 313–322. doi: 10.1017/S0140525X00062713

Olton, D. S., and Feustle, W. A. (1981). Hippocampal function required for nonspatial working memory. *Exp. Brain Res.* 41, 380–389.

Olton, D. S., and Samuelson, R. J. (1976). Remembrance of Places Passed - Spatial Memory in Rats. *J. Exp. Psychol. Anim. Behav. Process.* 2, 97–116. doi: 10.1037/0097-7403.2.2.97

Oules, B., Del Prete, D., Greco, B., Zhang, X., Lauritzen, I., Sevalle, J., et al. (2012). Ryanodine receptor blockade reduces amyloid-beta load and memory impairments in Tg2576 mouse model of Alzheimer disease. *J. Neurosci.* 32, 11820–11834. doi: 10.1523/JNEUROSCI.0875-12.2012

Ownby, R. L., Crocco, E., Acevedo, A., John, V., and Loewenstein, D. (2006). Depression and risk for Alzheimer disease: systematic review, meta-analysis, and metaregression analysis. *Arch. Gen. Psychiatry* 63, 530–538. doi: 10.1001/archpsyc.63.5.530

Palop, J. J., Jones, B., Kekonius, L., Chin, J., Yu, G. Q., Raber, J., et al. (2003). Neuronal depletion of calcium-dependent proteins in the dentate gyrus is tightly linked to Alzheimer's disease-related cognitive deficits. *Proc. Natl. Acad. Sci. U.S.A.* 100, 9572–9577. doi: 10.1073/pnas.1133381100

Papadopoulos, P., Rosa-Neto, P., Rochford, J., and Hamel, E. (2013). Pioglitazone improves reversal learning and exerts mixed cerebrovascular effects in a mouse model of Alzheimer's disease with combined amyloid-beta and cerebrovascular pathology. *PLoS ONE* 8:e68612. doi: 10.1371/journal.pone.0068612

Parasuraman, R., and Nestor, P. (1993). Attention and driving. Assessment in elderly individuals with dementia.*Clin. Geriatr. Med.* 9, 377–387.

Park, J. H., Widi, G. A., Gimbel, D. A., Harel, N. Y., Lee, D. H., and Strittmatter, S. M. (2006). Subcutaneous Nogo receptor removes brain amyloid-beta and improves spatial memory in Alzheimer's transgenic mice. *J. Neurosci.* 26, 13279–13286. doi: 10.1523/JNEUROSCI.4504-06.2006

Pattij, T., Janssen, M. C., Loos, M., Smit, A. B., Schoffelmeer, A. N., and Van Gaalen, M. M. (2007). Strain specificity and cholinergic modulation of visuospatial attention in three inbred mouse strains. *Genes Brain Behav.* 6, 579–587. doi: 10.1111/j.1601-183X.2006.00284.x

Pearlson, G. D., Ross, C. A., Lohr, W. D., Rovner, B. W., Chase, G. A., and Folstein, M. F. (1990). Association between family history of affective-disorder and the depressive syndrome of Alzheimers-disease. *Am. J. Psychiatry* 147, 452–456.

Perry, R. J., and Hodges, J. R. (1999). Attention and executive deficits in Alzheimer's disease. A critical review. *Brain* 122(Pt 3), 383–404. doi: 10.1093/brain/122.3.383

Perry, R. J., Watson, P., and Hodges, J. R. (2000). The nature and staging of attention dysfunction in early (minimal and mild) Alzheimer's disease: relationship to episodic and semantic memory impairment. *Neuropsychologia* 38, 252–271. doi: 10.1016/S0028-3932(99)00079-2

Pietropaolo, S., Feldon, J., and Yee, B. K. (2008). Age-dependent phenotypic characteristics of a triple transgenic mouse model of Alzheimer disease. *Behav. Neurosci.* 122, 733–747. doi: 10.1037/a0012520

Platt, T. L., Reeves, V. L., and Murphy, M. P. (2013). Transgenic models of Alzheimer's disease: better utilization of existing models through viral transgenesis. *Biochim. Biophys. Acta* 1832, 1437–1448. doi: 10.1016/j.bbadis.2013.04.017

Prut, L., Abramowski, D., Krucker, T., Levy, C. L., Roberts, A. J., Staufenbiel, M., et al. (2007). Aged APP23 mice show a delay in switching to the use of a strategy in the Barnes maze. *Behav. Brain Res.* 179, 107–110. doi: 10.1016/j.bbr.2007.01.017

Pugh, P. L., Richardson, J. C., Bate, S. T., Upton, N., and Sunter, D., (2007). Non-cognitive behaviours in an APP/PS1 transgenic model of Alzheimer's disease. *Behav. Brain Res.* 178, 18-28. doi: 10.1016/j.bbr.2006.11.044

Reiserer, R. S., Harrison, F. E., Syverud, D. C., and Mcdonald, M. P. (2007). Impaired spatial learning in the APPSwe + PSEN1DeltaE9 bigenic mouse model of Alzheimer's disease. *Genes Brain Behav.* 6, 54–65. doi: 10.1111/j.1601-183X.2006.00221.x

Richter, H., Ambree, O., Lewejohann, L., Herring, A., Keyvani, K., Paulus, W., et al. (2008). Wheel-running in a transgenic mouse model of Alzheimer's disease: protection or symptom? *Behav. Brain Res.* 190, 74–84. doi: 10.1016/j.bbr.2008.02.005

Riley, K. P., Jicha, G. A., Davis, D., Abner, E. L., Cooper, G. E., Stiles, N., et al. (2011). Prediction of preclinical Alzheimer's disease: longitudinal rates of change in cognition. *J. Alzheimers Dis.* 25, 707–717. doi: 10.3233/JAD-2011-102133

Riley, K. P., Snowdon, D. A., and Markesbery, W. R. (2002). Alzheimer's neurofibrillary pathology and the spectrum of cognitive function: findings from the Nun Study. *Ann. Neurol.* 51, 567–577. doi: 10.1002/ana.10161

Robbins, T. W. (1996). Dissociating executive functions of the prefrontal cortex. *Philos. Trans. R. Soc. Lond. B Biol. Sci.* 351, 1463–1470. discussion: 1470–1461. doi: 10.1098/rstb.1996.0131

Robbins, T. W. (2002). The 5-choice serial reaction time task: behavioural pharmacology and functional neurochemistry. *Psychopharmacology (Berl.)* 163, 362–380. doi: 10.1007/s00213-002-1154-7

Robinson, A. L., Heaton, R. K., Lehman, R. A., and Stilson, D. W. (1980). The utility of the Wisconsin Card Sorting Test in detecting and localizing frontal lobe lesions. *J. Consult. Clin. Psychol.* 48, 605–614. doi: 10.1037/0022-006X.48.5.605

Robinson, J. K., and Crawley, J. N. (1993). Intraventricular galanin impairs delayed nonmatching-to-sample performance in rats. *Behav. Neurosci.* 107, 458–467. doi: 10.1037/0735-7044.107.3.458

Robinson, J. L., Geser, F., Corrada, M. M., Berlau, D. J., Arnold, S. E., Lee, V. M., et al. (2011). Neocortical and hippocampal amyloid-beta and tau measures associate with dementia in the oldest-old. *Brain* 134, 3708–3715. doi: 10.1093/brain/awr308

Romberg, C., Bussey, T. J., and Saksida, L. M. (2013a). Paying more attention to attention: towards more comprehensive cognitive translation using mouse models of Alzheimer's disease. *Brain Res. Bull.* 92, 49–55. doi: 10.1016/j.brainresbull.2012.02.007

Romberg, C., Horner, A. E., Bussey, T. J., and Saksida, L. M. (2013b). A touch screen-automated cognitive test battery reveals impaired attention, memory abnormalities, and increased response inhibition in the TgCRND8 mouse model of Alzheimer's disease. *Neurobiol. Aging* 34, 731–744. doi: 10.1016/j.neurobiolaging.2012.08.006

Romberg, C., Mattson, M. P., Mughal, M. R., Bussey, T. J., and Saksida, L. M. (2011). Impaired attention in the 3xTgAD mouse model of Alzheimer's disease: rescue by donepezil (Aricept). *J. Neurosci.* 31, 3500–3507. doi: 10.1523/JNEUROSCI.5242-10.2011

Rosen, C., Hansson, O., Blennow, K., and Zetterberg, H. (2013). Fluid biomarkers in Alzheimer's disease - current concepts. *Mol. Neurodegener.* 8:20. doi: 10.1186/1750-1326-8-20

Rosen, C., and Zetterberg, H. (2013). Cerebrospinal fluid biomarkers for pathological processes in Alzheimer's disease. *Curr. Opin. Psychiatry* 26, 276–282. doi: 10.1097/YCO.0b013e32835f6747

Rosen, W. G., Mohs, R. C., and Davis, K. L. (1984). A new rating scale for Alzheimer's disease. *Am. J. Psychiatry* 141, 1356–1364.

Sabbagh, M. N., Cooper, K., Delange, J., Stoehr, J. D., Thind, K., Lahti, T., et al. (2010). Functional, global and cognitive decline correlates to accumulation of Alzheimer's pathology in MCI and AD. *Curr. Alzheimer Res.* 7, 280–286. doi: 10.2174/156720510791162340

Sabbagh, M. N., Corey-Bloom, J., Tiraboschi, P., Thomas, R., Masliah, E., and Thal, L. J. (1999). Neurochemical markers do not correlate with cognitive decline in the Lewy body variant of Alzheimer disease. *Arch. Neurol.* 56, 1458–1461. doi: 10.1001/archneur.56.12.1458

Sadowski, M., Pankiewicz, J., Scholtzova, H., Ji, Y., Quartermain, D., Jensen, C. H., et al. (2004). Amyloid-beta deposition is associated with decreased hippocampal glucose metabolism and spatial memory impairment in APP/PS1 mice. *J. Neuropathol. Exp. Neurol.* 63, 418–428. Available online at: http://journals.lww.com/jneuropath/Pages/default.aspx

Salmon, D. P., and Bondi, M. W. (2009). Neuropsychological assessment of dementia. *Annu. Rev. Psychol.* 60, 257–282. doi: 10.1146/annurev.psych.57.102904.190024

Salmon, D. P., Heindel, W. C., and Lange, K. L. (1999). Differential decline in word generation from phonemic and semantic categories during the course of Alzheimer's disease: implications for the integrity of semantic memory. *J. Int. Neuropsychol. Soc.* 5, 692–703. doi: 10.1017/S1355617799577126

Salmon, D. P., Thomas, R. G., Pay, M. M., Booth, A., Hofstetter, C. R., Thal, L. J., et al. (2002). Alzheimer's disease can be accurately diagnosed in very mildly impaired individuals. *Neurology* 59, 1022–1028. doi: 10.1212/WNL.59.7.1022

Sanchez-Mejia, R. O., Newman, J. W., Toh, S., Yu, G. Q., Zhou, Y., Halabisky, B., et al. (2008). Phospholipase A2 reduction ameliorates cognitive deficits in a mouse model of Alzheimer's disease. *Nat. Neurosci.* 11, 1311–1318. doi: 10.1038/nn.2213

Santacruz, K. S., Sonnen, J. A., Pezhouh, M. K., Desrosiers, M. F., Nelson, P. T., and Tyas, S. L. (2011). Alzheimer disease pathology in subjects without dementia in 2 studies of aging: the Nun Study and the Adult Changes in Thought Study. *J. Neuropathol. Exp. Neurol.* 70, 832–840. doi: 10.1097/NEN.0b013e31822e8ae9

Satlin, A., Volicer, L., Stopa, E. G., and Harper, D. (1995). Circadian locomotor activity and core-body temperature rhythms in Alzheimer's disease. *Neurobiol. Aging* 16, 765–771. doi: 10.1016/0197-4580(95)00059-N

Saura, C. A., Chen, G., Malkani, S., Choi, S. Y., Takahashi, R. H., Zhang, D., et al. (2005). Conditional inactivation of presenilin 1 prevents amyloid accumulation and temporarily rescues contextual and spatial working memory impairments in amyloid precursor protein transgenic mice. *J. Neurosci.* 25, 6755–6764. doi: 10.1523/JNEUROSCI.1247-05.2005

Schenk, D., Barbour, R., Dunn, W., Gordon, G., Grajeda, H., Guido, T., et al. (1999). Immunization with amyloid-beta attenuates Alzheimer-disease-like pathology in the PDAPP mouse. *Nature* 400, 173–177. doi: 10.1038/22124

Schmitt, F. A., Davis, D. G., Wekstein, D. R., Smith, C. D., Ashford, J. W., and Markesbery, W. R. (2000). "Preclinical" AD revisited: neuropathology of cognitively normal older adults. *Neurology* 55, 370–376. doi: 10.1212/WNL.55.3.370

Schmitt, F. A., and Wichems, C. H. (2006). A systematic review of assessment and treatment of moderate to severe Alzheimer's disease. *Prim. Care Companion J. Clin. Psychiatry* 8, 158–159. doi: 10.4088/PCC.v08n0306

Schmitt, F. S. M. (1994). *Handbook of Dementing Illnesses.* New York, NY: Marcel Dekker, Inc.

Seligman, M. E., Rosellini, R. A., and Kozak, M. J. (1975). Learned helplessness in the rat: time course, immunization, and reversibility. *J. Comp. Physiol. Psychol.* 88, 542–547. doi: 10.1037/h0076431

Senanarong, V., Cummings, J. L., Fairbanks, L., Mega, M., Masterman, D. M., O'connor, S. M., et al. (2004). Agitation in Alzheimer's disease is a manifestation of frontal lobe dysfunction. *Dement. Geriatr. Cogn. Disord.* 17, 14–20. doi: 10.1159/000074080

Shin, I. S., Carter, M., Masterman, D., Fairbanks, L., and Cummings, J. L. (2005). Neuropsychiatric symptoms and quality of life in Alzheimer disease. *Am. J. Geriatr. Psychiatry* 13, 469–474. doi: 10.1097/00019442-200506000-00005

Shukla, V., Zheng, Y. L., Mishra, S. K., Amin, N. D., Steiner, J., Grant, P., et al. (2013). A truncated peptide from p35, a Cdk5 activator, prevents Alzheimer's disease phenotypes in model mice. *FASEB J.* 27, 174–186. doi: 10.1096/fj.12-217497

Silver, M. H., Newell, K., Brady, C., Hedley-White, E. T., and Perls, T. T. (2002). Distinguishing between neurodegenerative disease and disease-free aging: correlating neuropsychological evaluations and neuropathological studies in centenarians. *Psychosom. Med.* 64, 493–501.

Simard, M., and Van Reekum, R. (1999). Memory assessment in studies of cognition-enhancing drugs for Alzheimer's disease. *Drugs Aging* 14, 197–230. doi: 10.2165/00002512-199914030-00004

Simon, A. M., Schiapparelli, L., Salazar-Colocho, P., Cuadrado-Tejedor, M., Escribano, L., Lopez De Maturana, R., et al. (2009). Overexpression of wild-type human APP in mice causes cognitive deficits and pathological features unrelated to Abeta levels. *Neurobiol. Dis.* 33, 369–378. doi: 10.1016/j.nbd.2008.11.005

Smith, C. (1985). Sleep states and learning: a review of the animal literature. *Neurosci. Biobehav. Rev.* 9, 157–168. doi: 10.1016/0149-7634(85)90042-9

Smith, G. E., Pankratz, V. S., Negash, S., Machulda, M. M., Petersen, R. C., Boeve, B. F., et al. (2007). A plateau in pre-Alzheimer memory decline: evidence for compensatory mechanisms? *Neurology* 69, 133–139. doi: 10.1212/01.wnl.0000265594.23511.16

Snyderman, D., and Rovner, B. (2009). Mental status exam in primary care: a review. *Am. Fam. Physician* 80, 809–814. Available online at: http://www.aafp.org/afp/2009/1015/p809

Song, C., and Leonard, B. E. (2005). The olfactory bulbectomised rat as a model of depression. *Neurosci. Biobehav. Rev.* 29, 627–647. doi: 10.1016/j.neubiorev.2005.03.010

Sood, A., Warren Beach, J., Webster, S. J., Terry, A. V., and Buccafusco, J. J. (2007). The effects of JWB1-84-1 on memory-related task performance by amyloid Abeta transgenic mice and by young and aged monkeys. *Neuropharmacology* 53, 588–600. doi: 10.1016/j.neuropharm.2007.06.028

Spreen, O., and Strauss, E. (1998). *A compendium of neuropsychological tests, 2nd Edn.* New York, NY: Oxford University Press.

Sterniczuk, R., Dyck, R. H., Laferla, F. M., and Antle, M. C. (2010). Characterization of the 3xTg-AD mouse model of Alzheimer's disease: Part 1. Circadian changes.*Brain Res.* 1348, 139–148. doi: 10.1016/j.brainres.2010.05.013

Stewart, S., Cacucci, F., and Lever, C. (2011). Which memory task for my mouse? A systematic review of spatial memory performance in the Tg2576 Alzheimer's mouse model. *J. Alzheimers Dis.* 26, 105–126. doi: 10.3233/JAD-2011-101827

Stopford, C. L., Thompson, J. C., Neary, D., Richardson, A. M., and Snowden, J. S. (2012). Working memory, attention, and executive function in Alzheimer's disease and frontotemporal dementia. *Cortex* 48, 429–446. doi: 10.1016/j.cortex.2010.12.002

Storandt, M. (1991). Neuropsychological assessment in Alzheimer's disease. *Exp. Aging Res.* 17, 100–101.

Storandt, M., Grant, E. A., Miller, J. P., and Morris, J. C. (2006). Longitudinal course and neuropathologic outcomes in original vs revised MCI and in pre-MCI. *Neurology* 67, 467–473. doi: 10.1212/01.wnl.0000228231.26111.6e

Storandt, M., and Hill, R. D. (1989). Very mild senile dementia of the Alzheimer type. II. Psychometric test performance. *Arch. Neurol.* 46, 383–386. doi: 10.1001/archneur.1989.00520400037017

Storandt, M., Kaskie, B., and Von Dras, D. D. (1998). Temporal memory for remote events in healthy aging and dementia. *Psychol. Aging* 13, 4–7. doi: 10.1037/0882-7974.13.1.4

Strauss, M. E., and Ogrocki, P. K. (1996). Confirmation of an association between family history of affective disorder and the depressive syndrome in Alzheimer's disease. *Am. J. Psychiatry* 153, 1340–1342.

Sturchler-Pierrat, C., Abramowski, D., Duke, M., Wiederhold, K. H., Mistl, C., Rothacher, S., et al. (1997). Two amyloid precursor protein transgenic mouse models with Alzheimer disease-like pathology. *Proc. Natl. Acad. Sci. U.S.A.* 94, 13287–13292. doi: 10.1073/pnas.94.24.13287

Tan, L. L., Wong, H. B., and Allen, H. (2005). The impact of neuropsychiatric symptoms of dementia on distress in family and professional caregivers in Singapore. *Int. Psychogeriatr.* 17, 253–263. doi: 10.1017/S1041610205001523

Thal, D. R., Rub, U., Orantes, M., and Braak, H. (2002). Phases of A beta-deposition in the human brain and its relevance for the development of AD. *Neurology* 58, 1791–1800. doi: 10.1212/WNL.58.12.1791

Thibault, O., Pancani, T., Landfield, P. W., and Norris, C. M. (2012). Reduction in neuronal L-type calcium channel activity in a double knock-in mouse model of Alzheimer's disease. *Biochim. Biophys. Acta* 1822, 546–549. doi: 10.1016/j.bbadis.2012.01.004

Tiraboschi, P., Hansen, L. A., Alford, M., Merdes, A., Masliah, E., Thal, L. J., et al. (2002). Early and widespread cholinergic losses differentiate dementia with Lewy bodies from Alzheimer disease. *Arch. Gen. Psychiatry* 59, 946–951. doi: 10.1001/archpsyc.59.10.946

Tiraboschi, P., Hansen, L. A., Thal, L. J., and Corey-Bloom, J. (2004). The importance of neuritic plaques and tangles to the development and evolution of AD. *Neurology* 62, 1984–1989. doi: 10.1212/01.WNL.0000129697.01779.0A

Tohda, C., Urano, T., Umezaki, M., Nemere, I., and Kuboyama, T. (2012). Diosgenin is an exogenous activator of 1,25D(3)-MARRS/Pdia3/ERp57 and improves Alzheimer's disease pathologies in 5XFAD mice. *Sci. Rep.* 2:535. doi: 10.1038/srep00535

Tomlinson, B. E., Blessed, G., and Roth, M. (1970). Observations on the brains of demented old people. *J. Neurol. Sci.* 11, 205–242. doi: 10.1016/0022-510X(70)90063-8

Trinchese, F., Liu, S., Battaglia, F., Walter, S., Mathews, P. M., and Arancio, O. (2004). Progressive age-related development of Alzheimer-like pathology in APP/PS1 mice. *Ann. Neurol.* 55, 801–814. doi: 10.1002/ana.20101

Tulving, E., and Markowitsch, H. J. (1998). Episodic and declarative memory: role of the hippocampus. *Hippocampus* 8, 198–204.

Tuokko, H., Morris, C., and Ebert, P. (2005). Mild cognitive impairment and everyday functioning in older adults. *Neurocase* 11, 40–47. doi: 10.1080/13554790490896802

Twamley, E. W., Ropacki, S. A. L., and Bondi, M. W. (2006). Neuropsychological and neuroimaging changes in preclinical Alzheimer's disease. *J. Int. Neuropsychol. Soc.* 12, 707–735. doi: 10.1017/S1355617706060863

Urano, T., and Tohda, C. (2010). Icariin improves memory impairment in Alzheimer's disease model mice (5xFAD) and attenuates amyloid beta-induced neurite atrophy. *Phytother. Res.* 24, 1658–1663. doi: 10.1002/ptr.3183

Van Dam, D., D'hooge, R., Staufenbiel, M., Van Ginneken, C., Van Meir, F., and De Deyn, P. P. (2003). Age-dependent cognitive decline in the APP23 model precedes amyloid deposition. *Eur. J. Neurosci.* 17, 388–396. doi: 10.1046/j.1460-9568.2003.02444.x

Van Der Poel, A. M. (1967). Ethological study of the behaviour of the albino rat in a passive-avoidance test. *Acta Physiol. Pharmacol. Neerl.* 14, 503–505.

Van Dorpe, J., Smeijers, L., Dewachter, I., Nuyens, D., Spittaels, K., Van Den Haute, C., et al. (2000). Prominent cerebral amyloid angiopathy in transgenic mice overexpressing the london mutant of human APP in neurons. *Am. J. Pathol.* 157, 1283–1298. doi: 10.1016/S0002-9440(10)64644-5

Van Someren, E. J., Hagebeuk, E. E., Lijzenga, C., Scheltens, P., De Rooij, S. E., Jonker, C., et al. (1996). Circadian rest-activity rhythm disturbances in Alzheimer's disease. *Biol. Psychiatry* 40, 259–270. doi: 10.1016/0006-3223(95)00370-3

Vanderwolf, C. H. (1964). Effect of combined medial thalamic and septal lesions on active-avoidance behavior. *J. Comp. Physiol. Psychol.* 58, 31–37. doi: 10.1037/h0042400

Vitiello, M. V., Bliwise, D. L., and Prinz, P. N. (1992). Sleep in Alzheimer's disease and the sundown syndrome. *Neurology* 42, 83–93. discussion: 93–84.

Vloeberghs, E., Van Dam, D., Coen, K., Staufenbiel, M., and De Deyn, P. P. (2006). Aggressive male APP23 mice modeling behavioral alterations in dementia. *Behav. Neurosci.* 120, 1380–1383. doi: 10.1037/0735-7044.120.6.1380

Vloeberghs, E., Van Dam, D., Engelborghs, S., Nagels, G., Staufenbiel, M., and De Deyn, P. P. (2004). Altered circadian locomotor activity in APP23 mice: a model for BPSD disturbances. *Eur. J. Neurosci.* 20, 2757–2766. doi: 10.1111/j.1460-9568.2004.03755.x

Volianskis, A., Kostner, R., Molgaard, M., Hass, S., and Jensen, M. S. (2010). Episodic memory deficits are not related to altered glutamatergic synaptic transmission and plasticity in the CA1 hippocampus of the APPswe/PS1deltaE9-deleted transgenic mice model of ss-amyloidosis. *Neurobiol. Aging* 31, 1173–1187. doi: 10.1016/j.neurobiolaging.2008.08.005

Webster, S. J., Bachstetter, A. D., and Van Eldik, L. J. (2013). Comprehensive behavioral characterization of an APP/PS-1 double knock-in mouse model of Alzheimer's disease. *Alzheimers. Res. Ther.* 5, 28. doi: 10.1186/alzrt182

Wechsler, D. (1997). *Wechsler Memory Scale. 3rd Edition Manual.* San Antonio, TX: The Psychological Corperation.

Weinberger, D. R., Berman, K. F., and Zec, R. F. (1986). Physiologic dysfunction of dorsolateral prefrontal cortex in schizophrenia. I. Regional cerebral blood flow evidence. *Arch. Gen. Psychiatry* 43, 114–124. doi: 10.1001/archpsyc.1986.01800020020004

Weintraub, S., Wicklund, A. H., and Salmon, D. P. (2012). The neuropsychological profile of Alzheimer disease. *Cold Spring Harb. Perspect. Med.* 2:a006171. doi: 10.1101/cshperspect.a006171

Welsh, K., Butters, N., Hughes, J., Mohs, R., and Heyman, A. (1991). Detection of abnormal memory decline in mild cases of Alzheimer's disease using CERAD neuropsychological measures. *Arch. Neurol.* 48, 278–281. doi: 10.1001/archneur.1991.00530150046016

Welsh, K. A., Butters, N., Hughes, J. P., Mohs, R. C., and Heyman, A. (1992). Detection and staging of dementia in Alzheimer's disease. Use of the neuropsychological measures developed for the consortium to establish a registry for Alzheimer's Disease. *Arch. Neurol.* 49, 448–452. doi: 10.1001/archneur.1992.00530290030008

Westerman, M. A., Cooper-Blacketer, D., Mariash, A., Kotilinek, L., Kawarabayashi, T., Younkin, L. H., et al. (2002). The relationship between Abeta and memory in the Tg2576 mouse model of Alzheimer's disease. *J. Neurosci.* 22, 1858–1867. Available online at: http://www.jneurosci.org/content/22/5/1858.long

Whitwell, J. L., Josephs, K. A., Murray, M. E., Kantarci, K., Przybelski, S. A., Weigand, S. D., et al. (2008). MRI correlates of neurofibrillary tangle pathology at autopsy: a voxel-based morphometry study. *Neurology* 71, 743–749. doi: 10.1212/01.wnl.0000324924.91351.7d

Wilcock, D. M., Rojiani, A., Rosenthal, A., Subbarao, S., Freeman, M. J., Gordon, M. N., et al. (2004). Passive immunotherapy against Abeta in aged APP-transgenic mice reverses cognitive deficits and depletes parenchymal amyloid deposits in spite of increased vascular amyloid and microhemorrhage. *J. Neuroinflammation* 1:24. doi: 10.1186/1742-2094-1-24

Wilkinson, R. T. (1963). Interaction of noise with knowledge of results and sleep deprivation. *J. Exp. Psychol.* 66, 332–337. doi: 10.1037/h0044161

Wisor, J. P., Edgar, D. M., Yesavage, J., Ryan, H. S., Mccormick, C. M., Lapustea, N., et al. (2005). Sleep and circadian abnormalities in a transgenic mouse model of Alzheimer's disease: a role for cholinergic transmission. *Neuroscience* 131, 375–385. doi: 10.1016/j.neuroscience.2004.11.018

Yassine, N., Lazaris, A., Dorner-Ciossek, C., Despres, O., Meyer, L., Maitre, M., et al. (2013). Detecting spatial memory deficits beyond blindness in tg2576 Alzheimer mice. *Neurobiol. Aging* 34, 716–730. doi: 10.1016/j.neurobiolaging.2012.06.016

Young, J. W., Light, G. A., Marston, H. M., Sharp, R., and Geyer, M. A. (2009). The 5-choice continuous performance test: evidence for a translational test of vigilance for mice. *PLoS ONE* 4:e4227. doi: 10.1371/journal.pone.0004227

Zhang, W., Hao, J., Liu, R., Zhang, Z., Lei, G., Su, C., et al. (2011). Soluble Abeta levels correlate with cognitive deficits in the 12-month-old APPswe/PS1dE9 mouse model of Alzheimer's disease. *Behav. Brain Res.* 222, 342–350. doi: 10.1016/j.bbr.2011.03.072

Zhuo, J. M., Prakasam, A., Murray, M. E., Zhang, H. Y., Baxter, M. G., Sambamurti, K., et al. (2008). An increase in Abeta42 in the prefrontal cortex is associated with a reversal-learning impairment in Alzheimer's disease model Tg2576 APPsw mice. *Curr. Alzheimer Res.* 5, 385–391. doi: 10.2174/156720508785132280

Zhuo, J. M., Prescott, S. L., Murray, M. E., Zhang, H. Y., Baxter, M. G., and Nicolle, M. M. (2007). Early discrimination reversal learning impairment and preserved spatial learning in a longitudinal study of Tg2576 APPsw mice. *Neurobiol. Aging* 28, 1248–1257. doi: 10.1016/j.neurobiolaging.2006.05.034

16

Longevity pathways and memory aging

Ilias Gkikas[1], Dionysia Petratou[1] and NektariosTavernarakis[1,2] *

[1] Institute of Molecular Biology and Biotechnology, Foundation for Research and Technology-Hellas, Heraklion, Crete, Greece
[2] Department of Basic Sciences, Faculty of Medicine, University of Crete, Heraklion, Crete, Greece

Edited by:
Shin Murakami, Touro University-California, USA

Reviewed by:
Douglas Gray, Ottawa Hospital Research Institute, Canada
Daniele Bano, Deutsches Zentrum für Neurodegenerative Erkrankungen, Germany
Marta Artal Sanz, University Pablo de Olavide, Spain

***Correspondence:**
Nektarios Tavernarakis, Institute of Molecular Biology and Biotechnology, Foundation for Research and Technology-Hellas, N. Plastira 100, Vassilika Vouton, P.O. Box 1385, Heraklion 71110, Crete, Greece
e-mail: tavernarakis@imbb.forth.gr

The aging process has been associated with numerous pathologies at the cellular, tissue, and organ level. Decline or loss of brain functions, including learning and memory, is one of the most devastating and feared aspects of aging. Learning and memory are fundamental processes by which animals adjust to environmental changes, evaluate various sensory signals based on context and experience, and make decisions to generate adaptive behaviors. Age-related memory impairment is an important phenotype of brain aging. Understanding the molecular mechanisms underlying age-related memory impairment is crucial for the development of therapeutic strategies that may eventually lead to the development of drugs to combat memory loss. Studies in invertebrate animal models have taught us much about the physiology of aging and its effects on learning and memory. In this review we survey recent progress relevant to conserved molecular pathways implicated in both aging and memory formation and consolidation.

Keywords: Alzheimer's disease, autophagy, dietary restriction, insulin/IGF-1 signaling, learning, mitochondria, neurodegeneration,TOR signaling

INTRODUCTION

During the past century, age-related memory impairments have emerged as one of the top public health threats. Both psychiatric and neurodegenerative disorders comprising schizophrenia, depression, Alzheimer's disease (AD), Parkinson's disease (PD), and Huntington's disease (HD) are associated with age-related memory impairment. In humans, cognitive decline starts in midlife and deepens with advancing age suggesting that the greatest risk factor is age itself. Thus, ultimately, prevention of these pathologies necessitates thorough understanding of the molecular mechanisms underlying their links with the aging process (Bishop et al., 2010).

Our knowledge of the molecular regulatory mechanisms of aging impinging on cognitive capacity is steadily increasing in recent years. Interestingly, analyses of vertebrate and invertebrate model systems suggest that molecular and genetic pathways regulating cognitive aging are highly conserved in yeast, flies, worms, and mammals (Barco et al., 2006; Ardiel and Rankin, 2010; Bishop et al., 2010; Kauffman et al., 2010). Accumulating evidence from these models suggest a dynamic association between cognitive functions and aging. Similarly to several phenotypes and biomarkers of aging, which can vary substantially among individuals, cognitive decline displays significant severity fluctuation within a population. Consequently, it is important to identify key regulators of both cognitive impairment and longevity pathways. A plethora of molecular and cellular studies indicate a strong entanglement between lifespan regulation pathways and cognitive decline or neurodegeneration. In this review, we survey the molecular mechanisms and genes associated with longevity that have also been implicated in cognitive aging (summarized in **Table 1**). We further focus on recent work in invertebrate model organisms linking learning and memory impairment with age.

REDUCED INSULIN/IGF-1 SIGNALING PROMOTES LEARNING ABILITY DURING AGING

The insulin/IGF-1 (IIS) signal transduction pathway and its downstream effectors have been found to influence lifespan in a wide range of diverse organisms, suggesting a tightly conserved role of these mechanisms in aging. Reduction of IIS signaling promotes longevity in *Caenorhabditis elegans* and flies (Kenyon et al., 1993; Kenyon, 2010; Partridge, 2010). Whether this function is conserved in mice and humans remains unclear (Clancy et al., 2001; Tatar et al., 2001; Bluher et al., 2003; Suh et al., 2008; Bokov et al., 2011). Main components of insulin signaling in *C. elegans* are the insulin homolog INS-1, its receptor DAF-2, and the PIP3-kinase (phosphatidylinositol-triphosphate kinase) homolog AGE-1. Insulin signaling has been implicated in learning and memory, and in neuronal aging. Reduction of IIS attenuates protein aggregation and insolubility, and prevents amyloid-beta toxic effects. These processes are tightly associated with impaired nervous system function and age-related neurodegenerative diseases (Florez-McClure et al., 2007; David et al., 2010; Keowkase et al., 2010; Zhang et al., 2011; Tamura et al., 2013). In mouse models of AD, reduced IGF1 signaling protects from disease-associated neuronal loss and behavioral impairment, allthough IGF1R haploinsufficiency does not necessarily extent lifespan in mice (Cohen et al., 2009; Bokov et al., 2011).

In *C. elegans,* IIS has been shown to influence thermotaxis learning (Kodama et al., 2006) and salt chemotaxis learning (Tomioka et al., 2006). Moreover, long-lived IIS mutants show improved ability to associate temperature with food at both young and old age (Murakami, 2007). By contrast, some of these mutants are impaired, at young age, in their ability to associate NaCl with the absence of food (Vellai et al., 2006), or to intergrate sensory stimuli, such as Cu^{2+} and diacetyl

Table 1 | Conserved signaling pathway genes and cognitive aging in worms and flies.

Pathway	Gene	Cognitive aging effect	
		Caenorhabditis elegans	***Drosophila melanogaster***
Insulin signaling	*ins-1/INS*	Regulates gustatory associative learning, thermotaxis, and chemotaxis learning	NA[1]
	daf-2/IGFR	Inhibits growth cone initiation, axon growth and neuronal regrowth; loss-of-function improves thermotaxis associative learning and blocks chemotaxis/sensory integration learning	NA
	age-1/PI3K	Mutations improve thermotaxis learning with age but cause defects in chemotaxis associative learning	NA
	daf-18/PTEN	Loss-of-function decreases chemotaxis, odorant associative, and sensory integration learning	Inhibits axon regeneration
	daf-16/FoXO	Neuroprotective, promotes regeneration and neuronal migration; loss-of-function reduces associative and sensory integration learning	NA
Dietary restriction	*eat-2/DR*	Loss-of-function increases temperature–food association and impairs LTM[2]	DR[3] decreases STM[4] at mid-age, enhances MTM[5] at young-age
TOR signaling	*rheb*	NA	Overexpression induces morphology defects, and decreases odor-sucrose MTM
	rictor	NA	Deficiency blocks LTM
Autophagy	*cdk-5*	NA	Olfactory learning and memory defects
	apl-1/APPL	Olfactory and gustatory learning defects, habituation delay	NA
	unc-51/atg-1	NA	Influence axonal and dendritic development affecting olfactory learning
Mitochondria	*sod-1*	NA	Memory impairment associated with less synapses and mitochondrial dysfunction
	ucp-4, ucp-2	Promote neuronal toxicity in Huntington's disease models	Susceptible to Parkinson's and Huntington's diseases
	ced-9/Debcl	NA	Ameliorate cognition
	clk-1	Developmental and behavioral defects	Influence rhythmic behaviors

[1] *No information available,* [2] *Long-term memory,* [3] *Dietary restriction,* [4] *Short-term memory,* [5] *Mid-term memory.*

perception, towards decision-making (Jiu et al., 2010). Moreover, long-lived *age-1* mutant animals display delayed age-related decline of isothermal tracking and locomotion. Similarly, *age-1* and *daf-2* mutants associate temperature and starvation more efficiently compared to wild type controls, while young adults of these muants show increased temperature–food association. The enhanced association capacity of *daf-2* mutants is dependent on the neuronal Ca^{2+}-sensor NCS-1, which modulates isothermal tracking in the amphid interneurons, a key component of the thermosensory circuit (Murakami et al., 2005). AGE-1 also acts in the benzaldehyde-sensing amphid wing C (AWC) sensory neurons to direct benzaldehyde–starvation associative plasticity (Lin et al., 2010). While, mutations in the *daf-2* IIS receptor improve memory performance in *C. elegans* early in adulthood, maintaining learning ability with age, no extension in long-term memory (LTM) during aging is evident. Reduced insulin signaling does not alter neuronal plasticity but rather establishes an association more rapidly and prolongs the duration of this association early in adulthood (Kauffman et al., 2010).

Neuronal cells not only degenerate with age but the nervous system also loses the ability to regenerate after injury. Genetic experiments indicate that axon regeneration in aging *C. elegans* motor neurons is repressed by elevated IIS, which inhibits both growth cone initiation and axon growth (but not axon guidance) in aged animals. IIS impairs regeneration by blocking the function of DAF-16, a FOXO transcription factor and downstream effector of IIS. DAF-16/FOXO is necessary and sufficient to promote neuronal regeneration in a cell-autonomous manner. (Byrne et al., 2014). DAF-16 has also been shown to promote developmental neuronal migration and to affect aspects of neuronal cell morphology, such as neurite outgrowth (Christensen et al., 2011; Kennedy et al., 2013). DLK-1, a mitogen activated kinase kinase kinase (MAPKKK) that regulates presynaptic development is downregulated by IIS. DAF-16 upregulates expression of *dlk-1* in a neuron-specific manner, to promote neuronal regeneration indipendently of lifespan (Byrne et al., 2014). In addition, DAF-16 and HSF-1, the *C. elegans* heat shock transcription factor ortholog, show neuroprotective characteristics since their activation can defer the morphological and functional defects that emerge on the synapses of touch receptor neurons with physiological aging (Toth et al., 2012).

The totality of these findings suggest that in addition to extending lifespan, reduced IIS signaling also promotes learning ability with age. However, this effect is not accompanied by maintenance or extension of long term-memory during aging. Instead, IIS signaling appears to play a more significant role in the retrieval rather than acquisition of memory.

DIETARY RESTRICTION AND LONG-TERM MEMORY

Dietary restriction (DR), a reduction in total food intake, has been shown to increase lifespan and reduce fecundity in a wide range of organisms such as yeast, nematodes, flies, and rodents (Masoro, 2005; Mair and Dillin, 2008; Piper and Bartke, 2008). Recent studies in primates indicate that DR prevents from aging-related pathologies like brain atrophy,but it is still under debate wether it extends lifespan (Colman et al., 2009; Mattison et al., 2012; Cava and Fontana, 2013; Colman et al., 2014). Little is known about the genes mediating these effects of DR. In *C. elegans*, knock-down of *mekk-3* a homolog of the mammalian mitogen-activated MEKK3-like kinase, recapitulates DR and extends lifespan. MEKK-3 deficiency leads to reprogramming of fatty acid metabolism and lowering reactive oxygen species (ROS) generation, through the nuclear hormone receptor NHR-49 and DAF-22, an ortholog of human sterol carrier protein SCP2 (Chamoli et al., 2014).

The *C. elegans* feeding-defective mutant *eat-2* has been utilized as a model of DR. *eat-2* mutants ingest food poorly and, as a consequence, are long-lived. Lifespan extension by *eat-2* mutations is at least in part mediated through a *daf-16*-independent pathway (Avery, 1993; Raizen et al., 1995; Lakowski and Hekimi, 1998; Panowski et al., 2007). DR has also been suggested to attenuate age-related cognitive decline in rats (Adams et al., 2008). In *C. elegans*, young adult *eat-2* mutants show increased consistency of isothermal tracking (temperature–food association; Murakami et al., 2005). Contrary to *daf-2*, *eat-2* mutants exhibit significantly impaired LTM during young adulthood, but maintain memory capacity longer with age. Although young *eat-2* mutants display normal benzaldehyde chemotaxis, they require more training to form long-term memories. The duration of short-term memory in *eat-2* animals is similar to wild type, contrary to significant short term associative memory extension observed in *daf-2* mutants (Kauffman et al., 2010).

Dietary restriction also affects learning performance during aging in *Drosophila melanogaster*. The performance of young and old flies in an aversive learning test, where an odor is associated with a noxius mechanical shock, has been examined. These experiments showed that dietary-restricted flies, that live on average 14% longer than rich-diet fed flies, appear to have a better learning ability, even at old age. Young, dietary restricted flies show enhanced mid-term memory but their short-term memory is not affected. By contrast, short-term memory of mid-aged flies is poorer, compared with flies that grew on rich diet. Mid-term memory performance of mid-aged and old flies is not improved (Burger et al., 2010). These results are consistent with findings in *C. elegans*, in that only long term-memory is affected by DR during aging (Kauffman et al., 2010). While DR and reduced IIS signaling both increase longevity, the two pathways influence cognitive ability of young adults in an opposing manner.The differential effects of IIS and DR on learning and memory decline with age are likely due to their differential regulation of expression levels and activity of CRH-1, the cyclic adenosine monophosphate (cAMP) response element-binding protein (CREB) transcription factor homolog in *C. elegans* (Kauffman et al., 2010).

MITOCHONDRIAL FUNCTION AND COGNITIVE AGING

Mitochondria play pivotal role in adenosine triphosphate (ATP) production, calcium homeostasis, and apoptosis regulation, and are the main source of endogenous ROS. The functionality of these organelles influences aging through multiple pathways that may be directly or indirectly relevant to cognitive decline. The link between mitochondrial dysfunction, neurodegeneration, and cognition has been a subject of intensive study in many metazoans, ranging from *C. elegans* to humans (Bishop et al., 2010; Aksenov et al., 2013). A growing body of evidence suggests that neuronal structure and function are particularly vulnerable to mitochondrial function impairment (Stein and Murphy, 2012). However, the contribution of mitochondria to selective neurodegeneration in a variety of neurodegenerative pathologies associated with cognitive decline remains a matter of debate.

Aging studies in invertebrate model organisms provide a common ground for mitopathology and cognitive research. Several conserved groups of genes influencing mitochondrial metabolism, neural plasticity and synaptic function show expression changes during aging. In *C. elegans*, loss of α-tubulin acetyltransferase gene *mec-17* causes axon degeneration, thereby leading to neuronal dysfunction. Axons lacking MEC-17 contain less mitochondria, display transport defects, and loss of synaptic integrity (Neumann and Hilliard, 2014). Atat1, the mouse homolog of MEC-17 is associated with the formation of dentate gyrus, which is essential for learning and memory (Kim et al., 2013). Moreover, studies in *C. elegans ric-7* mutants, where axonal mitochondria trafficking is impaired, suggest that mitochondria are important for protection of axons against degeneration (Rawson et al., 2014). During physiological aging, nematode touch receptor neurons display morphological and functional abnormalities, such as neurite outgrowth defects and reduced number of synapses. Positioning of mitochondria in branches required for neurite outgrowth and the accumulation of vesicles in neuronal processes suggests that trafficking deficiency underlies these age-related abnormalities (Toth et al., 2012). These morphological changes of neurons have been associated with a decline in cognition, learning, and memory during aging (Vohra et al., 2010; Kimata et al., 2012; Kim et al., 2013; Wang et al., 2013).

The nematode genome encodes five superoxide dismutases (SODs) that function in cytoplasm, mitochondria, and extracellularly. Specifically, SOD-1 regulates detoxification of syperoxide radicals in mitochondria and guards from accumulation of oxidative damage during aging (Harman, 1968; McCord and Fridovich,

1969; Yanase et al., 2009; Back et al., 2010). Nonetheless, lifespan extension in mutants overexpressing *sod-1* is not related with reduction of oxidative damage (Cabreiro et al., 2011). Transgenic *C. elegans* expressing the human G93A SOD1 variant, associated with familial amyotrophic lateral sclerosis (ALS), in motor neurons show motor defects and increased autophagy in an age-dependent manner (Aksenov et al., 2013; Li et al., 2013). SOD-1 overexpression has also been associated with mitochondrial swelling, and learning and memory impairment in flies, mice, and humans (Shin et al., 2004; Perluigi and Butterfield, 2012; Haddadi et al., 2014). For example, transgenic flies expressing a zinc-deficient SOD1 mutant display behavioral defects, including impairment of locomotion, associated with mitochondrial respiratory chain deficiency and matrix vacuolization, that is not accompanied by shortening of lifespan (Bahadorani et al., 2013). Moreover, SOD-1 activity and expression levels decline during normal aging of *Drosophila*. At the same time, knock-down of *sod-1* in the mushroom bodies deteriorates mid-term memory and LTM. These memory defects associate with reduced synapse formation and mitochondrial damage during *Drosophila* aging (Haddadi et al., 2014).

Converging evidence implicates members of the antiapoptotic BCL-2 family of proteins in neuronal injury and synapse deformation, through impairment of mitochondrial dynamics (Berman et al., 2009). CED-9, the *C. elegans* homolog of BCL-2, interacts with the mitofusin FZO-1 and the dymanin related protein EAT-3 to promote mitochondrial fusion under specific conditions. The *C. elegans eat-3* encodes a homolog of human OPA-1 which is associated with Dominant Optic Atrophy disorder (Breckenridge et al., 2009; Rolland et al., 2009). In *Drosophila*, the BCL-2 homologous proteins, Buffy and Debcl are involved in the permeabilization of mitochondria to cytochrome-*c* that is mediated by pro-death mitochondrial proteins including Reaper and Hid (Abdelwahid et al., 2011). Unlike in worms, Buffy inhibition results in normal flies, while knockdown of Debcl protects against polyglutamine (polyQ)-induced neurodegeneration through maintaining mitochondrial homeostasis. The Debcl ortholog in mice, Bax/Bak, was found to regulate neurogenesis in adult brain regions such as hippocampus and cerebellum and promote discrimination learning without affecting significantly spatial memory and learning (Senoo-Matsuda et al., 2005; Galindo et al., 2009; Sahay et al., 2011; Hardwick and Soane, 2013).

Neurons are particularly vulnerable to mitochondrial dysfunction. Interestingly, expression of the human mitochondrial uncoupling protein (UCP) *ucp2* in *Drosophila* dopaminergic neurons increases ATP production and locomotion activity, and results in neuroprotection against pathogenic stress associated with PD (Islam et al., 2012). Beyond neurons, enhanced expression of mitochondria UCPs in flies ameliorates HD phenotypes in glia cells by moderating ROS and ATP production (Besson et al., 2010). In *C. elegans*, depletion of UCP-4 exacerbates neuronal toxicity in animals expressing an expanded polyQ repeat protein in touch neurons, suggesting that similarly to flies, under normal conditions UCP-4 protects from neuronal injuries in worms (Parker et al., 2012). However, overexpression of *ucp-4* in worms does not extend lifespan (Sagi and Kim, 2012). Alterations in the expression of mitochondrial respiratory chain genes result in similar effects. For example, mutations in the *mev-1* and *gas-1* genes, encoding subunits of complex II and I of the respiratory chain, respectively, increase ROS production, shorten lifespan, and retard behavioral rates (Kayser et al., 2004). In another example, animals carrying mutations in mitochondria complex IV *sft-1* gene, show increased lifespan that is dependent on DAF-16 (Maxwell et al., 2013). Depletion of SURF1, the mouse ortholog of *sft-1*, also increases lifespan and improves cognitive function in mice (Lin et al., 2013a). Knockdown of *clk-1*, a gene required for ubiquinone biosynthesis reduces respiration rates and increases *C. elegans* lifespan, also delaying behavioral rates (Rea et al., 2007). Loss-of-function mutations in *clk-1* extend lifespan and slow development and behavioral rates (Takahashi et al., 2012). Similarly, knockdown of the mouse *clk-1* ortholog causes mild mitochondrial dysfunction and extends lifespan (Lapointe and Hekimi, 2008; Deepa et al., 2013). In *Drosophila*, reduced expression of complex I and IV genes specifically in adult neurons is sufficient to extend lifespan (Copeland et al., 2009). Furthermore, observations in *clk-1* mutants indicate that neurite outgrowth is inhibited in aged worms (Tank et al., 2011). The association between neuronal morphology and behavioral effects suggests that mitochondria dysfunction may, in part, underlie memory and learning decline during aging (Ardiel and Rankin, 2010; Kimata et al., 2012; Stein and Murphy, 2012). However, little is known about the molecular mechanisms that mediate the effects of alterations in mitochondrial metabolism on both cognitive capacity and longevity.

AUTOPHAGY AND PROTEIN HOMEOSTASIS IN LEARNING AND MEMORY

The autophagic pathway has also been implicated in aging and cognitive decline. Autophagic activity decreases during the course of aging and genes that control this process are strongly associated with lifespan regulation in flies and worms (Lionaki et al., 2013). In *Drosophila*, overexpression of autophagy-related genes in neurons enhances longevity, while their repression causes neuronal defects and shortening of lifespan (Simonsen et al., 2008). Similarly, increasing autophagy mediates lifespan extension in worms (Hansen et al., 2008). UNC-51, a nematode autophagy regulator also controls axonal and dendritic development and its homolog affects olfactory learning in flies (Mochizuki et al., 2011). Worms lacking UNC-51 display axonal membrane defects, indicating a role of autophagy in synaptic plasticity, which indirectly interferes with learning and memory (Sigmond et al., 2008; Ragagnin et al., 2013). In *Drosophila*, inhibition of the cyclin-dependent kinase 5 (cdk5) kinase ortholog decreases autophagy, shortens lifespan and causes structural defects in central brain regions associated with olfactory learning and memory (Trunova and Giniger, 2012). In both flies and worms, autophagy deficiency leads to abnormal accumulation of protein aggregates thus promoting pathological mechanisms associated with neurodegenerative disorders, such as HD and AD (Ling et al., 2009; Low et al., 2013). For example, accumulation of intracellular APL-1, a β-amyloid precursor protein, upon autophagy impairment, causes behavioral deficiencies, including olfactory and gustatory learning defects, and habituation delay in *C. elegans* (Ewald et al., 2012; Ewald and Li, 2012;

Chen et al., 2013). Accumulation of APL-1 also occurs during normal aging and can reach pathological levels contributing to the pathogenesis of AD (Nilsson et al., 2013).

Age-induced memory impairment studies in *Drosophila* suggest that cognitive aging is strongly associated with the autophagic pathway. Indeed, spermidine-induced autophagy reduces aggregation of ubiquitinated proteins and protects from age-related memory impairment, in the aged *Drosophila* brain (Gupta et al., 2013). Spermidine activates autophagy to also promote longevity in different metazoans ranging from *C. elegans* to mice (Eisenberg et al., 2009; Wang et al., 2012). Other studies suggest that spermidine may not act directly through autophagy to facilitate neuroprotection and memory during aging. Instead, spermidine administration may influence histone acetyltransferase activity to modulate autophagy (Simonsen and Tooze, 2009; Davis, 2013; Graff and Tsai, 2013). These findings indicate that although the protective effect of spermidine does require activation of the autophagy pathway, the involvement of additional regulatory pathways remains to be elucidated. In conclusion, the exact mechanism by which autophagy controls cognitive aging is multifaceted and remains poorly understood. Additional studies are required to elucidate the contribution of autophagy in both longevity and cognitive capacity maintenance during aging.

TOR SIGNALING AND LONG-TERM MEMORY

Reduced signaling through the target of rapamycin (TOR) kinase has been shown to extend lifespan in diverse organisms (Vellai et al., 2003; Jia et al., 2004; Kapahi et al., 2004; Kaeberlein et al., 2005; Powers et al., 2006; Kenyon, 2010). The evolutionarily conserved mTOR functions in two complexes, mTORC1 and mTORC2 (Hay and Sonenberg, 2004; Wullschleger et al., 2006; Guertin and Sabatini, 2007). Tight regulation of the upstream components of the TOR pathway is important for proper neural growth and function throughout development and adulthood in *C. elegans* (Goldsmith et al., 2010). Overexpression of the small GTPase RAS homolog enriched in brain (Rheb), an upstream activator of TOR, in *Drosophila* photoreceptor cells downregulates autophagy, causes axon guidance defects and induces cell death (Knox et al., 2007; Wang et al., 2009). Selective overexpression of Rheb in distinct subsets of central brain neurons results in enlarged cell bodies and projections. In addition, Rheb overexpression in the mushroom bodies decreases mid-term odor-sucrose memory (Brown et al., 2012).

In the PIP3/PTEN/Akt/TOR pathway phosphorylated Akt activates TOR to regulate cell cycle and protein synthesis. In flies, the PTEN/Akt pathway is implicated in axon regeneration (Song et al., 2012). Similarly, axon regeneration is evident after the loss of DAF-18/PTEN in young adult worms (Byrne et al., 2014). Reduced TORC2 activity causes LTM deterioration in fruit flies (Huang et al., 2013). Rapamycin, a protein synthesis inhibitor that acts through the TOR pathway (mainly mTORC1), blocks long-term facilitation (LTF) in *Aplysia californica* (Hu et al., 2006). Moreover, rapamycin completely disrupts pre-existing long-term synaptic plasticity in *Aplysia* (Hu et al., 2011). While rapamycin extends lifespan mainly by blocking the TOR pathway, it may exert its effects on cognition through a different mechanism (Neff et al., 2013).

The TOR pathway controls translation of 5′TOP mRNAs containing a 5′ terminal oligopyrimidine tract. 5′TOP mRNAs encode proteins of the translational machinery. Under physiological conditions, 5′TOP mRNAs are largely repressed. Serotonin, which activates the TOR pathway, aleviates this repression, in a rapamycin-sensitive manner (Garelick and Kennedy, 2011; Labban and Sossin, 2011). eEF2 (eukaryotic elongation factor 2) is implicated in LTF in *Aplysia*, but is differentially regulated by eEF2 kinase in the neurites and the soma of sensory neurons involved in LTF (Weatherill et al., 2011). TORC1 mediates regulation of phosphorylation of eEF2 through the eEF2K (Carroll et al., 2004). Both in *Aplysia*, and in rodents, eEF2K function is associated with increased memory processing, through enhancing expression of genes implicated in the regulation of syntaptic strength (Weatherill et al., 2011).

Similarly, long term administration of rapamycin eliminates neuronal demyelination and neurodegeneration observed during aging in senescence-accelerated OXYS rats, a strain characterized by overproduction of free radicals (Kolosova et al., 2013). In mouse models of AD, rapamycin administrated either prior or after the onset of AD symptoms, improves animal cognition, probably through the preservation of brain vascular integrity and function (Lin et al., 2013b). Moreover, chronic treatment with rapamycin enhances spatial learning and memory with age, as well as the ability to recall a memory, even when the administration takes place late in life (Halloran et al., 2012). However, short-term administration following the emergence of learning and memory defects with aging, is not accompanied by such positive effects. The improvement of cognitive ability with rapamycin is mediated through reduction of TOR signaling and of IL-1β levels in the hippocampus, the facilitation of NMDA signaling, and increased CREB phosphorylation (Majumder et al., 2012). Furthermore, increased phosphorylation of S6, a target of TOR, is observed in the prefrontal cortex, after the administration of rapamycin, in OXYS rats (Kolosova et al., 2013).

CONCLUSION

Understanding how neuronal aging and cognitive impairment are influenced by mechanisms that modulate lifespan is an ongoing challenge. Such well-studied mechanisms include the IIS signaling pathway, DR, mitochondrial dysfunction, autophagy, and the TOR signaling pathway. Accumulating evidence indicates that these pathways also impinge on age-related neuronal dysfunction and memory-impairment. Indeed, manipulation of these pathways in a variety of metazoans affects neuronal structure and function and consequently promotes age-related memory impairment. It is likely that the decline in different forms of memory is independently mediated by distinct aging mechanisms (**Figure 1**). Decreased IIS signaling promotes decision making and associative learning. However this is not a general rule and, instead, appears to be dependent on different types of association. Nonetheless, DAF-16 activation likely delays morphological changes that occur with aging and promotes neuronal regeneration. DR exerts negative effects on LTM but enhances association making and memory. DR effects on short-term and mid-term memory appear to be age dependent.

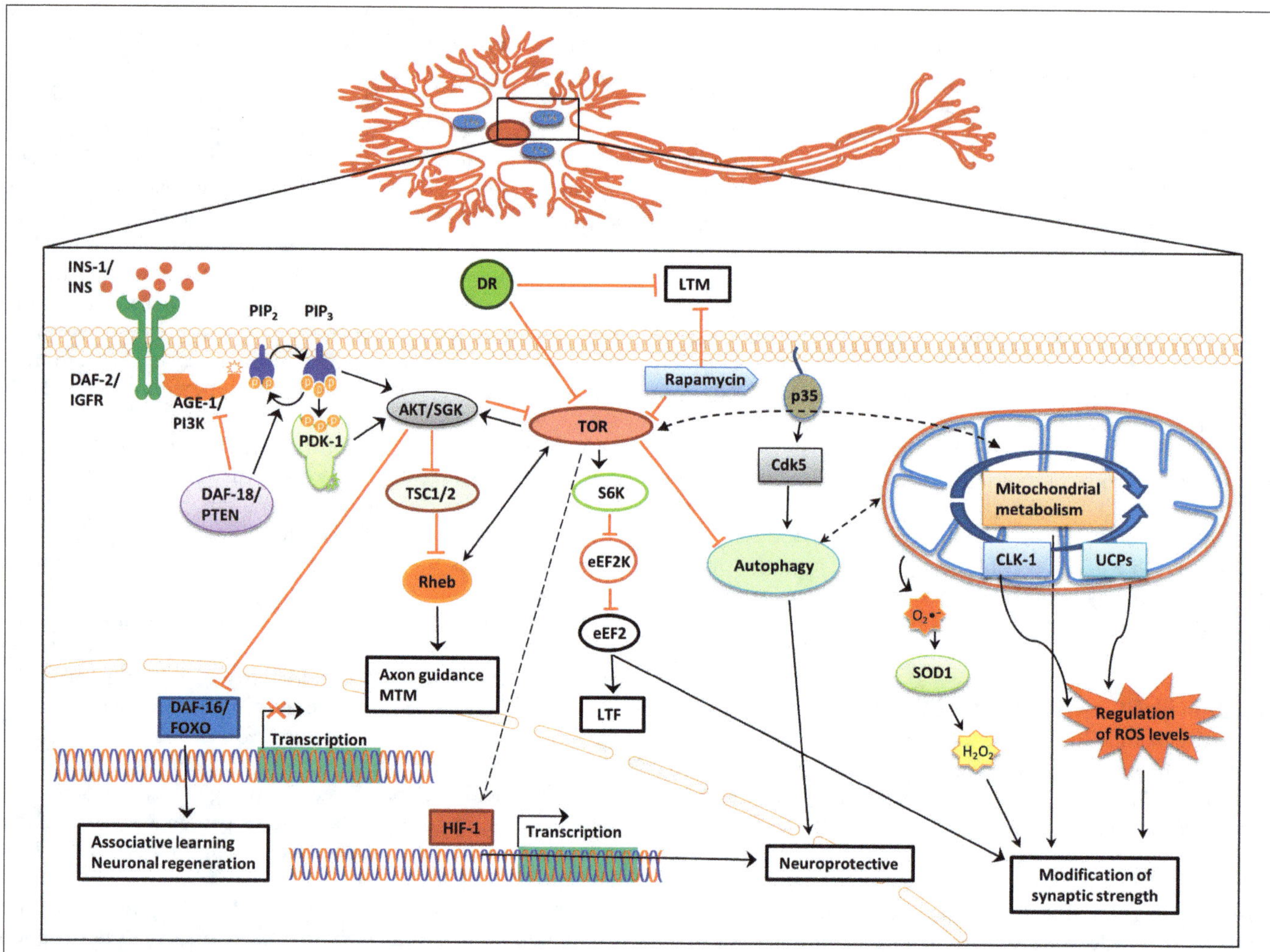

FIGURE 1 | Effects of IIS, DR, and TOR signaling, autophagy, and mitochondrial function on memory formation. In addition to extending lifespan, attenuation of IIS signaling, and subsequent de-repression of DAF-16 also reinforces associative learning and promotes axon regeneration and neuronal migration. Dietary restriction significantly impairs long-term memory, while it does not affect short-term memory. Blocking TOR signaling causes long-term-facilitation defects, while Rheb overexpression decreases mid-term memory and causes axon guidance defects. Regulation of autophagy through Cdk-5 affects lifespan and has also been associated with central nervous system structure defects, including olfactory learning and memory. Several mitochondrial genes promote neuroprotection. Impairment of mitochondrial function causes over production of ROS and concomitant synaptic deficiency. AGE-1/PI3K, phosphoinositide 3-kinase; AKT, protein kinase B; Cdk5, cyclin-dependent kinase 5; CLK-1, clock 1; DAF-2/IGFR, insulin-like growth factor receptor; DAF-16/FOXO, forkhead box O; DAF-18/PTEN, phosphatase and ensin homolog; DR, dietary restriction; eEF2, eukaryotic elongation factor 2; eEF2K, eukaryotic elongation factor 2 kinase; HIF-1, hypoxia-induced factor 1; INS, insulin; LTF, long-term facilitation; LTM, long-term memory; MTM, mid-term memory; PDK-1, 3-phosphoinositide-dependent kinase 1; PIP$_2$, phosphatidylinositol (4,5)-bisphosphate; PIP$_3$, phosphatidylinositol (3,4,5)-trisphosphate; Rheb, Ras homolog enriched in brain; S6K, ribosomal protein S6 kinase; SGK, serum- and glucocorticoid-inducible kinase; SOD1, superoxide dismutase 1; TSC1/2, tuberous sclerosis 1/2; TOR, target of rapamycin; UCPs, uncoupling proteins; Black arrow, direct stimulation; black dashed arrow, indirect stimulation; black dashed double head arrow, interplay; red arrow, inhibition.

The TOR pathway influences cognition by controlling protein biosynthesis, cell cycle, and metabolism (Garelick and Kennedy, 2011; Santos et al., 2011). Studies in invertebrates suggest that increased TOR signaling downregulates autophagy and causes axon guidance defects, while also promoting memory processing and synapse integrity. Conversely, in addition to increasing lifespan, downregulation of TOR signaling, mainly through rapamycin treatment, blocks LTM and LTF but also causes axon regeneration. In rodents rapamycin administration offsets the negative impact of aging on spatial learning and memory, increases memory recall ability, and enhances the vascular integrity of the brain. Moreover, morphological signs of AD and aging, such as neuronal demyelination and neurodegeneration are ameliorated. Activation of mTORC1 promotes mRNA translation, which likely enhances synapse formation. These distinct, but not necessarily conflicting results of manipulating TOR signaling could reflect a dose or compartment dependent regulation of cognition through TOR signaling.

In both worms and flies, activation of autophagy appears to promote lifespan and cognitive function. In mammals, little it is known about the role of autophagy during aging. However, recent studies in mice suggest that overexpression of autophagy-related gene Atg5 also increases lifespan (Pyo et al., 2013). Manipulation of mitochondria function during aging causes similar effects, either causing axon degeneration, or promoting axon integrity and stability (Keller et al., 2011; Fang et al., 2012). These ostensibly contradictory observations may suggest a neuron-specific function of mitochondria in aging. Despite recent progress and findings, several open questions need to be addressed. The involvement of epigenetic mechanisms and environmental conditions on nervous system aging is largely unknown. In addition, whether aging differentially affects subpopulations of neurons or different brain areas and to what extent remains unclear. While significant progress has been achieved towards deciphering the link between pathways that modulate both lifespan and aspects of neuronal function in invertebrate models, the relevance of these findings to neuronal aging and pathophysiology in higher organisms including humans has not been evaluated yet. Addressing these key issues will contribute towards developing informed strategies and therapeutic approaches aiming to battle age-related decline of nervous system performance and numerous neurodegenerative conditions associated with aging.

ACKNOWLEDGMENTS

We thank Maria Markaki for discussions and comments on the manuscript. Work in the authors' laboratory is funded by grants from the European Research Council (ERC), the European Commission Framework Programmes, and the Greek Ministry of Education. Ilias Gkikas is supported by the European Union Seventh Framework program through the Marie Curie Initial Training fellowship (Ageing Network – MarriAge). Dionysia Petratou is supported jointly by the European Union (European Social Fund – ESF) and Greek national program "THALES-MINOS" of the National Strategic Reference Framework (NSRF).

REFERENCES

Abdelwahid, E., Rolland, S., Teng, X., Conradt, B., Hardwick, J. M., and White, K. (2011). Mitochondrial involvement in cell death of non-mammalian eukaryotes. *Biochim. Biophys. Acta* 1813, 597–607. doi: 10.1016/j.bbamcr.2010.10.008

Adams, M. M., Shi, L., Linville, M. C., Forbes, M. E., Long, A. B., Bennett, C., et al. (2008). Caloric restriction and age affect synaptic proteins in hippocampal CA3 and spatial learning ability. *Exp. Neurol.* 211, 141–149. doi: 10.1016/j.expneurol.2008.01.016

Aksenov, V., Long, J., Liu, J., Szechtman, H., Khanna, P., Matravadia, S., et al. (2013). A complex dietary supplement augments spatial learning, brain mass, and mitochondrial electron transport chain activity in aging mice. *Age (Dordr.)* 35, 23–33. doi: 10.1007/s11357-011-9325-2

Ardiel, E. L., and Rankin, C. H. (2010). An elegant mind: learning and memory in *Caenorhabditis elegans*. *Learn. Mem.* 17, 191–201. doi: 10.1101/lm.960510

Avery, L. (1993). The genetics of feeding in *Caenorhabditis elegans*. *Genetics* 133, 897–917.

Back, P., Matthijssens, F., Vlaeminck, C., Braeckman, B. P., and Vanfleteren, J. R. (2010). Effects of sod gene overexpression and deletion mutation on the expression profiles of reporter genes of major detoxification pathways in *Caenorhabditis elegans*. *Exp. Gerontol.* 45, 603–610. doi: 10.1016/j.exger.2010.01.014

Bahadorani, S., Mukai, S. T., Rabie, J., Beckman, J. S., Phillips, J. P., and Hilliker, A. J. (2013). Expression of zinc-deficient human superoxide dismutase in *Drosophila* neurons produces a locomotor defect linked to mitochondrial dysfunction. *Neurobiol. Aging* 34, 2322–2330. doi: 10.1016/j.neurobiolaging.2013.03.024

Barco, A., Bailey, C. H., and Kandel, E. R. (2006). Common molecular mechanisms in explicit and implicit memory. *J. Neurochem.* 97, 1520–1533. doi: 10.1111/j.1471-4159.2006.03870.x

Berman, S. B., Chen, Y. B., Qi, B., McCaffery, J. M., Rucker, E. B. III, Goebbels, S., et al. (2009). Bcl-x L increases mitochondrial fission, fusion, and biomass in neurons. *J. Cell Biol.* 184, 707–719. doi: 10.1083/jcb.200809060

Besson, M. T., Dupont, P., Fridell, Y. W., and Lievens, J. C. (2010). Increased energy metabolism rescues glia-induced pathology in a *Drosophila* model of Huntington's disease. *Hum. Mol. Genet.* 19, 3372–3382. doi: 10.1093/hmg/ddq249

Bishop, N. A., Lu, T., and Yankner, B. A. (2010). Neural mechanisms of ageing and cognitive decline. *Nature* 464, 529–535. doi: 10.1038/nature08983

Bluher, M., Kahn, B. B., and Kahn, C. R. (2003). Extended longevity in mice lacking the insulin receptor in adipose tissue. *Science* 299, 572–574. doi: 10.1126/science.1078223

Bokov, A. F., Garg, N., Ikeno, Y., Thakur, S., Musi, N., DeFronzo, R. A., et al. (2011). Does reduced IGF-1R signaling in Igf1r$^{+/--}$ mice alter aging? *PLoS ONE* 6:e26891. doi: 10.1371/journal.pone.0026891

Breckenridge, D. G., Kang, B. H., and Xue, D. (2009). Bcl-2 proteins EGL-1 and CED-9 do not regulate mitochondrial fission or fusion in *Caenorhabditis elegans*. *Curr. Biol.* 19, 768–773. doi: 10.1016/j.cub.2009.03.022

Brown, H. L., Kaun, K. R., and Edgar, B. A. (2012). The small GTPase Rheb affects central brain neuronal morphology and memory formation in *Drosophila*. *PLoS ONE* 7:e44888. doi: 10.1371/journal.pone.0044888

Burger, J. M., Buechel, S. D., and Kawecki, T. J. (2010). Dietary restriction affects lifespan but not cognitive aging in *Drosophila melanogaster*. *Aging Cell* 9, 327–335. doi: 10.1111/j.1474-9726.2010.00560.x

Byrne, A. B., Walradt, T., Gardner, K. E., Hubbert, A., Reinke, V., and Hammarlund, M. (2014). Insulin/IGF1 signaling inhibits age-dependent axon regeneration. *Neuron* 81, 561–573. doi: 10.1016/j.neuron.2013.11.019

Cabreiro, F., Ackerman, D., Doonan, R., Araiz, C., Back, P., Papp, D., et al. (2011). Increased life span from overexpression of superoxide dismutase in *Caenorhabditis elegans* is not caused by decreased oxidative damage. *Free Radic. Biol. Med.* 51, 1575–1582. doi: 10.1016/j.freeradbiomed.2011.07.020

Carroll, M., Warren, O., Fan, X., and Sossin, W. S. (2004). 5-HT stimulates eEF2 dephosphorylation in a rapamycin-sensitive manner in *Aplysia* neurites. *J. Neurochem.* 90, 1464–1476. doi: 10.1111/j.1471-4159.2004.02634.x

Cava, E., and Fontana, L. (2013). Will calorie restriction work in humans? *Aging (Albany NY)* 5, 507–514.

Chamoli, M., Singh, A., Malik, Y., and Mukhopadhyay, A. (2014). A novel kinase regulates dietary restriction-mediated longevity in *Caenorhabditis elegans*. *Aging Cell.* doi: 10.1111/acel.12218 [Epub ahead of print].

Chen, C. H., Chen, Y. C., Jiang, H. C., Chen, C. K., and Pan, C. L. (2013). Neuronal aging: learning from *C. elegans*. *J. Mol. Signal.* 8, 14. doi: 10.1186/1750-2187-8-14

Christensen, R., de la Torre-Ubieta, L., Bonni, A., and Colon-Ramos, D. A. (2011). A conserved PTEN/FOXO pathway regulates neuronal morphology during *C. elegans* development. *Development* 138, 5257–5267. doi: 10.1242/dev.069062

Clancy, D. J., Gems, D., Harshman, L. G., Oldham, S., Stocker, H., Hafen, E., et al. (2001). Extension of life-span by loss of CHICO, a *Drosophila* insulin receptor substrate protein. *Science* 292, 104–106. doi: 10.1126/science.1057991

Cohen, E., Paulsson, J. F., Blinder, P., Burstyn-Cohen, T., Du, D., Estepa, G., et al. (2009). Reduced IGF-1 signaling delays age-associated proteotoxicity in mice. *Cell* 139, 1157–1169. doi: 10.1016/j.cell.2009.11.014

Colman, R. J., Anderson, R. M., Johnson, S. C., Kastman, E. K., Kosmatka, K. J., Beasley, T. M., et al. (2009). Caloric restriction delays disease onset and mortality in rhesus monkeys. *Science* 325, 201–204. doi: 10.1126/science.1173635

Colman, R. J., Beasley, T. M., Kemnitz, J. W., Johnson, S. C., Weindruch, R., and Anderson, R. M. (2014). Caloric restriction reduces age-related and all-cause mortality in rhesus monkeys. *Nat. Commun.* 5, 3557. doi: 10.1038/ncomms4557

Copeland, J. M., Cho, J., Lo, T., Hur, J. H., Bahadorani, S., Arabyan, T., et al. (2009). Extension of *Drosophila* life span by RNAi of the mitochondrial respiratory chain. *Curr. Biol.* 19, 1591–1598. doi: 10.1016/j.cub.2009.08.016

David, D. C., Ollikainen, N., Trinidad, J. C., Cary, M. P., Burlingame, A. L., and Kenyon, C. (2010). Widespread protein aggregation as an inherent part of aging in *C. elegans*. *PLoS Biol.* 8:e1000450. doi: 10.1371/journal.pbio.1000450

Davis, R. L. (2013). Spermidine cures flies of senior moments. *Nat. Neurosci.* 16, 1363–1364. doi: 10.1038/nn.3518

Deepa, S. S., Pulliam, D., Hill, S., Shi, Y., Walsh, M. E., Salmon, A., et al. (2013). Improved insulin sensitivity associated with reduced mitochondrial complex IV assembly and activity. *FASEB J.* 27, 1371–1380. doi: 10.1096/fj.12-221879

Eisenberg, T., Knauer, H., Schauer, A., Buttner, S., Ruckenstuhl, C., Carmona-Gutierrez, D., et al. (2009). Induction of autophagy by spermidine promotes longevity. *Nat. Cell Biol.* 11, 1305–1314. doi: 10.1038/ncb1975

Ewald, C. Y., Cheng, R., Tolen, L., Shah, V., Gillani, A., Nasrin, A., et al. (2012). Pan-neuronal expression of APL-1, an APP-related protein, disrupts olfactory, gustatory, and touch plasticity in *Caenorhabditis elegans. J. Neurosci.* 32, 10156–10169. doi: 10.1523/JNEUROSCI.0495-12.2012

Ewald, C. Y., and Li, C. (2012). *Caenorhabditis elegans* as a model organism to study APP function. *Exp. Brain Res.* 217, 397–411. doi: 10.1007/s00221-011-2905-7

Fang, Y., Soares, L., Teng, X., Geary, M., and Bonini, N. M. (2012). A novel *Drosophila* model of nerve injury reveals an essential role of Nmnat in maintaining axonal integrity. *Curr. Biol.* 22, 590–595. doi: 10.1016/j.cub.2012.01.065

Florez-McClure, M. L., Hohsfield, L. A., Fonte, G., Bealor, M. T., and Link, C. D. (2007). Decreased insulin-receptor signaling promotes the autophagic degradation of beta-amyloid peptide in *C. elegans. Autophagy* 3, 569–580.

Galindo, K. A., Lu, W. J., Park, J. H., and Abrams, J. M. (2009). The Bax/Bak ortholog in *Drosophila*, Debcl, exerts limited control over programmed cell death. *Development* 136, 275–283. doi: 10.1242/dev.019042

Garelick, M. G., and Kennedy, B. K. (2011). TOR on the brain. *Exp. Gerontol.* 46, 155–163. doi: 10.1016/j.exger.2010.08.030

Goldsmith, A. D., Sarin, S., Lockery, S., and Hobert, O. (2010). Developmental control of lateralized neuron size in the nematode *Caenorhabditis elegans. Neural Dev.* 5, 33. doi: 10.1186/1749-8104-5-33

Graff, J., and Tsai, L. H. (2013). Histone acetylation: molecular mnemonics on the chromatin. *Nat. Rev. Neurosci.* 14, 97–111. doi: 10.1038/nrn3427

Guertin, D. A., and Sabatini, D. M. (2007). Defining the role of mTOR in cancer. *Cancer Cell* 12, 9–22. doi: 10.1016/j.ccr.2007.05.008

Gupta, V. K., Scheunemann, L., Eisenberg, T., Mertel, S., Bhukel, A., Koemans, T. S., et al. (2013). Restoring polyamines protects from age-induced memory impairment in an autophagy-dependent manner. *Nat. Neurosci.* 16, 1453–1460. doi: 10.1038/nn.3512

Haddadi, M., Jahromi, S. R., Sagar, B. K., Patil, R. K., Shivanandappa, T., and Ramesh, S. R. (2014). Brain aging, memory impairment and oxidative stress: a study in *Drosophila melanogaster. Behav. Brain Res.* 259, 60–69. doi: 10.1016/j.bbr.2013.10.036

Halloran, J., Hussong, S. A., Burbank, R., Podlutskaya, N., Fischer, K. E., Sloane, L. B., et al. (2012). Chronic inhibition of mammalian target of rapamycin by rapamycin modulates cognitive and non-cognitive components of behavior throughout lifespan in mice. *Neuroscience* 223, 102–113. doi: 10.1016/j.neuroscience.2012.06.054

Hansen, M., Chandra, A., Mitic, L. L., Onken, B., Driscoll, M., and Kenyon, C. (2008). A role for autophagy in the extension of lifespan by dietary restriction in *C. elegans. PLoS Genet.* 4:e24. doi: 10.1371/journal.pgen.0040024

Hardwick, J. M., and Soane, L. (2013). Multiple functions of BCL-2 family proteins. *Cold Spring Harb. Perspect. Biol.* 5. doi: 10.1101/cshperspect.a008722

Harman, D. (1968). Free radical theory of aging: effect of free radical reaction inhibitors on the mortality rate of male LAF mice. *J. Gerontol.* 23, 476–482. doi: 10.1093/geronj/23.4.476

Hay, N., and Sonenberg, N. (2004). Upstream and downstream of mTOR. *Genes Dev.* 18, 1926–1945. doi: 10.1101/gad.1212704

Hu, J. Y., Baussi, O., Levine, A., Chen, Y., and Schacher, S. (2011). Persistent long-term synaptic plasticity requires activation of a new signaling pathway by additional stimuli. *J. Neurosci.* 31, 8841–8850. doi: 10.1523/JNEUROSCI.1358-11.2011

Hu, J. Y., Wu, F., and Schacher, S. (2006). Two signaling pathways regulate the expression and secretion of a neuropeptide required for long-term facilitation in *Aplysia. J. Neurosci.* 26, 1026–1035. doi: 10.1523/JNEUROSCI.4258-05.2006

Huang, W., Zhu, P. J., Zhang, S., Zhou, H., Stoica, L., Galiano, M., et al. (2013). mTORC2 controls actin polymerization required for consolidation of long-term memory. *Nat. Neurosci.* 16, 441–448. doi: 10.1038/nn.3351

Islam, R., Yang, L., Sah, M., Kannan, K., Anamani, D., Vijayan, C., et al. (2012). A neuroprotective role of the human uncoupling protein 2 (hUCP2) in a *Drosophila* Parkinson's disease model. *Neurobiol. Dis.* 46, 137–146. doi: 10.1016/j.nbd.2011.12.055

Jia, K., Chen, D., and Riddle, D. L. (2004). The TOR pathway interacts with the insulin signaling pathway to regulate *C. elegans* larval development, metabolism and life span. *Development* 131, 3897–3906. doi: 10.1242/dev.01255

Jiu, Y. M., Yue, Y., Yang, S., Liu, L., Yu, J. W., Wu, Z. X., et al. (2010). Insulin-like signaling pathway functions in integrative response to an olfactory and a gustatory stimuli in *Caenorhabditis elegans. Protein Cell* 1, 75–81. doi: 10.1007/s13238-010-0003-4

Kaeberlein, M., Powers, R. W. III, Steffen, K. K., Westman, E. A., Hu, D., Dang, N., et al. (2005). Regulation of yeast replicative life span by TOR and Sch9 in response to nutrients. *Science* 310, 1193–1196. doi: 10.1126/science.1115535

Kapahi, P., Zid, B. M., Harper, T., Koslover, D., Sapin, V., and Benzer, S. (2004). Regulation of lifespan in *Drosophila* by modulation of genes in the TOR signaling pathway. *Curr. Biol.* 14, 885–890. doi: 10.1016/j.cub.2004.03.059

Kauffman, A. L., Ashraf, J. M., Corces-Zimmerman, M. R., Landis, J. N., and Murphy, C. T. (2010). Insulin signaling and dietary restriction differentially influence the decline of learning and memory with age. *PLoS Biol.* 8:e1000372. doi: 10.1371/journal.pbio.1000372

Kayser, E. B., Sedensky, M. M., Morgan, P. G., and Hoppel, C. L. (2004). Mitochondrial oxidative phosphorylation is defective in the long-lived mutant clk-1. *J. Biol. Chem.* 279, 54479–54486. doi: 10.1074/jbc.M403066200

Keller, L. C., Cheng, L., Locke, C. J., Muller, M., Fetter, R. D., and Davis, G. W. (2011). Glial-derived prodegenerative signaling in the *Drosophila* neuromuscular system. *Neuron* 72, 760–775. doi: 10.1016/j.neuron.2011.09.031

Kennedy, L. M., Pham, S. C., and Grishok, A. (2013). Nonautonomous regulation of neuronal migration by insulin signaling, DAF-16/FOXO, and PAK-1. *Cell Rep.* 4, 996–1009. doi: 10.1016/j.celrep.2013.07.045

Kenyon, C., Chang, J., Gensch, E., Rudner, A., and Tabtiang, R. (1993). A *C. elegans* mutant that lives twice as long as wild type. *Nature* 366, 461–464. doi: 10.1038/366461a0

Kenyon, C. J. (2010). The genetics of ageing. *Nature* 464, 504–512. doi: 10.1038/nature08980

Keowkase, R., Aboukhatwa, M., and Luo, Y. (2010). Fluoxetine protects against amyloid-beta toxicity, in part via daf-16 mediated cell signaling pathway, in *Caenorhabditis elegans. Neuropharmacology* 59, 358–365. doi: 10.1016/j.neuropharm.2010.04.008

Kim, G. W., Li, L., Gorbani, M., You, L., and Yang, X. J. (2013). Mice lacking alpha-tubulin acetyltransferase 1 are viable but display alpha-tubulin acetylation deficiency and dentate gyrus distortion. *J. Biol. Chem.* 288, 20334–20350. doi: 10.1074/jbc.M113.464792

Kimata, T., Sasakura, H., Ohnishi, N., Nishio, N., and Mori, I. (2012). Thermotaxis of *C. elegans* as a model for temperature perception, neural information processing and neural plasticity. *Worm* 1, 31–41. doi: 10.4161/worm.19504

Knox, S., Ge, H., Dimitroff, B. D., Ren, Y., Howe, K. A., Arsham, A. M., et al. (2007). Mechanisms of TSC-mediated control of synapse assembly and axon guidance. *PLoS ONE* 2:e375. doi: 10.1371/journal.pone.0000375

Kodama, E., Kuhara, A., Mohri-Shiomi, A., Kimura, K. D., Okumura, M., Tomioka, M., et al. (2006). Insulin-like signaling and the neural circuit for integrative behavior in *C. elegans. Genes Dev.* 20, 2955–2960. doi: 10.1101/gad.1479906

Kolosova, N. G., Vitovtov, A. O., Muraleva, N. A., Akulov, A. E., Stefanova, N. A., and Blagosklonny, M. V. (2013). Rapamycin suppresses brain aging in senescence-accelerated OXYS rats. *Aging (Albany NY)* 5, 474–484.

Labban, M., and Sossin, W. S. (2011). Translation of 5′ terminal oligopyrimidine tract (5′TOP) mRNAs in *Aplysia californica* is regulated by the target of rapamycin (TOR). *Biochem. Biophys. Res. Commun.* 404, 816–821. doi: 10.1016/j.bbrc.2010.12.066

Lakowski, B., and Hekimi, S. (1998). The genetics of caloric restriction in *Caenorhabditis elegans. Proc. Natl. Acad. Sci. U.S.A.* 95, 13091–13096. doi: 10.1073/pnas.95.22.13091

Lapointe, J., and Hekimi, S. (2008). Early mitochondrial dysfunction in long-lived Mclk1$^{+/--}$ mice. *J. Biol. Chem.* 283, 26217–26227. doi: 10.1074/jbc.M803287200

Li, J., Huang, K. X., and Le, W. D. (2013). Establishing a novel *C. elegans* model to investigate the role of autophagy in amyotrophic lateral sclerosis. *Acta pharmacol. Sin.* 34, 644–650. doi: 10.1038/aps.2012.190

Lin, A. L., Pulliam, D. A., Deepa, S. S., Halloran, J. J., Hussong, S. A., Burbank, R. R., et al. (2013a). Decreased in vitro mitochondrial function is associated with enhanced brain metabolism, blood flow, and memory in Surf1-deficient mice. *J. Cereb. Blood Flow Metab.* 33, 1605–1611. doi: 10.1038/jcbfm.2013.116

Lin, A. L., Zheng, W., Halloran, J. J., Burbank, R. R., Hussong, S. A., Hart, M. J., et al. (2013b). Chronic rapamycin restores brain vascular integrity and function through NO synthase activation and improves memory in symptomatic mice modeling Alzheimer's disease. *J. Cereb. Blood Flow Metab.* 33, 1412–1421. doi: 10.1038/jcbfm.2013.82

Lin, C. H., Tomioka, M., Pereira, S., Sellings, L., Iino, Y., and van der Kooy, D. (2010). Insulin signaling plays a dual role in *Caenorhabditis elegans* memory acquisition and memory retrieval. *J. Neurosci.* 30, 8001–8011. doi: 10.1523/JNEUROSCI.4636-09.2010

Ling, D., Song, H. J., Garza, D., Neufeld, T. P., and Salvaterra, P. M. (2009). Abeta42-induced neurodegeneration via an age-dependent autophagic-lysosomal injury in *Drosophila. PLoS ONE* 4:e4201. doi: 10.1371/journal.pone.0004201

Lionaki, E., Markaki, M., and Tavernarakis, N. (2013). Autophagy and ageing: insights from invertebrate model organisms. *Ageing Res. Rev.* 12, 413–428. doi: 10.1016/j.arr.2012.05.001

Low, P., Varga, A., Pircs, K., Nagy, P., Szatmari, Z., Sass, M., et al. (2013). Impaired proteasomal degradation enhances autophagy via hypoxia signaling in *Drosophila. BMC Cell Biol.* 14, 29. doi: 10.1186/1471-2121-14-29

Mair, W., and Dillin, A. (2008). Aging and survival: the genetics of life span extension by dietary restriction. *Annu. Rev. Biochem.* 77, 727–754. doi: 10.1146/annurev.biochem.77.061206.171059

Majumder, S., Caccamo, A., Medina, D. X., Benavides, A. D., Javors, M. A., Kraig, E., et al. (2012). Lifelong rapamycin administration ameliorates age-dependent cognitive deficits by reducing IL-1beta and enhancing NMDA signaling. *Aging Cell* 11, 326–335. doi: 10.1111/j.1474-9726.2011.00791.x

Masoro, E. J. (2005). Overview of caloric restriction and ageing. *Mech. Ageing Dev.* 126, 913–922. doi: 10.1016/j.mad.2005.03.012

Mattison, J. A., Roth, G. S., Beasley, T. M., Tilmont, E. M., Handy, A. M., Herbert, R. L., et al. (2012). Impact of caloric restriction on health and survival in rhesus monkeys from the NIA study. *Nature* 489, 318–321. doi: 10.1038/nature11432

Maxwell, S., Harding, J., Brabin, C., Appleford, P. J., Brown, R., Delaney, C., et al. (2013). The SFT-1 and OXA-1 respiratory chain complex assembly factors influence lifespan by distinct mechanisms in *C. elegans. Longev. Healthspan* 2, 9. doi: 10.1186/2046-2395-2-9

McCord, J. M., and Fridovich, I. (1969). Superoxide dismutase. An enzymic function for erythrocuprein (hemocuprein). *J. Biol. Chem.* 244, 6049–6055.

Mochizuki, H., Toda, H., Ando, M., Kurusu, M., Tomoda, T., and Furukubo-Tokunaga, K. (2011). Unc-51/ATG1 controls axonal and dendritic development via kinesin-mediated vesicle transport in the *Drosophila* brain. *PLoS ONE* 6:e19632. doi: 10.1371/journal.pone.0019632

Murakami, H., Bessinger, K., Hellmann, J., and Murakami, S. (2005). Aging-dependent and -independent modulation of associative learning behavior by insulin/insulin-like growth factor-1 signal in *Caenorhabditis elegans. J. Neurosci.* 25, 10894–10904. doi: 10.1523/JNEUROSCI.3600-04.2005

Murakami, S. (2007). *Caenorhabditis elegans* as a model system to study aging of learning and memory. *Mol. Neurobiol.* 35, 85–94. doi: 10.1007/BF02700625

Neff, F., Flores-Dominguez, D., Ryan, D. P., Horsch, M., Schroder, S., Adler, T., et al. (2013). Rapamycin extends murine lifespan but has limited effects on aging. *J. Clin. Invest.* 123, 3272–3291. doi: 10.1172/JCI67674

Neumann, B., and Hilliard, M. A. (2014). Loss of MEC-17 Leads to microtubule instability and axonal degeneration. *Cell Rep.* 6, 93–103. doi: 10.1016/j.celrep.2013.12.004

Nilsson, P., Loganathan, K., Sekiguchi, M., Matsuba, Y., Hui, K., Tsubuki, S., et al. (2013). Abeta secretion and plaque formation depend on autophagy. *Cell Rep.* 5, 61–69. doi: 10.1016/j.celrep.2013.08.042

Panowski, S. H., Wolff, S., Aguilaniu, H., Durieux, J., and Dillin, A. (2007). PHA-4/Foxa mediates diet-restriction-induced longevity of *C. elegans. Nature* 447, 550–555. doi: 10.1038/nature05837

Parker, J. A., Vazquez-Manrique, R. P., Tourette, C., Farina, F., Offner, N., Mukhopadhyay, A., et al. (2012). Integration of beta-catenin, sirtuin, and FOXO signaling protects from mutant huntingtin toxicity. *J. Neurosci.* 32, 12630–12640. doi: 10.1523/JNEUROSCI.0277-12.2012

Partridge, L. (2010). The new biology of ageing. *Philos. Trans. R. Soc. Lond. B Biol. Sci.* 365, 147–154. doi: 10.1098/rstb.2009.0222

Perluigi, M., and Butterfield, D. A. (2012). Oxidative stress and Down syndrome: a route toward Alzheimer-like dementia. *Curr. Gerontol. Geriatr. Res.* 2012, 724904. doi: 10.1155/2012/724904

Piper, M. D., and Bartke, A. (2008). Diet and aging. *Cell Metab.* 8, 99–104. doi: 10.1016/j.cmet.2008.06.012

Powers, R. W. III, Kaeberlein, M., Caldwell, S. D., Kennedy, B. K., and Fields, S. (2006). Extension of chronological life span in yeast by decreased TOR pathway signaling. *Genes Dev.* 20, 174–184. doi: 10.1101/gad.1381406

Pyo, J. O., Yoo, S. M., Ahn, H. H., Nah, J., Hong, S. H., Kam, T. I., et al. (2013). Overexpression of Atg5 in mice activates autophagy and extends lifespan. *Nat. Commun.* 4, 2300. doi: 10.1038/ncomms3300

Ragagnin, A., Guillemain, A., Grant, N. J., and Bailly, Y. J. R. (2013). "Neuronal autophagy and prion proteins," in *Autophagy - A Double-Edged Sword - Cell Survival or Death?*, ed. Y. Bailly (Croatia: InTech), 377–419.

Raizen, D. M., Lee, R. Y., and Avery, L. (1995). Interacting genes required for pharyngeal excitation by motor neuron MC in *Caenorhabditis elegans. Genetics* 141, 1365–1382.

Rawson, R. L., Yam, L., Weimer, R. M., Bend, E. G., Hartwieg, E., Horvitz, H. R., et al. (2014). Axons degenerate in the absence of mitochondria in *C. elegans. Curr. Biol.* 24, 760–765. doi: 10.1016/j.cub.2014.02.025

Rea, S. L., Ventura, N., and Johnson, T. E. (2007). Relationship between mitochondrial electron transport chain dysfunction, development, and life extension in *Caenorhabditis elegans. PLoS Biol.* 5:e259. doi: 10.1371/journal.pbio.0050259

Rolland, S. G., Lu, Y., David, C. N., and Conradt, B. (2009). The BCL-2-like protein CED-9 of *C. elegans* promotes FZO-1/Mfn1,2- and EAT-3/Opa1-dependent mitochondrial fusion. *J. Cell Biol.* 186, 525–540. doi: 10.1083/jcb.200905070

Sagi, D., and Kim, S. K. (2012). An engineering approach to extending lifespan in *C. elegans. PLoS Genet.* 8:e1002780. doi: 10.1371/journal.pgen.1002780

Sahay, A., Scobie, K. N., Hill, A. S., O'Carroll, C. M., Kheirbek, M. A., Burghardt, N. S., et al. (2011). Increasing adult hippocampal neurogenesis is sufficient to improve pattern separation. *Nature* 472, 466–470. doi: 10.1038/nature09817

Santos, R. X., Correia, S. C., Cardoso, S., Carvalho, C., Santos, M. S., and Moreira, P. I. (2011). Effects of rapamycin and TOR on aging and memory: implications for Alzheimer's disease. *J. Neurochem.* 117, 927–936. doi: 10.1111/j.1471-4159.2011.07262.x

Senoo-Matsuda, N., Igaki, T., and Miura, M. (2005). Bax-like protein Drob-1 protects neurons from expanded polyglutamine-induced toxicity in *Drosophila. EMBO J.* 24, 2700–2713. doi: 10.1038/sj.emboj.7600721

Shin, J. H., London, J., Le Pecheur, M., Hoger, H., Pollak, D., and Lubec, G. (2004). Aberrant neuronal and mitochondrial proteins in hippocampus of transgenic mice overexpressing human Cu/Zn superoxide dismutase 1. *Free Radic. Biol. Med.* 37, 643–653. doi: 10.1016/j.freeradbiomed.2004.05.019

Sigmond, T., Feher, J., Baksa, A., Pasti, G., Palfia, Z., Takacs-Vellai, K., et al. (2008). Qualitative and quantitative characterization of autophagy in *Caenorhabditis elegans* by electron microscopy. *Methods Enzymol.* 451, 467–491. doi: 10.1016/S0076-6879(08)03228-X

Simonsen, A., Cumming, R. C., Brech, A., Isakson, P., Schubert, D. R., and Finley, K. D. (2008). Promoting basal levels of autophagy in the nervous system enhances longevity and oxidant resistance in adult *Drosophila. Autophagy* 4, 176–184.

Simonsen, A., and Tooze, S. A. (2009). Coordination of membrane events during autophagy by multiple class III PI3-kinase complexes. *J. Cell Biol.* 186, 773–782. doi: 10.1083/jcb.200907014

Song, Y., Ori-McKenney, K. M., Zheng, Y., Han, C., Jan, L. Y., and Jan, Y. N. (2012). Regeneration of *Drosophila* sensory neuron axons and dendrites is regulated by the Akt pathway involving Pten and microRNA bantam. *Genes Dev.* 26, 1612–1625. doi: 10.1101/gad.193243.112

Stein, G. M., and Murphy, C. T. (2012). The intersection of aging, longevity pathways, and learning and memory in *C. elegans. Front. Genet.* 3:259. doi: 10.3389/fgene.2012.00259

Suh, Y., Atzmon, G., Cho, M. O., Hwang, D., Liu, B., Leahy, D. J., et al. (2008). Functionally significant insulin-like growth factor I receptor mutations in centenarians. *Proc. Natl. Acad. Sci. U.S.A.* 105, 3438–3442. doi: 10.1073/pnas.0705467105

Takahashi, M., Ogawara, M., Shimizu, T., and Shirasawa, T. (2012). Restoration of the behavioral rates and lifespan in clk-1 mutant nematodes in response to exogenous coenzyme Q(10). *Exp. Gerontol.* 47, 276–279. doi: 10.1016/j.exger.2011.12.012

Tamura, T., Sone, M., Nakamura, Y., Shimamura, T., Imoto, S., Miyano, S., et al. (2013). A restricted level of PQBP1 is needed for the best longevity of *Drosophila. Neurobiol. Aging* 34, 356.e311–356.e320. doi: 10.1016/j.neurobiolaging.2012.07.015

Tank, E. M. H., Rodgers, K. E., and Kenyon, C. (2011). Spontaneous age-related neurite branching in *Caenorhabditis elegans. J. Neurosci.* 31, 9279–9288. doi: 10.1523/JNEUROSCI.6606-10.2011

Tatar, M., Kopelman, A., Epstein, D., Tu, M. P., Yin, C. M., and Garofalo, R. S. (2001). A mutant *Drosophila* insulin receptor homolog that extends life-span and impairs neuroendocrine function. *Science* 292, 107–110. doi: 10.1126/science.1057987

Tomioka, M., Adachi, T., Suzuki, H., Kunitomo, H., Schafer, W. R., and Iino, Y. (2006). The insulin/PI 3-kinase pathway regulates salt chemotaxis learning in *Caenorhabditis elegans. Neuron* 51, 613–625. doi: 10.1016/j.neuron.2006.07.024

Toth, M. L., Melentijevic, I., Shah, L., Bhatia, A., Lu, K., Talwar, A., et al. (2012). Neurite sprouting and synapse deterioration in the aging *Caenorhabditis elegans* nervous system. *J. Neurosci.* 32, 8778–8790. doi: 10.1523/JNEUROSCI.1494-11.2012

Trunova, S., and Giniger, E. (2012). Absence of the Cdk5 activator p35 causes adult-onset neurodegeneration in the central brain of *Drosophila. Dis. Model. Mech.* 5, 210–219. doi: 10.1242/dmm.008847

Vellai, T., McCulloch, D., Gems, D., and Kovacs, A. L. (2006). Effects of sex and insulin/insulin-like growth factor-1 signaling on performance in an associative learning paradigm in *Caenorhabditis elegans. Genetics* 174, 309–316. doi: 10.1534/genetics.106.061499

Vellai, T., Takacs-Vellai, K., Zhang, Y., Kovacs, A. L., Orosz, L., and Muller, F. (2003). Genetics: influence of TOR kinase on lifespan in *C. elegans. Nature* 426, 620. doi: 10.1038/426620a

Vohra, B. P., Sasaki, Y., Miller, B. R., Chang, J., DiAntonio, A., and Milbrandt, J. (2010). Amyloid precursor protein cleavage-dependent and -independent axonal degeneration programs share a common nicotinamide mononucleotide adenylyltransferase 1-sensitive pathway. *J. Neurosci.* 30, 13729–13738. doi: 10.1523/JNEUROSCI.2939-10.2010

Wang, I. F., Guo, B. S., Liu, Y. C., Wu, C. C., Yang, C. H., Tsai, K. J., et al. (2012). Autophagy activators rescue and alleviate pathogenesis of a mouse model with proteinopathies of the TAR DNA-binding protein 43. *Proc. Natl. Acad. Sci. U.S.A.* 109, 15024–15029. doi: 10.1073/pnas.1206362109

Wang, T., Lao, U., and Edgar, B. A. (2009). TOR-mediated autophagy regulates cell death in *Drosophila* neurodegenerative disease. *J. Cell Biol.* 186, 703–711. doi: 10.1083/jcb.200904090

Wang, Y., Yin, H., Li, J., Zhang, Y., Han, B., Zeng, Z., et al. (2013). Amelioration of beta-amyloid-induced cognitive dysfunction and hippocampal axon degeneration by curcumin is associated with suppression of CRMP-2 hyperphosphorylation. *Neurosci. Lett.* 557(Pt B), 112–117. doi: 10.1016/j.neulet.2013.10.024

Weatherill, D. B., McCamphill, P. K., Pethoukov, E., Dunn, T. W., Fan, X., and Sossin, W. S. (2011). Compartment-specific, differential regulation of eukaryotic elongation factor 2 and its kinase within *Aplysia* sensory neurons. *J. Neurochem.* 117, 841–855. doi: 10.1111/j.1471-4159.2011.07251.x

Wullschleger, S., Loewith, R., and Hall, M. N. (2006). TOR signaling in growth and metabolism. *Cell* 124, 471–484. doi: 10.1016/j.cell.2006.01.016

Yanase, S., Onodera, A., Tedesco, P., Johnson, T. E., and Ishii, N. (2009). SOD-1 deletions in *Caenorhabditis elegans* alter the localization of intracellular reactive oxygen species and show molecular compensation. *J. Gerontol. A Biol. Sci. Med. Sci.* 64, 530–539. doi: 10.1093/gerona/glp020

Zhang, T., Mullane, P. C., Periz, G., and Wang, J. (2011). TDP-43 neurotoxicity and protein aggregation modulated by heat shock factor and insulin/IGF-1 signaling. *Hum. Mol. Genet.* 20, 1952–1965. doi: 10.1093/hmg/ddr076

17

Emerging functional similarities and divergences between *Drosophila* Spargel/dPGC-1 and mammalian PGC-1 protein

Subhas Mukherjee[1†], Mohammed A. Basar[1], Claudette Davis[1,2] and Atanu Duttaroy[1*]

[1] Department of Biology, Howard University, Washington, DC, USA
[2] Biology Undergraduate Program, College of Science, George Mason University, Fairfax, VA, USA

Edited by:
Shin Murakami, Touro University-California, USA

Reviewed by:
Johannes Bauer, Southern Methodist University, USA
Margarida Matos, Faculdade de Ciencias da Universidade de Lisboa, Portugal

***Correspondence:**
Atanu Duttaroy, Department of Biology, Howard University, 415, College Street, NW, Washington, DC 20059, USA
e-mail: aduttaroy@howard.edu

†Present address:
Subhas Mukherjee, Department of Pathology and Laboratory Medicine, Winship Cancer Institute, Emory University School of Medicine, Atlanta, USA

Peroxisome Proliferator Activated Receptor Gamma Co-activator-1 (PGC-1) is a well-conserved protein among all chordates. Entire *Drosophila* species subgroup carries a *PGC-1* homolog in their genome called *spargel/dPGC-1* showing very little divergence. Recent studies have reported that significant functional similarities are shared between vertebrate and invertebrate PGC-1's based on their role in mitochondrial functions and biogenesis, gluconeogenesis, and most likely in transcription and RNA processing. With the help of genetic epistasis analysis, we established that *Drosophila* Spargel/dPGC-1 affects cell growth process as a terminal effector in the Insulin-TOR signaling pathway. The association between Spargel/dPGC-1 and Insulin signaling could also explain its role in the aging process. Here we provided a further comparison between Spargel/dPGC-1 and PGC-1 focusing on nuclear localization, oxidative stress resistance, and a possible role of Spargel/dPGC-1 in oogenesis reminiscing the role of Spargel in reproductive aging like many Insulin signaling partners. This led us to hypothesize that the discovery of newer biological functions in *Drosophila* Spargel/dPGC-1 will pave the way to uncover novel functional equivalents in mammals.

Keywords: *Drosophila*, PGC-1, mitochondria, oogenesis, RNA processing

Homeothermic mammals utilize the Peroxisome Proliferator Activated Receptor Gamma Co-activator 1 (PGC-1) as a thermogenic regulator (maintains body temperature) to protect against excessive cold or excess calorie intake (Puigserver et al., 1998). Thus PGC-1 is expressed in tissues with high metabolic requirement and it is linked to multiple metabolic pathways such as gluconeogenesis, adipogenesis, myogenesis, and mitogenesis (Handschin and Spiegelman, 2006). Apart from metabolism, PGC-1 might play a central role in maintaining oxidative homeostasis (Austin and St-Pierre, 2012). Homologs of *PGC-1* were found in all chordates including the fish genomes (Lin et al., 2005) where body temperature regulation isn't necessary (with the exception of a few marine species). Among invertebrate models, only *Drosophila* carries a single *PGC-1* homolog in its genome (Gershman et al., 2007) whereas other invertebrate models such as yeast and *C. elegans* do not carry any *PGC-1* homologous sequence (Lin et al., 2005). *Drosophila PGC-1*, designated as *spargel/dPGC-1* (Tiefenbock et al., 2010), is well conserved in distantly related *Drosophila* species subgroups with its C-terminal RS and RRM domains (**Figure 1A**). Two notable differences between PGC-1 and Spargel/dPGC-1 are: the C-terminal FDSLL domain of PGC-1 is replaced with FEALL in all *Drosophila* species (Gershman et al., 2007; Tiefenbock et al., 2010; Bugger et al., 2011), and the larger size of Spargel/dPGC-1 protein as it carries ~300 more amino acids than PGC-1 (**Figure 1A**). Although nuclear receptors are generally known to interact with the leucine rich motifs (LXXLL) (Matsuda et al., 2004), the FEALLL variant of this motif in *Drosophila* is able to interact with the nuclear receptors as well (Wang et al., 2007). In light of the fact that significant functional overlap exists between the three PGC-1 homologs in mice PGC-1α, PGC-1β and PRC, which makes it difficult to tease apart their relative roles *in vivo*, we propose that the presence of a single *Drosophila PGC-1* homolog will provide an enormous advantage to study the function of this essential transcriptional coactivator in an alternate model. Within the last few years, significant functional homologies have surfaced between mammalian PGC-1 and *Drosophila* Spargel/dPGC-1, which called for a discussion of this topic in greater detail.

ENERGY METABOLISM

As a transcriptional coactivator PGC-1 activates many nuclear receptor, which in turn regulate the transcription activity of variety of nuclear genes (Puigserver and Spiegelman, 2003). Similarly, Spargel/dPGC-1 regulates the expression of mitochondrial oxidative phosphorylation (OXPHOS) genes through *NRF1* (Nuclear Respiratory Factor) homolog *delg* (Tiefenbock et al., 2010). *Spargel/dPGC-1* gain of function (overexpression) correlates with an increased rate of mitochondrial oxygen consumption (Rera et al., 2011) and ATP production (Mukherjee and Duttaroy, 2013), enhanced mitochondrial DNA content, increased enzyme activity and protein production in the mitochondrial matrix (Rera et al., 2011). These observations are reminiscent of the effect of PGC-1α on mitochondrial biogenesis, functional capacity and energy metabolism (Liu and Lin, 2011). Thus, regulation of

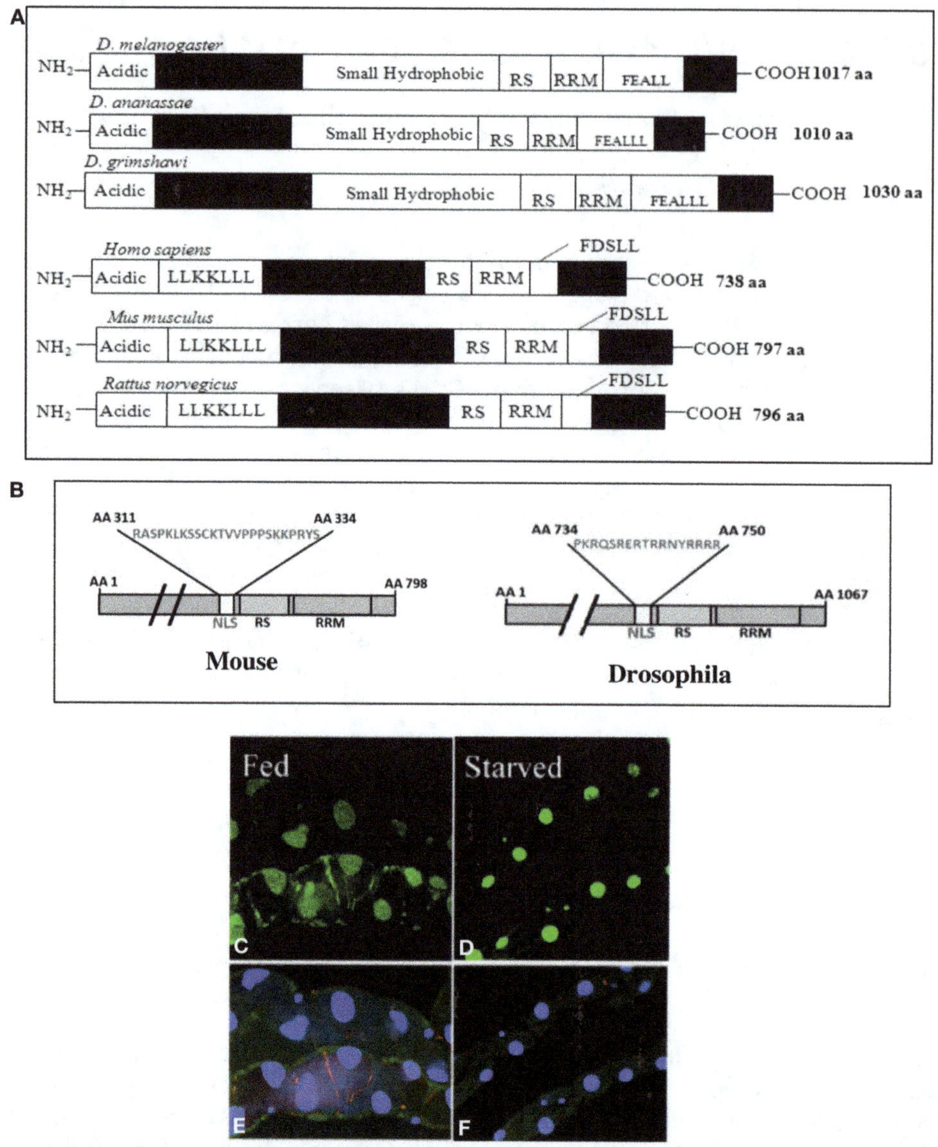

FIGURE 1 | (A) Comparison of the Spargel/dPGC-1 protein structure in 3 widely divergent subgroups of *Drosophila melanogaster*, *D. ananassae*, and *D. grimshawi* (van der Linde and Houle, 2008). Vertebrate PGC-1 is about 300 amino acids shorter in length than the Spargel/dPGC-1. Filled boxes represent regions of non-homology. **(B)** An authentic Nuclear Localization Signal (NLS) has been found in mammalian PGC-1 with the help of NLS Predict Software. **(C)** Nuclear localization of Spargel is documented in the gut tissue with a Spargel-GFP protein (green). Following 48 h of starvation, the gut turns thinner and Insulin signaling is reduced, but it imposes no effect on nuclear localization of the Spargel-GFP protein **(D)**. **(E,F)** DAPI staining of the same gut tissue.

mitochondrial function is truly an ancestral function for PGC-1 group of proteins.

INTRACELLULAR LOCALIZATION

Serine-Arginine (SR) repeats and RNA Recognition Motifs (RRM) are classical hallmarks of "RNA processing domains." Furthermore, localization of PGC-1 in the nuclear compartment where it is concentrated in nuclear speckles along with splicing factor α-U1 and SR splicing factor SC-35 are irrefutable evidence that PGC-1 is involved in the splicing complex (Monsalve et al., 2000). We recently demonstrated that a Spargel-GFP fusion protein also localizes itself in the nucleus forming distinct punctate structures (Mukherjee and Duttaroy, 2013). An authentic Nuclear Localization Signal (NLS) was uncovered in Spargel/dPGC-1 with the help of a NLS predict software (Mukherjee and Duttaroy, 2013) that most likely assists in Spargel/dPGC-1 localization into the nucleus. With the help of the same software we now located a NLS between the amino acids 311–334 in mammalian PGC-1 (score 0.93) (**Figure 1B**), which should also justify the presence of PGC-1 protein in the nucleus (Monsalve et al., 2000).

An earlier study claimed that activation of Insulin signaling is important for transport of Spargel/dPGC-1 protein from cytoplasm to the nucleus (Tiefenbock et al., 2010) and Spargel/dPGC-1 is now established as a member of the

Insulin-TOR signaling pathway (Mukherjee and Duttaroy, 2013). Nutrient availability controls the Insulin/TOR signaling pathway from TOR downstream (Takano et al., 2001) therefore, under starvation condition, Insulin mediated signal transduction is reduced. We rationalized that if Insulin signaling is essential for nuclear localization of Spargel/dPGC-1 then reduction of this signal should sequester the protein to the cytosol. To test this prediction, gut malphigian tubule preparations were obtained from flies following two days of starvation (only water given to prevent dehydration) and analyzed for Spargel expression. Since the localization of Spargel/dPGC-1 is still restricted to the nucleus following starvation (**Figures 1C–F**) this supports that cellular localization of Spargel/dPGC-1 occurs independent of Insulin signaling.

Spargel/dPGC-1 DOESN'T INFLUENCE ANTIOXIDANT ENZYMES

The apparent involvement of PGC-1 in oxidative metabolism has been established from the following: PGC-1 activates Nuclear Respiratory Factor1 (*NRF1*); muscle specific overexpression of PGC-1α induces specific antioxidants like *Sod2* and *GpX* transcription activity (St-Pierre et al., 2006) whereas ablation of PGC-1α in cultured cell cause down regulation of a whole panel of antioxidants including *SOD1, SOD2, GpX, UCP1,* and *UCP2,* resulting in hypersensitivity to hydrogen peroxide induced oxidative stress (St-Pierre et al., 2006). Another interesting observation is that cells from patients with Friedrich's Ataxia show coordinated suppression of PGC-1 and antioxidant enzymes (Coppola et al., 2009). It was inferred from these observations that PGC-1 controls mitochondrial reactive oxygen species (ROS) by regulating the antioxidant defense system (Austin and St-Pierre, 2012).

We attempted to validate this prediction in a whole animals model by utilizing the *Drosophila spargel* mutant hypomorph, srl^1 (Tiefenbock et al., 2010) and a *spargel* transgenic line that is capable of overexpressing Spargel/dPGC-1 (Mukherjee and Duttaroy, 2013). For systemic oxidative stress generation, we used methyl violgen (commercially known as "paraquat") that is stable at room temperature. Male and female flies overexpressing Spargel were exposed to 20 mM paraquat and both survived better than the control (**Figures 2A,B**). After 48 h of paraquat treatment, Spargel/dPGC-1 overexpression helped 50% males to remain viable, where as in control flies 50% survival was attained within 24 h. Female flies appear slightly more sensitive to paraquat treatment although a significant difference still persists with respect to the control (**Figures 2A,B**). This increased resistance to oxidative stress in Spargel/dPGC-1 overexpressing flies makes it tempting to conclude that Spargel/dPGC-1 is also involved in oxidative stress resistance and imposes the same effect on antioxidant defense enzymes like PGC-1. However, this expectation may not be true since the expression of two front line antioxidant defense enzymes SOD2 and SOD1 remain unchanged when Spargel/dPGC-1 is overexpressed (gain of function) or reduced in srl^1 hypomorphs (**Figure 2C**). Since these experiments were performed on whole animals as opposed to cultured cells, it might be necessary to check the status of these antioxidant enzymes in *PGC-1KO* mice. Secondly,

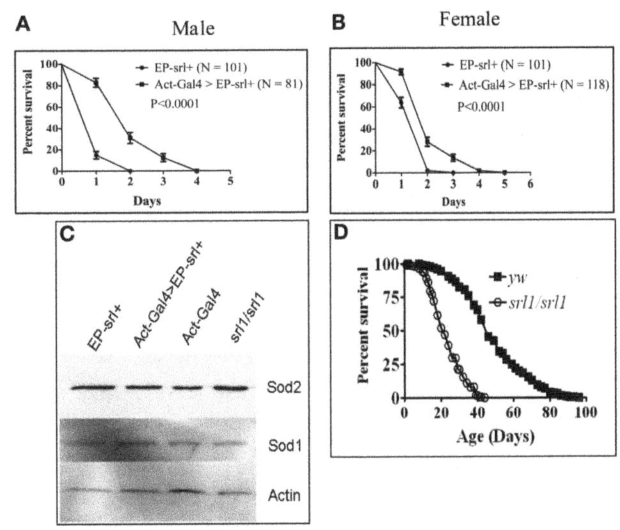

FIGURE 2 | Spargel gain of function was achieved by activating an *EP-srl*$^+$ transgene ubiquitously with the help of *Actin-GAL4* driver (see Kapahi et al., 2004, for detail). Percent survival was measured following exposure to 20 mM paraquat made in 1% sucrose solution. **(A,B)** Male and female flies overexpressing Spargel/dPGC-1 survive longer in paraquat than the control indicating that Spargel/dPGC-1 overexpression cause increased resistance to oxidative stress, **(C)** Spargel/dPGC-1 overexpression or its ablation in srl^1 does not alter the expression of SOD2 and SOD1 antioxidant enzymes, **(D)** Reduced Spargel/dPGC-1 in srl^1 cause significant reduction in life span.

since it is involved in the Insulin-TOR signaling (Mukherjee and Duttaroy, 2013), Spargel/dPGC-1 might utilize other stress resistance pathways (which remain to be tested) such as FoxO or Jnk as opposed to antioxidant enzymes. Incidentally, a recent study in *Drosophila* showed that *Wolbachea* induced metabolic stress promotes mitogenesis through activation of Spargel/dPGC-1 (Chen et al., 2012). Clearly, more needs to be done to understand the relationship between Spargel/dPGC-1 and stress resistance.

GROWTH, LONGEVITY, AND AGING

Insulin-TOR signaling pathway is involved in systemic regulation of growth, longevity and aging in all taxa (Hietakangas and Cohen, 2009; Partridge et al., 2011). In the absence of Insulin, PGC-1 expression is elevated in liver and gluconeogenesis is initiated (Puigserver et al., 2003). Therefore liver-specific knock down of PGC-1 shows higher insulin sensitivity in mice (Koo et al., 2004). On the contrary, absence of PGC-1 in skeletal muscles imposes no effect on insulin sensitivity (Zechner et al., 2010). Thus one can assume that the metabolic role of PGC-1 and its relationship with Insulin/TOR signaling became more tissue specific during the course of evolution.

The requirement of Spargel/dPGC-1 in the Insulin-TOR signaling pathway (Tiefenbock et al., 2010; Mukherjee and Duttaroy, 2013) automatically connects it to the cell growth process. Spargel/dPGC-1 is a terminal effector of this pathway hence reduced *spargel* expression results in growth retardation with smaller body size and developmental delays, though Spargel/dPGC-1 overexpression has no immediate effect on growth (Rera et al., 2011; Mukherjee and Duttaroy, 2013).

With respect to longevity, members of the Insulin-TOR signaling pathway extend life span in *C. elegans* (Vellai et al., 2003; Kenyon, 2010; Partridge et al., 2011), *Drosophila* (Clancy et al., 2001; Tatar et al., 2001; Kapahi et al., 2004) and mice (Fontana et al., 2010; Kenyon, 2010) by delaying the aging process. Mutant forms of *Insulin receptor (InR)*, the Insulin receptor substrate *chico* and TOR all extend longevity, whereas for *FoxO* lifespan extension happens through its overexpression. Spargel/dPGC-1's action on longevity is apparent as reduced Spargel/dPGC-1 expression cause significant shortening of life span (**Figure 2D**). Reduced ROS production and stem cell over proliferation were cited as two major reasons for Spargel/dPGC-1 mediated extension of lifespan (Rera et al., 2011), though the gain of function effects are specific to the intestinal stem cells as opposed to the Insulin and TOR mediated lifespan extensions, which are largely ubiquitous. So, research on *Drosophila* is pioneering for understanding the aging aspects of the PGC-1 group of proteins, and we are anxiously awaiting studies on how the mammalian PGC-1 protein influences aging.

To summarize, the effects of Spargel/dPGC-1 on growth and survival are positive, like all the other members of the Insulin/TOR signaling pathway (Mukherjee and Duttaroy, 2013). So, *spargel/dPGC-1* loss of function is lethal (Duttaroy et al., in preparation), *spargel/dPGC-1* hypomorphs have a much shorter life span (**Figure 2D**) where as ubiquitous gain of Spargel/dPGC-1 function does not extend lifespan (Rera et al., 2011). Thus, Spargel/dPGC-1 completes the function of Insulin-TOR pathway leading to survival.

IS Spargel/dPGC-1 ESSENTIAL FOR FEMALE FERTILITY?

Reduced Spargel/dPGC-1 expression causes only a few viable adults to appear from srl^1 homozygous mothers, indicating that fecundity is seriously compromised in srl^1 hypomorphic females though the fertility of srl^1 males remain unchanged (**Table 1**). The growth retardation effect of srl^1 could be the reason for the appearance of dysgenic ovaries, which carry about half the number of ovarioles compared to the wild type (**Figures 3A,B**). A simple time course analysis of oogenesis revealed that srl^1 ovaries develop slowly. In 24 h post eclosion (PE) wild type ovarioles reach up to stage 10/11 whereas ovarioles in srl^1 are lagging behind in stage 6/7. By 48 h mature oocytes appear in the wild type ovarioles, whereas most srl^1 ovarioles are observed around stage 10 during this time (**Figure 3C**). Efforts are underway to pin down the requirement of Spargel/dPGC-1 during oogenesis through its selective ablation in the ovaries. Interestingly, decreased female fecundity results from oogenesis defects in *InR* and *chico* mutants (Tatar et al., 2001; Partridge et al., 2011). These observations suggested a correlation between Insulin signaling and reproductive aging. Incidentally, the effect of srl^1 mutant on

Table 1 | Fertility of srl^1 females.

Genotype	Fecundity (# of adults)
y w	361
y w; srl^1 female X *y w* male	8
y w; srl^1 male X *y w* female	296
y w; srl^1 female X *y w, srl*^{1} male	0

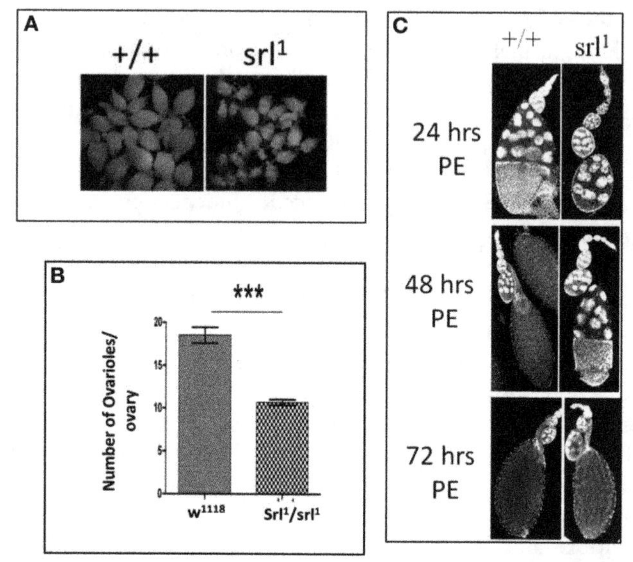

FIGURE 3 | Possible requirement of Spargel/dPGC-1 during oogenesis. **(A)** Mature ovaries from *spargel* hypomorph srl^1 females are much smaller in size with respect to the control ovaries of same age, **(B)** Quantification of number of ovarioles suggest srl^1 ovaries carry about 40% less number of ovarioles with respect to the wild type ovaries. **(C)** Time course analysis of oogenesis shows srl^1 ovaries matures more slowly in comparison to the wild type ovaries (PE, post eclosion). $^{***}P < 0.001$.

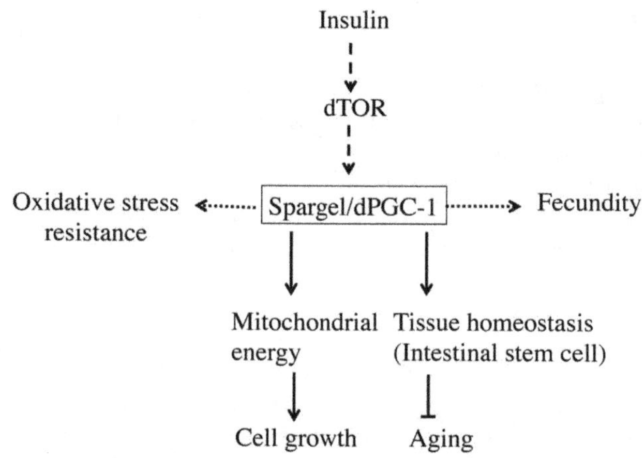

FIGURE 4 | Spargel/dPGC-1 plays a central role in maintaining homeostasis. Spargel/dPGC-1 is acting downstream of Insulin/TOR signaling pathway. At this position, Spargel/dPGC-1 is regulating the mitochondrial energy flow into the system leading to cell growth. In addition, Spargel/dPGC-1 provides oxidative stress resistance. Though unlike mammals, this stress resistance does not confer SOD1 and SOD2 protein expression. Spargel/dPGC-1 also affects *Drosophila* fecundity possibly through oogenesis. Moreover, Spargel/dPGC-1 regulates tissue homeostasis by controlling over proliferation of intestinal stem cells in older flies.

female fecundity and oogenesis appears to suggest that Spargel could be important for reproductive aging.

In summary, the PGC-1 group of proteins retained many important biological functions between vertebrates and invertebrates, though many are still unknown. The overarching hypothesis of this article is that Spargel/dPGC-1 can pave the way to uncover newer biological functions, which can be tested in mammalian PGC-1 (**Figure 4**). Given the amount of functional overlaps already existing between PGC-1 and Spargel/dPGC-1, some of these similarities may be of immediate interest, including the role of the PGC-1 group of proteins on transcription and RNA processing and finding PGC-1 interacting proteins involved in growth and metabolism. Available genetic tools and genomic reagents in *Drosophila* should come in handy for exploring the functionality of this omnipotent transcription co-activator.

ACKNOWLEDGMENTS

We thank the *Drosophila* Stock Center in Bloomington, Indiana for the fly stocks. Thanks are due to Dr. Nathan Smith for careful reading of the manuscript.

REFERENCES

Austin, S., and St-Pierre, J. (2012). PGC1alpha and mitochondrial metabolism–emerging concepts and relevance in ageing and neurodegenerative disorders. *J. Cell Sci.* 125, 4963–4971. doi: 10.1242/jcs.113662

Bugger, H., Guzman, C., Zechner, C., Palmeri, M., Russell, K. S., and Russell, R. R. 3rd. (2011). Uncoupling protein downregulation in doxorubicin-induced heart failure improves mitochondrial coupling but increases reactive oxygen species generation. *Cancer Chemother. Pharmacol.* 67, 1381–1388. doi: 10.1007/s00280-010-1441-7

Chen, S., Oliveira, M. T., Sanz, A., Kemppainen, E., Fukuoh, A., Schlicht, B., et al. (2012). A cytoplasmic suppressor of a nuclear mutation affecting mitochondrial functions in Drosophila. *Genetics* 192, 483–493. doi: 10.1534/genetics.112.143719

Clancy, D. J., Gems, D., Harshman, L. G., Oldham, S., Stocker, H., Hafen, E., et al. (2001). Extension of life-span by loss of CHICO, a Drosophila insulin receptor substrate protein. *Science* 292, 104–106. doi: 10.1126/science.1057991

Coppola, G., Marmolino, D., Lu, D., Wang, Q., Cnop, M., Rai, M., et al. (2009). Functional genomic analysis of frataxin deficiency reveals tissue-specific alterations and identifies the PPARgamma pathway as a therapeutic target in Friedreich's ataxia. *Hum. Mol. Genet.* 18, 2452–2461. doi: 10.1093/hmg/ddp183

Fontana, L., Partridge, L., and Longo, V. D. (2010). Extending healthy life span–from yeast to humans. *Science* 328, 321–326. doi: 10.1126/science.1172539

Gershman, B., Puig, O., Hang, L., Peitzsch, R. M., Tatar, M., and Garofalo, R. S. (2007). High-resolution dynamics of the transcriptional response to nutrition in Drosophila: a key role for dFOXO. *Physiol. Genomics* 29, 24–34. doi: 10.1152/physiolgenomics.00061.2006

Handschin, C., and Spiegelman, B. M. (2006). Peroxisome proliferator-activated receptor gamma coactivator 1 coactivators, energy homeostasis, and metabolism. *Endocr. Rev.* 27, 728–735. doi: 10.1210/er.2006-0037

Hietakangas, V., and Cohen, S. M. (2009). Regulation of tissue growth through nutrient sensing. *Annu. Rev. Genet.* 43, 389–410. doi: 10.1146/annurev-genet-102108-134815

Kapahi, P., Zid, B. M., Harper, T., Koslover, D., Sapin, V., and Benzer, S. (2004). Regulation of lifespan in Drosophila by modulation of genes in the TOR signaling pathway. *Curr. Biol.* 14, 885–890. doi: 10.1016/j.cub.2004.03.059

Kenyon, C. J. (2010). The genetics of ageing. *Nature* 464, 504–512. doi: 10.1038/nature08980

Koo, S. H., Satoh, H., Herzig, S., Lee, C. H., Hedrick, S., Kulkarni, R., et al. (2004). PGC-1 promotes insulin resistance in liver through PPAR-alpha-dependent induction of TRB-3. *Nat. Med.* 10, 530–534. doi: 10.1038/nm1044

Lin, J., Handschin, C., and Spiegelman, B. M. (2005). Metabolic control through the PGC-1 family of transcription coactivators. *Cell Metab.* 1, 361–370. doi: 10.1016/j.cmet.2005.05.004

Liu, C., and Lin, J. D. (2011). PGC-1 coactivators in the control of energy metabolism. *Acta Biochim. Biophys. Sin. (Shanghai)* 43, 248–257. doi: 10.1093/abbs/gmr007

Matsuda, S., Harries, J. C., Viskaduraki, M., Troke, P. J., Kindle, K. B., Ryan, C., et al. (2004). A conserved alpha-helical motif mediates the binding of diverse nuclear proteins to the SRC1 interaction domain of CBP. *J. Biol. Chem.* 279, 14055–14064. doi: 10.1074/jbc.M310188200

Monsalve, M., Wu, Z., Adelmant, G., Puigserver, P., Fan, M., and Spiegelman, B. M. (2000). Direct coupling of transcription and mRNA processing through the thermogenic coactivator PGC-1. *Mol. Cell* 6, 307–316. doi: 10.1016/S1097-2765(00)00031-9

Mukherjee, S., and Duttaroy, A. (2013). Spargel/dPGC-1 is a new downstream effector in the insulin-TOR signaling pathway in Drosophila. *Genetics* 195, 433–441. doi: 10.1534/genetics.113.154583

Partridge, L., Alic, N., Bjedov, I., and Piper, M. D. (2011). Ageing in Drosophila: the role of the insulin/Igf and TOR signalling network. *Exp. Gerontol.* 46, 376–381. doi: 10.1016/j.exger.2010.09.003

Puigserver, P., Rhee, J., Donovan, J., Walkey, C. J., Yoon, J. C., Oriente, F., et al. (2003). Insulin-regulated hepatic gluconeogenesis through FOXO1-PGC-1alpha interaction. *Nature* 423, 550–555. doi: 10.1038/nature01667

Puigserver, P., and Spiegelman, B. M. (2003). Peroxisome proliferator-activated receptor-gamma coactivator 1 alpha (PGC-1 alpha): transcriptional coactivator and metabolic regulator. *Endocr. Rev.* 24, 78–90. doi: 10.1210/er.2002-0012

Puigserver, P., Wu, Z., Park, C. W., Graves, R., Wright, M., and Spiegelman, B. M. (1998). A cold-inducible coactivator of nuclear receptors linked to adaptive thermogenesis. *Cell* 92, 829–839. doi: 10.1016/S0092-8674(00)81410-5

Rera, M., Bahadorani, S., Cho, J., Koehler, C. L., Ulgherait, M., Hur, J. H., et al. (2011). Modulation of longevity and tissue homeostasis by the Drosophila PGC-1 homolog. *Cell Metab.* 14, 623–634. doi: 10.1016/j.cmet.2011.09.013

St-Pierre, J., Drori, S., Uldry, M., Silvaggi, J. M., Rhee, J., Jager, S., et al. (2006). Suppression of reactive oxygen species and neurodegeneration by the PGC-1 transcriptional coactivators. *Cell* 127, 397–408. doi: 10.1016/j.cell.2006.09.024

Takano, A., Usui, I., Haruta, T., Kawahara, J., Uno, T., Iwata, M., et al. (2001). Mammalian target of rapamycin pathway regulates insulin signaling via subcellular redistribution of insulin receptor substrate 1 and integrates nutritional signals and metabolic signals of insulin. *Mol. Cell. Biol.* 21, 5050–5062. doi: 10.1128/MCB.21.15.5050-5062.2001

Tatar, M., Kopelman, A., Epstein, D., Tu, M. P., Yin, C. M., and Garofalo, R. S. (2001). A mutant Drosophila insulin receptor homolog that extends life-span and impairs neuroendocrine function. *Science* 292, 107–110. doi: 10.1126/science.1057987

Tiefenbock, S. K., Baltzer, C., Egli, N. A., and Frei, C. (2010). The Drosophila PGC-1 homologue Spargel coordinates mitochondrial activity to insulin signalling. *EMBO J.* 29, 171–183. doi: 10.1038/emboj.2009.330

van der Linde, K., and Houle, D. (2008). A supertree analysis and literature review of the genus Drosophila and closely related genera (Diptera, Drosophilidae). *Insect. Syst. Evol.* 39, 241–267. doi: 10.1163/187631208788784237

Vellai, T., Takacs-Vellai, K., Zhang, Y., Kovacs, A. L., Orosz, L., and Muller, F. (2003). Genetics: influence of TOR kinase on lifespan in *C. elegans*. *Nature* 426, 620. doi: 10.1038/426620a

Wang, J., Li, Y., Zhang, M., Liu, Z., Wu, C., Yuan, H., et al. (2007). A zinc finger HIT domain-containing protein, ZNHIT-1, interacts with orphan nuclear hormone receptor Rev-erbbeta and removes Rev-erbbeta-induced inhibition of apoCIII transcription. *FEBS J.* 274, 5370–5381. doi: 10.1111/j.1742-4658.2007.06062.x

Zechner, C., Lai, L., Zechner, J. F., Geng, T., Yan, Z., Rumsey, J. W., et al. (2010). Total skeletal muscle PGC-1 deficiency uncouples mitochondrial derangements from fiber type determination and insulin sensitivity. *Cell Metab.* 12, 633–642. doi: 10.1016/j.cmet.2010.11.008

18

Insulin signaling in the aging of healthy and proteotoxically stressed mechanosensory neurons

Courtney Scerbak[1,2], Elena M. Vayndorf[1]*, J. Alex Parker[3], Christian Neri[4,5], Monica Driscoll[6] and Barbara E. Taylor[1,2]*

[1] Institute of Arctic Biology, University of Alaska Fairbanks, Fairbanks, AK, USA
[2] Department of Biology and Wildlife, University of Alaska Fairbanks, Fairbanks, AK, USA
[3] Department of Neuroscience, CRCHUM, University of Montreal, Montreal, QC, Canada
[4] Laboratory of Neuronal Cell Biology and Pathology, Centre National de la Recherche Scientifique, UMR 8652, Paris, France
[5] Sorbonnes Universités, UPMC Univ Paris 06, Paris, France
[6] Nelson Biological Laboratories, Department of Molecular Biology and Biochemistry, Rutgers, The State University of New Jersey, Piscataway, NJ, USA

Edited by:
Shin Murakami, Touro University California, USA

Reviewed by:
Eirini Lionaki, Foundation for Research and Technology-Hellas, Greece
Veena Prahlad, University of Iowa, USA
Mark A. McCormick, Buck Institute for Research on Aging, USA

***Correspondence:**
Elena M. Vayndorf, Institute of Arctic Biology, University of Alaska Fairbanks, 902 North Koyukuk Drive, Irving Building I Room 313, Fairbanks, AK 99775-7000, USA
e-mail: evayndorf@alaska.edu;
Barbara E. Taylor, Department of Biology and Wildlife, Institute of Arctic Biology, University of Alaska Fairbanks, 902 Koyokuk Drive, Irving Building I Room 313, Fairbanks, AK 99775-7000, USA
e-mail: betaylor@alaska.edu

Insulin signaling is central to cellular metabolism and organismal aging. However, the role of insulin signaling in natural and proteotoxically stressed aging neurons has yet to be fully described. We studied aging of *Caenorbaditis elegans* mechanosensory neurons expressing a neurotoxic expanded polyglutamine transgene (polyQ128), or lacking this proteotoxicity stressor (polyQ0), under conditions in which the insulin signaling pathway was disrupted by RNA interference (RNAi). We describe specific changes in lifespan, mechanosensory neuronal morphologies, and mechansensory function following RNAi treatment targeting the insulin signaling pathway. Overall, we confirmed that transcription factor DAF-16 is neuroprotective in the proteotoxically stressed model, though not strikingly in the naturally aging model. Decreased insulin signaling through *daf-2* RNAi improved mechanosensory function in both models and decreased protein aggregation load in polyQ128, yet showed opposing effects on accumulation of neuronal aberrations in both strains. Decreased *daf-2* signaling slightly enhanced mechanosensation while greatly enhancing branching of the mechanosensory neuron axons and dendrites in polyQ0 animals, suggesting that branching is an adaptive response in natural aging. These effects in polyQ0 did not appear to involve DAF-16, suggesting the existence of a non-canonical DAF-2 pathway for the modulation of morphological adaptation. However, in polyQ128 animals, decreased *daf-2* signaling significantly enhanced mechanosensation while decreasing neuronal aberrations. Unlike other interventions that reduce the strength of insulin signaling, *daf-2* RNAi dramatically redistributed large polyQ128 aggregates to the cell body, away from neuronal processes. Our results suggest that insulin signaling strength can differentially affect specific neurons aging naturally or under proteotoxic stress.

Keywords: neuronal aging, insulin signaling, proteotoxicity, Huntington's Disease, *Caenorhabditis elegans*

INTRODUCTION

The insulin/insulin-like growth factor (IGF) signaling pathway is involved in longevity and stress response across species (Broughton and Partridge, 2009). Signaling through this evolutionarily conserved pathway can promote longevity through increased expression of cellular stress and metabolism genes, including those encoding stress-response, chaperone, and antioxidant proteins (Kenyon, 1993; Hsu et al., 2003; Taguchi et al., 2007; Cohen et al., 2009). The progression of neurodegenerative disorders, such as Huntington's, Alzheimer's, and Parkinson's diseases, has been linked to insulin signaling in both invertebrate and mammalian model systems (Dillin and Cohen, 2011). In addition, decreased insulin signaling has protective effects against neurodegenerative-associated proteotoxicity across species (Freude et al., 2009; Killick et al., 2009).

The *Caenorhabditis elegans* insulin signaling pathway is regulated by insulin-like signaling ligands, INS-1 through INS-39, that modulate the activity of the DAF-2 tyrosine kinase receptor (**Figure 1**). DAF-2 is orthologous to the mammalian insulin/IGF receptor. This receptor activates a protein kinase signaling pathway, which, through phosphorylation of downstream transcription factor DAF-16 by AKT protein kinase, regulates functions similar to receptor kinases in the insulin signaling pathway in humans. Under high signaling conditions, DAF-16 is phosphorylated to prevent nuclear entry and hence transcription. Under low signaling conditions, DAF-16 is free from inhibitory phosphorylation and can regulate the expression of many different genes contributing to metabolism and physiological defense and homeostasis responses (Mukhopadhyay et al., 2006). This insulin signaling pathway has many branch points, including AKT, and

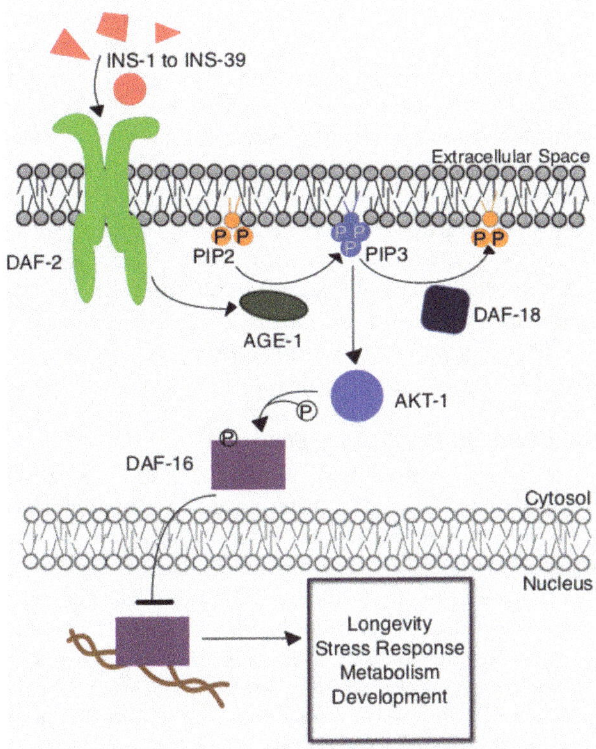

FIGURE 1 | The insulin signaling pathway in *Caenorhabditis elegans*. Upon insulin ligand binding to the DAF-2 insulin receptor in *C. elegans*, AGE-1 (homolog to mammalian PI3-K) is activated and converts PIP_2 to PIP_3 at the cellular membrane. PIP_3 activates the central kinase AKT-1 (ortholog to mammalian PKB), which phosphorylates DAF-16, the *C. elegans* FOXO transcription factor, preventing its entry into the nucleus where it would otherwise regulate the expression of genes contributing to longevity, stress response, and metabolism. The DAF-18 (homolog to mammalian PTEN) phosphatase negatively regulates the system by decreasing the amount of PIP_3 present at the membrane by reconverting it to PIP_2.

there is some variation in the identities of proteins involved in nematodes, flies, and mice, three organisms in which the role of insulin signaling in aging has been investigated. Nevertheless, this central, conserved insulin signaling pathway is critical for appropriate cellular metabolism and maintenance of overall organismal health.

Various mutations in genes modulating the *C. elegans* insulin signaling pathway have been shown to directly regulate lifespan. For example, *daf-2* insulin receptor mutants live twice as long as wildtype animals (Kenyon, 1993), *age-1* PI3K mutants live longer than wildtype animals (Friedman and Johnson, 1988), and the lack of the *daf-16* FOXO transcription factor gene shortens lifespan (Oh et al., 2006). Longevity effects can result from limiting insulin signaling in only the neurons or intestinal cells (Libina et al., 2003). In mammals, the effect of reduced insulin signaling on overall health and lifespan is complex, but combined evidence from many studies points to the potential of insulin signaling reduction to extend lifespan (Taguchi and White, 2008). In mice, reduced neuronal or whole animal expression of IRS2, a kinase activated by the insulin receptor, increases lifespan (Taguchi et al., 2007). In humans, various studies have detected an association between longevity and single nucleotide polymorphisms in genes involved in insulin signaling, including the DAF-16-related transcription factor inhibited by insulin signaling (FOXO3A), the insulin receptor (IGF1R), and a central protein kinase (AKT-1) (Newman and Murabito, 2013). Excellent reviews comparing insulin signaling in various model systems have been published (Taguchi and White, 2008; Broughton and Partridge, 2009; Neri, 2012).

C. elegans exhibit many important neuronal components found in humans, including, but not limited to, neurotransmitters, ligand receptors, and ion channels; thus, these animals are a powerful model for studying neuronal aging and neurodegeneration *in vivo*. Neurodegenerative disorders, such as Huntington's, Alzheimer's, and Parkinson's diseases, result in the progressive loss of structure and function of neurons with age. Of these protein aggregation-associated neurodegenerative diseases, Huntington's disease is caused by the expansion of CAG trinucleotide repeats in the huntingtin gene, which results in an expansion of the length of polyglutamine residues at the N-terminus of the huntingtin protein. Expanded polyglutamine repeats in mutated huntingtin lead to neuronal protein aggregation, impairments in movement and cognitive function, and psychological disorders. Multiple Huntington's disease model strains of *C. elegans* have been developed (Faber et al., 1999; Parker et al., 2001, 2005; Morley et al., 2002). In the model strain used in this study, touch-receptor neuron-specific expression of a transgene encoding the first 57 amino acids of human huntingtin with 128 polyglutamine repeats impairs function, without neuronal death (Parker et al., 2001, 2005). Thus, this model may feature conserved events associated with dysfunction that typify early disease stages in humans.

Aging is the primary risk factor for multiple neurodegenerative diseases, yet the intersection of natural neuronal aging and neurodegenerative states is not well understood. As a consequence of sensing and responding to the environment, the nervous system is known to play a role in physiological aging (Alcedo et al., 2013). In normal, healthy aging, *C. elegans* mechanosensory and other neuron classes develop morphological aberrations, including new outgrowths from the soma, novel process branching, and dendritic restructuring (Pan et al., 2011; Tank et al., 2011; Toth et al., 2012). Neuronal insulin signaling appears to be involved in this natural aging process; the link between normal aging and decline under disease conditions is relatively unexplored. To address this relationship, we studied and compared morphological features of aging mechanosensory neurons with and without a neurotoxic expanded polyglutamine transgene, under conditions in which genes of the canonical insulin signaling pathway were disrupted by neuron-targeted RNA interference (RNAi). Our findings suggest that insulin signaling strength can differentially affect specific neurons aging naturally or under conditions of disrupted proteostasis. Under conditions of polyglutamine expansion stress, insulin receptor DAF-2 appears to act through DAF-16/FOXO. However, under conditions of normal aging, DAF-2 activates a non-canonical pathway that acts independently to induce neuroprotection.

MATERIALS AND METHODS

STRAINS

The *C. elegans* Huntington's disease model strain used was derived from two previously engineered strains. Strain ID1 (*igls1* [$P_{mec\text{-}7}$*yfp*, $P_{mec\text{-}3}$*htt57Q128::cfp*, *lin-15(+)*]) (polyQ128) contains the first 57 amino acids of human huntingtin fused to CFP-labeled expanded polyglutamine tract (Q128) expressed in the 6 mechanosensory neurons as well as in PVD and FLP neurons (Parker et al., 2001). These polyQ128 animals show functional deficiencies in touch response and accumulation of huntingtin protein aggregates in mechanosensory neurons, without cell death (Parker et al., 2001). Strain TU3270 (*uIs57* [$P_{unc\text{-}119}$*SID-1*, $P_{unc\text{-}119}$*yfp*, $P_{mec\text{-}6}$*mec-6*]) overexpresses the transmembrane channel SID-1 pan-neuronally, allowing the dsRNA from RNAi treatment to enter all neurons (Calixto et al., 2010). TU3270 and ID1 were crossed to generate ZB4062 *igIs1*[$P_{mec\text{-}7}$*yfp*, $P_{mec\text{-}3}$*htt57Q128::cfp*, *lin-15(+)*]; *uIs57* [$P_{unc\text{-}119}$*SID-1*, $P_{unc\text{-}119}$*yfp*, $P_{mec\text{-}6}$*mec-6*], a polyQ128-expressing strain with neurons susceptible to RNAi. We also crossed a healthy transgenic model, ZB154 (*zdIs5* [$P_{mec\text{-}4}$*GFP*, *lin-15(+)*]), to TU3270 to generate ZB4064 *zdIs5* [$P_{mec\text{-}4}$*GFP*, *lin-15(+)*]; *uIs57* [$P_{unc\text{-}119}$*SID-1*, $P_{unc\text{-}119}$*yfp*, $P_{mec\text{-}6}$*mec-6*] to render mechanosensory neurons susceptible to RNAi treatment (polyQ0).

WORM MAINTENANCE

Standard methods were used for strain maintenance, bacterial culturing, and animal manipulation (Brenner, 1974). Stock animals were cultured at room temperature (about 22°C) on nematode growth media (NGM) agar plates seeded with live bacteria (*E. coli* strain OP50-1).

RNA INTERFERENCE TREATMENTS

We prepared RNAi plates using 4× concentrated live HT115 *E. coli* bacteria from the Ahringer Library induced at room temperature for 2 days on agar plates. For each batch of RNAi experiments, we performed a control experiment comparing the amount of nerve ring fluorescence knockdown following GFP treatment to empty vector (L4440) in age-matched animals to confirm neuronal RNAi sensitivity of the strain used (Supplemental Figure 1). Only experiments that showed a significant (unpaired *t*-test, $p < 0.05$) knockdown of GFP were used for further RNAi studies. We performed RNAi treatments at 25°C protected from light with age-synchronous populations created using timed egg lay. To perform each egg lay, adult worms laid eggs on each of the described RNAi treatment plates for 4 h. Animals in all RNAi experiments were transferred by hand each day of adulthood to fresh RNAi plates. We performed and analyzed RNAi experiments "blinded" to the intervention so that the experimenter was not aware of the genetic identity of the RNAi treatment given to each population of animals. We repeated each experiment at least 3 times. We selected day 5 of adulthood as a time point for analysis in the following experiments based on Toth et al. (2012) who reported a significant difference in mechanosensory neuronal morphology between day 1 and day 5 of adulthood.

LIFESPAN ANALYSIS

Following the production of age-synchronous populations, we transferred approximately 50 animals from each RNAi treatment group everyday of adulthood to fresh, seeded RNAi treatment small plates and checked for survival by visual observation or gentle prodding with a platinum wire. Animals with protruding intestines, those that bore live young, or that crawled off the plates were censored. Survival experiments always included all 6 RNAi treatment groups (L4440 empty vector, *daf-2*, *age-1*, *daf-18*, *akt-1*, *daf-16*) at once for, usually, one strain at a time, and were repeated at least twice. We used Kaplan–Meier log-rank survival statistics to analyze differences in mean survival between RNAi treatment groups and $p < 0.05$ was noted as significant.

MECHANOSENSORY RESPONSE ASSAY

We generated synchronous populations as described above, maintained cultures at 25°C, and transferred each day of adulthood to fresh RNAi treatment plates. On day 5 of adulthood we scored individuals for motility class. Individuals were grouped into 3 classes: A class indicates normal, voluntary sinusoidal movement, B class indicates locomotion following gentle prodding, and C class indicates inability to locomote. We then tested individuals for their ability to respond to touch by gently touching alternatively on the anterior and posterior end with an eyelash pick, 5 times each (**Figure 2B**). Animals responded either by moving (or attempting to move) in the opposite direction of the touch or by showing no movement. We scored animals (0–5) based on the number of positive responses to touch out of 5 touches at the anterior and 5 touches at the posterior. We also recorded the mobility of each animal. We then imaged the mechanosensory neurons of the tested individuals as described below.

NEURONAL MORPHOLOGY IMAGING

Following the mechanosensory response assay on day 5 of adulthood, we mounted animals between 2 cover slips using 2 μL of 36% w/v Pluronic™ solution dissolved in water and imaged using the 20× objective of an Axiovert S100 inverted fluorescent microscope. Using constant microscope settings, we collected images of the 6 mechanosensory neurons of each individual and their associated huntingtin protein aggregates, if present, using FITC and CFP filters, respectively. We discarded animals after imaging, so data presented is cross-sectional rather than longitudinal. We repeated mechanosensory response assays and neuronal morphology imaging for each strain and RNAi treatment group at least 3 times. We examined the images of 6 mechanosensory neurons of each individual for morphological aberrations, namely cell body outgrowths, cell body guidance errors, and process branching (Toth et al., 2012).

PROTEIN AGGREGATE QUANTIFICATION AND DATA ANALYSIS

For polyQ128 experiments, we analyzed huntingtin aggregates (fused with CFP) with ImageJ, using a custom macroinstruction that includes quantification of the total area of aggregates seen in each cell. For comparisons of mechanosensory response

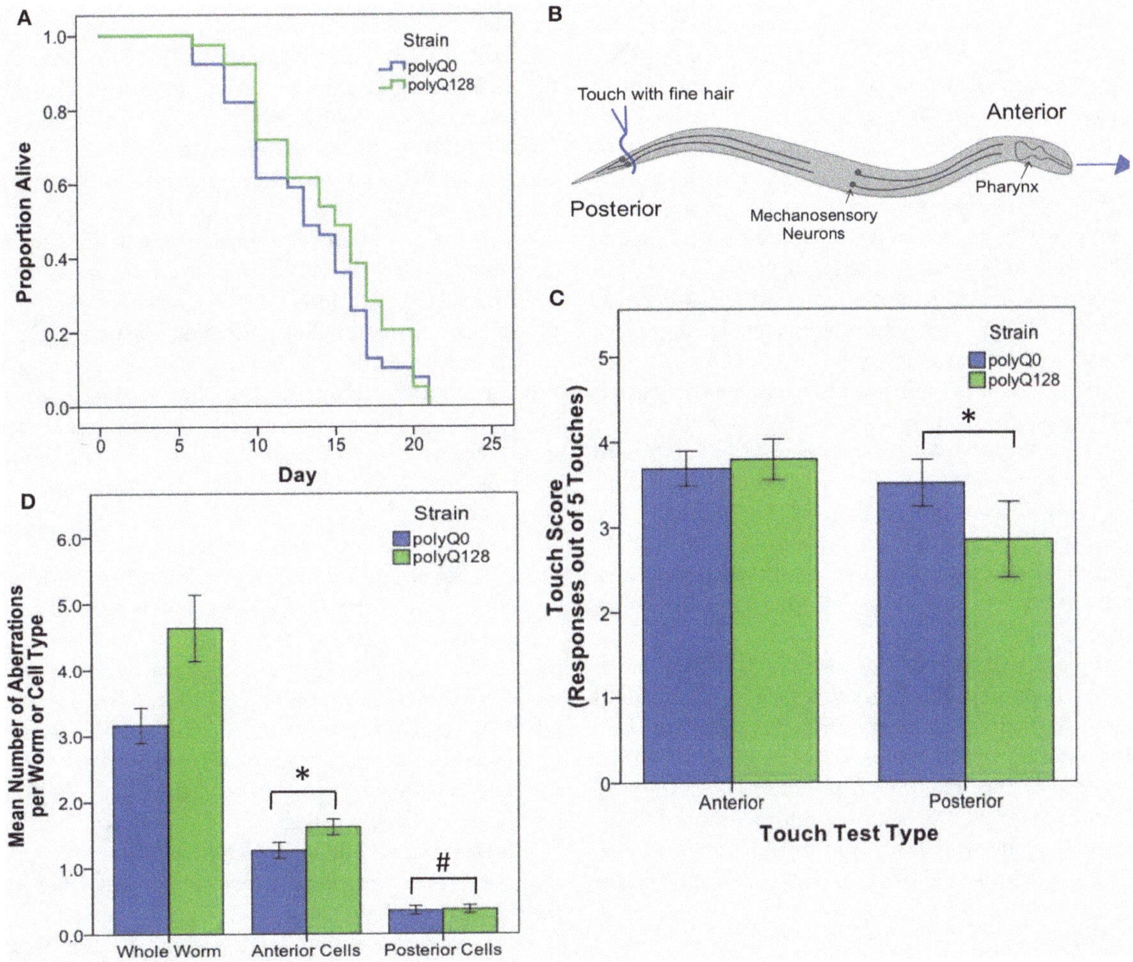

FIGURE 2 | PolyQ0 and polyQ128 exhibit basal differences in mechanosensory neuron morphology and function without altered lifespan. (A) Kaplan–Meier survival curves for one representative survival experiment shown for empty vector (L4440) treated polyQ0 and polyQ128 animals. Mean and median lifespan do not differ between the two strains. **(B)** Schematic of posterior touch test; an animal is touched at the tail and normally moves forward, gaining 1 positive response to touch (out of 5). For anterior touch test, animals are touched at the head and scored for backwards movement. Mechanosensory neurons (PLMs and ALMs) and pharynx shown. **(C)** Anterior and posterior touch test scores for empty vector control individuals. Each bar represents the mean number of positive responses out of 5 to soft touch. **(D)** Total number of aberrations (e.g., number of outgrowths and branches and presence of abnormal cell body and punctae) per worm and cell type for each empty vector control group. Whole worm bars represent the mean values of the sum of all 4 neurons scored (ALML, ALMR, PLML, and PLMR) for each individual. Anterior and posterior bars represent the mean values for individual anterior (ALML or ALMR) or posterior (PLML or PLMR) neurons. *Denotes significance of $p < 0.01$ and #denotes significance of $p < 0.10$ following Mann–Whitney U comparison. Each bar shows mean ± SE for $N = 69$ (polyQ0) and $N = 84$ (polyQ128) animals.

and neuronal morphology between empty vector control polyQ0 and polyQ128 strains, we used a Mann–Whitney U comparison. For the mechanosensory response assays, neuronal morphology imaging, and protein aggregate counts following RNAi treatments, we used a generalized linear model with a log link function (Poisson regression) and Wald tests for significance of treatment effects. For total aggregate area measurements, we used a One-Way ANOVA with Tukey's pairwise comparisons. SPSS (Version 20) statistical software was used to perform, the analyses. A *p*-value of less than 0.05 was considered statistically significant. Values presented in the text represent mean ± standard error.

RESULTS

NEURON AND SYSTEMIC RNAi KNOCKDOWN OF INSULIN SIGNALING PROTEINS ALTERS polyQ0 AND polyQ128 *C. ELEGANS* LIFESPAN

To initiate analysis of the influence of key insulin signaling pathway genes on normal aging and polyQ128-induced neuronal deficits in mid-adult life, we constructed *C. elegans* strains by genetic crosses with fluorescent mechanosensory (or touch) neuron reporters that express the *sid-1* double stranded (ds) RNA transporter pan-neuronally. This *sid-1* compensates for the lack of a neuronal dsRNA transporter, enabling genes expressed in neurons to be targeted by RNAi (Calixto et al., 2010). Moreover, *sid-1* overexpression in neurons can diminish non-neuronal RNAi effects, such that the *sid-1(+)* neurons act as a sink for double stranded RNA (Calixto et al., 2010). We studied one strain that was free of proteotoxic stress (hereafter referred to as polyQ0), and one that expresses the first 57 amino acids of human huntingtin protein with expanded polyglutamines fluorescently labeled with CFP (polyQ128) (Parker et al., 2001). In these strains, we can measure neuronal function via mechanosensory touch response assays, visualize neuronal morphology structures, and directly observe polyQ128 aggregates. We first confirmed that polyQ0 and Huntington's disease model (polyQ128) strain neurons were sensitive to RNAi treatment by feeding as detected by GFP knockdown in the nerve ring (Supplemental Figure 1). Indeed, GFP knockdown was efficient in both strains, supporting that our intended studies on insulin signaling pathway genes could effectively target mechanosensory neurons.

Interestingly, healthy polyQ0 and proteotoxically stressed polyQ128 empty vector (L4440) treated animals exhibited similar, not significantly different, mean lifespan (**Figure 2A**). Thus, increased polyglutamine load in mechanosensory neurons does not confer decreased lifespan, consistent with previous work showing mechanosensory neurons are dispensable for viability and lifespan (Chalfie et al., 1985). However, empty vector treated control polyQ128 animals do exhibit signs of abnormal function as measured by motility, touch response, and accumulation of mechanosensory neuronal aberrations (**Table 1, Figures 2C,D**), agreeing with previous work (Parker et al., 2001). Specifically, polyQ128 posterior touch response is significantly decreased (Mann–Whitney U, $p < 0.01$) and neuronal aberrations are increased at the whole worm (Mann–Whitney U, $p < 0.01$), anterior cells (Mann–Whitney U, $p < 0.01$), and posterior cells level (Mann–Whitney U, $p = 0.04$) when compared to age-matched polyQ0 individuals. This suggests that increased polyglutamine load in the mechanosensory neurons negatively affects the function and healthspan of polyQ128 animals.

Table 1 | Effect of RNAi treatment on polyQ0 and polyQ128 motility.

Strain	RNAi treatment	Number per motility class			Total *N*
		A	*B*	*C*	
polyQ0	Empty vector	65	4	0	69
	daf-2	53	0	0	53
	age-1	67	4	0	71
	daf-18	47	2	0	49
	akt-1	50	1	0	51
	daf-16	48	3	0	51
polyQ128	Empty vector	69	15	0	84
	daf-2	87	6	0	93
	age-1	77	18	0	95
	daf-18	47	0	0	47
	akt-1	31	15	1	47
	daf-16	51	20	1	72

Number of individuals falling into A, B, or C class motility for each treatment group is shown. A class indicates normal, voluntary sinusoidal movement, B class indicates locomotion following gentle prodding, and C class indicates inability to locomote. Overall, polyQ128 animals have higher incidence of B class motility than polyQ0. Only polyQ128 daf-18(RNAi) results in a significant difference in motility compared to control.

Because several previously published mutant and RNAi experiments did not utilize *sid-1* enhanced neuronal RNAi targeting, and thus would not have assayed neuronal knockdown effects, we also confirmed RNAi effects on longevity under the conditions we used for our studies. We found that knockdown of insulin signaling pathway genes in neurons and other tissues altered healthy polyQ0 life as previously reported, with *daf-2*, *age-1*, and *akt-1* RNAi interventions lengthening lifespan, and *daf-16* RNAi shortening it (**Figure 3A** and **Table 2**). Insulin signaling pathway interventions in the polyQ128 strain (*daf-2*, *age-1*) similarly increased mean lifespan, while *daf-16* RNAi treatment decreased mean lifespan (**Figure 3B** and **Table 2**). In the 3 biological replicates of *akt-1* RNAi in polyQ128 animals, lifespan impact was variable.

To further address whether there might be differences in general viability between polyQ0 and polyQ128 strains, we compared percent change in mean lifespan between polyQ0 and polyQ128 animals for each RNAi treatment group. We found no significant differences in relative percent changes between healthy transgenic and polyQ128 animals for the same RNAi treatment (*t*-tests, $p > 0.05$), except for *daf-16* RNAi, which approached significance in the polyQ128 background (**Figure 3C**; $p = 0.07$). We also measured endogenous reactive oxygen species (ROS) as detected by the membrane permeable 2′, 7′-Dichlorofluorescin diacetate (DCF-DA, Sigma) following RNAi treatments and found that RNAi treatment targeted at insulin signaling pathway proteins from embryo did not consistently significantly affect young adult (day 1) endogenous ROS levels in both healthy transgenic and polyQ128 strains (data not shown). However, *daf-16* RNAi treatment through mid-life in polyQ128 worms significantly increased endogenous ROS levels across all biological replicates.

We conclude that RNAi interventions in our polyQ0 and polyQ128 strains are efficacious and exert similar general influences on aging biology in polyQ0 and polyQ128 strains. Disruption of a small set of sensory neurons by the proteotoxic stress of polyQ128 is not sufficient to grossly impair whole animal function, although there are some functional impairment and increased morphological aberrations. However, we note that in middle-aged adults, *daf-16* RNAi is associated with elevated ROS levels and decreased mid-life viability specifically in the polyQ128 strain, raising the possibility that the combination of small scale neuronal proteostasis disruption can influence entire organism decline when DAF-16-dependent defenses are impaired.

DECREASED INSULIN SIGNALING THROUGH RNAi KNOCKDOWN INFLUENCES HEALTHY MECHANOSENSORY NEURON MORPHOLOGY AND FUNCTION

Previous studies on morphological aging of mechanosensory neurons indicated that manipulation of the insulin signaling pathway can change accumulation of neuronal aberrations (Pan et al., 2011; Tank et al., 2011; Toth et al., 2012). These studies differed in details of methods and outcomes, and did not address *akt-1* or *daf-18* activities. Moreover, these studies left open the

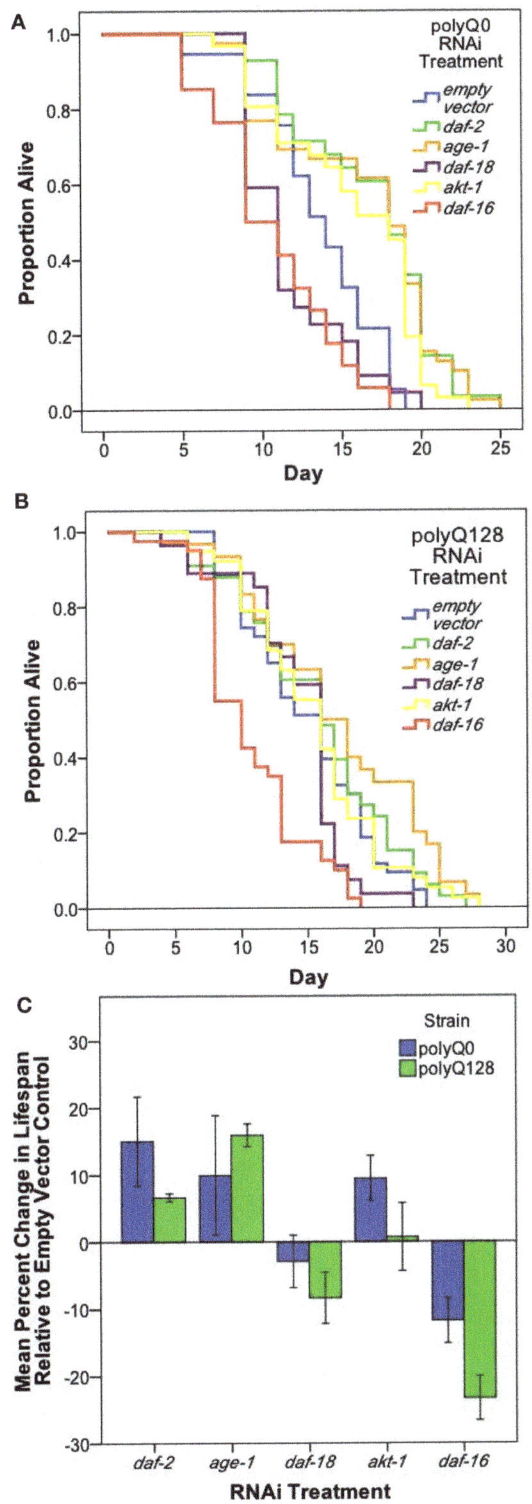

FIGURE 3 | Neuronal and systemic insulin signaling mediates lifespan of both healthy (polyQ0) and proteotoxically stressed (polyQ128) animals. Kaplan–Meier survival curves for one representative survival experiment shown for polyQ0 **(A)** and polyQ128 **(B)** animals with RNAi knockdown of the indicated insulin signaling pathway gene. Mean lifespan, sample size, and significance reported as Replicate 1 for each strain in *(Continued)*

FIGURE 3 | Continued
Table 2. (C) Mean percent change in lifespan with RNAi treatment for polyQ0 and polyQ128 animals pooled across biological replicates. Only *daf-16* RNAi showed a significant impact on lifespan for polyQ128 animals when compared to polyQ128 empty vector controls (23.3 ± 4.1% for 3 replicates of 45–50 animals). Each bar represents mean ± SE.

question of how morphological features relate to function. To address these gaps and discrepancies, we measured neuronal morphology and touch response as a surrogate for mechanosensory function when components of the insulin signaling pathway were knocked down in polyQ0 animals. We performed touch response tests (**Figure 4A**) and then imaged mechanosensory neurons of characterized animals for changes in morphology (**Figures 4B,C**) at mid-life (day 5 of adulthood; described in detail in Materials and Methods). Total neuronal aberrations include all morphological aberrations observed in an individual or cell type, including soma outgrowths, abnormal cell somas, process branching, and process punctae (**Figure 4B**).

Our analysis of touch sensory function revealed that both anterior and posterior touch responses in *daf-2* RNAi were better than empty vector at day 5 of adult life (**Figure 4A**; Wald test, $p < 0.01$ for anterior and posterior scores). *daf-16* RNAi preferentially decreased posterior touch ($p < 0.01$), revealing an interesting difference between anterior and posterior mechanosensory neurons. We found that RNAi knockdown of *age-1*, *daf-18*, and *akt-1* did not alter touch responses as compared to empty vector.

A striking result from our analysis of morphological aberrations at day 5 of adulthood is that *daf-2* RNAi increased the occurrence of total neuronal aberrations as compared to control (from 3.2 ± 0.23 to 4.7 ± 0.26 per individual) in both anterior and posterior neurons (**Figure 4C**). We found that this increase was driven exclusively by process branching, which was the only specific neuronal aberration observed to change with *daf-2* RNAi (**Figure 4D**; from 12.8 ± 3.40 to 32.7 ± 3.80% in anterior cells and 14.5 ± 3.20 to 39.4 ± 3.70% in posterior cells). *age-1* RNAi also increased total aberrations (from 3.2 ± 0.23 to 4.4 ± 0.23 per individual) (**Figure 4C**) and novel branching in anterior neurons (**Figure 4D**; from 12.8 ± 3.40 to 25.3 ± 3.40% in anterior cells and 14.5 ± 3.20 to 26.7 ± 3.30% in posterior cells), whereas *daf-18*, *akt-1*, and *daf-16* interventions did not induce statistically significant changes in overall aberrations or in the hyper-branching phenotype. Our findings suggest that *daf-2* disruption, and lowered insulin signaling could differentially effect different morphologies, and raise the question as to whether branching might be an indication of a neuroprotective response (see Discussion).

TOUCH RESPONSE, MECHANOSENSORY NEURONAL MORPHOLOGY, AND PROTEIN AGGREGATE ACCUMULATION ARE AFFECTED BY INSULIN SIGNALING IN A MODEL STRAIN OF HUNTINGTON'S DISEASE PATHOGENESIS

We next examined functionality and morphological aberrations in the polyQ128 strain in which mechanosensory neurons are exposed to a chronic proteotoxic stress that promotes early dysfunction (Parker et al., 2001). As previously noted,

Table 2 | Effects of RNAi treatment targeting insulin signaling on polyQ0 and polyQ128 animals' mean lifespan.

Strain	RNAi treatment	Replicate 1		Replicate 2		Replicate 3	
		N	Mean lifespan days ± *SE*	*N*	Mean lifespan days ± *SE*	*N*	Mean lifespan days ± *SE*
polyQ0	Empty vector	50	13.7 ± 0.56	60	14.3 ± 0.58	55	13.5 ± 0.66
	daf-2	40	16.8 ± 0.83*	*N/A*	*N/A*	48	16.3 ± 1.04*
	age-1	51	16.3 ± 0.82*	59	16.9 ± 0.61*	*N/A*	*N/A*
	daf-18	30	11.7 ± 0.70	60	14.8 ± 0.57	50	13.5 ± 0.62
	akt-1	40	15.8 ± 0.79*	60	16.2 ± 0.52*	48	13.4 ± 0.50
	daf-16	46	11.0 ± 0.61*	60	12.1 ± 0.53*	51	12.9 ± 0.68
polyQ128	Empty vector	50	15.2 ± 0.71	50	15.1 ± 0.61	56	13.4 ± 0.55
	daf-2	51	16.1 ± 0.94	50	16.2 ± 0.89*	*N/A*	*N/A*
	age-1	40	17.9 ± 1.01*	*N/A*	*N/A*	59	15.0 ± 0.89*
	daf-18	38	15.6 ± 0.79	50	14.5 ± 0.66	59	11.4 ± 0.42*
	akt-1	47	15.8 ± 0.79	25	14.4 ± 1.15	56	11.4 ± 0.44*
	daf-16	48	10.9 ± 0.60*	50	12.8 ± 0.63*	61	10.4 ± 0.39*

*Mean lifespan in days ± SE of each RNAi treatment replicate for the polyQ0 and polyQ128 strains are shown. Each replicate of 6 treatments (empty vector control, DAF-2, AGE-1, DAF-18, AKT-1, and DAF-16) was run one strain at a time. Entries with * are significantly different ($p < 0.05$) from the strain- and replicate-matched empty vector control following Kaplan–Meier log-rank survival statistics. Replicate with missing data (N/A) was censored from experiment.*

empty vector treated polyQ128 animals exhibit increased aberrant neuronal morphology and decreased touch response compared to age-matched, empty vector treated wildtype animals (**Figures 3C,D**).

We tested touch response in polyQ128 animals subjected to RNAi for insulin signaling pathway components (**Figure 5A**). *daf-2* RNAi had a neuroprotective effect on both anterior (Wald test, $p < 0.001$) and posterior touch sensitivity (Wald test, $p < 0.001$). Interestingly, however, all other RNAi knockdown interventions (*age-1*, *daf-18*, *akt-1*, and *daf-16*) had generally deleterious effects on touch sensitivity in the polyQ128 background, with a particularly significant change in posterior touch response in polyQ128 animals compared with empty vector (L4440).

We then examined neuronal morphology in the polyQ128 strain following RNAi of the insulin signaling pathway genes (**Figure 5B**). We found that numbers of aberrations in the polyQ128 strain were reduced upon *daf-2* RNAi when compared to empty vector (from 4.78 ± 0.21 to 2.94 ± 0.15 per individual, Wald test, $p < 0.001$). In contrast, *age-1* RNAi, modestly increased aberrations (from 4.3 ± 0.2 to 5.4 ± 0.1 per individual), as did *akt-1* and *daf-16* interventions in anterior mechanosensory neurons. Thus for polyQ128-expressing neurons, morphological aberrations generally inversely correlate with function: low abnormality abundance corresponds to enhanced mechanosensory function.

In polyQ128 animals, the huntingtin:polyQ128 protein is fused with CFP and can be visualized as aggregates in our strain (**Figure 5C**). We therefore also examined the number and size of fluorescent aggregates in mechanosensory neurons following RNAi knockdown of insulin signaling components (**Figure 5D**). Under conditions of *daf-2* RNAi we found that mean numbers of aggregates were lowered compared to wildtype (Wald test, $p < 0.01$ for whole individuals, anterior cells, and posterior cells). Mean aggregate area was unchanged for *daf-2* RNAi (Supplemental Figure 2), suggesting that less aggregated protein persists in mid-life mechanosensory neurons when DAF-2 signals are reduced. Conversely, we found modest increases in aggregate number and size for *age-1*, *akt-1*, and *daf-16* knockdown (**Figure 5D** and Supplemental Figure 2). Importantly, Parker et al. (2005) showed no difference in huntingtin expression of the polyQ128 animals in *age-1* and *daf-16* genetic mutants. This suggests that our findings of altered protein aggregation in the polyQ128 strain is likely not due to changed huntingtin expression, but rather is more likely attributed to cellular responses of the expanded polyglutamine protein (**Figure 5**).

Interestingly, we noted a striking difference in the localization of polyQ128 protein aggregates in posterior and anterior cells for *daf-2* RNAi (**Figures 5E,F**). In *daf-2* RNAi treated animals, 80–90% of the detected aggregates localized in the cell body of anterior and posterior cells whereas other insulin signaling pathway knockdowns were associated with a majority (50–60%) of aggregates localized within the process of these cells, similar to empty vector controls. We also note that aggregates were never observed in outgrowths without also being present in the cell body. This dramatic difference of aggregate localization in *daf-2* RNAi animals suggests that subcellular distribution of protein aggregates is regulated by a DAF-2 non-canonical pathway.

RNAi KNOCKDOWN OF *daf-2* RETURNS polyQ128 MECHANOSENSORY NEURON MORPHOLOGY TO HEALTHY LEVELS

At the whole worm and anterior and posterior cell levels, *daf-2* RNAi knockdown in the neurons of polyQ128 worms lowers the occurrence of total neuronal aberrations to levels observed in polyQ0 empty vector treated animals (Wald test, $p < 0.01$). However, *daf-2* RNAi polyQ128 touch response is still significantly lower than polyQ0 empty vector treated animals (Wald test, $p < 0.01$).

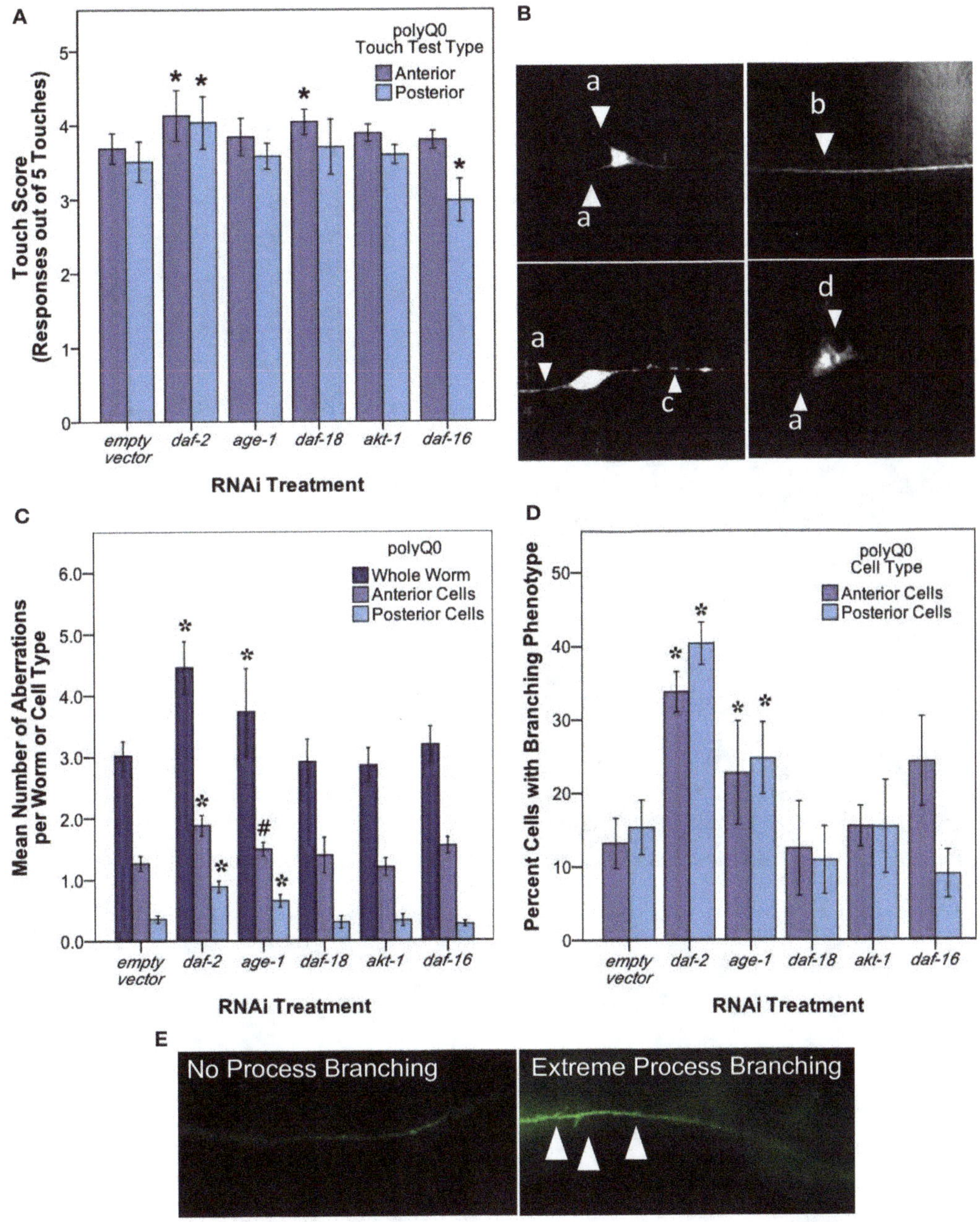

FIGURE 4 | *daf-2* RNAi mediates mechanosensory neuron morphology and function in polyQ0 animals. (A) Anterior and posterior touch test scores of polyQ0 animals following RNAi treatment. Each bar represents the mean number of positive responses to 5 soft touches. **(B)** Representative examples of outgrowths (a), branching (b), punctae (c), and abnormal cell body (d) phenotypes seen in aging mechanosensory neurons of polyQ0 and polyQ128 individuals. **(C)** Mean number of neuronal aberrations per whole animal (sum of all 4 neurons scored in an individual) and individual cell type (anterior [ALML or ALMR] and posterior [PLML or PLMR]). **(D)** Percentage of neurons with branching phenotype for each RNAi treatment. Neurons with this phenotype may have more than one branch (data not shown). **(E)** Representative images of mechanosensory neuron processes and process branching (white arrows) in polyQ0 animals. *Denotes significance of $p < 0.01$ and #denotes significance of $p < 0.10$ relative to appropriate empty vector control following a generalized linear model with a log link function (Poisson regression) and Wald tests for significance of treatment effects. Each bar represents mean ± SE for $N = 49–70$ animals.

DISCUSSION

SUMMARY OF FINDINGS

To begin to address the relationship between natural and proteotoxically challenged neuronal aging in a physiological context, we took advantage of high resolution *in vivo* analyses of *C. elegans* mechanosensory neuron morphology and function. We compared mid-life morphological and functional features of mechanosensory neurons that aged without, or

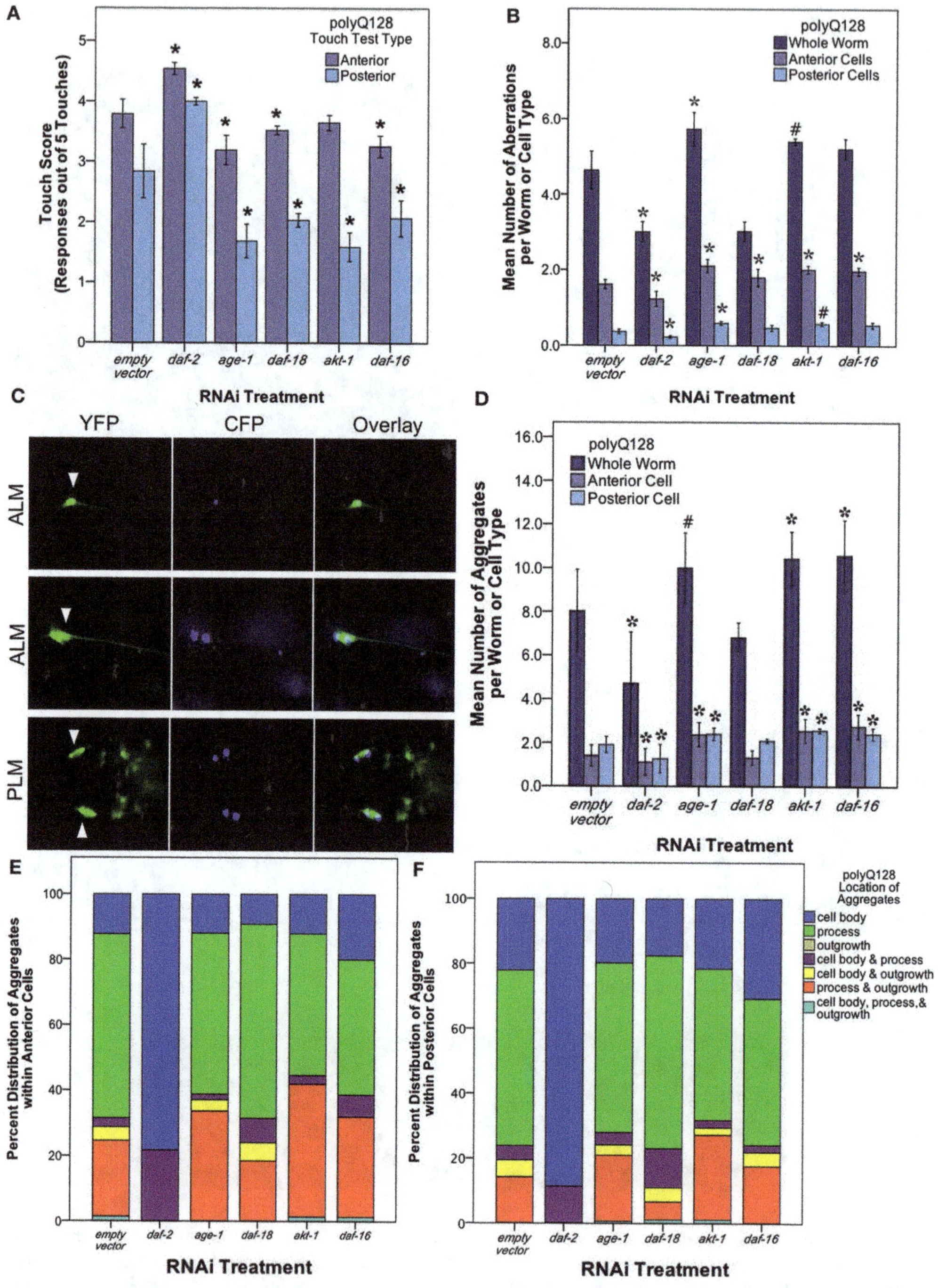

FIGURE 5 | The insulin signaling pathway mediates mechanosensory neuron morphology and function in polyQ128 animals. (A) Anterior and posterior touch test scores, representing the number of positive responses to 5 soft touches, following RNAi treatment for indicated insulin signaling pathway gene of polyQ128 animals. **(B)** Mean number of neuronal aberrations per whole animal (sum of all 4 neurons scored in an individual) and individual cell type (anterior [ALML or ALMR] and posterior [PLML or PLMR]). **(C)** Representative image of polyQ128 aggregate (CFP, blue panels) accumulation within anterior (ALM) and posterior neurons (PLM) (YFP, green panels). White arrows in YFP panels indicate the location of the cell body of each neuron. **(D)** The effect of RNAi treatment on the number of distinct CFP-labeled extended polyglutamine huntingtin protein aggregates in whole animal and anterior and posterior neurons of polyQ128 animals. **(E)** Sub-cellular localization of poyQ128 aggregates within anterior neurons of polyQ128 animals that contained aggregates. **(F)** Location of polyQ128 aggregates in posterior neurons of polyQ128 animals. *Denotes significance of $p < 0.01$ and #denotes significance of $p < 0.10$ relative to appropriate empty vector control following generalized linear model analysis with a log link function (Poisson regression) and Wald tests for significance of treatment effects. Each bar represents mean ± SE.

with, the proteotoxic stressor polyQ128, under RNAi conditions that mimic systemic, including neurons, low or high activation of the insulin signaling pathway. Our data suggest that insulin signaling plays complex roles in neuronal maintenance in both healthy (polyQ0) and degenerate (polyQ128) neurons, with distinct outcomes on individual neurons notable even among the similar group of 6 mechanosensory neurons. Our data on individual neurons highlight remarkable neuronal diversity of responses to cellular signaling. Comparison of how the insulin signaling pathway impacts natural and proteotoxic-associated decline reveals some interesting differences in these two processes.

We conclude that RNAi down-regulation of the *daf-2* insulin receptor plays a role in morphological aging of mechanosensory neurons in both normally aging (polyQ0) and proteotoxically stressed (polyQ128) animals. Anterior and posterior neurons can be differentially affected by altered neuronal insulin signaling (**Table 3**). Importantly, our data suggest that decreased insulin signaling in normally aging systems (polyQ0) actually enhances some process aberrations in middle aged adults, with a focused impact on formation of ectopic branches on axons and dendrites. That *daf-2* mechanosensory function is improved raises the possibility that the structural aberrations (branching) we observe actually reflect consequences of a defensive response that enhances or protects neuronal health during aging (**Figure 4**). *age-1* may contribute partially to this process in polyQ0 animals, but evidence for the involvement of other pathway components is not compelling in our study. We also find that *daf-2* RNAi knockdown has distinctive impact on the proteotoxically stressed polyQ128 mechanosensory neurons: morphological aberrations are lower; and aggregates are fewer in number and smaller in size, with a striking subcellular restriction of aggregates to the cell body, as compared to empty vector controls. Somewhat surprisingly, other insulin signaling pathway disruptions have relatively modest impact on cell function, aggregate morphology, and aggregate distribution in polyQ128 animals; we found that *age-1* RNAi, which extends overall lifespan, did not confer dramatic changes in mechanosensory neurons, and often correlated with *daf-16* RNAi in inducing modest effects. Our data raise the possibility that, under conditions of extreme proteotoxic stress, neurons utilize a non-canonical *daf-2* pathway to enhance neuroprotection.

EXTENDING UNDERSTANDING OF THE INFLUENCE OF INSULIN SIGNALING ON HEALTHY AGING MECHANOSENSORY NEURONS

daf-2 insulin receptor

Mechanosensory neuron morphology changes with age in wildtype animals (Pan et al., 2011; Tank et al., 2011; Toth et al., 2012). Overall, genetic mutants and systemic RNAi treatments have suggested that *daf-2* mutants maintain youthful, aberration-free phenotypes longer than wildtype animals. Toth et al. (2012) distinguished among specific abnormality classes to measure decreases in cell body outgrowths and wavy process phenotypes, with a trend toward delaying branching in posterior mechanosensory neurons. Tank et al. (2011) showed that 10 day old *daf-2(e1370)* mutants had decreased process branching. Using a neuron-targeted *daf-2* RNAi approach, we measured an increase in neuronal aberrations at day 5 of adulthood, the vast majority of which are novel branches (**Figures 4D,E**). Because we find increased aberrations in *daf-2* RNAi coincident with a period of enhanced function (**Figure 4A**), we raise the question

Table 3 | RNAi treatments targeting the insulin signaling pathway differentially effect polyQ128 specific mechanosensory neuronal aberrations.

Specific types of aberrations per	Cell type	RNAi treatment on polyQ128 animals										
		Empty vector ($N_{anterior}$ = 226; $N_{posterior}$ = 217)	(*daf-2* $N_{anterior}$ = 199; $N_{posterior}$ = 202)		*age-1* ($N_{anterior}$ = 185; $N_{posterior}$ = 185)		*daf-18* ($N_{anterior}$ = 92; $N_{posterior}$ = 94)		*akt-1* ($N_{anterior}$ = 93; $N_{posterior}$ = 92)		*daf-16* ($N_{anterior}$ = 143; $N_{posterior}$ = 140)	
		Mean ± *SE*	Mean ± *SE*	p-value	Mean ± *SE*	p-value	Mean ± *SE*	p-value	Mean ± *SE*	p-value	Mean ± *SE*	p-value
Number of cell body outgrowths	Anterior	1.11 ± 0.05	0.86 ± 0.04	*0.00	1.32 ± 0.06	*0.01	1.21 ± 0.08	*n.s.*	1.24 ± 0.08	*n.s.*	1.29 ± 0.06	*0.03
	Posterior	0.01 ± 0.01	0.01 ± 0.03	*n.s.*	0.03 ± 0.03	*n.s.*	0.01 ± 0.01	*n.s.*	0.00 ± 0.00	*n.s.*	0.01 ± 0.01	*n.s.*
Number of branches	Anterior	0.15 ± 0.03	0.09 ± 0.02	*0.05	0.16 ± 0.03	*n.s.*	0.23 ± 0.05	*n.s.*	0.10 ± 0.03	*n.s.*	0.13 ± 0.03	*n.s.*
	Posterior	0.07 ± 0.02	0.05 ± 0.02	*n.s.*	0.08 ± 0.02	*n.s.*	0.05 ± 0.02	*n.s.*	0.03 ± 0.02	*n.s.*	0.05 ± 0.02	*n.s.*
Presence of punctae	Anterior	0.14 ± 0.02	0.04 ± 0.02	*0.00	0.37 ± 0.02	*0.00	0.27 ± 0.03	*0.02	0.39 ± 0.03	*0.00	0.33 ± 0.02	*0.00
	Posterior	0.71 ± 0.03	0.90 ± 0.03	*0.00	0.59 ± 0.04	*0.02	0.65 ± 0.05	*n.s.*	0.55 ± 0.05	*0.01	0.58 ± 0.04	*0.01
Presence of abnormal cell body	Anterior	0.13 ± 0.01	0.03 ± 0.01	*0.00	0.19 ± 0.01	*n.s.*	0.10 ± 0.02	*n.s.*	0.15 ± 0.02	*n.s.*	0.11 ± 0.01	*n.s.*
	Posterior	0.00 ± 0.01	0.02 ± 0.01	*0.02	0.03 ± 0.01	*0.01	0.02 ± 0.02	*n.s.*	0.00 ± 0.02	*n.s.*	0.03 ± 0.01	*0.02

Table depicts mean number and significant difference for anterior (ALML or ALMR) and posterior (PLML or PLMR) mechanosensory neurons following RNAi treatment for each specific neuronal aberration observed (i.e., cell body outgrowths, process branching, presence of process punctae, and cell body abnormality). p-values indicate significance compared to appropriate empty vector control following generalized linear model analysis. Sample sizes for anterior ($N_{anterior}$) and posterior ($N_{posterior}$) neurons of each RNAi treatment are shown. Example outgrowths (A), branching (B), punctae (C), and abnormal cell body (D) are shown in ***Figure 4B****. *Denotes significance of $p < 0.05$.*

of whether mid-life branching might be a manifestation of a normal neuronal defense mechanism that actually improves sensory capacity, although this issue remains to be resolved with single animal functional imaging. This finding is also significant in that it suggests that all changes in morphology seen with age or treatments are not the same mechanistically and that some phenotypes, such as process branching, may be protective to neurons. Differences from other studies (Pan et al., 2011; Tank et al., 2011; Toth et al., 2012) could arise from differences in methods for reducing *daf-2* expression (with RNAi knockdown being distinct from modulation of specific amino acid resides in receptor reduction-of-function mutants) and different timing of scoring during adult life.

age-1 PI3 kinase and other insulin signaling molecules

We found that *age-1* RNAi modestly increased branching of mechanosensory neuron processes at day 5 of adult life, but did not alter touch sensitivity. The latter observation establishes that morphological phenotype and function are not always linked. *akt-1*, *daf-18*, and *daf-16* RNAi interventions did not alter the trajectory of age-associated morphological change in otherwise healthy neurons. The role of *age-1, akt-1*, and *daf-18* in morphological aging of the mechanosensory neurons has not been previously reported. Overall, *age-1* knockdown can have an effect on mechanosensory neuron morphological aging (**Figures 4D,E**) but impact on function is not large at mid-life. Other pathways that run in parallel may be important in mid-adult life (Tank et al., 2011).

daf-16

For natural aging of mechanosensory neurons, we find that *daf-16* RNAi exerts a small but statistically significant effect on day 5 adult posterior touch response, but not on aberrations. Tank et al. (2011) also came to the conclusion that aberrations for day 10 branching in a *daf-16* deletion mutant were similar to wildtype; whereas Pan et al. (2011) and Toth et al. (2012) noted a small increase in aberrations in *daf-16* mutants at days 9 and 10 (note the latter study, like ours, found no change at adult day 5). Still, time course studies do not support a profound impact of *daf-16* disruption on morphological aging of the mechanosensory neurons. *daf-16* appears to be needed for *daf-2(rf)*-mediated suppression of excess branching, though cell autonomy of this activity is disputed (Pan et al., 2011; Tank et al., 2011).

Overall, although compelling data support that insulin signaling a factor in natural aging of mechanosensory neurons, with reduced signaling correlating with reduced function, other pathways likely influence the process as well (Tank et al., 2011).

DISTINCTIVE OUTCOMES OF daf-2 RNAi IN THE PROTEOTOXICALLY STRESSED HUNTINGTON'S DISEASE MODEL STRAIN

daf-2

In middle-aged polyQ128 animals, we found that *daf-2* RNAi improved mechanosensory function, limited the number of morphological aberrations, and decreased overall aggregate number and size, compared to empty vector controls (**Figure 5**). Thus, reduced insulin receptor signaling through DAF-2 confers neuroprotection that is associated with diminished polyQ128 aggregate load in this model. Our data are consistent with studies in other disease models (Cohen et al., 2010) implicating *daf-2* in enhanced proteostasis during toxic protein challenge.

age-1 PI3 kinase and other insulin signaling molecules

We found that *age-1* RNAi modestly impairs touch sensitivity at a time point at which the mean number of aberrations and of aggregates are elevated relative to empty vector controls (**Figure 4**). Unexpectedly, *akt-1* and *daf-16* RNAi, which should have opposing impacts on the signal transduction pathway, induce similar outcomes in these proteotoxically challenged mechanosensory neurons. Because *age-1* RNAi [and sometimes *akt-1* (Hertweck et al., 2004)] extend lifespan (**Table 2**), dysfunction is not the anticipated outcome of such interventions. We emphasize two points here: first, our data raise the possibility that the most commonly outlined downstream pathway for DAF-2 signaling may not be the operative signaling pathway for the mechansensory neuron proteotoxicity pathway; and second, as it has previously been noted that other healthspan phenotypes differentially affected by *daf-2* vs. *age*-1 mutations. For example, in *age-1* mutants the biphasic profile for rate of increase in lipofuscin/age pigments during adulthood shows a temporal shift (delay in onset without change in time course), whereas for *daf-2* mutants the rate of lipofuscin accumulation remains low across adulthood (Gerstbrein et al., 2005). In other words, *daf-2* is more effective in preventing long term elevation in age pigment accumulation, while *age-1* delays onset of accumulation. This anomaly is a precedent for differential health outcomes following closely related insulin signaling pathway interventions.

In previous work, Morley et al. (2002) found that *C. elegans* expressing polyQ82 in body wall muscle show slower development of aggregates and motility defects with *age-1* RNAi and *age-1* mutants. While those authors showed the opposite effect of *age-1* RNAi on polyQ accumulation and toxicity compared to our study using a different cell type, they stressed the importance of threshold stresses in their interpretation. We note that our model carries an elevated polyglutamine load (polyQ128) as compared to polyQ82. In humans, longer polyglutamine expansion in huntingtin is well known to result in earlier onset of Huntington's disease and lower life expectancy.

daf-16

As expected, we observed *daf-16* RNAi confers diminished mechanosensory function together with increased anterior aberration and increased number and size of aggregates. Our results are consistent with previous studies showing that *daf-16* deficiency is associated with exacerbated polyQ128 proteotoxicity in young adult mechanosensory neurons (Parker et al., 2005, 2012; Lejeune et al., 2012) and with enhanced proteotoxicity in a polyQ82 model (Morley et al., 2002) and an Alzheimer's disease model (Cohen et al., 2009).

Overall, changes in anterior and posterior cell function, morphology, and protein aggregation load and localization (**Figures 4, 5**) correlate with whole animal observations (**Figure 3**) in both polyQ0 and polyQ128 strains. However, with polyQ128 *daf-16* RNAi we observed decreased anterior and posterior mechanosensory function (**Figure 5A**) and increased protein aggregate area and number in whole animal and both cell types (**Figure 5D** and Supplemental Figure 2), while only anterior mechanosensory neurons (ALML or ALMR) increased significantly in total neuronal aberrations (**Figure 5B**). This maintenance of neuronal morphology with worsened function and protein aggregation suggests other mechanisms can mediate these endpoints.

daf-2 RNAi UNIQUELY CHANGES DISTRIBUTION OF polYQ128 AGGREGATE LOAD

A striking observation of *daf-2* RNAi animals is a profound difference in the distribution of polyQ128 aggregates (**Figures 5E,F**). *daf-2* RNAi is the only intervention we tested that induces localization of CFP-labeled polyQ128 aggregates nearly exclusively to the neuron cell body. Most aggregates we concentrated in only a few dots, which resembled perinuclear lysosomes. Although this subcellular domain restriction remains to be definitively identified, our observations suggest that for both anterior and posterior mechanosensory neurons, *daf-2* may exert neuroprotection by sequestering aggregates to prevent them from interfering with other cellular functions. The lower aggregate size suggests that enhanced degradation may occur when DAF-2 signaling is low. Our data also suggest that DAF-2 signaling could influence axonal transport of aggregate proteins or their retention in the cell body. Since we did not observe the cell body restricted pattern of *age-1* RNAi, a non-canonical downstream signaling pathway might be responsible for the observed effect.

NEURONS AGING UNDER EXTREME AGGREGATE CHALLENGE EXHIBIT DIFFERENCES FROM NATURAL AGING

It is striking that the *daf-2* RNAi polyQ128 neuronal aberration level is below that of polyQ128 empty vector controls (**Figure 5B**), and similar to that of polyQ0 empty vector controls (**Figure 4C**), while polyQ0 *daf-2* RNAi increases aberrations. Together with stresses induced by polyQ128, low insulin signaling (*daf-2* and *age-1* RNAi treatment) is associated both with protection from and an increase in morphological restructuring. Without extreme proteotoxic challenge at mid-life (as in polyQ0), however, neuronal aberrations are more apparent when insulin signaling is low. One possibility to explain these differences between *daf-2* RNAi in the naturally aging (polyQ0) and proteotoxically stressed (polyQ128) models is that hormetic consequences induced by polyQ128 are involved in suppression of aberrations. Alternatively, the aberrations in polyQ0 may be a manifestation of cellular maintenance that cannot be executed in the face of extreme polyQ128 challenge. An interesting question is whether additional neuron classes in the polyQ128 animals are affected by the expression of polyQ aggregates in the mechanosensory neurons or whether these effects are cell autonomous.

A second striking difference between natural aging and aging under extreme proteotoxic stress resides in *daf-16* RNAi treatment effects. In polyQ0 animals, *daf-16* RNAi impairs posterior touch sensation, but does not markedly alter neuronal morphology (only affecting anterior touch sensitivity). In contrast, in polyQ128 animals, *daf-16* RNAi results in both impaired touch response and increased neuronal aberrations. Also, *daf-16* RNAi in polyQ128, aggregate load increases and lifespan decreases proportionally more than in polyQ0. This suggests that polyQ128 expression in mechanosensory neurons induces stress signaling to other body tissues to disrupt the overall health of the animal.

A potential mechanism for the differences in effects of manipulating insulin signaling in polyQ0 and polyQ128 is increased basal insulin signaling in polyQ128 as a result of its protein load. However, we propose this is unlikely to be the mechanism underlying the observed differences. We see no difference in lifespan between empty vector control (L4440) treated polyQ0 and polyQ128 lifespan (**Figure 2A**). This is not surprising given that mechanosensory neurons do not seem to modulate lifespan (Chalfie et al., 1985). Further, microarray analysis of polyQ128 FACS-purified P_{mec-3} cells (mechanosensory neurons) showed no apparent dysregulation of genes in the insulin signaling pathway compared to non-toxic huntingtin:polyglutamine-expressing controls (Tourette and Neri, personal communication). Thus, the differences in neuron morphology and function seen in empty vector control treated polyQ0 and polyQ128 animals are likely due to some mechanism other than insulin signaling.

We have seen that with age, the effects on touch response and mechanosensory morphology are negatively correlated in polyQ0 and polyQ128 models (Vayndorf et al., in preparation). We showed that this correlation between increased morphological aberrations and decreased function remains in all RNAi treated polyQ128 animals (**Figure 5**). However, when polyQ0 animals receive RNAi treatment targeting components of the insulin signaling pathway, touch response and accumulation of aberrant morphology are no longer negatively correlated (**Figure 4**). Interestingly, while only *daf-2* RNAi showed overall significant effects on mechanosensory morphology and function in polyQ0 animals, RNAi treatment of polyQ128 animals yielded a higher number of significant changes. Also, we observed empty vector control polyQ128 animals decreased touch response and increased changes in neuronal morphology when compared to polyQ0 animals. Perhaps the decreased baseline neuronal function and worsened baseline neuronal morphology of the polyQ128 animals makes them more susceptible to changes in expression of insulin signaling pathway proteins, whereas naturally aging animals have more ability to compensate with other signaling pathways when there are changes in insulin signaling protein expression.

Overall, our findings suggest that improving neuronal aging outcomes and neuronal dysfunction associated with elevated protein aggregate stress may not be as simple as decreasing classical insulin signaling. This is not surprising because there are 40 insulin ligands with different expression levels in various cell types all vying for binding sites at the *C. elegans* insulin receptor, DAF-2. Others have shown that this insulin network is complex and works together to respond to varying stresses (Ritter et al., 2013), including protein misfolding and dysfunction like in our polyQ128 model. In addition, in mammalian and cell culture models, huntingtin is a phosphorylation substrate for AKT/PKB (Humbert et al., 2002; Dong et al., 2012). AKT can be modified and even cleaved into an inactive form in a rat model of Huntington's disease (Colin et al., 2005). Thus, in systems with endogenous huntingtin, unlike *C. elegans*, complex interactions between insulin signaling, expanded polyglutamine huntingtin aggregation, and neuronal morphology and function may be operative. Further genetic studies of the huntingtin polyQ128 model in *C. elegans* have the potential to elucidate mechanisms that influence morphological changes during neuronal aging.

ACKNOWLEDGMENTS

The authors would like to thank Dr. Marton Toth for the *zdIs5* strain, Leena Shah for helping with the strain crosses, Dr. Kriya Dunlap and Theresia Schnurr for training on and use of the microplate reader, and Jason Neuswanger for statistical consulting and the ImageJ macro used for aggregate analysis. Work was supported by NIH NINDS 2U54NS041069-06AI (Elena M. Vayndorf), NIH 8P20GM103395-12 (Barbara E. Taylor), ANR-08-MNPS-024-01 (Christian Neri), and NIH 1R01AG046358, R21 NS076868-01 (Monica Driscoll).

REFERENCES

Alcedo, J., Flatt, T., and Pasyukova, E. G. (2013). Neuronal inputs and outputs of aging and longevity. *Front. Genet.* 4:71. doi: 10.3389/fgene.2013.00071

Brenner, S. (1974). The genetics of *Caenorhabditis elegans*. *Genetics* 77, 71–94.

Broughton, S., and Partridge, L. (2009). Insulin/IGF-like signalling, the central nervous system and aging. *Biochem. J.* 418, 1–12. doi: 10.1042/BJ20082102

Calixto, A., Chelur, D., Topalidou, I., Chen, X., and Chalfie, M. (2010). Enhanced neuronal RNAi in *C. elegans* using SID-1. *Nat. Methods* 7, 554–559. doi: 10.1038/nmeth.1463

Chalfie, M., Sulston, J. E., White, J. G., Southgate, E., Thomson, J. N., and Brenner, S. (1985). The neural circuit for touch sensitivity in *Caenorhabditis elegans*. *J. Neurosci.* 5, 956–964.

Cohen, E., Du, D., Joyce, D., Kapernick, E. A., Volovik, Y., Kelly, J. W., et al. (2010). Temporal requirements of insulin/IGF-1 signaling for proteotoxicity protection. *Aging Cell* 9, 126–134. doi: 10.1111/j.1474-9726.2009.00541.x

Cohen, E., Paulsson, J. F., Blinder, P., Burstyn-Cohen, T., Du, D., Estepa, G., et al. (2009). Reduced IGF-1 signaling delays age-associated proteotoxicity in mice. *Cell* 139, 1157–1169. doi: 10.1016/j.cell.2009.11.014

Colin, E., Régulier, E., Perrin, V., Dürr, A., Brice, A., Aebischer, P., et al. (2005). Akt is altered in an animal model of Huntington's disease and in patients. *Eur. J. Neurosci.* 21, 1478–1488. doi: 10.1111/j.1460-9568.2005.03985.x

Dillin, A., and Cohen, E. (2011). Ageing and protein aggregation-mediated disorders: from invertebrates to mammals. *Philos. Trans. R. Soc. Lond. B Biol. Sci.* 366, 94–98. doi: 10.1098/rstb.2010.0271

Dong, G., Callegari, E., Gloeckner, C. J., Ueffing, M., and Wang, H. (2012). Mass spectrometric identification of novel posttranslational modification sites in Huntingtin. *Proteomics* 12, 2060–2064. doi: 10.1002/pmic.201100380

Faber, P. W., Alter, J. R., MacDonald, M. E., and Hart, A. C. (1999). Polyglutamine-mediated dysfunction and apoptotic death of a *Caenorhabditis elegans* sensory neuron. *Proc. Natl. Acad. Sci. U.S.A.* 96, 179–84. doi: 10.1073/pnas.96.1.179

Freude, S., Hettich, M. M., Schumann, C., Stöhr, O., Koch, L., Köhler, C., et al. (2009). Neuronal IGF-1 resistance reduces Abeta accumulation and protects against premature death in a model of Alzheimer's disease. *FASEB J.* 23, 3315–3324. doi: 10.1096/fj.09-132043

Friedman, D. B., and Johnson, T. E. (1988). Three mutants that extend both mean and maximum life span of the nematode, *Caenorhabditis elegans*, define the age-1 gene. *J. Gerontol.* 43, B102–B109. doi: 10.1093/geronj/43.4.B102

Gerstbrein, B., Stamatas, G., Kollias, N., and Driscoll, M. (2005). *In vivo* spectrofluorimetry reveals endogenous biomarkers that report healthspan and dietary restriction in *Caenorhabditis elegans*. *Aging Cell* 4, 127–137. doi: 10.1111/j.1474-9726.2005.00153.x

Hertweck, M., Göbel, C., and Baumeister, R. (2004). *C. elegans* SGK-1 is the critical component in the Akt/PKB kinase complex to control stress response and life span. *Dev. Cell* 6, 577–588. doi: 10.1016/S1534-5807(04)00095-4

Hsu, A.-L., Murphy, C. T., and Kenyon, C. (2003). Regulation of aging and age-related disease by DAF-16 and heat-shock factor. *Science* 300, 1142–1145. doi: 10.1126/science.1083701

Humbert, S., Bryson, E. A., Cordelie, F. P., Connors, N. C., Datta, S. R., Finkbeiner, S., et al. (2002). The IGF-1/Akt pathway is neuroprotective in huntington' s disease and involves huntingtin phosphorylation by akt. *Dev. Cell* 2, 831–837. doi: 10.1016/S1534-5807(02)00188-0

Kenyon, C. J. (1993). A *C. elegans* mutant that lives twice as long as wild type. *Nature* 366, 461–464. doi: 10.1038/366461a0

Killick, R., Scales, G., Leroy, K., Causevic, M., Hooper, C., Irvine, E. E., et al. (2009). Deletion of Irs2 reduces amyloid deposition and rescues behavioural deficits in APP transgenic mice. *Biochem. Biophys. Res. Commun.* 386, 257–262. doi: 10.1016/j.bbrc.2009.06.032

Lejeune, F., Mesrob, L., Parmentier, F., Bicep, C., Vazquez, R., Parker, A., et al. (2012). Large-scale functional RNAi screen in *C. elegans* identifies genes that regulate the dysfunction of mutant polyglutamine neurons. *BMC Genomics* 13:91. doi: 10.1186/1471-2164-13-91

Libina, N., Berman, J. R., and Kenyon, C. (2003). Tissue-specific activities of C. elegans DAF-16 in the regulation of lifespan. *Cell* 115, 489–502. doi: 10.1016/S0092-8674(03)00889-4

Morley, J. F., Brignull, H. R., Weyers, J. J., and Morimoto, R. I. (2002). The threshold for polyglutamine-expansion protein aggregation and cellular toxicity is dynamic and influenced by aging in *Caenorhabditis elegans*. *Proc. Natl. Acad. Sci. U.S.A.* 99, 10417–10422. doi: 10.1073/pnas.152161099

Mukhopadhyay, A., Oh, S. W., and Tissenbaum, H. A. (2006). Worming pathways to and from DAF-16/FOXO. *Exp. Gerontol.* 41, 928–934. doi: 10.1016/j.exger.2006.05.020

Neri, C. (2012). Role and therapeutic potential of the pro-longevity factor foxo and its regulators in neurodegenerative disease. *Front. Pharmacol.* 3:15. doi: 10.3389/fphar.2012.00015

Newman, A. B., and Murabito, J. M. (2013). The epidemiology of longevity and exceptional survival. *Epidemiol. Rev.* 35, 1–17. doi: 10.1093/epirev/mxs013

Oh, S. W., Mukhopadhyay, A., Dixit, B. L., Raha, T., Green, M. R., and Tissenbaum, H. A. (2006). Identification of direct DAF-16 targets controlling longevity, metabolism and diapause by chromatin immunoprecipitation. *Nat. Genet.* 38, 251–257. doi: 10.1038/ng1723

Pan, C.-L., Peng, C.-Y., Chen, C.-H., and McIntire, S. (2011). Genetic analysis of age-dependent defects of the *Caenorhabditis elegans* touch receptor neurons. *Proc. Natl. Acad. Sci. U.S.A.* 108, 9274–9279. doi: 10.1073/pnas.1011711108

Parker, J. A., Arango, M., Abderrahmane, S., Lambert, E., Tourette, C., Catoire, H., et al. (2005). Resveratrol rescues mutant polyglutamine cytotoxicity in nematode and mammalian neurons. *Nat. Genet.* 37, 349–350. doi: 10.1038/ng1534

Parker, J. A., Connolly, J. B., Wellington, C., Hayden, M., Dausset, J., and Neri, C. (2001). Expanded polyglutamines in *Caenorhabditis elegans* cause axonal abnormalities and severe dysfunction of PLM mechanosensory neurons without cell death. *Proc. Natl. Acad. Sci. U.S.A.* 98, 13318–13323. doi: 10.1073/pnas.231476398

Parker, J. A., Vazquez-Manrique, R. P., Tourette, C., Farina, F., Offner, N., Mukhopadhyay, A., et al. (2012). Integration of β-catenin, sirtuin, and FOXO signaling protects from mutant huntingtin toxicity. *J. Neurosci.* 32, 12630–12640. doi: 10.1523/JNEUROSCI.0277-12.2012

Ritter, A. D., Shen, Y., Fuxman Bass, J., Jeyaraj, S., Deplancke, B., Mukhopadhyay, A., et al. (2013). Complex expression dynamics and robustness in *C. elegans* insulin networks. *Genome Res.* 23, 954–965. doi: 10.1101/gr.150466.112

Taguchi, A., Wartschow, L. M., and White, M. F. (2007). Brain IRS2 signaling coordinates life span and nutrient homeostasis. *Science* 317, 369–372. doi: 10.1126/science.1142179

Taguchi, A., and White, M. F. (2008). Insulin-like signaling, nutrient homeostasis, and life span. *Annu. Rev. Physiol.* 70, 191–212. doi: 10.1146/annurev.physiol.70.113006.100533

Tank, E. M. H., Rodgers, K. E., and Kenyon, C. (2011). Spontaneous age-related neurite branching in caenorhabditis elegans. *J. Neurosci.* 31, 9279–9288. doi: 10.1523/JNEUROSCI.6606-10.2011

Toth, M. L., Melentijevic, I., Shah, L., Bhatia, A., Lu, K., Talwar, A., et al. (2012). Neurite sprouting and synapse deterioration in the aging caenorhabditis elegans nervous system. *J. Neurosci.* 32, 8778–8790. doi: 10.1523/JNEUROSCI.1494-11.2012

19

Use of *Caenorhabditis elegans* as a model to study Alzheimer's disease and other neurodegenerative diseases

Adanna G. Alexander[1,2†], Vanessa Marfil[1†] and Chris Li[1,2*]

[1] Department of Biology, City College of New York, New York, NY, USA
[2] Department of Biology, The Graduate Center, City University of New York, New York, NY, USA

Edited by:
Shin Murakami, Touro University-California, USA

Reviewed by:
Patrick Hu, University of Michigan, USA
Yelena V. Budovskaya, University of Amsterdam, Netherlands

***Correspondence:**
Chris Li, Department of Biology, City College of New York, New York, NY, USA
e-mail: cli@sci.ccny.cuny.edu

†Adanna G. Alexander and Vanessa Marfil have contributed equally to this work.

Advances in research and technology has increased our quality of life, allowed us to combat diseases, and achieve increased longevity. Unfortunately, increased longevity is accompanied by a rise in the incidences of age-related diseases such as Alzheimer's disease (AD). AD is the sixth leading cause of death, and one of the leading causes of dementia amongst the aged population in the USA. It is a progressive neurodegenerative disorder, characterized by the prevalence of extracellular Aβ plaques and intracellular neurofibrillary tangles, derived from the proteolysis of the amyloid precursor protein (APP) and the hyperphosphorylation of microtubule-associated protein tau, respectively. Despite years of extensive research, the molecular mechanisms that underlie the pathology of AD remain unclear. Model organisms, such as the nematode, *Caenorhabditis elegans*, present a complementary approach to addressing these questions. *C. elegans* has many advantages as a model system to study AD and other neurodegenerative diseases. Like their mammalian counterparts, they have complex biochemical pathways, most of which are conserved. Genes in which mutations are correlated with AD have counterparts in *C. elegans*, including an *APP*-related gene, *apl-1*, a tau homolog, *ptl-1*, and presenilin homologs, such as *sel-12* and *hop-1*. Since the neuronal connectivity in *C. elegans* has already been established, *C. elegans* is also advantageous in modeling learning and memory impairments seen during AD. This article addresses the insights *C. elegans* provide in studying AD and other neurodegenerative diseases. Additionally, we explore the advantages and drawbacks associated with using this model.

Keywords: *apl-1, C. elegans,* Alzheimer's disease, ALS, Parkinson disease, model systems

INTRODUCTION TO ALZHEIMER'S DISEASE

Alzheimer's disease (AD) is the 6th leading cause of death in the US and affects more than 35 million people worldwide (Alzheimer's Disease International, 2014). AD is a neurodegenerative disease characterized by a progressive loss of memory. Most cases of AD occur sporadically in aged people (>60 years, late-onset AD) without a clear inheritance pattern. However, in 5% of the cases (familial or early onset AD) AD symptoms appear earlier and are linked with gene mutations. Both forms of AD have two main neuropathologic features: the presence of extra-neuronal amyloid plaques, often referred to as senile plaques, and intraneuronal neurofibrillary tangles (Kidd, 1964; Luse and Smith, 1964; Terry et al., 1964; Krigman et al., 1965). Amyloid plaques are aggregates of the beta-amyloid peptide (Aβ), a cleavage product of the amyloid precursor protein (APP; Glenner and Wong, 1984; Masters et al., 1985; Kang et al., 1987). Hyperphosphorylation of the microtubule associated protein tau causes its polymerization into paired helical filaments (PHFs) and, presumably, its formation into neurofibrillary tangles (Goedert et al., 1989a).

Mutations in the *APP* gene and/or the enzymes involved in APP processing (γ-secretase components presenilins, PSEN1 and PSEN2; Chartier-Harlin et al., 1991; Goate et al., 1991; Murrell et al., 1991; Levy-Lahad et al., 1995; Rogaev et al., 1995; Sherrington et al., 1995) are correlated with early onset AD. These mutations increase the levels of toxic Aβ species and promote neurodegeneration. By contrast, a recently identified mutation in *APP* affects cleavage of APP, causing less Aβ production and conferring neuroprotective benefits (Jonsson et al., 2012). Despite the significant advances made using *APP* transgenic and knock-out models in mammals, unraveling the cellular role of APP has been difficult. Alternative animal models provide complementary approaches to dissecting the function of APP and tau. In this review, we discuss the latest uses of the nematode *Caenorhabditis elegans* as a model system for the study of AD. We also include a brief review of a few representative examples of how *C. elegans* is being utilized to model other neurodegenerative diseases.

C. elegans AS A MODEL FOR ALZHEIMER'S DISEASE

Caenorhabditis elegans is a free-living, non-parasitic nematode that was first introduced as a model organism by Sydney Brenner in 1963 (Brenner, 1974). It is a small (1 mm in length), transparent roundworm, which makes it easy for manipulation, and has a short life cycle of 3 days from egg to adult at 25°C (Brenner, 1974). Under suitable growing conditions, hatched animals develop through four larval stages (L1–L4), each punctuated by a molt, to arise as an adult hermaphrodite with 959 somatic cells (Sulston and Horvitz, 1977). Its life span is between 2 and

3 weeks, which facilitates the study of its biology. Completion of the *C. elegans* genome sequence in 1998 (*C. elegans* Sequencing Consortium, 1998) demonstrated that roughly 38% of worm genes have a human ortholog, such as *APP* and *tau* (Shaye and Greenwald, 2011). Hence, *C. elegans* has many excellent advantages as an *in vivo* model for the study of AD and other neurodegenerative diseases.

MOLECULAR PATHWAYS OF APP. SIMILARITIES AND DIFFERENCES BETWEEN MAMMALS AND *C. elegans*

FUNCTION AND PROCESSING OF APP: NON-AMYLOIDOGENIC AND AMYLOIDOGENIC Aβ PATHWAY

The APP family of proteins contains three members, APP, APLP1, and APLP2 (Wasco et al., 1992, 1993; Sprecher et al., 1993; Sandbrink et al., 1994; Slunt et al., 1994), which are characterized by a large extracellular region containing conserved E1 and E2 domains, a single transmembrane domain, and a small cytosolic domain (Kang et al., 1987). APLP1 and APLP2 do not contain the Aβ sequence and, hence, do not produce Aβ (**Figure 1A**; Wasco et al., 1992, 1993). The APP gene family is required for viability and brain development. *APP* mouse knockouts were viable, but had behavioral and cognitive defects (Ring et al., 2007). While knockout of APLP1 resulted in postnatal growth defects (Heber et al., 2000), mice in which APLP2 was inactivated appeared wild type (von Koch et al., 1997). Double knockouts of APLP2 and either APP or APLP1, however, resulted in postnatal lethality (von Koch et al., 1997; Heber et al., 2000); the lethality of *APP/APLP2* double knockouts could be rescued by knock-in of an APP extracellular fragment, sAPPα (Weyer et al., 2011), suggesting that sAPPα is sufficient for viability. The triple knockout caused lethality and a type II lissencephaly and cortical disorganization (Herms et al., 2004). Collectively, these results suggest that APP family members have essential and redundant functions during development, including proper brain development, and these functions do not require Aβ.

In mammals, APP is processed through two proteolytic pathways, only one of which produces Aβ (**Figure 1B**; Haass et al., 1992, 1994a,b). In the non-amyloidogenic pathway, APP is first cleaved by an α-secretase within the Aβ sequence to release an extracellular fragment, sAPPα (**Figure 1B**). The remaining APP fragment (known as APP-CTFα or C83) is then cleaved by the γ-secretase complex to release the APP intracellular domain (AICD) to the cytosol. By contrast, in the amyloidogenic pathway, after cleavage by the β-secretase (BACE) to release sAPPβ, the remaining APP fragment (known as APP-CTFβ or C99) is then cleaved by the γ-secretase complex, liberating Aβ to the lumen and AICD to the cytosol (Gu et al., 2001; Sastre et al., 2001; Weidemann et al., 2002). This latter pathway is likely favored in AD patients.

Mammalian γ-secretase is a protease complex consisting of several components: presenilins 1 and 2 (PSEN1 and PSEN2), nicastrin (NCT), anterior pharynx defective (APH-1), and the presenilin enhancer (PEN-2; Yu et al., 2000; Francis et al., 2002). PSEN1 and PSEN2 are the catalytic components of the γ-secretase complex. NCT works as a stabilizing cofactor required for γ-secretase complex assembly and trafficking (Li et al., 2003; Zhang et al., 2005) and PEN-2 and APH-1 have a role in the maturation process of PSEN1 and PSEN2 (Luo et al., 2003). Besides APP, the γ-secretase complex is also involved in the proteolysis of Notch receptors, and the first identification of any PEN-2 or APH-1 ortholog was in *C. elegans* as the result of a genetic screen for modifiers of the Notch pathway (Francis et al., 2002; Goutte et al., 2002). Within the γ-secretase complex, only mutations in PSEN1 and PSEN2 have been associated with early onset AD (Levy-Lahad et al., 1995; Rogaev et al., 1995; Sherrington et al., 1995).

PROCESSING OF *C. elegans* APL-1

In *C. elegans* there is only one APP-related gene, *apl-1*. Like human APP (Kang et al., 1987), APL-1 contains a large extracellular region whose conserved E1 and E2 domains share 46 and 49% sequence similarity to human APP, respectively, a transmembrane domain, and a relatively small cytosolic domain, which shares 71% sequence similarity to human APP (**Figure 1A**; Daigle and Li, 1993). Notably, unlike APP but similar to APLP1 and APLP2, APL-1 does not contain the Aβ sequence (Daigle and Li, 1993).

Two α-secretase proteins are present in *C. elegans*, SUP-17 and ADM-4 (Jarriault and Greenwald, 2005). They work redundantly in the cleavage of the *C. elegans* Notch homologs, LIN-12 and GLP-1 (Jarriault and Greenwald, 2005). However, no experiments thus far have tested whether SUP-17 or ADM-4 cleaves APL-1. No BACE ortholog has been identified by bioinformatic searches and no β-secretase activity that cleaves human APP has been detected in *C. elegans*, suggesting that APL-1 is only processed by the α/γ-secretase processing pathway (Link, 2006). α-secretase cleavage of APL-1 releases the extracellular fragment, sAPL-1; subsequent cleavage of APL-1-CTFα by the γ-secretase complex liberates the intracellular domain (AICD; **Figure 1B**).

The initial characterizations of human PSEN1 (then called S182) and PSEN2 (first named E5-1) described them as novel proteins with multiple transmembrane domains (Rogaev et al., 1995; Sherrington et al., 1995). The cellular functions of the presenilins were determined by their homology to the *C. elegans* protein, SEL-12 (Levitan and Greenwald, 1995). The two *C. elegans* Notch genes, *lin-12* and *glp-1*, are involved in many cell fate decisions during development, including vulval cell specification and germline development (Greenwald et al., 1983; Lambie and Kimble, 1991; Newman et al., 1995; Levitan et al., 1996) *sel-12*/PSEN was identified in a genetic screen to isolate suppressors of a dominant Lin-12/Notch multivulva phenotype (Levitan and Greenwald, 1995). Loss of *sel-12*/PSEN suppressed the Lin-12/Notch multivulva phenotype and produced a defect in egg laying that was rescued by introducing human PSEN1 or PSEN2, suggesting a conserved function between human and *C. elegans* presenilins (Levitan and Greenwald, 1995; Levitan et al., 1996). Like human PSENs (Thinakaran et al., 1996), SEL-12/PSEN is cleaved to attain its final topology (Li and Greenwald, 1996). A *C. elegans* PSEN gene family was identified and includes *sel-12*, *hop-1*, and *spe-4* (L'Hernault and Arduengo, 1992; Levitan and Greenwald, 1995; Li and Greenwald, 1997; Westlund et al., 1999); *spe-4* is exclusively expressed in male gonadal cells and will not be further discussed (Arduengo et al., 1998). Knockdown of *hop-1*/PSEN in *sel-12*/PSEN mutants showed maternal effect lethality, germline defects, and missing anterior pharynx, defects associated with loss of *glp-1*/Notch function, suggesting

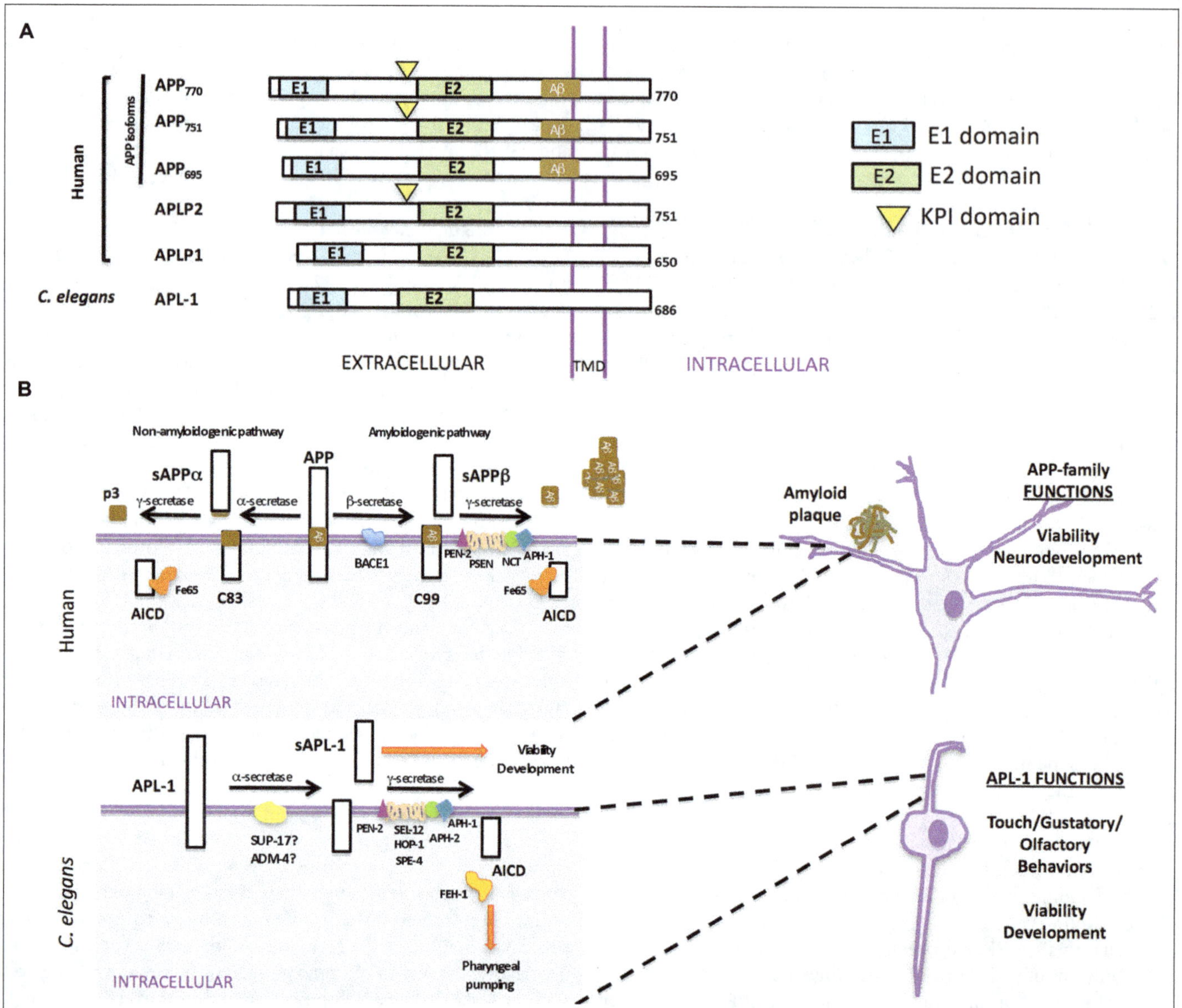

FIGURE 1 | Similarities and differences between human APP and *Caenorhabditis elegans* APL-1. (A) Schematic representation of human APP isoforms, other members of the APP family (APLP1 and APLP2), and *C. elegans* APL-1. **(B)** Comparison between human APP proteolytic pathways (top) and *C. elegans* APL-1 proteolytic pathway (bottom). *Top.* APP can be cleaved by two different pathways. In the anti-amyloidogenic pathway, APP is first cleaved by the α-secretase to release an extracellular fragment sAPPα. The remaining APP fragment (APP-CTFα or C83) is then cleaved by the γ-secretase complex to release p3 extracellularly and the APP intracellular domain (AICD) to the cytosol. In the amyloidogenic pathway, β-secretase first cleaves APP, releasing the sAPPβ fragment. The APP-CTFβ (C99) fragment is subsequently cleaved by the γ-secretase complex, liberating the AICD to the cytosol and Aβ to the lumen. Aβ will aggregate to form amyloid plaques. *Bottom.* In *C. elegans*, APL-1 is first cleaved by the α-secretase homologs SUP-17/ADM-4, liberating the extracellular sAPL-1 that is known to regulate worm viability and development. The γ-secretase complex will then cleave the remaining APL-1-CTF to release AICD into the cytosol. General functions of the APP family and APL-1 are indicated.

that *sel-12* and *hop-1* function redundantly in the LIN-12 and GLP-1/Notch pathways (Westlund et al., 1999). Similarly, mice carrying a null mutation in *PSEN1* showed embryonic lethality, skeletal defects, and disrupted somite boundaries (Shen et al., 1997), similar to the phenotypes seen in Notch1 knockouts (Krebs et al., 2000, 2003, 2004; Duarte et al., 2004; Gale et al., 2004).

In screening for novel mutants showing the *glp-1*/Notch phenotype of defective anterior pharynx, Goutte et al. (2000, 2002) identified two genes, *aph-1* and *aph-2*, which encodes the *C. elegans* NCT ortholog. Independently, Francis et al. (2002) screened for enhancers of *sel-12*/PSEN activity and identified *pen-2*. *aph-2*/NCT, *pen-2*, and *aph-1* are all required for proper Notch signaling. Human PSEN, NCT, Aph1α2, and PEN-2 were subsequently shown to physically associate and cooperatively regulate the maturation of individual components to form a proteolytically active γ-secretase complex (Kimberly et al., 2003).

FUNCTION AND REGULATION OF APL-1

Like the mammalian APP family (Slunt et al., 1994; Lorent et al., 1995; Thinakaran et al., 1995), *apl-1* is expressed in multiple tissue types. *apl-1* expression is observed in neurons, supporting cells, and head muscles throughout development, while expression in vulval muscles, vulval cells, and hypodermal seam cells is not detected until the L4 stage to adult (Hornsten et al., 2007; Niwa et al., 2008).

Inactivation of *apl-1*, such as with the *yn10* null allele, results in a completely penetrant lethality during the first to second larval (L1–L2) transition due to a molting defect (Hornsten et al., 2007). *apl-1* activity is also necessary for later larval transitions, as RNAi knockdown of *apl-1* in an RNAi-sensitized background showed animals with molting defects during the L3–L4 and L4 to adult transitions (Wiese et al., 2010). This lethality was rescued by microinjection of an *apl-1* genomic fragment or cDNA. Hence, similar to the mammalian APP family, *apl-1* has an essential function. High levels of *apl-1* expression caused an incompletely penetrant L1 lethality (70% lethality), shortened body length, and morphogenetic, reproductive, and locomotory defects (Hornsten et al., 2007; Ewald et al., 2012b). These results indicate that levels of APL-1 must be tightly regulated as loss of APL-1 as well as high levels of APL-1 result in lethality. When *sel-12*/PSEN activity was reduced in transgenic animals with APL-1 overexpression, the 70% lethality was partially rescued, suggesting that SEL-12/PSEN regulates APL-1 cleavage and/or trafficking (Hornsten et al., 2007). The underlying basis of the loss- and gain-of-function *apl-1* lethality is still unclear, but is not dependent on activation of CED-3/caspase or necrotic cell death pathways (Hornsten et al., 2007). Characterization of *apl-1* function may provide insights into the general function and pathways of APP, of which much is still unknown.

The *apl-1(yn5)* mutant, which contains a deletion of the region encoding the APL-1 transmembrane and cytosolic domains, produces only the extracellular domain of APL-1 (APL-1EXT) and is viable. Because APL-1EXT is not further cleaved by α-secretase, APL-1EXT is slightly larger than sAPL-1 and is expressed at high levels in *apl-1(yn5)* mutants (Hornsten et al., 2007). Hence, the APL-1 extracellular domain is sufficient for viability, similar to the rescue of APP/APLP2 double mutants by the knock-in of sAPPα (Weyer et al., 2011). However, although *apl-1(yn5)* mutants are viable, they display several phenotypes, including a slower developmental progression, decreased body length, reproductive defects, and temperature-sensitive lethality (Hornsten et al., 2007; Ewald et al., 2012b). Because these defects can be phenocopied by microinjection of APL-1EXT transgenes into wild-type animals, the phenotypes are due to overexpression of APL-1EXT and not due to loss of APL-1 signaling through its cytoplasmic domain (Ewald et al., 2012b). Interestingly, pan-neuronal expression of APL-1EXT, but not expression from muscle or hypodermal cells, is sufficient to rescue the lethality observed in *apl-1* null mutants (Hornsten et al., 2007), suggesting that the cells (i.e., neurons) from which sAPL-1 is released as well as the extracellular milieu in which sAPL-1 travels is functionally relevant. We suggest that high levels of sAPP may also contribute to the pathology seen in AD patients. Down's syndrome patients, whose chromosome 21 trisomy includes trisomy of APP, display a high incidence of AD and intellectual disability (Zigman, 2013), perhaps contributed in small part by the high levels of APP expression.

Decreasing *apl-1* activity by RNAi resulted in hypersensitivity to aldicarb, an acetylcholinesterase inhibitor (Wiese et al., 2010). Using *apl-1* knockouts to test different *apl-1* deletion constructs, Wiese et al. (2010) determined that lack of sAPL-1 is responsible for the aldicarb hypersensitivity. These findings are consistent with mammalian studies, which show that a lack of APP and APLP2 impairs synaptic function at cholinergic neuromuscular junctions (Wang et al., 2005).

Heterochronic genes, whose differential spatiotemporal expression ensures proper progression through larval stages and transition into adulthood (Chalfie et al., 1981; Ambros and Horvitz, 1984), regulate expression of *apl-1* in hypodermal seam cells (Niwa et al., 2008). Loss of *let-7* microRNA (miRNA) function caused precocious seam cell development and vulval bursting at the adult stage, leading to death (Reinhart et al., 2000). These *let-7* phenotypes can be rescued by knockdown of *apl-1* (Niwa et al., 2008). *apl-1*, however, is not a direct target of *let-7* miRNA. NHR-25/Ftz-F1, which is a nuclear hormone receptor (NHR) that is required for completion of larval molts (Asahina et al., 2000; Gissendanner and Sluder, 2000), binds an enhancer element in the promoter of *apl-1* to regulate *apl-1* expression in seam cells (Niwa and Hada, 2010). *nhr-25*/Ftz-F1 transcripts are possible targets of the *let-7* family of miRNAs for downregulation (Hayes et al., 2006). Regulation of continued *apl-1* expression in adult seam cells and other cell types is unknown.

Pathways through which apl-1 functions

The *apl-1(yn5)* phenotypes require activity of the DAF-16/FOXO transcription factor, which is negatively regulated by the insulin pathway. *C. elegans* has only one insulin/IGF-1 receptor, DAF-2 (Kimura et al., 1997). Under favorable environmental conditions, such as when adequate food is present, signaling through the insulin pathway activates a conserved PI 3-kinase/AKT cascade (Morris et al., 1996; Kimura et al., 1997; Paradis and Ruvkun, 1998; Paradis et al., 1999), which causes phosphorylation of DAF-16/FOXO, thereby allowing reproductive development (Larsen et al., 1995; Gems et al., 1998; Henderson and Johnson, 2001). Phosphorylation of DAF-16/FOXO causes its sequestration in the cytoplasm (Lin et al., 2001), thereby preventing it from entering the nucleus to activate its target genes (Henderson and Johnson, 2001; Lee et al., 2001), which regulate longevity (Lin et al., 1997; Ogg et al., 1997), stress resistance (McElwee et al., 2003, 2004; Murphy et al., 2003), and dauer formation (Riddle et al., 1981; Vowels and Thomas, 1992). Environmental conditions also affect other metabolic functions, such as reproductive behavior, which is inhibited under starvation conditions (Seidel and Kimble, 2011), and body size. Starvation survival behavior is regulated by DAF-16/FOXO activity (Lee and Ashrafi, 2008) and the insulin (So et al., 2011) and DAF-7/TGFβ (Savage-Dunn et al., 2003) pathways work in parallel to regulate body length via *daf-16*/FOXO activity.

The slowed development, decreased body size, and decreased reproductive rates of *apl-1(yn5)* mutants are dependent on *daf-16*/FOXO activity. At 20°C, mutants with decreased insulin signaling or *apl-1(yn5)* mutants showed a delayed developmental progression and shorter body length, which were enhanced when insulin signaling was decreased in *apl-1(yn5)* mutants [i.e., *daf-2(e1370); apl-1(yn5)* double mutants]; at 25°C, the *apl-1(yn5)* mutants with decreased insulin signaling went into L1 arrest (Ewald et al., 2012b). By contrast, when *daf-16*/FOXO activity was removed from *apl-1(yn5)* mutants, the delayed developmental progression, decreased reproductive rate, and smaller body length of *apl-1(yn5)* single mutants were suppressed. Furthermore, loss of *daf-16*/FOXO activity in *apl-1(yn5)* mutants with decreased insulin signaling rescued the short body length and L1 arrest phenotypes (Ewald et al., 2012b). These results suggest that sAPL-1 signals in a parallel pathway to the insulin pathway or modulates the DAF-2/insulin/IGF-1 pathway to activate *daf-16*/FOXO activity to affect developmental progression, reproductive rates, and body length (**Figure 2**). Mammalian sAPP may have similar roles in development.

Activity of the *daf-12*/NHR signals in multiple pathways to integrate environmental stimuli with metabolic needs and can modulate the insulin pathway as well as function in an independent pathway (Gerisch et al., 2001; Dumas et al., 2010). Decreasing *daf-12*/NHR activity in *apl-1(yn5)* mutants rescued the slow development, low reproductive rate, and decreased body length phenotypes (Ewald et al., 2012b). Hence, decreased insulin signaling and signaling through a parallel *daf-12*/NHR pathway converge to activate *daf-16*/FOXO for the phenotypes seen in *apl-1(yn5)* mutants. Noteworthy, levels of insulin/IGF-1 receptors are decreased in AD brains (Steen et al., 2005), and APP processing and Aβ production *in vitro* was modulated by insulin signaling (Gasparini et al., 2001). Analogous to *C. elegans*, sAPP may also act to modulate the insulin pathway.

Pan-neuronal APL-1 expression affects learning

In transgenic mice expressing human or mouse APP, animals showed an increased lethality and learning defects that were not correlated with Aβ deposition (Hsiao et al., 1995); similarly, doubly transgenic mice carrying transgenes with APP and PSEN1 mutations showed learning defects that were not correlated with the number of Aβ plaques (Holcomb et al., 1999). The mechanisms underlying these defects are unclear. Use of the *C. elegans* model could be informative. *C. elegans* has many sensory modalities, including smell and taste. They respond to volatile and water soluble chemicals by moving toward or away from chemoattractive or chemorepulsive stimuli, respectively. Many chemoattractants and chemorepellants have been identified and the neural circuits mediating the chemosensory response identified (Bargmann and Horvitz, 1991). For instance, when *C. elegans* is given the choice between a neutral compound and a chemoattractant, such as benzaldehyde, animals will move toward benzaldehyde; this response is mediated by the AWC neurons (Bargmann et al., 1993); similarly, ASEL, a gustatory neuron, mediates chemoattraction to sodium acetate (Bargmann and Horvitz, 1991; Pierce-Shimomura et al., 2001).

Although *apl-1* is not expressed in AWC neurons and the morphology of sensory neurons appears wild type with GFP markers, the overall chemoattractive response to benzaldyhyde and sodium acetate was decreased in *apl-1(yn10/+)* heterozygotes and transgenic animals that overexpress APL-1 [e.g., *ynIs79* (P*apl-1::apl-1::GFP*)] (Ewald et al., 2012a). The chemotaxis response was restored in APL-1 overexpression lines [e.g., *ynIs79* (P*apl-1::apl-1::GFP*)] when insulin signaling was decreased, but not when *daf-16*/FOXO activity was decreased, suggesting that *daf-16*/FOXO activity is needed for normal chemotaxis in transgenic lines overexpressing APL-1 (**Figure 2**). Pan-neuronal expression of APL-1 or targeted overexpression of APL-1 in the AWC or ASEL neurons resulted in wild-type chemotaxis responses (Ewald et al., 2012a). By contrast, ectopic expression of *apl-1* with the *snb-1* promoter, which drives pan-neuronal and multi-cell type expression, resulted in no chemotaxis response to benzaldehyde or sodium acetate (Ewald et al., 2012a). When signaling through the DAF-2/insulin/IGF-1 receptor, DAF-12/NHR, or DAF-7/TGFβ was decreased, the chemotaxis response toward benzaldehyde and sodium acetate in these transgenic lines was restored, indicating that the loss of the chemotaxis response due to ectopic *apl-1* signaling in cells outside the nervous system is dependent on insulin and TGFβ signaling.

In addition to chemosensory responses, *C. elegans* is also capable of associative chemosensory plasticity (Wen et al., 1997). For example, when benzaldehyde was paired with starvation for as short as 30 min, *C. elegans* showed a significant reduction in preference for benzaldehyde; persistence of this plasticity was positively correlated with the length of pairing time (Colbert and Bargmann, 1995; Tomioka et al., 2006; Lin et al., 2010), suggestive of stable memory formation. Both chemotaxis and associative plasticity are dependent on insulin signaling (Tomioka et al., 2006; Lin et al., 2010). Little associative plasticity, however, was observed after pairing benzaldehyde with starvation for 60 min in animals with pan-neuronal APL-1 expression (Ewald et al., 2012a). The plasticity could be restored when *daf-16*/FOXO, *daf-12*/NHR, or *daf-7*/TGFβ activity was decreased, indicating that the impaired associative plasticity with pan-neuronal APL-1 expression requires *daf-16*/FOXO, *daf-12*/NHR, and *daf-7*/TGFβ activity (Ewald et al., 2012a).

Touch habituation is another sensory characteristic affected by pan-neuronal APL-1 expression. When a gentle touch is applied to the head of the animal, *C. elegans* responds by moving backward; conversely, when touched on the tail, the animal moves forward (Chalfie and Sulston, 1981). This response to gentle body touch is mediated by six mechanosensory touch neurons (Chalfie et al., 1985). After six cycles of alternating head/tail touches, wild-type animals habituated and became unresponsive (Ewald et al., 2012a). *apl-1(yn10/+)* heterozygotes or transgenic animals that overexpress APL-1 showed touch habituation. By contrast, animals with pan-neuronal APL-1 expression were slow to habituate and required more alternating head/tail touch cycles before becoming habituated (Ewald et al., 2012a). Collectively, these results indicate that pan-neuronal overexpression of APL-1 causes learning defects. These results parallel those seen in mammalian models in which overexpression of APP leads to cognitive defects, independent of Aβ aggregates (Hsiao et al., 1995; Simón et al., 2009), thereby suggesting that sAPP activity, in addition to Aβ aggregates, contributes to cognitive

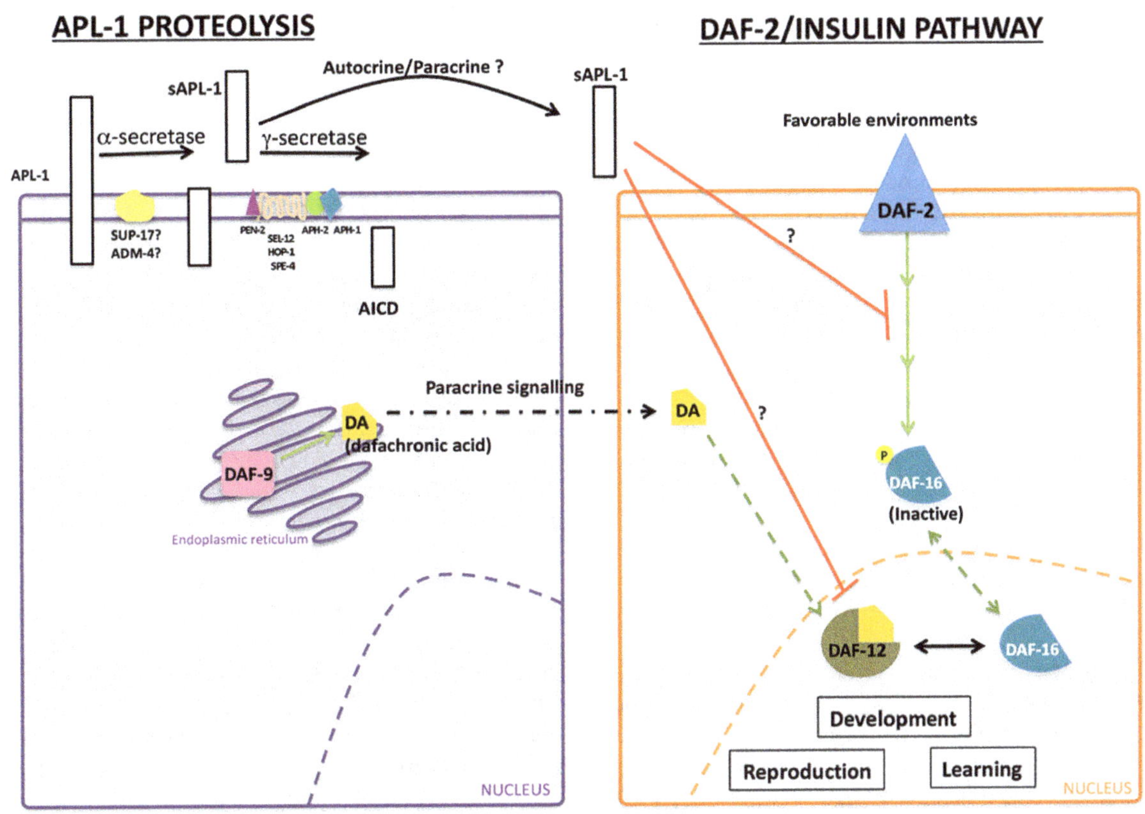

FIGURE 2 | Interaction between sAPL-1 and DAF-2 insulin/IGF-1 receptor and DAF-12/NHR pathways. Schematic representation of APL-1 proteolytic pathway and how sAPL-1 may modulate DAF-2 insulin/IGF-1 receptor and DAF-12/NHR signaling pathways. APL-1 is cleaved by the α/γ-secretase pathway in *C. elegans*. Released sAPL-1 could act as a signaling molecule in the same cell (autocrine regulation) or in neighboring cells (paracrine regulation) to inhibit *daf-2* insulin/IGF-1 receptor and *daf-12*/NHR pathways to affect worm viability and development. The exact mechanism by which sAPL-1inhibits *daf-2* insulin/IGF-1 receptor and *daf-12*/NHR is still unknown and labeled as a question mark (see Ewald et al., 2012b).

defects. Whether these cognitive defects depend on the DAF-16/FOXO transcription factor and/or TGFβ signaling remains to be tested.

APL-1 TRAFFICKING IS IMPORTANT FOR SYNAPTIC TRANSMISSION

APL-1, like APP (Koo et al., 1990), is transported from the cell body to synapses (Wiese et al., 2010). UNC-108, which is a neuronally expressed GTPase and localizes to the Golgi complex and early endosomes (Mangahas et al., 2008; Edwards et al., 2009), is involved in the maturation of dense core vesicles (Borgonovo et al., 2006; Mangahas et al., 2008; Edwards et al., 2009; Sumakovic et al., 2009) and the packaging of APL-1 into mature dense core vesicles (Wiese et al., 2010). Both UNC-116/kinesin-1 and UNC-104/KIF1A/kinesin-3 are involved in the anterograde transport of APL-1 (Wiese et al., 2010; Arimoto et al., 2011), but only UNC-116/kinesin-1 and dynein motors are responsible for the retrograde transport of APL-1 back to the cell body (Arimoto et al., 2011). The rates of anterograde and retrograde transport of APL-1 vesicles are 1.1 μm/s and 1.6 μm/s, respectively (Arimoto et al., 2011). Hence, APL-1 is transported similarly as in mammalian models where kinesin-1 is responsible for APP axonal transport (Koo et al., 1990). Surprisingly, mutations in *unc-116*/kinesin-1 and *unc-104*/KIF1A/kinesin-3 both caused decreased levels of APL-1 expression without affecting transcript levels, suggesting that without transport motors, APL-1 does not accumulate in cell bodies because of protein degradation (Wiese et al., 2010; Arimoto et al., 2011). APL-1 is also internalized from the cell surface of neurons via a RAB-5-dependent endocytosis (Wiese et al., 2010).

AICD INTRACELLULAR TRAFFICKING

The Fe65 family of proteins binds the cytoplasmic YENPTY sequence of APP, APLP1, and APLP2, via their PTB2 domain (Guénette et al., 1996; Zambrano et al., 1997; Duilio et al., 1998; Russo et al., 1998). Likewise, the sole family member ortholog in *C. elegans*, FEH-1, has a WW domain and PTB1 and PTB2 domains, which closely resemble those of the Fe65 family, and the PTB2 domain of FEH-1 interacts with APL-1 (Zambrano et al., 2002).

FEH-1 is expressed in pharyngeal muscle and neuronal processes and is necessary for survival. Inactivation of *feh-1* caused an incompletely penetrant embryonic lethality. Survivors showed little pharyngeal pumping and were unable to feed, thereby resulting in L1 arrest (Zambrano et al., 2002). Decreasing *feh-1* activity or decreasing *feh-1* dosage caused pharyngeal pumping rates to increase, suggesting that the rate of pharyngeal pumping is *feh-1* dosage dependent. However, the functional significance of FEH-1 and APL-1 interactions is unclear as *apl-1(yn5)* mutants, which do not have an AICD domain, and *apl-1(yn10/+)* heterozygotes do not have defective pumping rates (Ewald et al., 2012b).

INVESTIGATING THE AMYLOID HYPOTHESIS OF AD IN *C. elegans*

Aβ peptide, the cleavage product of APP believed to underlie the pathology of AD (Glenner and Wong, 1984; Masters et al., 1985; Gorevic et al., 1986; Selkoe et al., 1986), is not present in APL-1 (Daigle and Li, 1993) nor does *C. elegans* possess β-secretase activity to produce Aβ (Link, 2006). Nevertheless, *C. elegans* provides a powerful *in vivo* genetic system to study the effects of neurotoxic Aβ through transgene analysis (Shankar et al., 2008). Many transgenic strains have been generated in which a signal sequence followed by the human Aβ sequence is expressed in all cells, in all neurons, in specific subsets of neurons, or in muscle cells (**Figure 4**). These strains produce either $A\beta_{1-42}$ or $A\beta_{3-42}$.

AD is a late onset neurodegenerative disease. *C. elegans* expressing human $A\beta_{3-42}$ in muscle tissue (Link, 1995; Link et al., 2001) showed an age-dependent paralysis at 20°C (Cohen et al., 2006; McColl et al., 2009); paralysis occurred more rapidly and more severely when $A\beta_{1-42}$ was produced at 25°C (McColl et al., 2009). The level of muscle paralysis was significantly decreased when insulin signaling was decreased (Cohen et al., 2006). Furthermore, inhibiting *daf-16*/FOXO and *hsf-1,* which encodes a heat shock protein transcription factor (Hsu et al., 2003; Morley and Morimoto, 2004), reversed the effects of decreased insulin signaling (Cohen et al., 2006). Hence, the paralysis effects of Aβ correlates with age and is dependent on insulin signaling.

Since aggregated Aβ is toxic to neurons (Glenner and Wong, 1984; Masters et al., 1985; Gorevic et al., 1986; Selkoe et al., 1986) and causes muscle paralysis in *C. elegans,* molecules and pathways that can prevent the formation or promote the disassembly of Aβ aggregates can be screened for in *C. elegans.* For instance, when *C. elegans* extracts are incubated with aggregated human $A\beta_{3-42}$ in the presence or absence of protease inhibitors, disaggregation occurred, but disaggregation did not occur when extracts were either heated to denature proteins or incubated with proteinases (Bieschke et al., 2009). Hence, an unidentified protein or protein complex in *C. elegans* extracts can disaggregate $A\beta_{3-42}$ aggregates.

Several orthologs to human heat shock (HSP) chaperone proteins were found to interact directly with $A\beta_{3-42}$ in *C. elegans. C. elegans* HSP-16 proteins, HSP-16-1, HSP-16-2, and HSP-16–48, orthologs of αB-crystallin, bound intracellular $A\beta_{3-42}$ monomers and soluble $A\beta_{3-42}$ oligomers, but not fibrillar $A\beta_{3-42}$ (Fonte et al., 2002). Moreover, *hsp-16* transcript levels were upregulated in $A\beta_{3-42}$ transgenic lines, but whether these chaperone proteins protect against or promote Aβ paralysis is unclear (Fonte et al., 2002). By contrast, increased expression of the HSP70 chaperones had a protective role by suppressing paralysis (Fonte et al., 2008). These results are consistent with human studies showing that HSP70 and αB-crystallin were upregulated in AD brains (Hamos et al., 1991; Perez et al., 1991; Shinohara et al., 1993; Renkawek et al., 1994; Yoo et al., 2001) and binds Aβ (Liang, 2000).

Transgenic lines in which Aβ is expressed in glutamatergic neurons showed age-dependent neurodegeneration, whereby 7-day adults showed 75% glutamatergic neurodegeneration (Treusch et al., 2011). This degeneration was suppressed when genes involved in clathrin-mediated endocytosis, such as *unc-11, unc-26, Y44E3A.4, C. elegans RTS1* ortholog, *C. elegans ADE12* ortholog, and human *CRMI,* were co-expressed with Aβ, and enhanced when a *PBS2/MAP2K4* mitogen-activated protein kinase transgene was co-expressed with Aβ in glutamatergic neurons (Treusch et al., 2011). Interestingly, mutations in the *C. elegans* human REST ortholog *spr-4,* which suppressed the *sel-12*/PSEN egg-laying defect (Lakowski et al., 2003), also enhanced the degeneration seen in the transgenic animals expressing Aβ in glutamatergic neurons (Lu et al., 2014). Modifying clathrin-mediated endocytosis in rat cortical neurons was similarly neuroprotective against Aβ aggregates (Treusch et al., 2011). In addition, early stage AD brains showed higher expression of REST target genes, while late stage AD and frontotemporal dementia (FTD) brains showed lower expression (Lu et al., 2014). Hence, REST may confer neuroprotective benefits in *C. elegans* and in humans (Lu et al., 2014).

The *C. elegans* Aβ model also proves useful in screens to identify drugs that disaggregate Aβ. The drug PBT2, an 8-hydroxy quinoline analog, reversed AD phenotypes in mice within days (Adlard et al., 2008). Similarly, *C. elegans* expressing inducible $A\beta_{1-42}$, which become paralyzed within 48 h after induction, were protected against paralysis when exposed to PBT2 (McColl et al., 2012).

C. elegans lrp-1 FUNCTIONS SIMILARLY TO LRP2/MEGALIN, AN LDL RECEPTOR FAMILY MEMBER

In mammals, the LDL receptor family is responsible for many functions, including binding ligands for internalization and degradation and cholesterol metabolism (Brown and Goldstein, 1986; Mahley, 1988; Herz et al., 1992; Willnow et al., 1994). Binding of LRP1 to sAPP770 or full-length APP770, one of the APP isoforms (**Figure 1**), causes its internalization and degradation (Kounnas et al., 1995; Knauer et al., 1996); disrupting cell surface APP internalization with an LRP-antagonist increases sAPPα processing and full-length APP at the cell surface and decreases Aβ formation, suggesting that LRP1-APP interactions favor APP processing through the amyloidogenic pathway (Ulery et al., 2000). Apolipoprotein E and LRP2/megalin have also been implicated in Aβ clearance (Zlokovic et al., 1996; Deane et al., 2004; Carro et al., 2005).

C. elegans LRP-1 most closely resembles mammalian LRP2/megalin (Yochem and Greenwald, 1993; Yochem et al., 1999). *C. elegans* does not have the ability to synthesize cholesterol and, therefore, must rely on dietary sources (Hieb and Rothstein, 1968). Inactivation of *lrp-1* resulted in late larval lethality due to molting defects during the L3–L4 transition (Yochem et al., 1999). When wild-type *C. elegans* were grown in the absence of cholesterol, the molting defects of the *lrp-1* knockouts were phenocopied (Yochem et al., 1998; Wiese et al., 2012), suggesting that LRP-1 is involved in cholesterol uptake from the environment. LRP-1 is expressed in the epithelial hypodermal cells, hyp6 and hyp7, where it localizes to their apical surface (Yochem et al., 1999) and where *apl-1* is also expressed in adults (Niwa et al., 2008). Similarly, its mammalian counterpart, LRP2/megalin, is mainly expressed at the apical surface of epithelial cells (Cui et al., 1996; Morales et al., 1996; Willnow et al., 1996; Nielsen et al., 1998; Zheng et al., 1998; Hermo et al., 1999; Mizuta et al., 1999).

LRP2/megalin interacts with different domains of APP (Zlokovic et al., 1996; Pietrzik et al., 2004; Carro et al., 2005; Yoon et al., 2005; Cam and Bu, 2006). A physical interaction between APL-1 and LRP-1 has not been determined. Expression of LRP-1 with an N-terminal domain truncation did not rescue the lethality of *apl-1* null mutants, suggesting that sAPL-1 is not activating an *lrp-1* pathway (Hornsten et al., 2007). When *lrp-1* expression is decreased or when wild-type animals are deprived of dietary cholesterol, neurotransmission is affected (Wiese et al., 2012). However, *apl-1* null mutants die at an earlier stage in development than *lrp-1* null mutants, suggesting that *apl-1* functions in earlier developmental pathways that are necessary for survival.

C. elegans AS A MODEL FOR OTHER NEURODEGENERATIVE DISEASES

PTL-1 AS A TAU MODEL

Accumulation of neurofibrillary tangles in cell bodies is another hallmark characteristic of AD and other neurodegenerative disorders. The major component of these tangles is tau, which belongs to the family of microtubule-associated proteins (MAPs) that includes MAP2 and MAP4 (Lee et al., 1988; Lewis et al., 1988; Goedert et al., 1989b; Chapin and Bulinski, 1991). MAPs share characteristic homology domains, including a proline-rich domain and a region of a variable number of tandem amino acid repeats (**Figure 3A**; Goedert et al., 1988, 1989a,b, 1992a; Lee et al., 1988; Lewis et al., 1988; Aizawa et al., 1990). Tau is the predominant MAP expressed in axons, while MAP2 is expressed in dendrites (Matus et al., 1981; Binder et al., 1985) and MAP4 is expressed in dividing cells (Bulinski and Borisy, 1980). MAPs bind microtubules and are responsible for promoting microtubule assembly and stability (reviewed in Amos and Schlieper, 2005). MAP family members appear to have redundant functions; mice in which tau was knocked out were viable, but showed increased levels of MAP1A (Harada et al., 1994), suggesting that upregulation of MAP1A can compensate for the lack of tau *in vivo*. Tau phosphorylation affects its ability to bind microtubules and can cause a conformational change that favors tubulin assembly (**Figure 3B**; Feijoo et al., 2005). Aberrant hyperphosphorylation of tau, however, impairs its ability to bind microtubules, thus resulting in their disassembly (Lindwall and Cole, 1984; Biernat et al., 1993; Bramblett et al., 1993). In addition, phosphorylated tau self-aggregates into PHFs and presumably generates the intracellular neurofibrillary tangles characteristic of AD patients (**Figure 3B**; Goedert et al., 1992b; Alonso et al., 1996, 1997, 2001; Billingsley and Kincaid, 1997).

Because of the functional redundancy of MAPs, their specific functions have been difficult to determine. *C. elegans* has only one tau homolog protein with tau-like repeats 1 (PTL-1; Goedert et al., 1996; McDermott et al., 1996). PTL-1 exists as two isoforms, PTL-1A and PTL-1B, with five or four tandem repeats, respectively (Goedert et al., 1996; **Figure 3A**). They have a high level of sequence homology with mammalian tau, especially in the C-terminal microtubule binding region (Goedert et al., 1996; McDermott et al., 1996). Both PTL-1A and PTL-1B bound microtubules *in vitro* and induced tubulin polymerization (Goedert et al., 1996; McDermott et al., 1996). PTL-1 is initially expressed embryonically in the epidermis of elongating embryos and in head neurons; in larval and adult animals PTL-1 is expressed mainly in the mechanosensory neurons mediating gentle body touch (**Figure 3B**; Goedert et al., 1996; Gordon et al., 2008), although transcriptional fusions show a wider expression pattern in neurons and stomatointestinal cells (Gordon et al., 2008).

Loss of *ptl-1*/tau results in an incompletely penetrant lethality at the same stage of embryogenesis (Gordon et al., 2008) at which PTL-1/tau expression is first observed (Goedert et al., 1996). *ptl-1*/tau mutants that escaped lethality showed normal development, but had a shortened lifespan, and although the overall integrity of microtubule structure appeared unaffected at the light microscopic level, there was a significant reduction in gentle touch sensitivity as compared to wild-type (Gordon et al., 2008; Chew et al., 2013). These touch defects were enhanced in mutants with defects in β- and α-tubulin, indicating that the absence of full-length PTL-1/tau disrupts mechanosensation, but it does so independently of tubulin (Gordon et al., 2008). In mutants in which only the C-terminal microtubule binding repeats of PTL-1/tau are deleted, touch sensitivity was identical to that of wild-type (Chew et al., 2013), suggesting that the N-terminal domain of PTL-1/tau is sufficient for gentle touch responses.

As *C. elegans* ages, mechanosensory touch neurons exhibit age-related morphological changes: cell bodies initially elaborate branches and axons subsequently display blebbing and branching (Pan et al., 2011; Tank et al., 2011; Toth et al., 2012). Strikingly, mechanosensory touch neurons in *ptl-1*/tau mutants displayed these aging characteristics at higher incidences and at an earlier stage than wild-type animals; GABAergic neurons also showed age-related phenotypes, such as ectopic branching (Chew et al., 2013). Expression of a human tau isoform (htau40) in *ptl-1*/tau mutants rescued the touch insensitivity, but not the morphological aging defects, indicating that htau40 shares some functional conservation with PTL-1/tau (Chew et al., 2013). Interestingly, when *ptl-1*/tau was expressed in Sf9 cells, cells projected neurite-like processes that were positive for PTL-1/tau immunoreactivity (Goedert et al., 1996) and that were indistinguishable from those visualized when htau40 was expressed in Sf9 cells (Knops et al., 1991; Chen et al., 1992). Although wild-type PTL-1/tau has not been reported to aggregate into fibrils, PTL-1/tau, like human tau, clearly has an essential role in maintaining neuronal integrity, controlling neuronal aging, and affecting lifespan (Goedert et al., 1996; Gordon et al., 2008). While there are no known mutations in tau that are associated with AD, tau mutations are associated with FTD with parkinsonism (FTPD-17), another form of dementia (Hutton et al., 1998; Poorkaj et al., 1998; Spillantini et al., 1998; see Section "Frontotemporal Dementia").

FRONTOTEMPORAL DEMENTIA

Frontotemporal dementia (FTD) is a group of neurodegenerative disorders characterized by severe brain frontotemporal lobar degeneration (reviewed in Rabinovici and Miller, 2010). In some cases it may be hard to distinguish between FTD and AD; however,

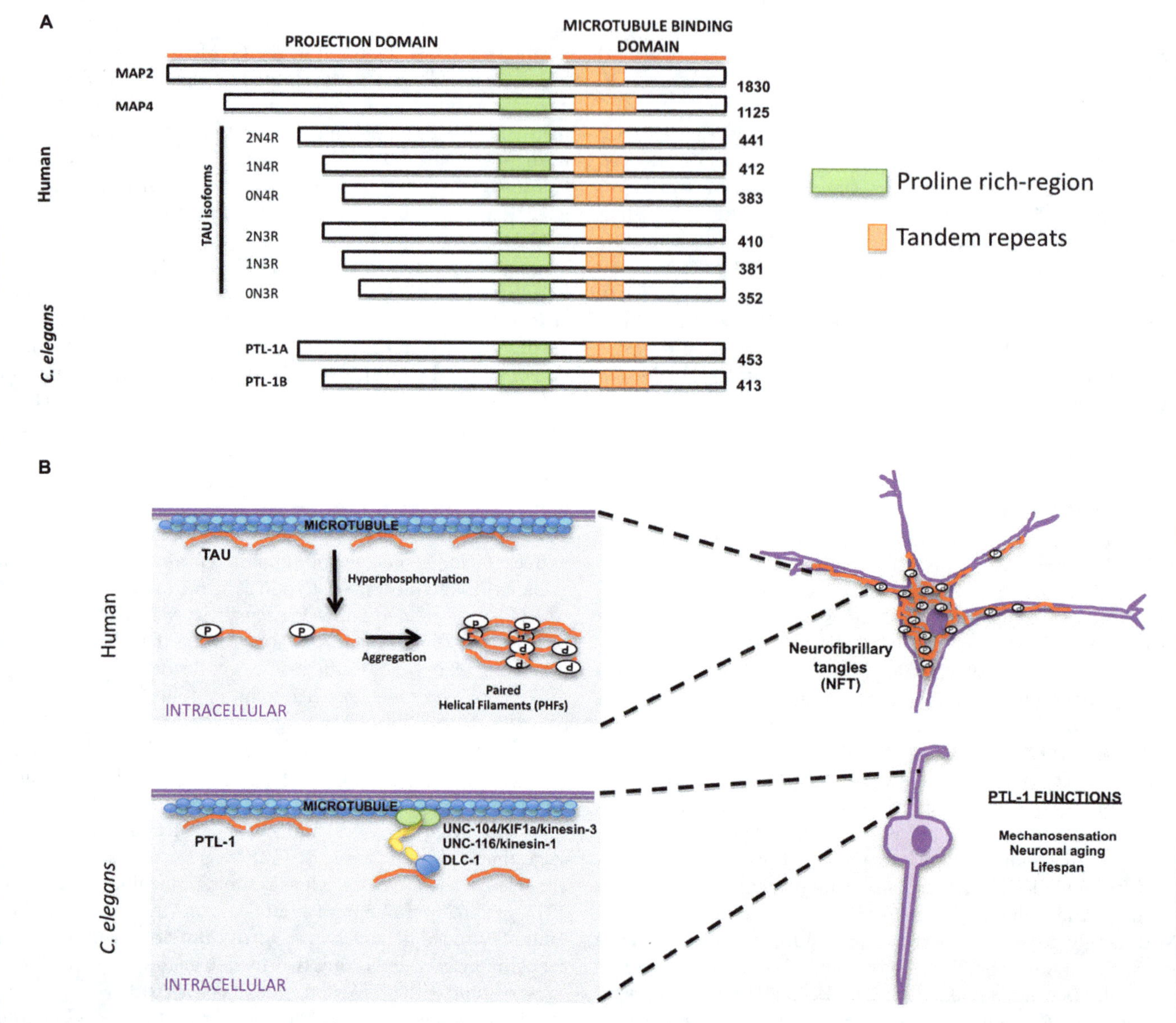

FIGURE 3 | Similarities and differences between human tau and *Caenorhabditis elegans* PTL-1. (A) Schematic representation of human microtubule binding proteins (MAPs) family, including tau isoforms and *C. elegans* PTL-1 isoforms. **(B)** Comparison between tau functions in humans (top) and C. *elegans* PTL-1/tau functions (bottom). *Top.* Tau has a physiological role in promoting and maintaining microtubule stability. In pathological conditions tau is hyperphosphorylated and self-aggregates into paired helical filaments (PHFs) that can form intracellular neurofibrillary tangles (NFT). *Bottom. C. elegans* PTL-1/tau binds microtubules and induces microtubule assembly. It also affects synaptic transport through motor proteins UNC-104/KIF1a/kinesin-3, UNC-116/kinesin-1, and DLC-1/dynein. PTL-1/tau is also important for *C. elegans* mechanosensation and aging.

FTD usually develops earlier in life and is more likely to have a genetic component (Lindau et al., 2000; Pasquier, 2005). Many mutations can cause FTD with or without motor neuron disease (Cruts et al., 2012). Two mutations have been well characterized and are associated with specific types of FTD: tau-positive FTD linked to chromosome 17 (FTD-17) and FTD caused by TDP43 proteinopathy (FTD-TDP43). Patients with FTD-17 suffer behavioral changes and often Parkinson-like motor problems. While mutations in the tau gene *MAPT* are not described in familial or sporadic AD, *MAPT* tau mutations are linked with FTD-17 (Hutton et al., 1998; Poorkaj et al., 1998; Spillantini et al., 1998).

Several transgenic lines expressing human tau harboring FTD-17 mutations (htau-FTD-17) have been generated in *C. elegans* (**Figure 4B**) (see also Section "PTL-1 as a Tau Model"; Kraemer et al., 2003; Miyasaka et al., 2005; Brandt et al., 2009; Fatouros et al., 2012). Pan-neuronal transgene expression of wild type or htau-FTD-17 caused an uncoordinated phenotype that progressively worsened with age, an accumulation of insoluble tau, and neurodegeneration (Kraemer et al., 2003). Similarly, expression of htau-FTD-17 in touch neurons resulted in a decrease in the touch response due to neuritic abnormalities and tau accumulation (Miyasaka et al., 2005). Using these *C. elegans* models of

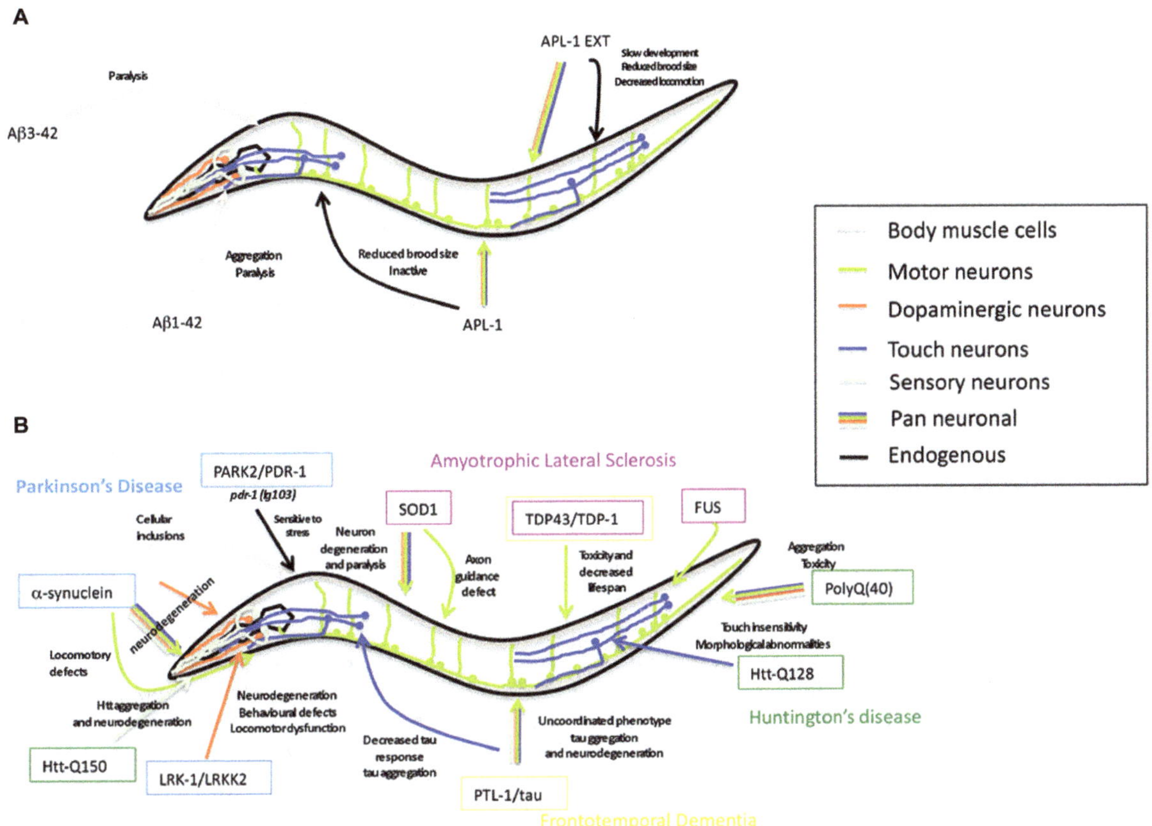

FIGURE 4 | *Caenorhabditis elegans* as a transgenic model for AD and other neurodegenerative diseases. (A) Summary of the Alzheimer's disease models in *C. elegans* expressing human Aβ peptide or *C. elegans* full-length APL-1 or APL-1 extracellular domain (APL-1 EXT). Arrow color represents the tissues where transgenes were expressed. Phenotypes observed are next to the arrow. **(B)** Summary of the *C. elegans* models for Parkinson's disease (PD), amyotrophic lateral sclerosis (ALS), frontotemporal dementia (FTD), and Huntington's disease (HD). Genes modeling PD are shown in blue boxes, ALS in pink boxes, FTD in yellow boxes, and HD in green boxes. Arrow color represents tissues where transgenes were expressed. Phenotypes observed are written close to the arrow.

tauopathy in forward genetic screens, Kraemer and co-workers identified two new factors, SUT-1 and SUT-2, that may participate in the pathological pathway activated by tau (Kraemer et al., 2003; Kraemer and Schellenberg, 2007; Guthrie et al., 2009). Moreover, down-regulation of the human SUT-2 homolog (MSUT-2) in mammalian cell lines caused a marked decrease in tau aggregation, suggesting that MSUT-2 may be a good candidate target for FTD therapies (Wheeler et al., 2010; Guthrie et al., 2011). More recently, Fatouros et al. (2012) generated two htau-FTD-17 transgenic models: one with a pro-aggregant mutated form of human tau (deletion of K280) and a second with mutated forms of human tau (I277P and I308P) that prevented tau aggregation. The tau (ΔK280) transgenic line had high levels of tau aggregation, which caused uncoordinated movement in adults, axonal defects, and alterations in presynaptic structures (Fatouros et al., 2012); the locomotory defects could be partially suppressed by a compound of the aminothioenopyridazine (ATPZ) class cmp16, suggesting that this compound may be neuroprotective (Fatouros et al., 2012). The tau (I277P and I308P) transgenic lines had low levels of tau aggregates and displayed only mild phenotypes with significantly less morphological abnormalities.

Accumulation of TDP-43 [transactive response (TAR) DNA-binding protein] is found in ~50% of the cases of FTD (The Association for Frontotemporal Degeneration, 2014) and has numerous genetic causes. However, only one case has been reported with mutations in the TDP-43 gene (Borroni et al., 2009). *C. elegans* models overexpressing human TDP-43 or its *C. elegans* ortholog TDP-1 recapitulates some of the FTD phenotypes, including neurotoxicity and protein aggregation (see also Section "Amyotrophic Lateral Sclerosis").

C9orf72 encodes a protein that regulates endosomal trafficking and autophagy in primary neurons and neuronal cells (Farg et al., 2014). It is expressed in multiple tissue types, including cerebellar cortex and spinal cord (DeJesus-Hernandez et al., 2011). Hexanucleotide (GGGGCC) repeat expansions in a non-coding region of C9orf72 are found in patients with amyotrophic lateral sclerosis (ALS) and FTD (DeJesus-Hernandez et al., 2011; Renton et al., 2011; Majounie et al., 2012), providing the first genetic link between the two diseases, although it remains unclear how C9orf72 hexanucleotide expansion triggers ALS and FTD pathology. Mutations in the *C. elegans* C9ORF72 ortholog *alfa-1* caused age-dependent motility defects, leading to paralysis and degeneration of GABAergic motoneurons (Therrien et al., 2013), suggesting that a loss-of-function mechanism is involved in the C9ORF72-dependent pathogenesis.

PARKINSON'S DISEASE

Parkinson's disease (PD) is a progressive neurodegenerative disorder that affects the control of body movements. The impaired motor control in PD is the result of the death of dopaminergic (DA) neurons (Hughes et al., 1992; Fahn and Sulzer, 2004). The disease is characterized by the accumulation of α-synuclein into neuronal inclusions called Lewy bodies (Lewy, 1912; Tretiakoff, 1919). Most PD cases are of unknown cause. However, ~5–10% of PD cases are familial (Wood-Kaczmar et al., 2006) and include mutations in the following genes: α-synuclein, parkin (PRKN), leucine-rich repeat kinase 2 (LRRK2), PTEN-induced putative kinase 1 (PINK1), and ATP13A2 (Hardy, 2010).

α-synuclein is a presynaptic neuronal protein whose cellular function is not well understood, but may include controlling the supply of synaptic vesicles in neuronal terminals and regulating dopamine release. It is a small acidic protein (14 kDa) whose sequence can be divided into three domains: the N-terminal α-helical domain (amino acids 1–65), the central hydrophobic domain (residues 66–95), and the acidic carboxyl-terminal domain (residues 96–140; Recchia et al., 2004). Three mutations in the α-helical domain (A53T, A30P, E46K) are linked with autosomal dominant early onset PD, suggesting that these mutations can predispose to oligomer and fibril formation (Polymeropoulos et al., 1997; Krüger et al., 1998; Conway et al., 2000a,b,c; Zarranz et al., 2004). Because *C. elegans* has no α-synuclein ortholog, *C. elegans* models are based on transgenic worms overexpressing wild-type or mutant forms of human α-synuclein (**Figure 4B**). Although different transgenic lines showed some differences, most lines with pan-neuronal or DA neuronal expression of wild-type or mutated α-synuclein (A53T and/or A30P mutations) displayed locomotory defects and degeneration of dopamine neurons (Lakso et al., 2003; Kuwahara et al., 2006; Cao et al., 2010). Furthermore, downregulating the activity of the nuclease EndoG decreased α-synuclein toxicity in DA neurons (Büttner et al., 2013). EndoG is a mitochondria-specific endonuclease that mediates cellular death by apoptosis (Li et al., 2001). When cell death is induced, EndoG translocates from the mitochondria to the nucleus to fragment DNA (Li et al., 2001). Approximately 50% of the dopamine neurons expressing α-synuclein degenerate, whereas a mutation in *cps-6*, which encodes the *C. elegans* EndoG ortholog, rescues this degeneration (Büttner et al., 2013). Similar results were found in yeast, flies, and human cells suggesting that EndoG is a conserved requirement for α-synuclein toxicity (Büttner et al., 2013).

C. elegans models of α-synuclein overexpression-induced toxicity have also been examined by whole genome RNAi knockdown and microarray screenings (Vartiainen et al., 2006; Hamamichi et al., 2008; Kuwahara et al., 2008; van Ham et al., 2008). These screens highlighted the importance of endocytosis for ameliorating α-synuclein-dependent neurotoxicity (Kuwahara et al., 2008). Transgenic lines expressing α-synuclein specifically in body wall muscle cells produced inclusions as animals aged, resembling a feature of neurons in patients with PD; the number of inclusions decreased when genes affecting different biological processes, such as vesicle and lysosomal trafficking (W08D2.5/ATP13A2), lipid metabolism, and lifespan control (*sir-2.1*, *lagr-1*), were knocked down (van Ham et al., 2008). In a genome-wide microarray analysis to identify genes that were modulated in *C. elegans* overexpressing wild-type or A53T human α-synuclein, seven genes encoding components of the ubiquitin-proteasome machinery and 35 mitochondrial function genes were found to be upregulated, while nine genes encoding histones H1, H2B, and H4 were down regulated (Vartiainen et al., 2006). These data provide support for the role of the proteasome complex and mitochondrial proteins in mediating neurotoxicity.

Parkin (human PARK2) is a component of an ubiquitin E3 ligase that is part of the proteasome complex (Shimura et al., 2000). Mutations in PARK2 have been associated with early onset recessive forms of PD (Kitada et al., 1998; Poorkaj et al., 2004). *C. elegans* has a parkin ortholog, PDR-1. A truncated form of PDR-1(Δaa24–247) encoded by the in-frame deletion null allele *pdr-1*(*lg103*) had altered solubility and propensity to aggregate when expressed in cell lines, resembling parkin mutant proteins in PD (Springer et al., 2005). Furthermore, *pdr-1* mutants were hypersensitive to different proteotoxic stress conditions, suggesting that PDR-1/PARK2 mutations act to block the proteostasis machinery, thereby making it easier for proteins to abnormally fold and aggregate (Springer et al., 2005).

Mutations in LRRK2/leucine-rich repeat kinase 2 are the most common known cause of late-onset PD. LRRK2 belongs to the LRRK family; gain-of-function LRRK2 mutations interfere with chaperone-mediated autophagic functions and presumably decrease levels of α-synuclein degradation (Orenstein et al., 2013). Transgenic worms overexpressing pathogenic mutant forms of LRRK2 in DA neurons caused DA neurodegeneration (Liu et al., 2011; Yao et al., 2013). Interestingly, treatment of the transgenic worms with kinase inhibitors resulted in arrested neurodegeneration, suggesting that LRRK2 kinase activity is important for its pathogenesis (Liu et al., 2011; Yao et al., 2013).

Many studies have reported a link between toxin exposure and increased risk of PD. *C. elegans* has been used to test different toxins and help elucidate the mechanism by which they produce neurotoxicity. Administration of the 6-hydroxydopamine (6-OHDA) neurotoxin to *C. elegans* produced specific degeneration of dopamine neurons (Nass et al., 2002). By performing forward genetic and high-throughput chemical screens, mutations within the dopamine transporter *dat-1* were found to suppress 6-OHDA sensitivity (Nass et al., 2005) and bromocriptine, quinpirole, and acetaminophen, and plant extracts from *Bacopa monnieri* and *Uncaria tomentosa* were found to be neuroprotective (Marvanova and Nichols, 2007; Locke et al., 2008; Ruan et al., 2010; Jadiya et al., 2011; Shi et al., 2013). These data demonstrate that pathological characteristics of PD can be recapitulated in *C. elegans* models and used to investigate the mechanism by which α-synuclein and other PD proteins produce neurotoxicity and cause motor defects.

AMYOTROPHIC LATERAL SCLEROSIS

Amyotrophic lateral sclerosis is a neurodegenerative disease characterized by the death of motor neurons in brain and spinal cord and progressive paralysis of the body (Hardiman et al., 2011). Approximately 10% of ALS cases are familial and associated with mutations in several genes. The most common mutation in familial ALS is found in the superoxide dismutase enzyme (SOD1) with more than 160 different mutations identified (Wroe et al., 2008). SOD1 is a ubiquitously expressed protein that converts the toxic radical superoxide anion to hydrogen peroxide. Although it is not clear yet how SOD1 mutations causes motor neuron degeneration, toxicity is likely generated by a gain-of-function mechanism (Valentine et al., 2005) and associated with misfolding and aggregation of the enzyme (Pasinelli and Brown, 2006).

Transgenic lines expressing mutant human SOD1 proteins have been successfully generated in *C. elegans* and recapitulate the motor neuron degeneration and paralysis characteristic of ALS patients (**Figure 4B**) (Witan et al., 2008; Gidalevitz et al., 2009; Wang et al., 2009; Li et al., 2014). The locomotion defect caused by pan-neuronal expression of the SOD1(G85R) mutant isoform was reduced when insulin signaling was decreased (Boccitto et al., 2012), suggesting that decreased insulin signaling increases the capacity of cells to prevent the accumulation of toxic non-soluble proteins and opening the possibility of finding new therapeutic targets. Similarly, when wild-type or mutant SOD1(G93A) was expressed exclusively in GABAergic motor neurons, animals showed an age-dependent paralysis and accumulation of wild-type and mutant SOD1(G93A), although defects were more severe in the mutant lines; interestingly, the SOD1 aggregates were soluble in the wild-type SOD1 lines and insoluble in the SOD1(G93A) lines (Li et al., 2014). In addition, motor neurons showed axonal guidance defects during development and caspase-independent cell death in adulthood in the wild-type and SOD1(G93A) lines (Li et al., 2014).

Other genes associated with ALS have also been modeled using *C. elegans*. TDP-43 [TAR DNA-binding protein] is a 43 kDa RNA binding protein identified as the main component of ubiquitinated protein aggregates (Tsuda et al., 2008; Murakami et al., 2012; Vaccaro et al., 2012a,b; Han et al., 2013; Therrien et al., 2013) found in patients with sporadic ALS (Neumann et al., 2006) and also in some cases of FTD (see Section "Frontotemporal Dementia"). TDP-43 is normally located in the nucleus of neurons, but dominant mutations in TDP-43 cause aberrant localization of TDP-43 in the cytoplasm, thereby preventing it from functioning in the nucleus (Gitcho et al., 2008; Kabashi et al., 2008; Sreedharan et al., 2008; Van Deerlin et al., 2008; Yokoseki et al., 2008; Ash et al., 2010). *C. elegans* has one TDP-43 ortholog, TDP-1. TDP-1 controls longevity and oxidative stress in the worm by regulating the insulin pathway (Vaccaro et al., 2012b). Overexpression of *tdp-1*/TDP-43 resulted in toxicity and decreased lifespan, analogous to the phenotypes found in ALS patients (Vaccaro et al., 2012b). In transgenic worms expressing TDP-43 harboring ALS-associated mutations, proteotoxicity affecting neuronal functions was induced. Similar results were found when the RNA binding protein FUS with ALS-related mutations was expressed in the nematode (Murakami et al., 2012; Vaccaro et al., 2012b).

Excess exposure to some pesticides and chemicals, such as the metalloid selenium, have been implicated in the etiology of ALS (Vinceti et al., 2009; Kamel et al., 2012; Malek et al., 2012). Exposure to high levels of sodium selenite in the worm induced neurodegeneration and resulted in paralysis (Estevez et al., 2012, 2014). When insulin pathway activity was reduced, the adverse effects of environmental selenium exposure was altered (Estevez et al., 2014). Overall, the *C. elegans* models have highlighted the possible importance of the insulin and autophagy pathways in the generation of ALS.

HUNTINGTON'S DISEASE

Huntington's disease (HD) is a progressive neurodegenerative disorder inherited through autosomal dominant mutations of the *IT15* gene. *ITI5* encodes the huntingtin protein, whose functions remain unknown (The Huntington's Disease Collaborative Research Group, 1993). The mutations result in an N-terminal polyglutamine (polyQ) expansion (Goldberg et al., 1996; Mangiarini et al., 1996). In normal individuals, up to 34 repeats have been reported, whereas in HD afflicted individuals, up to 100 polyQ repeats have been recorded (The Huntington's Disease Collaborative Research Group, 1993). The huntingtin-polyQ (HdhQ) proteins form aggregates, whose toxicity is determined by the length of the polyQ expansion and which cause swollen, disorganized, and ribosome-deficient endoplasmic reticulum and chromatin irregularities (Martindale et al., 1998). Eventually, cellular defects caused by the aggregates culminate in HD symptoms, which include involuntary movement, cognitive impairment, and loss of neurons in the striatum and deep layers of the frontal cortex (Martin and Gusella, 1986).

Although *C. elegans* does not have a huntingtin homolog, transgenic *C. elegans* models that express an N-terminal human huntingtin (htt) fragment with different numbers of CAG repeats have been used to model HD and identify genes that prevent polyQ aggregates (**Figure 4B**). The models generally express the repeats in specific neurons, such as the ASH sensory neurons, which are multi-modal sensory neurons that mediate avoidance to chemo- and mechanosensory stimuli. In transgenic animals expressing htt171 with 150 CAG repeats (htt171-Q150), 13% of the ASH neurons began to lose function after 8 days, suggesting an age-dependent degeneration (Faber et al., 1999). This loss of ASH function was reversed in a *ced-3*/caspase (Faber et al., 1999) or *hda-3*/HDAC (Bates et al., 2006) mutant background, suggesting that processes characteristic of apoptotic cell death and histone deacetylases play a role in HD (Dragunow et al., 1995). By contrast, the number of htt171-Q150 aggregates and neurodegeneration were enhanced when genes mediating autophagy, CREB, CREB binding proteins, and *pqe-1* were disrupted, suggesting that autophagy and activation of CREB target genes decreases htt171-Q150 aggregation and are neuroprotective (Faber et al., 2002; Bates et al., 2006; Jia et al., 2007). Transgenic animals expressing fewer CAG repeats (2, 23, and 95 polyQ) showed normal ASH function (Faber et al., 1999). The onset of behavioral defects are consistent with most cases of HD, in which symptoms usually appear during midlife (Vonsattel et al., 1985; Martin and Gusella, 1986; Strong et al., 1993; The Huntington's Disease Collaborative Research Group, 1993; Gusella and MacDonald, 1995) and fewer than 10% of reported cases occur before the age of 21 (Farrer and Conneally, 1985; van Dijk et al., 1986; Nance, 1997; Siesling et al., 1997).

In a different HD model, htt57-Q128 was expressed in the touch mechanosensory neurons (Parker et al., 2001). These transgenic animals did not show neurodegeneration, but had a significantly reduced response to posterior touch and a milder defect in anterior touch response (Parker et al., 2001). The touch neurons contained polyQ aggregates and morphological abnormalities primarily along axonal processes (Parker et al., 2001). The touch insensitivity could be rescued by activating Sir2 sirtuins (Parker et al., 2005), which act through the DAF-16/FOXO transcription factor to promote longevity (Tissenbaum and Guarente, 2001). Similarly, in neuronal cell lines derived from knockin HdhQ111 mice, activation of sirtuins reduced the level of cell death (Parker et al., 2005). Additionally, in an RNAi based screen for genes that suppressed htt57-Q128 defects, identified *C. elegans* genes were also upregulated in the striatum of mouse HD models (Lejeune et al., 2012). Thus, *C. elegans* is a useful model to identify additional genes that may protect against or contribute to defects caused by polyQ expansions.

RNAi knockdown of *dnj-27*/ERdj5, an ER luminal protein upregulated in response to ER stress, exacerbated the impaired mobility observed when a Q40 transgene is expressed in body wall muscles, suggesting that *dnj-27* interacts with polyQ and protects against polyQ induced paralysis (Muñoz-Lobato et al., 2014).

C. elegans has the advantage that it is transparent, allowing visualization of the formation of that aggregates, including aggregates made by shorter polyQ tracts, whereas only longer tracts are visible in mammals (Brignull et al., 2006). To determine the threshold number of polyQ repeats needed to elicit a morphological and behavioral response, varying lengths of polyQ repeats were tested in *C. elegans*. Pan-neuronal expression of more than 40 polyQ led to variable protein aggregation and paralysis (Brignull et al., 2006). These data suggest that 40 polyQ may be the critical number of repeats to elicit HD symptoms and are consistent with unaffected humans who have up to 34 polyQ repeats and HD patients who have as few as 42 repeats (The Huntington's Disease Collaborative Research Group, 1993).

Overall, *C. elegans* HD models illustrate that human huntingtin polyQs disrupt the morphology and function of sensory neurons. The genetic and RNAi screens highlight candidate genes that may be involved in HD pathogenesis in mammalian models and provide insights into genes that may serve a protective role against polyQ toxicity. In addition to HD, other diseases caused by polyQ repeats include spinocerebellar ataxias and spinal and bulbar muscular atrophy (Orr and Zoghbi, 2007). Hence, using *C. elegans* provides another approach toward determining how polyQ pathogenicity contributes to neurodegeneration.

ADVANTAGES AND LIMITATIONS OF THE *C. elegans* MODEL

The use of *C. elegans* to study AD and other neurodegenerative diseases has, as many other models, many advantages as well as some drawbacks. Major advantages of *C. elegans* include the ability to perform forward genetic, RNAi, and high throughput chemical screens and the ease of generating transgenic lines. These benefits have been effective in informing the role of APP and the presenilins and identifying components of the γ-secretase complex. The function of APP and the pathways in which it acts are still unclear. *C. elegans* presents a complementary system to understand the function and pathways of an APP-related protein, APL-1. Furthermore, overexpression of APL-1 by mutation or by transgene induces phenotypes that converge on the insulin/DAF-16/FOXO pathways, similar to what has been found in mammals. Although APL-1 does not contain the Aβ sequence and *C. elegans* does not have β-secretase activity, transgenic lines that produce Aβ expression pan-neuronally or in muscle are being used to identify pathways that detoxify the Aβ aggregates, some of which also involve the insulin/DAF-16/FOXO pathways. Whether these models are relevant to human pathology or whether the pathways will be conserved in humans are unknown; however, they present alternative approaches to understanding neurodegenerative diseases for which there are currently few effective therapies. Human tau, as well as mutant tau isoforms, have also been expressed in the worm to recapitulate AD and FTD phenotypes. Recent findings have shown that PTL-1 regulates neuronal aging in the worm. These findings may be important to link aging and tau pathology in AD and FTD patients. Although *C. elegans* transgene models have many advantages, they also have several disadvantages. In *C. elegans*, transgenes are present as extrachromosomal arrays and are not integrated into the genome as they are in other systems; a few copies to several hundred copies of the transgene are present in the arrays, so the level of overexpression can be much higher than what is found *in vivo*. Fortunately, methods for single copy insertions have now been developed (Frøkjaer-Jensen et al., 2008).

AD is considered a multifactorial disease in which other risk factors, such as neuroinflammation, head trauma, and diabetes, may be important in the development of the disease. The *C. elegans* nervous system is simple compared to the human nervous system. This simplicity allows researchers to study neuronal function and neural circuits in a tractable system. However, the complex network of connections and cell interactions found in humans is not mimicked in *C. elegans* and this complexity may underlie some of the pathology of neurodegenerative diseases. Nevertheless, most of the pathways and signaling molecules in *C. elegans* are conserved between worms and mammals. The goal is to translate some of the *C. elegans* insights into understanding the pathology of AD and other neurodegenerative diseases and designing effective strategies to treat the diseases.

ACKNOWLEDGMENTS

We thank Collin Ewald for reviewing our manuscript. This work was supported by grants from the NIH and NSF.

REFERENCES

Adlard, P. A., Cherny, R. A., Finkelstein, D. I., Gautier, E., Robb, E., Cortes, M., et al. (2008). Rapid restoration of cognition in Alzheimer's transgenic mice with 8-hydroxy quinoline analogs is associated with decreased interstitial Abeta. *Neuron* 59, 43–55. doi: 10.1016/j.neuron.2008.06.018

Aizawa, H., Emori, Y., Murofushi, H., Kawasaki, H., Sakai, H., and Suzuki, K. (1990). Molecular cloning of a ubiquitously distributed microtubule-associated protein with Mr 190,000. *J. Biol. Chem.* 265, 13849–13855.

Alonso, A., Zaidi, T., Novak, M., Grundke-Iqbal, I., and Iqbal, K. (2001). Hyperphosphorylation induces self-assembly of tau into tangles of paired helical filaments/straight filaments. *Proc. Natl. Acad. Sci. U.S.A.* 98, 6923–6928. doi: 10.1073/pnas.121119298

Alonso, A. C., Grundke-Iqbal, I., and Iqbal, K. (1996). Alzheimer's disease hyperphosphorylated tau sequesters normal tau into tangles of filaments and disassembles microtubules. *Nat. Med.* 2, 783–787. doi: 10.1038/nm0796-783

Alonso, A. D., Grundke-Iqbal, I., Barra, H. S., and Iqbal, K. (1997). Abnormal phosphorylation of tau and the mechanism of Alzheimer neurofibrillary degeneration: sequestration of microtubule-associated proteins 1 and 2 and the disassembly of microtubules by the abnormal tau. *Proc. Natl. Acad. Sci. U.S.A.* 94, 298–303. doi: 10.1073/pnas.94.1.298

Alzheimer's Disease International. (2014). *World Alzheimer report 2013 [Online].* Available at: http://www.alz.co.uk/ (accessed March 05, 2014).

Ambros, V., and Horvitz, H. R. (1984). Heterochronic mutants of the nematode *Caenorhabditis elegans. Science* 226, 409–416. doi: 10.1126/science.6494891

Amos, L. A., and Schlieper, D. (2005). Microtubules and maps. *Adv. Protein Chem.* 71, 257–298. doi: 10.1016/S0065-3233(04)71007-4

Arduengo, P. M., Appleberry, O. K., Chuang, P., and L'hernault, S. W. (1998). The presenilin protein family member SPE-4 localizes to an ER/Golgi derived organelle and is required for proper cytoplasmic partitioning during *Caenorhabditis elegans* spermatogenesis. *J. Cell Sci.* 111, 3645–3654.

Arimoto, M., Koushika, S. P., Choudhary, B. C., Li, C., Matsumoto, K., and Hisamoto, N. (2011). The *Caenorhabditis elegans* JIP3 protein UNC-16 functions as an adaptor to link kinesin-1 with cytoplasmic dynein. *J. Neurosci.* 31, 2216–2224. doi: 10.1523/JNEUROSCI.2653-10.2011

Asahina, M., Ishihara, T., Jindra, M., Kohara, Y., Katsura, I., and Hirose, S. (2000). The conserved nuclear receptor Ftz-F1 is required for embryogenesis, moulting and reproduction in *Caenorhabditis elegans. Genes Cells* 5, 711–723. doi: 10.1046/j.1365-2443.2000.00361.x

Ash, P. E., Zhang, Y. J., Roberts, C. M., Saldi, T., Hutter, H., Buratti, E., et al. (2010). Neurotoxic effects of TDP-43 overexpression in *C. elegans. Hum. Mol. Genet.* 19, 3206–3218. doi: 10.1093/hmg/ddq230

Bargmann, C. I., Hartwieg, E., and Horvitz, H. R. (1993). Odorant-selective genes and neurons mediate olfaction in *C. elegans. Cell* 74, 515–527. doi: 10.1016/0092-8674(93)80053-H

Bargmann, C. I., and Horvitz, H. R. (1991). Chemosensory neurons with overlapping functions direct chemotaxis to multiple chemicals in *C. elegans. Neuron* 7, 729–742. doi: 10.1016/0896-6273(91)90276-6

Bates, E. A., Victor, M., Jones, A. K., Shi, Y., and Hart, A. C. (2006). Differential contributions of *Caenorhabditis elegans* histone deacetylases to huntingtin polyglutamine toxicity. *J. Neurosci.* 26, 2830–2838. doi: 10.1523/JNEUROSCI.3344-05.2006

Biernat, J., Gustke, N., Drewes, G., Mandelkow, E. M., and Mandelkow, E. (1993). Phosphorylation of Ser262 strongly reduces binding of tau to microtubules: distinction between PHF-like immunoreactivity and microtubule binding. *Neuron* 11, 153–163. doi: 10.1016/0896-6273(93)90279-Z

Bieschke, J., Cohen, E., Murray, A., Dillin, A., and Kelly, J. W. (2009). A kinetic assessment of the *C. elegans* amyloid disaggregation activity enables uncoupling of disassembly and proteolysis. *Protein Sci.* 18, 2231–2241. doi: 10.1002/pro.234

Billingsley, M. L., and Kincaid, R. L. (1997). Regulated phosphorylation and dephosphorylation of tau protein: effects on microtubule interaction, intracellular trafficking and neurodegeneration. *Biochem. J.* 323, 577–591.

Binder, L. I., Frankfurter, A., and Rebhun, L. I. (1985). The distribution of tau in the mammalian central nervous system. *J. Cell Biol.* 101, 1371–1378. doi: 10.1083/jcb.101.4.1371

Boccitto, M., Lamitina, T., and Kalb, R. G. (2012). Daf-2 signaling modifies mutant SOD1 toxicity in *C. elegans. PLoS ONE* 7:e33494. doi: 10.1371/journal.pone.0033494

Borgonovo, B., Ouwendijk, J., and Solimena, M. (2006). Biogenesis of secretory granules. *Curr. Opin. Cell Biol.* 18, 365–370. doi: 10.1016/j.ceb.2006.06.010

Borroni, B., Bonvicini, C., Alberici, A., Buratti, E., Agosti, C., Archetti, S., et al. (2009). Mutation within TARDBP leads to frontotemporal dementia without motor neuron disease. *Hum. Mutat.* 30, E974–E983. doi: 10.1002/humu.21100

Bramblett, G. T., Goedert, M., Jakes, R., Merrick, S. E., Trojanowski, J. Q., and Lee, V. M. (1993). Abnormal tau phosphorylation at Ser396 in Alzheimer's disease recapitulates development and contributes to reduced microtubule binding. *Neuron* 10, 1089–1099. doi: 10.1016/0896-6273(93)90057-X

Brandt, R., Gergou, A., Wacker, I., Fath, T., and Hutter, H. (2009). A *Caenorhabditis elegans* model of tau hyperphosphorylation: induction of developmental defects by transgenic overexpression of Alzheimer's disease-like modified tau. *Neurobiol. Aging* 30, 22–33. doi: 10.1016/j.neurobiolaging.2007.05.011

Brenner, S. (1974). The genetics of *Caenorhabditis elegans. Genetics* 77, 71–94.

Brignull, H. R., Moore, F. E., Tang, S. J., and Morimoto, R. I. (2006). Polyglutamine proteins at the pathogenic threshold display neuron-specific aggregation in a pan-neuronal *Caenorhabditis elegans* model. *J. Neurosci.* 26, 7597–7606. doi: 10.1523/JNEUROSCI.0990-06.2006

Brown, M. S., and Goldstein, J. L. (1986). A receptor-mediated pathway for cholesterol homeostasis. *Science* 232, 34–47. doi: 10.1126/science.3513311

Bulinski, J. C., and Borisy, G. G. (1980). Microtubule-associated proteins from cultured HeLa cells. Analysis of molecular properties and effects on microtubule polymerization. *J. Biol. Chem.* 255, 11570–11576.

Büttner, S., Habernig, L., Broeskamp, F., Ruli, D., Vögtle, F. N., Vlachos, M., et al. (2013). Endonuclease G mediates α-synuclein cytotoxicity during Parkinson's disease. *EMBO J.* 32, 3041–3054. doi: 10.1038/emboj.2013.228

C. elegans Sequencing Consortium. (1998). Genome sequence of the nematode *C. elegans*: a platform for investigating biology. *Science* 282, 2012–2018.

Cam, J. A., and Bu, G. (2006). Modulation of beta-amyloid precursor protein trafficking and processing by the low density lipoprotein receptor family. *Mol. Neurodegener.* 1:8. doi: 10.1186/1750-1326-1-8

Cao, P., Yuan, Y., Pehek, E. A., Moise, A. R., Huang, Y., Palczewski, K., et al. (2010). Alpha-synuclein disrupted dopamine homeostasis leads to dopaminergic neuron degeneration in *Caenorhabditis elegans. PLoS ONE* 5:e9312. doi: 10.1371/journal.pone.0009312

Carro, E., Spuch, C., Trejo, J. L., Antequera, D., and Torres-Aleman, I. (2005). Choroid plexus megalin is involved in neuroprotection by serum insulin-like growth factor I. *J. Neurosci.* 25, 10884–10893. doi: 10.1523/JNEUROSCI.2909-05.2005

Chalfie, M., Horvitz, H. R., and Sulston, J. E. (1981). Mutations that lead to reiterations in the cell lineages of *C. elegans. Cell* 24, 59–69. doi: 10.1016/0092-8674(81)90501-8

Chalfie, M., and Sulston, J. (1981). Developmental genetics of the mechanosensory neurons of *Caenorhabditis elegans. Dev. Biol.* 82, 358–370. doi: 10.1016/0012-1606(81)90459-0

Chalfie, M., Sulston, J. E., White, J. G., Southgate, E., Thomson, J. N., and Brenner, S. (1985). The neural circuit for touch sensitivity in *Caenorhabditis elegans. J. Neurosci.* 5, 956–964.

Chapin, S. J., and Bulinski, J. C. (1991). Non-neuronal 210 × 10^3 Mr microtubule-associated protein (MAP4) contains a domain homologous to the microtubule-binding domains of neuronal MAP2 and tau. *J. Cell Sci.* 98, 27–36.

Chartier-Harlin, M. C., Crawford, F., Houlden, H., Warren, A., Hughes, D., Fidani, L., et al. (1991). Early-onset Alzheimer's disease caused by mutations at codon 717 of the beta-amyloid precursor protein gene. *Nature* 353, 844–846. doi: 10.1038/353844a0

Chen, J., Kanai, Y., Cowan, N. J., and Hirokawa, N. (1992). Projection domains of MAP2 and tau determine spacings between microtubules in dendrites and axons. *Nature* 360, 674–677. doi: 10.1038/360674a0

Chew, Y. L., Fan, X., Götz, J., and Nicholas, H. R. (2013). PTL-1 regulates neuronal integrity and lifespan in *C. elegans. J. Cell Sci.* 126, 2079–2091. doi: 10.1242/jcs.jcs124404

Cohen, E., Bieschke, J., Perciavalle, R. M., Kelly, J. W., and Dillin, A. (2006). Opposing activities protect against age-onset proteotoxicity. *Science* 313, 1604–1610. doi: 10.1126/science.1124646

Colbert, H. A., and Bargmann, C. I. (1995). Odorant-specific adaptation pathways generate olfactory plasticity in *C. elegans. Neuron* 14, 803–812. doi: 10.1016/0896-6273(95)90224-4

Conway, K. A., Harper, J. D., and Lansbury, P. T. (2000a). Fibrils formed *in vitro* from alpha-synuclein and two mutant forms linked to Parkinson's disease are typical amyloid. *Biochemistry* 39, 2552–2563. doi: 10.1021/bi991447r

Conway, K. A., Lee, S. J., Rochet, J. C., Ding, T. T., Harper, J. D., Williamson, R. E., et al. (2000b). Accelerated oligomerization by Parkinson's disease linked alpha-synuclein mutants. *Ann. N. Y. Acad. Sci.* 920, 42–45. doi: 10.1111/j.1749-6632.2000.tb06903.x

Conway, K. A., Lee, S. J., Rochet, J. C., Ding, T. T., Williamson, R. E., and Lansbury, P. T. (2000c). Acceleration of oligomerization, not fibrillization, is a shared property of both alpha-synuclein mutations linked to early-onset Parkinson's disease: implications for pathogenesis and therapy. *Proc. Natl. Acad. Sci. U.S.A.* 97, 571–576. doi: 10.1073/pnas.97.2.571

Cruts, M., Theuns, J., and Van Broeckhoven, C. (2012). Locus-specific mutation databases for neurodegenerative brain diseases. *Hum. Mutat.* 33, 1340–1344. doi: 10.1002/humu.22117

Cui, S., Verroust, P. J., Moestrup, S. K., and Christensen, E. I. (1996). Megalin/gp330 mediates uptake of albumin in renal proximal tubule. *Am. J. Physiol.* 271, F900–F907.

Daigle, I., and Li, C. (1993). apl-1, a *Caenorhabditis elegans* gene encoding a protein related to the human beta-amyloid protein precursor. *Proc. Natl. Acad. Sci. U.S.A.* 90, 12045–12049. doi: 10.1073/pnas.90.24.12045

Deane, R., Wu, Z., Sagare, A., Davis, J., Du Yan, S., Hamm, K., et al. (2004). LRP/amyloid beta-peptide interaction mediates differential brain efflux of Abeta isoforms. *Neuron* 43, 333–344. doi: 10.1016/j.neuron.2004.07.017

DeJesus-Hernandez, M., Mackenzie, I. R., Boeve, B. F., Boxer, A. L., Baker, M., Rutherford, N. J., et al. (2011). Expanded GGGGCC hexanucleotide repeat in noncoding region of C9ORF72 causes chromosome 9p-linked FTD and ALS. *Neuron* 72, 245–256. doi: 10.1016/j.neuron.2011.09.011

Dragunow, M., Faull, R. L., Lawlor, P., Beilharz, E. J., Singleton, K., Walker, E. B., et al. (1995). In situ evidence for DNA fragmentation in Huntington's disease striatum and Alzheimer's disease temporal lobes. *Neuroreport* 6, 1053–1057. doi: 10.1097/00001756-199505090-00026

Duarte, A., Hirashima, M., Benedito, R., Trindade, A., Diniz, P., Bekman, E., et al. (2004). Dosage-sensitive requirement for mouse Dll4 in artery development. *Genes Dev.* 18, 2474–2478. doi: 10.1101/gad.1239004

Duilio, A., Faraonio, R., Minopoli, G., Zambrano, N., and Russo, T. (1998). Fe65L2: a new member of the Fe65 protein family interacting with the intracellular domain of the Alzheimer's beta-amyloid precursor protein. *Biochem. J.* 330, 513–519.

Dumas, K. J., Guo, C., Wang, X., Burkhart, K. B., Adams, E. J., Alam, H., et al. (2010). Functional divergence of dafachronic acid pathways in the control of C. elegans development and lifespan. *Dev. Biol.* 340, 605–612. doi: 10.1016/j.ydbio.2010.02.022

Edwards, S. L., Charlie, N. K., Richmond, J. E., Hegermann, J., Eimer, S., and Miller, K. G. (2009). Impaired dense core vesicle maturation in *Caenorhabditis elegans* mutants lacking Rab2. *J. Cell Biol.* 186, 881–895. doi: 10.1083/jcb.200902095

Estevez, A. O., Morgan, K. L., Szewczyk, N. J., Gems, D., and Estevez, M. (2014). The neurodegenerative effects of selenium are inhibited by FOXO and PINK1/PTEN regulation of insulin/insulin-like growth factor signaling in *Caenorhabditis elegans. Neurotoxicology* 41C, 28–43. doi: 10.1016/j.neuro.2013.12.012

Estevez, A. O., Mueller, C. L., Morgan, K. L., Szewczyk, N. J., Teece, L., Miranda-Vizuete, A., et al. (2012). Selenium induces cholinergic motor neuron degeneration in *Caenorhabditis elegans. Neurotoxicology* 33, 1021–1032. doi: 10.1016/j.neuro.2012.04.019

Ewald, C. Y., Cheng, R., Tolen, L., Shah, V., Gillani, A., Nasrin, A., et al. (2012a). Pan-neuronal expression of APL-1, an APP-related protein, disrupts olfactory, gustatory, and touch plasticity in *Caenorhabditis elegans. J. Neurosci.* 32, 10156–10169. doi: 10.1523/JNEUROSCI.0495-12.2012

Ewald, C. Y., Raps, D. A., and Li, C. (2012b). APL-1, the Alzheimer's Amyloid precursor protein in *Caenorhabditis elegans*, modulates multiple metabolic pathways throughout development. *Genetics* 191, 493–507. doi: 10.1534/genetics.112.138768

Faber, P. W., Alter, J. R., Macdonald, M. E., and Hart, A. C. (1999). Polyglutamine-mediated dysfunction and apoptotic death of a *Caenorhabditis elegans* sensory neuron. *Proc. Natl. Acad. Sci. U.S.A.* 96, 179–184. doi: 10.1073/pnas.96.1.179

Faber, P. W., Voisine, C., King, D. C., Bates, E. A., and Hart, A. C. (2002). Glutamine/proline-rich PQE-1 proteins protect *Caenorhabditis elegans* neurons from huntingtin polyglutamine neurotoxicity. *Proc. Natl. Acad. Sci. U.S.A.* 99, 17131–17136. doi: 10.1073/pnas.262544899

Fahn, S., and Sulzer, D. (2004). Neurodegeneration and neuroprotection in Parkinson disease. *NeuroRx* 1, 139–154. doi: 10.1602/neurorx.1.1.139

Farg, M. A., Sundaramoorthy, V., Sultana, J. M., Yang, S., Atkinson, R. A., Levina, V., et al. (2014). C9ORF72, implicated in amytrophic lateral sclerosis and frontotemporal dementia, regulates endosomal trafficking. *Hum. Mol. Genet.* 23, 3579–3595. doi: 10.1093/hmg/ddu068

Farrer, L. A., and Conneally, P. M. (1985). A genetic model for age at onset in Huntington disease. *Am. J. Hum. Genet.* 37, 350–357.

Fatouros, C., Pir, G. J., Biernat, J., Koushika, S. P., Mandelkow, E., Mandelkow, E. M., et al. (2012). Inhibition of tau aggregation in a novel *Caenorhabditis elegans* model of tauopathy mitigates proteotoxicity. *Hum. Mol. Genet.* 21, 3587–3603. doi: 10.1093/hmg/dds190

Feijoo, C., Campbell, D. G., Jakes, R., Goedert, M., and Cuenda, A. (2005). Evidence that phosphorylation of the microtubule-associated protein Tau by SAPK4/p38delta at Thr50 promotes microtubule assembly. *J. Cell Sci.* 118, 397–408. doi: 10.1242/jcs.01655

Fonte, V., Kapulkin, W. J., Kapulkin, V., Taft, A., Fluet, A., Friedman, D., et al. (2002). Interaction of intracellular beta amyloid peptide with chaperone proteins. *Proc. Natl. Acad. Sci. U.S.A.* 99, 9439–9444. doi: 10.1073/pnas.152313999

Fonte, V., Kipp, D. R., Yerg, J., Merin, D., Forrestal, M., Wagner, E., et al. (2008). Suppression of *in vivo* beta-amyloid peptide toxicity by overexpression of the HSP-16.2 small chaperone protein. *J. Biol. Chem.* 283, 784–791. doi: 10.1074/jbc.M703339200

Francis, R., Mcgrath, G., Zhang, J., Ruddy, D. A., Sym, M., Apfeld, J., et al. (2002). aph-1 and pen-2 are required for Notch pathway signaling, gamma-secretase cleavage of betaAPP, and presenilin protein accumulation. *Dev. Cell* 3, 85–97. doi: 10.1016/S1534-5807(02)00189-2

Frøkjaer-Jensen, C., Davis, M. W., Hopkins, C. E., Newman, B. J., Thummel, J. M., Olesen, S. P., et al. (2008). Single-copy insertion of transgenes in *Caenorhabditis elegans. Nat. Genet.* 40, 1375–1383. doi: 10.1038/ng.248

Gale, N. W., Dominguez, M. G., Noguera, I., Pan, L., Hughes, V., Valenzuela, D. M., et al. (2004). Haploinsufficiency of delta-like 4 ligand results in embryonic lethality due to major defects in arterial and vascular development. *Proc. Natl. Acad. Sci. U.S.A.* 101, 15949–15954. doi: 10.1073/pnas.0407290101

Gasparini, L., Gouras, G. K., Wang, R., Gross, R. S., Beal, M. F., Greengard, P., et al. (2001). Stimulation of beta-amyloid precursor protein trafficking by insulin reduces intraneuronal beta-amyloid and requires mitogen-activated protein kinase signaling. *J. Neurosci.* 21, 2561–2570.

Gems, D., Sutton, A. J., Sundermeyer, M. L., Albert, P. S., King, K. V., Edgley, M. L., et al. (1998). Two pleiotropic classes of daf-2 mutation affect larval arrest, adult behavior, reproduction and longevity in *Caenorhabditis elegans. Genetics* 150, 129–155.

Gerisch, B., Weitzel, C., Kober-Eisermann, C., Rottiers, V., and Antebi, A. (2001). A hormonal signaling pathway influencing *C. elegans* metabolism, reproductive development, and life span. *Dev. Cell* 1, 841–851. doi: 10.1016/S1534-5807(01)00085-5

Gidalevitz, T., Krupinski, T., Garcia, S., and Morimoto, R. I. (2009). Destabilizing protein polymorphisms in the genetic background direct phenotypic expression of mutant SOD1 toxicity. *PLoS Genet.* 5:e1000399. doi: 10.1371/journal.pgen.1000399

Gissendanner, C. R., and Sluder, A. E. (2000). nhr-25, the *Caenorhabditis elegans* ortholog of ftz-f1, is required for epidermal and somatic gonad development. *Dev. Biol.* 221, 259–272. doi: 10.1006/dbio.2000.9679

Gitcho, M. A., Baloh, R. H., Chakraverty, S., Mayo, K., Norton, J. B., Levitch, D., et al. (2008). TDP-43 A315T mutation in familial motor neuron disease. *Ann. Neurol.* 63, 535–538. doi: 10.1002/ana.21344

Glenner, G. G., and Wong, C. W. (1984). Alzheimer's disease and Down's syndrome: sharing of a unique cerebrovascular amyloid fibril protein. *Biochem. Biophys. Res. Commun.* 122, 1131–1135. doi: 10.1016/0006-291X(84)91209-9

Goate, A., Chartier-Harlin, M. C., Mullan, M., Brown, J., Crawford, F., Fidani, L., et al. (1991). Segregation of a missense mutation in the amyloid precursor protein gene with familial Alzheimer's disease. *Nature* 349, 704–706. doi: 10.1038/349704a0

Goedert, M., Baur, C. P., Ahringer, J., Jakes, R., Hasegawa, M., Spillantini, M. G., et al. (1996). PTL-1, a microtubule-associated protein with tau-like repeats from the nematode *Caenorhabditis elegans. J. Cell Sci.* 109, 2661–2672.

Goedert, M., Cohen, E. S., Jakes, R., and Cohen, P. (1992a). p42 MAP kinase phosphorylation sites in microtubule-associated protein tau are dephosphorylated by protein phosphatase 2A1. Implications for Alzheimer's disease [corrected]. *FEBS Lett.* 312, 95–99. doi: 10.1016/0014-5793(92)81418-L

Goedert, M., Spillantini, M. G., Cairns, N. J., and Crowther, R. A. (1992b). Tau proteins of Alzheimer paired helical filaments: abnormal phosphorylation of all six brain isoforms. *Neuron* 8, 159–168. doi: 10.1016/0896-6273(92)90117-V

Goedert, M., Spillantini, M. G., Jakes, R., Rutherford, D., and Crowther, R. A. (1989a). Multiple isoforms of human microtubule-associated protein tau:

sequences and localization in neurofibrillary tangles of Alzheimer's disease. *Neuron* 3, 519–526. doi: 10.1016/0896-6273(89)90210-9

Goedert, M., Spillantini, M. G., Potier, M. C., Ulrich, J., and Crowther, R. A. (1989b). Cloning and sequencing of the cDNA encoding an isoform of microtubule-associated protein tau containing four tandem repeats: differential expression of tau protein mRNAs in human brain. *EMBO J.* 8, 393–399.

Goedert, M., Wischik, C. M., Crowther, R. A., Walker, J. E., and Klug, A. (1988). Cloning and sequencing of the cDNA encoding a core protein of the paired helical filament of Alzheimer disease: identification as the microtubule-associated protein tau. *Proc. Natl. Acad. Sci. U.S.A.* 85, 4051–4055. doi: 10.1073/pnas.85.11.4051

Goldberg, Y. P., Kalchman, M. A., Metzler, M., Nasir, J., Zeisler, J., Graham, R., et al. (1996). Absence of disease phenotype and intergenerational stability of the CAG repeat in transgenic mice expressing the human Huntington disease transcript. *Hum. Mol. Genet.* 5, 177–185. doi: 10.1093/hmg/5.2.177

Gordon, P., Hingula, L., Krasny, M. L., Swienckowski, J. L., Pokrywka, N. J., and Raley-Susman, K. M. (2008). The invertebrate microtubule-associated protein PTL-1 functions in mechanosensation and development in *Caenorhabditis elegans*. *Dev. Genes Evol.* 218, 541–551. doi: 10.1007/s00427-008-0250-z

Gorevic, P. D., Goñi, F., Pons-Estel, B., Alvarez, F., Peress, N. S., and Frangione, B. (1986). Isolation and partial characterization of neurofibrillary tangles and amyloid plaque core in Alzheimer's disease: immunohistological studies. *J. Neuropathol. Exp. Neurol.* 45, 647–664. doi: 10.1097/00005072-198611000-00004

Goutte, C., Hepler, W., Mickey, K. M., and Priess, J. R. (2000). aph-2 encodes a novel extracellular protein required for GLP-1-mediated signaling. *Development* 127, 2481–2492.

Goutte, C., Tsunozaki, M., Hale, V. A., and Priess, J. R. (2002). APH-1 is a multipass membrane protein essential for the Notch signaling pathway in *Caenorhabditis elegans* embryos. *Proc. Natl. Acad. Sci. U.S.A.* 99, 775–779. doi: 10.1073/pnas.022523499

Greenwald, I. S., Sternberg, P. W., and Horvitz, H. R. (1983). The lin-12 locus specifies cell fates in *Caenorhabditis elegans*. *Cell* 34, 435–444. doi: 10.1016/0092-8674(83)90377-X

Gu, Y., Misonou, H., Sato, T., Dohmae, N., Takio, K., and Ihara, Y. (2001). Distinct intramembrane cleavage of the beta-amyloid precursor protein family resembling gamma-secretase-like cleavage of Notch. *J. Biol. Chem.* 276, 35235–35238. doi: 10.1074/jbc.C100357200

Gusella, J. F., and MacDonald, M. E. (1995). Huntington's disease: CAG genetics expands neurobiology. *Curr. Opin. Neurobiol.* 5, 656–662. doi: 10.1016/0959-4388(95)80072-7

Guthrie, C. R., Greenup, L., Leverenz, J. B., and Kraemer, B. C. (2011). MSUT2 is a determinant of susceptibility to tau neurotoxicity. *Hum. Mol. Genet.* 20, 1989–1999. doi: 10.1093/hmg/ddr079

Guthrie, C. R., Schellenberg, G. D., and Kraemer, B. C. (2009). SUT-2 potentiates tau-induced neurotoxicity in *Caenorhabditis elegans*. *Hum. Mol. Genet.* 18, 1825–1838. doi: 10.1093/hmg/ddp099

Guénette, S. Y., Chen, J., Jondro, P. D., and Tanzi, R. E. (1996). Association of a novel human FE65-like protein with the cytoplasmic domain of the beta-amyloid precursor protein. *Proc. Natl. Acad. Sci. U.S.A.* 93, 10832–10837. doi: 10.1073/pnas.93.20.10832

Haass, C., Hung, A. Y., Selkoe, D. J., and Teplow, D. B. (1994a). Mutations associated with a locus for familial Alzheimer's disease result in alternative processing of amyloid beta-protein precursor. *J. Biol. Chem.* 269, 17741–17748.

Haass, C., Koo, E. H., Teplow, D. B., and Selkoe, D. J. (1994b). Polarized secretion of beta-amyloid precursor protein and amyloid beta-peptide in MDCK cells. *Proc. Natl. Acad. Sci. U.S.A.* 91, 1564–1568. doi: 10.1073/pnas.91.4.1564

Haass, C., Koo, E. H., Mellon, A., Hung, A. Y., and Selkoe, D. J. (1992). Targeting of cell-surface beta-amyloid precursor protein to lysosomes: alternative processing into amyloid-bearing fragments. *Nature* 357, 500–503. doi: 10.1038/357500a0

Hamamichi, S., Rivas, R. N., Knight, A. L., Cao, S., Caldwell, K. A., and Caldwell, G. A. (2008). Hypothesis-based RNAi screening identifies neuroprotective genes in a Parkinson's disease model. *Proc. Natl. Acad. Sci. U.S.A.* 105, 728–733. doi: 10.1073/pnas.0711018105

Hamos, J. E., Oblas, B., Pulaski-Salo, D., Welch, W. J., Bole, D. G., and Drachman, D. A. (1991). Expression of heat shock proteins in Alzheimer's disease. *Neurology* 41, 345–350. doi: 10.1212/WNL.41.3.345

Han, S. M., El Oussini, H., Scekic-Zahirovic, J., Vibbert, J., Cottee, P., Prasain, J. K., et al. (2013). VAPB/ALS8 MSP ligands regulate striated muscle energy metabolism critical for adult survival in *Caenorhabditis elegans*. *PLoS Genet.* 9:e1003738. doi: 10.1371/journal.pgen.1003738

Harada, A., Oguchi, K., Okabe, S., Kuno, J., Terada, S., Ohshima, T., et al. (1994). Altered microtubule organization in small-calibre axons of mice lacking tau protein. *Nature* 369, 488–491. doi: 10.1038/369488a0

Hardiman, O., Van Den Berg, L. H., and Kiernan, M. C. (2011). Clinical diagnosis and management of amyotrophic lateral sclerosis. *Nat. Rev. Neurol.* 7, 639–649. doi: 10.1038/nrneurol.2011.153

Hardy, J. (2010). Genetic analysis of pathways to Parkinson disease. *Neuron* 68, 201–206. doi: 10.1016/j.neuron.2010.10.014

Hayes, G. D., Frand, A. R., and Ruvkun, G. (2006). The mir-84 and let-7 paralogous microRNA genes of *Caenorhabditis elegans* direct the cessation of molting via the conserved nuclear hormone receptors NHR-23 and NHR-25. *Development* 133, 4631–4641. doi: 10.1242/dev.02655

Heber, S., Herms, J., Gajic, V., Hainfellner, J., Aguzzi, A., Rülicke, T., et al. (2000). Mice with combined gene knock-outs reveal essential and partially redundant functions of amyloid precursor protein family members. *J. Neurosci.* 20, 7951–7963.

Henderson, S. T., and Johnson, T. E. (2001). daf-16 integrates developmental and environmental inputs to mediate aging in the nematode *Caenorhabditis elegans*. *Curr. Biol.* 11, 1975–1980. doi: 10.1016/S0960-9822(01)00594-2

Hermo, L., Lustig, M., Lefrancois, S., Argraves, W. S., and Morales, C. R. (1999). Expression and regulation of LRP-2/megalin in epithelial cells lining the efferent ducts and epididymis during postnatal development. *Mol. Reprod. Dev.* 53, 282–293. doi: 10.1002/(SICI)1098-2795(199907)53:3<282::AID-MRD4>3.0.CO;2-A

Herms, J., Anliker, B., Heber, S., Ring, S., Fuhrmann, M., Kretzschmar, H., et al. (2004). Cortical dysplasia resembling human type 2 lissencephaly in mice lacking all three APP family members. *EMBO J.* 23, 4106–4115. doi: 10.1038/sj.emboj.7600390

Herz, J., Clouthier, D. E., and Hammer, R. E. (1992). LDL receptor-related protein internalizes and degrades uPA-PAI-1 complexes and is essential for embryo implantation. *Cell* 71, 411–421. doi: 10.1016/0092-8674(92)90511-A

Hieb, W. F., and Rothstein, M. (1968). Sterol requirement for reproduction of a free-living nematode. *Science* 160, 778–780. doi: 10.1126/science.160.3829.778

Holcomb, L. A., Gordon, M. N., Jantzen, P., Hsiao, K., Duff, K., and Morgan, D. (1999). Behavioral changes in transgenic mice expressing both amyloid precursor protein and presenilin-1 mutations: lack of association with amyloid deposits. *Behav. Genet.* 29, 177–185. doi: 10.1023/A:1021691918517

Hornsten, A., Lieberthal, J., Fadia, S., Malins, R., Ha, L., Xu, X., et al. (2007). APL-1, a *Caenorhabditis elegans* protein related to the human beta-amyloid precursor protein, is essential for viability. *Proc. Natl. Acad. Sci. U.S.A.* 104, 1971–1976. doi: 10.1073/pnas.0603997104

Hsiao, K. K., Borchelt, D. R., Olson, K., Johannsdottir, R., Kitt, C., Yunis, W., et al. (1995). Age-related CNS disorder and early death in transgenic FVB/N mice overexpressing Alzheimer amyloid precursor proteins. *Neuron* 15, 1203–1218. doi: 10.1016/0896-6273(95)90107-8

Hsu, A. L., Murphy, C. T., and Kenyon, C. (2003). Regulation of aging and age-related disease by DAF-16 and heat-shock factor. *Science* 300, 1142–1145. doi: 10.1126/science.1083701

Hughes, A. J., Ben-Shlomo, Y., Daniel, S. E., and Lees, A. J. (1992). What features improve the accuracy of clinical diagnosis in Parkinson's disease: a clinicopathologic study. *Neurology* 42, 1142–1146. doi: 10.1212/WNL.42.6.1142

Hutton, M., Lendon, C. L., Rizzu, P., Baker, M., Froelich, S., Houlden, H., et al. (1998). Association of missense and 5′-splice-site mutations in tau with the inherited dementia FTDP-17. *Nature* 393, 702–705. doi: 10.1038/31508

Jadiya, P., Khan, A., Sammi, S. R., Kaur, S., Mir, S. S., and Nazir, A. (2011). Anti-Parkinsonian effects of *Bacopa monnieri*: insights from transgenic and pharmacological *Caenorhabditis elegans* models of Parkinson's disease. *Biochem. Biophys. Res. Commun.* 413, 605–610. doi: 10.1016/j.bbrc.2011.09.010

Jarriault, S., and Greenwald, I. (2005). Evidence for functional redundancy between *C. elegans* ADAM proteins SUP-17/Kuzbanian and ADM-4/TACE. *Dev. Biol.* 287, 1–10. doi: 10.1016/j.ydbio.2005.08.014

Jia, K., Hart, A. C., and Levine, B. (2007). Autophagy genes protect against disease caused by polyglutamine expansion proteins in *Caenorhabditis elegans*. *Autophagy* 3, 21–25. doi: 10.4161/auto.3528

Jonsson, T., Atwal, J. K., Steinberg, S., Snaedal, J., Jonsson, P. V., Bjornsson, S., et al. (2012). A mutation in APP protects against Alzheimer's disease and age-related cognitive decline. *Nature* 488, 96–99. doi: 10.1038/nature11283

Kabashi, E., Valdmanis, P. N., Dion, P., Spiegelman, D., Mcconkey, B. J., Vande Velde, C., et al. (2008). TARDBP mutations in individuals with sporadic and familial amyotrophic lateral sclerosis. *Nat. Genet.* 40, 572–574. doi: 10.1038/ng.132

Kamel, F., Umbach, D. M., Bedlack, R. S., Richards, M., Watson, M., Alavanja, M. C., et al. (2012). Pesticide exposure and amyotrophic lateral sclerosis. *Neurotoxicology* 33, 457–462. doi: 10.1016/j.neuro.2012.04.001

Kang, J., Lemaire, H. G., Unterbeck, A., Salbaum, J. M., Masters, C. L., Grzeschik, K. H., et al. (1987). The precursor of Alzheimer's disease amyloid A4 protein resembles a cell-surface receptor. *Nature* 325, 733–736. doi: 10.1038/325733a0

Kidd, M. (1964). Alzheimer's disease–An electron microscopical study. *Brain* 87, 307–320. doi: 10.1093/brain/87.2.307

Kimberly, W. T., Lavoie, M. J., Ostaszewski, B. L., Ye, W., Wolfe, M. S., and Selkoe, D. J. (2003). Gamma-secretase is a membrane protein complex comprised of presenilin, nicastrin, Aph-1, and Pen-2. *Proc. Natl. Acad. Sci. U.S.A.* 100, 6382–6387. doi: 10.1073/pnas.1037392100

Kimura, K. D., Tissenbaum, H. A., Liu, Y., and Ruvkun, G. (1997). daf-2, an insulin receptor-like gene that regulates longevity and diapause in *Caenorhabditis elegans*. *Science* 277, 942–946. doi: 10.1126/science.277.5328.942

Kitada, T., Asakawa, S., Hattori, N., Matsumine, H., Yamamura, Y., Minoshima, S., et al. (1998). Mutations in the parkin gene cause autosomal recessive juvenile parkinsonism. *Nature* 392, 605–608. doi: 10.1038/33416

Knauer, M. F., Orlando, R. A., and Glabe, C. G. (1996). Cell surface APP751 forms complexes with protease nexin 2 ligands and is internalized via the low density lipoprotein receptor-related protein (LRP). *Brain Res.* 740, 6–14. doi: 10.1016/S0006-8993(96)00711-1

Knops, J., Kosik, K. S., Lee, G., Pardee, J. D., Cohen-Gould, L., and Mcconlogue, L. (1991). Overexpression of tau in a nonneuronal cell induces long cellular processes. *J. Cell Biol.* 114, 725–733. doi: 10.1083/jcb.114.4.725

Koo, E. H., Sisodia, S. S., Archer, D. R., Martin, L. J., Weidemann, A., Beyreuther, K., et al. (1990). Precursor of amyloid protein in Alzheimer disease undergoes fast anterograde axonal transport. *Proc. Natl. Acad. Sci. U.S.A.* 87, 1561–1565. doi: 10.1073/pnas.87.4.1561

Kounnas, M. Z., Moir, R. D., Rebeck, G. W., Bush, A. I., Argraves, W. S., Tanzi, R. E., et al. (1995). LDL receptor-related protein, a multifunctional ApoE receptor, binds secreted beta-amyloid precursor protein and mediates its degradation. *Cell* 82, 331–340. doi: 10.1016/0092-8674(95)90320-8

Kraemer, B. C., and Schellenberg, G. D. (2007). SUT-1 enables tau-induced neurotoxicity in *C. elegans*. *Hum. Mol. Genet.* 16, 1959–1971. doi: 10.1093/hmg/ddm143

Kraemer, B. C., Zhang, B., Leverenz, J. B., Thomas, J. H., Trojanowski, J. Q., and Schellenberg, G. D. (2003). Neurodegeneration and defective neurotransmission in a *Caenorhabditis elegans* model of tauopathy. *Proc. Natl. Acad. Sci. U.S.A.* 100, 9980–9985. doi: 10.1073/pnas.1533448100

Krebs, L. T., Shutter, J. R., Tanigaki, K., Honjo, T., Stark, K. L., and Gridley, T. (2004). Haploinsufficient lethality and formation of arteriovenous malformations in Notch pathway mutants. *Genes Dev.* 18, 2469–2473. doi: 10.1101/gad.1239204

Krebs, L. T., Xue, Y., Norton, C. R., Shutter, J. R., Maguire, M., Sundberg, J. P., et al. (2000). Notch signaling is essential for vascular morphogenesis in mice. *Genes Dev.* 14, 1343–1352.

Krebs, L. T., Xue, Y., Norton, C. R., Sundberg, J. P., Beatus, P., Lendahl, U., et al. (2003). Characterization of Notch3-deficient mice: normal embryonic development and absence of genetic interactions with a Notch1 mutation. *Genesis* 37, 139–143. doi: 10.1002/gene.10241

Krigman, M. R., Feldman, R. G., and Bensch, K. (1965). Alzheimer's presenile dementia. A histochemical and electron microscopic study. *Lab. Invest.* 14, 381–396.

Krüger, R., Kuhn, W., Müller, T., Woitalla, D., Graeber, M., Kösel, S., et al. (1998). Ala30Pro mutation in the gene encoding alpha-synuclein in Parkinson's disease. *Nat. Genet.* 18, 106–108. doi: 10.1038/ng0298-106

Kuwahara, T., Koyama, A., Gengyo-Ando, K., Masuda, M., Kowa, H., Tsunoda, M., et al. (2006). Familial Parkinson mutant alpha-synuclein causes dopamine neuron dysfunction in transgenic *Caenorhabditis elegans*. *J. Biol. Chem.* 281, 334–340. doi: 10.1074/jbc.M504860200

Kuwahara, T., Koyama, A., Koyama, S., Yoshina, S., Ren, C. H., Kato, T., et al. (2008). A systematic RNAi screen reveals involvement of endocytic pathway in neuronal dysfunction in alpha-synuclein transgenic *C. elegans*. *Hum. Mol. Genet.* 17, 2997–3009. doi: 10.1093/hmg/ddn198

L'Hernault, S. W., and Arduengo, P. M. (1992). Mutation of a putative sperm membrane protein in *Caenorhabditis elegans* prevents sperm differentiation but not its associated meiotic divisions. *J. Cell Biol.* 119, 55–68. doi: 10.1083/jcb.119.1.55

Lakowski, B., Eimer, S., Göbel, C., Böttcher, A., Wagler, B., and Baumeister, R. (2003). Two suppressors of sel-12 encode C2H2 zinc-finger proteins that regulate presenilin transcription in *Caenorhabditis elegans*. *Development* 130, 2117–2128. doi: 10.1242/dev.00429

Lakso, M., Vartiainen, S., Moilanen, A. M., Sirviö, J., Thomas, J. H., Nass, R., et al. (2003). Dopaminergic neuronal loss and motor deficits in *Caenorhabditis elegans* overexpressing human alpha-synuclein. *J. Neurochem.* 86, 165–172. doi: 10.1046/j.1471-4159.2003.01809.x

Lambie, E. J., and Kimble, J. (1991). Two homologous regulatory genes, lin-12 and glp-1, have overlapping functions. *Development* 112, 231–240.

Larsen, P. L., Albert, P. S., and Riddle, D. L. (1995). Genes that regulate both development and longevity in *Caenorhabditis elegans*. *Genetics* 139, 1567–1583.

Lee, B. H., and Ashrafi, K. (2008). A TRPV channel modulates *C. elegans* neurosecretion, larval starvation survival, and adult lifespan. *PLoS Genet.* 4:e1000213. doi: 10.1371/journal.pgen.1000213

Lee, R. Y., Hench, J., and Ruvkun, G. (2001). Regulation of *C. elegans* DAF-16 and its human ortholog FKHRL1 by the daf-2 insulin-like signaling pathway. *Curr. Biol.* 11, 1950–1957. doi: 10.1016/S0960-9822(01)00595-4

Lee, V. M., Otvos, L., Carden, M. J., Hollosi, M., Dietzschold, B., and Lazzarini, R. A. (1988). Identification of the major multiphosphorylation site in mammalian neurofilaments. *Proc. Natl. Acad. Sci. U.S.A.* 85, 1998–2002. doi: 10.1073/pnas.85.6.1998

Lejeune, F. X., Mesrob, L., Parmentier, F., Bicep, C., Vazquez-Manrique, R. P., Parker, J. A., et al. (2012). Large-scale functional RNAi screen in *C. elegans* identifies genes that regulate the dysfunction of mutant polyglutamine neurons. *BMC Genomics* 13:91. doi: 10.1186/1471-2164-13-91.

Levitan, D., Doyle, T. G., Brousseau, D., Lee, M. K., Thinakaran, G., Slunt, H. H., et al. (1996). Assessment of normal and mutant human presenilin function in *Caenorhabditis elegans*. *Proc. Natl. Acad. Sci. U.S.A.* 93, 14940–14944. doi: 10.1073/pnas.93.25.14940

Levitan, D., and Greenwald, I. (1995). Facilitation of lin-12-mediated signalling by sel-12, a *Caenorhabditis elegans* S182 Alzheimer's disease gene. *Nature* 377, 351–354. doi: 10.1038/377351a0

Levy-Lahad, E., Wasco, W., Poorkaj, P., Romano, D. M., Oshima, J., Pettingell, W. H., et al. (1995). Candidate gene for the chromosome 1 familial Alzheimer's disease locus. *Science* 269, 973–977. doi: 10.1126/science.7638622

Lewis, S. A., Wang, D. H., and Cowan, N. J. (1988). Microtubule-associated protein MAP2 shares a microtubule binding motif with tau protein. *Science* 242, 936–939. doi: 10.1126/science.3142041

Lewy, F. H. (1912). Handbuch der Neurologie. (Berlin: Springer), 920–933.

Li, J., Li, T., Zhang, X., Tang, Y., Yang, J., and Le, W. (2014). Human superoxide dismutase 1 overexpression in motor neurons of *Caenorhabditis elegans* causes axon guidance defect and neurodegeneration. *Neurobiol. Aging* 35, 837–846. doi: 10.1016/j.neurobiolaging.2013.09.003

Li, L. Y., Luo, X., and Wang, X. (2001). Endonuclease G is an apoptotic DNase when released from mitochondria. *Nature* 412, 95–99. doi: 10.1038/35083620

Li, T., Ma, G., Cai, H., Price, D. L., and Wong, P. C. (2003). Nicastrin is required for assembly of presenilin/gamma-secretase complexes to mediate Notch signaling and for processing and trafficking of beta-amyloid precursor protein in mammals. *J. Neurosci.* 23, 3272–3277.

Li, X., and Greenwald, I. (1996). Membrane topology of the *C. elegans* SEL-12 presenilin. *Neuron* 17, 1015–1021. doi: 10.1016/S0896-6273(00)80231-7

Li, X., and Greenwald, I. (1997). HOP-1, a *Caenorhabditis elegans* presenilin, appears to be functionally redundant with SEL-12 presenilin and to facilitate LIN-12 and GLP-1 signaling. *Proc. Natl. Acad. Sci. U.S.A.* 94, 12204–12209. doi: 10.1073/pnas.94.22.12204

Liang, J. J. (2000). Interaction between beta-amyloid and lens alphaB-crystallin. *FEBS Lett.* 484, 98–101. doi: 10.1016/S0014-5793(00)02136-0

Lin, C. H., Tomioka, M., Pereira, S., Sellings, L., Iino, Y., and Van Der Kooy, D. (2010). Insulin signaling plays a dual role in *Caenorhabditis elegans* memory acquisition and memory retrieval. *J. Neurosci.* 30, 8001–8011. doi: 10.1523/JNEUROSCI.4636-09.2010

Lin, K., Dorman, J. B., Rodan, A., and Kenyon, C. (1997). daf-16: an HNF-3/forkhead family member that can function to double the life-span of *Caenorhabditis elegans*. *Science* 278, 1319–1322. doi: 10.1126/science.278.5341.1319

Lin, K., Hsin, H., Libina, N., and Kenyon, C. (2001). Regulation of the *Caenorhabditis elegans* longevity protein DAF-16 by insulin/IGF-1 and germline signaling. *Nat. Genet.* 28, 139–145. doi: 10.1038/88850

Lindau, M., Almkvist, O., Kushi, J., Boone, K., Johansson, S. E., Wahlund, L. O., et al. (2000). First symptoms–frontotemporal dementia versus Alzheimer's disease. *Dement. Geriatr. Cogn. Disord.* 11, 286–293. doi: 10.1159/000017251

Lindwall, G., and Cole, R. D. (1984). Phosphorylation affects the ability of tau protein to promote microtubule assembly. *J. Biol. Chem.* 259, 5301–5305.

Link, C. D. (1995). Expression of human beta-amyloid peptide in transgenic *Caenorhabditis elegans*. *Proc. Natl. Acad. Sci. U.S.A.* 92, 9368–9372. doi: 10.1073/pnas.92.20.9368

Link, C. D. (2006). *C. elegans* models of age-associated neurodegenerative diseases: lessons from transgenic worm models of Alzheimer's disease. *Exp. Gerontol.* 41, 1007–1013. doi: 10.1016/j.exger.2006.06.059

Link, C. D., Johnson, C. J., Fonte, V., Paupard, M., Hall, D. H., Styren, S., et al. (2001). Visualization of fibrillar amyloid deposits in living, transgenic *Caenorhabditis elegans* animals using the sensitive amyloid dye, X-34. *Neurobiol. Aging* 22, 217–226. doi: 10.1016/S0197-4580(00)00237-2

Liu, Z., Hamamichi, S., Lee, B. D., Yang, D., Ray, A., Caldwell, G. A., et al. (2011). Inhibitors of LRRK2 kinase attenuate neurodegeneration and Parkinson-like phenotypes in *Caenorhabditis elegans* and *Drosophila* Parkinson's disease models. *Hum. Mol. Genet.* 20, 3933–3942. doi: 10.1093/hmg/ddr312

Locke, C. J., Fox, S. A., Caldwell, G. A., and Caldwell, K. A. (2008). Acetaminophen attenuates dopamine neuron degeneration in animal models of Parkinson's disease. *Neurosci. Lett.* 439, 129–133. doi: 10.1016/j.neulet.2008.05.003

Lorent, K., Overbergh, L., Moechars, D., De Strooper, B., Van Leuven, F., and Van Den Berghe, H. (1995). Expression in mouse embryos and in adult mouse brain of three members of the amyloid precursor protein family, of the alpha-2-macroglobulin receptor/low density lipoprotein receptor-related protein and of its ligands apolipoprotein E, lipoprotein lipase, alpha-2-macroglobulin and the 40,000 molecular weight receptor-associated protein. *Neuroscience* 65, 1009–1025. doi: 10.1016/0306-4522(94)00555-J

Lu, T., Aron, L., Zullo, J., Pan, Y., Kim, H., Chen, Y., et al. (2014). REST and stress resistance in ageing and Alzheimer's disease. *Nature* 507, 448–454. doi: 10.1038/nature13163

Luo, W. J., Wang, H., Li, H., Kim, B. S., Shah, S., Lee, H. J., et al. (2003). PEN-2 and APH-1 coordinately regulate proteolytic processing of presenilin 1. *J. Biol. Chem.* 278, 7850–7854. doi: 10.1074/jbc.C200648200

Luse, S. A., and Smith, K. R. (1964). The ultrastructure of senile plaques. *Am. J. Pathol.* 44, 553–563.

Mahley, R. W. (1988). Apolipoprotein E: cholesterol transport protein with expanding role in cell biology. *Science* 240, 622–630. doi: 10.1126/science.3283935

Majounie, E., Abramzon, Y., Renton, A. E., Keller, M. F., Traynor, B. J., and Singleton, A. B. (2012). Large C9orf72 repeat expansions are not a common cause of Parkinson's disease. *Neurobiol. Aging* 33, e2521–e2522. doi: 10.1016/j.neurobiolaging.2012.05.007

Malek, A. M., Barchowsky, A., Bowser, R., Youk, A., and Talbott, E. O. (2012). Pesticide exposure as a risk factor for amyotrophic lateral sclerosis: a meta-analysis of epidemiological studies: pesticide exposure as a risk factor for ALS. *Environ. Res.* 117, 112–119. doi: 10.1016/j.envres.2012.06.007

Mangahas, P. M., Yu, X., Miller, K. G., and Zhou, Z. (2008). The small GTPase Rab2 functions in the removal of apoptotic cells in *Caenorhabditis elegans*. *J. Cell Biol.* 180, 357–373. doi: 10.1083/jcb.200708130

Mangiarini, L., Sathasivam, K., Seller, M., Cozens, B., Harper, A., Hetherington, C., et al. (1996). Exon 1 of the HD gene with an expanded CAG repeat is sufficient to cause a progressive neurological phenotype in transgenic mice. *Cell* 87, 493–506. doi: 10.1016/S0092-8674(00)81369-0

Martin, J. B., and Gusella, J. F. (1986). Huntington's disease. Pathogenesis and management. *N. Engl. J. Med.* 315, 1267–1276. doi: 10.1056/NEJM198611133152006

Martindale, D., Hackam, A., Wieczorek, A., Ellerby, L., Wellington, C., Mccutcheon, K., et al. (1998). Length of huntingtin and its polyglutamine tract influences localization and frequency of intracellular aggregates. *Nat. Genet.* 18, 150–154. doi: 10.1038/ng0298-150

Marvanova, M., and Nichols, C. D. (2007). Identification of neuroprotective compounds of *Caenorhabditis elegans* dopaminergic neurons against 6-OHDA. *J. Mol. Neurosci.* 31, 127–137.

Masters, C. L., Simms, G., Weinman, N. A., Multhaup, G., Mcdonald, B. L., and Beyreuther, K. (1985). Amyloid plaque core protein in Alzheimer disease and Down syndrome. *Proc. Natl. Acad. Sci. U.S.A.* 82, 4245–4249. doi: 10.1073/pnas.82.12.4245

Matus, A., Bernhardt, R., and Hugh-Jones, T. (1981). High molecular weight microtubule-associated proteins are preferentially associated with dendritic microtubules in brain. *Proc. Natl. Acad. Sci. U.S.A.* 78, 3010–3014. doi: 10.1073/pnas.78.5.3010

McColl, G., Roberts, B. R., Gunn, A. P., Perez, K. A., Tew, D. J., Masters, C. L., et al. (2009). The *Caenorhabditis elegans* A beta 1-42 model of Alzheimer disease predominantly expresses A beta 3-42. *J. Biol. Chem.* 284, 22697–22702. doi: 10.1074/jbc.C109.028514

McColl, G., Roberts, B. R., Pukala, T. L., Kenche, V. B., Roberts, C. M., Link, C. D., et al. (2012). Utility of an improved model of amyloid-beta ($A\beta_{1-42}$) toxicity in *Caenorhabditis elegans* for drug screening for Alzheimer's disease. *Mol. Neurodegener.* 7:57. doi: 10.1186/1750-1326-7-57

McDermott, J. B., Aamodt, S., and Aamodt, E. (1996). ptl-1, a *Caenorhabditis elegans* gene whose products are homologous to the tau microtubule-associated proteins. *Biochemistry* 35, 9415–9423. doi: 10.1021/bi952646n

McElwee, J., Bubb, K., and Thomas, J. H. (2003). Transcriptional outputs of the *Caenorhabditis elegans* forkhead protein DAF-16. *Aging Cell* 2, 111–121. doi: 10.1046/j.1474-9728.2003.00043.x

McElwee, J. J., Schuster, E., Blanc, E., Thomas, J. H., and Gems, D. (2004). Shared transcriptional signature in *Caenorhabditis elegans* Dauer larvae and long-lived daf-2 mutants implicates detoxification system in longevity assurance. *J. Biol. Chem.* 279, 44533–44543. doi: 10.1074/jbc.M406207200

Miyasaka, T., Ding, Z., Gengyo-Ando, K., Oue, M., Yamaguchi, H., Mitani, S., et al. (2005). Progressive neurodegeneration in *C. elegans* model of tauopathy. *Neurobiol. Dis.* 20, 372–383. doi: 10.1016/j.nbd.2005.03.017

Mizuta, K., Saito, A., Watanabe, T., Nagura, M., Arakawa, M., Shimizu, F., et al. (1999). Ultrastructural localization of megalin in the rat cochlear duct. *Hear. Res.* 129, 83–91. doi: 10.1016/S0378-5955(98)00221-4

Morales, C. R., Igdoura, S. A., Wosu, U. A., Boman, J., and Argraves, W. S. (1996). Low density lipoprotein receptor-related protein-2 expression in efferent duct and epididymal epithelia: evidence in rats for its *in vivo* role in endocytosis of apolipoprotein J/clusterin. *Biol. Reprod.* 55, 676–683. doi: 10.1095/biolreprod55.3.676

Morley, J. F., and Morimoto, R. I. (2004). Regulation of longevity in *Caenorhabditis elegans* by heat shock factor and molecular chaperones. *Mol. Biol. Cell* 15, 657–664. doi: 10.1091/mbc.E03-07-0532

Morris, J. Z., Tissenbaum, H. A., and Ruvkun, G. (1996). A phosphatidylinositol-3-OH kinase family member regulating longevity and diapause in *Caenorhabditis elegans*. *Nature* 382, 536–539. doi: 10.1038/382536a0

Murakami, T., Yang, S. P., Xie, L., Kawano, T., Fu, D., Mukai, A., et al. (2012). ALS mutations in FUS cause neuronal dysfunction and death in *Caenorhabditis elegans* by a dominant gain-of-function mechanism. *Hum. Mol. Genet.* 21, 1–9. doi: 10.1093/hmg/ddr417

Murphy, C. T., Mccarroll, S. A., Bargmann, C. I., Fraser, A., Kamath, R. S., Ahringer, J., et al. (2003). Genes that act downstream of DAF-16 to influence the lifespan of *Caenorhabditis elegans*. *Nature* 424, 277–283. doi: 10.1038/nature01789

Murrell, J., Farlow, M., Ghetti, B., and Benson, M. D. (1991). A mutation in the amyloid precursor protein associated with hereditary Alzheimer's disease. *Science* 254, 97–99. doi: 10.1126/science.1925564

Muñoz-Lobato, F., Rodríguez-Palero, M. J., Naranjo-Galindo, F. J., Shephard, F., Gaffney, C. J., Szewczyk, N. J., et al. (2014). Protective role of DNJ-27/ERdj5 in *Caenorhabditis elegans* models of human neurodegenerative diseases. *Antioxid. Redox. Signal.* 20, 217–235. doi: 10.1089/ars.2012.5051

Nance, M. A. (1997). Genetic testing of children at risk for Huntington's disease. US Huntington Disease Genetic Testing Group. *Neurology* 49, 1048–1053. doi: 10.1212/WNL.49.4.1048

Nass, R., Hahn, M. K., Jessen, T., Mcdonald, P. W., Carvelli, L., and Blakely, R. D. (2005). A genetic screen in *Caenorhabditis elegans* for dopamine neuron insensitivity to 6-hydroxydopamine identifies dopamine transporter mutants impacting transporter biosynthesis and trafficking. *J. Neurochem.* 94, 774–785. doi: 10.1111/j.1471-4159.2005.03205.x

Nass, R., Hall, D. H., Miller, D. M., and Blakely, R. D. (2002). Neurotoxin-induced degeneration of dopamine neurons in *Caenorhabditis elegans. Proc. Natl. Acad. Sci. U.S.A.* 99, 3264–3269. doi: 10.1073/pnas.042497999

Neumann, M., Sampathu, D. M., Kwong, L. K., Truax, A. C., Micsenyi, M. C., Chou, T. T., et al. (2006). Ubiquitinated TDP-43 in frontotemporal lobar degeneration and amyotrophic lateral sclerosis. *Science* 314, 130–133. doi: 10.1126/science.1134108

Newman, A. P., White, J. G., and Sternberg, P. W. (1995). The *Caenorhabditis elegans* lin-12 gene mediates induction of ventral uterine specialization by the anchor cell. *Development* 121, 263–271.

Nielsen, R., Birn, H., Moestrup, S. K., Nielsen, M., Verroust, P., and Christensen, E. I. (1998). Characterization of a kidney proximal tubule cell line, LLC-PK1, expressing endocytotic active megalin. *J. Am. Soc. Nephrol.* 9, 1767–1776.

Niwa, R., and Hada, K. (2010). Identification of a spatio-temporal enhancer element for the Alzheimer's amyloid precursor protein-like-1 gene in the nematode *Caenorhabditis elegans. Biosci. Biotechnol. Biochem.* 74, 2497–2500. doi: 10.1271/bbb.100450

Niwa, R., Zhou, F., Li, C., and Slack, F. J. (2008). The expression of the Alzheimer's amyloid precursor protein-like gene is regulated by developmental timing microRNAs and their targets in *Caenorhabditis elegans. Dev. Biol.* 315, 418–425. doi: 10.1016/j.ydbio.2007.12.044

Ogg, S., Paradis, S., Gottlieb, S., Patterson, G. I., Lee, L., Tissenbaum, H. A., et al. (1997). The Fork head transcription factor DAF-16 transduces insulin-like metabolic and longevity signals in *C. elegans. Nature* 389, 994–999. doi: 10.1038/40194

Orenstein, S. J., Kuo, S. H., Tasset, I., Arias, E., Koga, H., Fernandez-Carasa, I., et al. (2013). Interplay of LRRK2 with chaperone-mediated autophagy. *Nat. Neurosci.* 16, 394–406. doi: 10.1038/nn.3350

Orr, H. T., and Zoghbi, H. Y. (2007). Trinucleotide repeat disorders. *Annu. Rev. Neurosci.* 30, 575–621. doi: 10.1146/annurev.neuro.29.051605.113042

Pan, C. L., Peng, C. Y., Chen, C. H., and Mcintire, S. (2011). Genetic analysis of age-dependent defects of the *Caenorhabditis elegans* touch receptor neurons. *Proc. Natl. Acad. Sci. U.S.A.* 108, 9274–9279. doi: 10.1073/pnas.1011711108

Paradis, S., Ailion, M., Toker, A., Thomas, J. H., and Ruvkun, G. (1999). A PDK1 homolog is necessary and sufficient to transduce AGE-1 PI3 kinase signals that regulate diapause in *Caenorhabditis elegans. Genes Dev.* 13, 1438–1452. doi: 10.1101/gad.13.11.1438

Paradis, S., and Ruvkun, G. (1998). *Caenorhabditis elegans* Akt/PKB transduces insulin receptor-like signals from AGE-1 PI3 kinase to the DAF-16 transcription factor. *Genes Dev.* 12, 2488–2498. doi: 10.1101/gad.12.16.2488

Parker, J. A., Arango, M., Abderrahmane, S., Lambert, E., Tourette, C., Catoire, H., et al. (2005). Resveratrol rescues mutant polyglutamine cytotoxicity in nematode and mammalian neurons. *Nat. Genet.* 37, 349–350. doi: 10.1038/ng1534

Parker, J. A., Connolly, J. B., Wellington, C., Hayden, M., Dausset, J., and Neri, C. (2001). Expanded polyglutamines in *Caenorhabditis elegans* cause axonal abnormalities and severe dysfunction of PLM mechanosensory neurons without cell death. *Proc. Natl. Acad. Sci. U.S.A.* 98, 13318–13323. doi: 10.1073/pnas.231476398

Pasinelli, P., and Brown, R. H. (2006). Molecular biology of amyotrophic lateral sclerosis: insights from genetics. *Nat. Rev. Neurosci.* 7, 710–723. doi: 10.1038/nrn1971

Pasquier, F. (2005). Telling the difference between frontotemporal dementia and Alzheimer's disease. *Curr. Opin. Psychiatry* 18, 628–632. doi: 10.1097/01.yco.0000185988.05741.2a

Perez, N., Sugar, J., Charya, S., Johnson, G., Merril, C., Bierer, L., et al. (1991). Increased synthesis and accumulation of heat shock 70 proteins in Alzheimer's disease. *Mol. Brain Res.* 11, 249–254. doi: 10.1016/0169-328X(91)90033-T

Pierce-Shimomura, J. T., Faumont, S., Gaston, M. R., Pearson, B. J., and Lockery, S. R. (2001). The homeobox gene lim-6 is required for distinct chemosensory representations in *C. elegans. Nature* 410, 694–698. doi: 10.1038/35070575

Pietrzik, C. U., Yoon, I. S., Jaeger, S., Busse, T., Weggen, S., and Koo, E. H. (2004). FE65 constitutes the functional link between the low-density lipoprotein receptor-related protein and the amyloid precursor protein. *J. Neurosci.* 24, 4259–4265. doi: 10.1523/JNEUROSCI.5451-03.2004

Polymeropoulos, M. H., Lavedan, C., Leroy, E., Ide, S. E., Dehejia, A., Dutra, A., et al. (1997). Mutation in the alpha-synuclein gene identified in families with Parkinson's disease. *Science* 276, 2045–2047. doi: 10.1126/science.276.5321.2045

Poorkaj, P., Bird, T. D., Wijsman, E., Nemens, E., Garruto, R. M., Anderson, L., et al. (1998). Tau is a candidate gene for chromosome 17 frontotemporal dementia. *Ann. Neurol.* 43, 815–825. doi: 10.1002/ana.410430617

Poorkaj, P., Nutt, J. G., James, D., Gancher, S., Bird, T. D., Steinbart, E., et al. (2004). parkin mutation analysis in clinic patients with early-onset Parkinson [corrected] disease. *Am. J. Med. Genet. A* 129A, 44–50. doi: 10.1002/ajmg.a.30157

Rabinovici, G. D., and Miller, B. L. (2010). Frontotemporal lobar degeneration: epidemiology, pathophysiology, diagnosis and management. *CNS Drugs* 24, 375–398. doi: 10.2165/11533100-000000000-00000

Recchia, A., Debetto, P., Negro, A., Guidolin, D., Skaper, S. D., and Giusti, P. (2004). Alpha-synuclein and Parkinson's disease. *FASEB J.* 18, 617–626. doi: 10.1096/fj.03-0338rev

Reinhart, B. J., Slack, F. J., Basson, M., Pasquinelli, A. E., Bettinger, J. C., Rougvie, A. E., et al. (2000). The 21-nucleotide let-7 RNA regulates developmental timing in *Caenorhabditis elegans. Nature* 403, 901–906. doi: 10.1038/35002607

Renkawek, K., Voorter, C. E., Bosman, G. J., Van Workum, F. P., and De Jong, W. W. (1994). Expression of alpha B-crystallin in Alzheimer's disease. *Acta Neuropathol.* 87, 155–160. doi: 10.1007/BF00296185

Renton, A. E., Majounie, E., Waite, A., Simón-Sánchez, J., Rollinson, S., Gibbs, J. R., et al. (2011). A hexanucleotide repeat expansion in C9ORF72 is the cause of chromosome 9p21-linked ALS-FTD. *Neuron* 72, 257–268. doi: 10.1016/j.neuron.2011.09.010

Riddle, D. L., Swanson, M. M., and Albert, P. S. (1981). Interacting genes in nematode dauer larva formation. *Nature* 290, 668–671. doi: 10.1038/290668a0

Ring, S., Weyer, S. W., Kilian, S. B., Waldron, E., Pietrzik, C. U., Filippov, M. A., et al. (2007). The secreted beta-amyloid precursor protein ectodomain APPs alpha is sufficient to rescue the anatomical, behavioral, and electrophysiological abnormalities of APP-deficient mice. *J. Neurosci.* 27, 7817–7826. doi: 10.1523/JNEUROSCI.1026-07.2007

Rogaev, E. I., Sherrington, R., Rogaeva, E. A., Levesque, G., Ikeda, M., Liang, Y., et al. (1995). Familial Alzheimer's disease in kindreds with missense mutations in a gene on chromosome 1 related to the Alzheimer's disease type 3 gene. *Nature* 376, 775–778. doi: 10.1038/376775a0

Ruan, Q., Harrington, A. J., Caldwell, K. A., Caldwell, G. A., and Standaert, D. G. (2010). VPS41, a protein involved in lysosomal trafficking, is protective in *Caenorhabditis elegans* and mammalian cellular models of Parkinson's disease. *Neurobiol. Dis.* 37, 330–338. doi: 10.1016/j.nbd.2009.10.011

Russo, T., Faraonio, R., Minopoli, G., De Candia, P., De Renzis, S., and Zambrano, N. (1998). Fe65 and the protein network centered around the cytosolic domain of the Alzheimer's beta-amyloid precursor protein. *FEBS Lett.* 434, 1–7. doi: 10.1016/S0014-5793(98)00941-7

Sandbrink, R., Masters, C. L., and Beyreuther, K. (1994). Similar alternative splicing of a non-homologous domain in beta A4-amyloid protein precursor-like proteins. *J. Biol. Chem.* 269, 14227–14234.

Sastre, M., Steiner, H., Fuchs, K., Capell, A., Multhaup, G., Condron, M. M., et al. (2001). Presenilin-dependent gamma-secretase processing of beta-amyloid precursor protein at a site corresponding to the S3 cleavage of Notch. *EMBO Rep.* 2, 835–841. doi: 10.1093/embo-reports/kve180

Savage-Dunn, C., Maduzia, L. L., Zimmerman, C. M., Roberts, A. F., Cohen, S., Tokarz, R., et al. (2003). Genetic screen for small body size mutants in *C. elegans* reveals many TGFbeta pathway components. *Genesis* 35, 239–247. doi: 10.1002/gene.10184

Seidel, H. S., and Kimble, J. (2011). The oogenic germline starvation response in *C. elegans. PLoS ONE* 6:e28074. doi: 10.1371/journal.pone.0028074

Selkoe, D. J., Abraham, C. R., Podlisny, M. B., and Duffy, L. K. (1986). Isolation of low-molecular-weight proteins from amyloid plaque fibers in

Alzheimer's disease. *J. Neurochem.* 46, 1820–1834. doi: 10.1111/j.1471-4159.1986.tb08501.x

Shankar, G. M., Li, S., Mehta, T. H., Garcia-Munoz, A., Shepardson, N. E., Smith, I., et al. (2008). Amyloid-beta protein dimers isolated directly from Alzheimer's brains impair synaptic plasticity and memory. *Nat. Med.* 14, 837–842. doi: 10.1038/nm1782

Shaye, D. D., and Greenwald, I. (2011). OrthoList: a compendium of *C. elegans* genes with human orthologs. *PLoS ONE* 6:e20085. doi: 10.1371/journal.pone.0020085

Shen, J., Bronson, R. T., Chen, D. F., Xia, W., Selkoe, D. J., and Tonegawa, S. (1997). Skeletal and CNS defects in Presenilin-1-deficient mice. *Cell* 89, 629–639. doi: 10.1016/S0092-8674(00)80244-5

Sherrington, R., Rogaev, E. I., Liang, Y., Rogaeva, E. A., Levesque, G., Ikeda, M., et al. (1995). Cloning of a gene bearing missense mutations in early-onset familial Alzheimer's disease. *Nature* 375, 754–760. doi: 10.1038/375754a0

Shi, Z., Lu, Z., Zhao, Y., Wang, Y., Zhao-Wilson, X., Guan, P., et al. (2013). Neuroprotective effects of aqueous extracts of *Uncaria tomentosa*: insights from 6-OHDA induced cell damage and transgenic *Caenorhabditis elegans* model. *Neurochem. Int.* 62, 940–947. doi: 10.1016/j.neuint.2013.03.001

Shimura, H., Hattori, N., Kubo, S., Mizuno, Y., Asakawa, S., Minoshima, S., et al. (2000). Familial Parkinson disease gene product, parkin, is a ubiquitin-protein ligase. *Nat. Genet.* 25, 302–305. doi: 10.1038/77060

Shinohara, H., Inaguma, Y., Goto, S., Inagaki, T., and Kato, K. (1993). Alpha B crystallin and HSP28 are enhanced in the cerebral cortex of patients with Alzheimer's disease. *J. Neurol. Sci.* 119, 203–208. doi: 10.1016/0022-510X(93)90135-L

Siesling, S., Vegter-Van Der Vlis, M., and Roos, R. A. (1997). Juvenile Huntington disease in the Netherlands. *Pediatr. Neurol.* 17, 37–43. doi: 10.1016/S0887-8994(97)00069-6

Simón, A. M., Schiapparelli, L., Salazar-Colocho, P., Cuadrado-Tejedor, M., Escribano, L., López De Maturana, R., et al. (2009). Overexpression of wild-type human APP in mice causes cognitive deficits and pathological features unrelated to Abeta levels. *Neurobiol. Dis.* 33, 369–378. doi: 10.1016/j.nbd.2008.11.005

Slunt, H. H., Thinakaran, G., Von Koch, C., Lo, A. C., Tanzi, R. E., and Sisodia, S. S. (1994). Expression of a ubiquitous, cross-reactive homologue of the mouse beta-amyloid precursor protein (APP). *J. Biol. Chem.* 269, 2637–2644.

So, S., Miyahara, K., and Ohshima, Y. (2011). Control of body size in *C. elegans* dependent on food and insulin/IGF-1 signal. *Genes Cells* 16, 639–651. doi: 10.1111/j.1365-2443.2011.01514.x

Spillantini, M. G., Crowther, R. A., Kamphorst, W., Heutink, P., and Van Swieten, J. C. (1998). Tau pathology in two Dutch families with mutations in the microtubule-binding region of tau. *Am. J. Pathol.* 153, 1359–1363. doi: 10.1016/S0002-9440(10)65721-5

Sprecher, C. A., Grant, F. J., Grimm, G., O'hara, P. J., Norris, F., Norris, K., et al. (1993). Molecular cloning of the cDNA for a human amyloid precursor protein homolog: evidence for a multigene family. *Biochemistry* 32, 4481–4486. doi: 10.1021/bi00068a002

Springer, W., Hoppe, T., Schmidt, E., and Baumeister, R. (2005). A *Caenorhabditis elegans* Parkin mutant with altered solubility couples alpha-synuclein aggregation to proteotoxic stress. *Hum. Mol. Genet.* 14, 3407–3423. doi: 10.1093/hmg/ddi371

Sreedharan, J., Blair, I. P., Tripathi, V. B., Hu, X., Vance, C., Rogelj, B., et al. (2008). TDP-43 mutations in familial and sporadic amyotrophic lateral sclerosis. *Science* 319, 1668–1672. doi: 10.1126/science.1154584

Steen, E., Terry, B. M., Rivera, E. J., Cannon, J. L., Neely, T. R., Tavares, R., et al. (2005). Impaired insulin and insulin-like growth factor expression and signaling mechanisms in Alzheimer's disease – is this type 3 diabetes? *J. Alzheimers Dis.* 7, 63–80.

Strong, T. V., Tagle, D. A., Valdes, J. M., Elmer, L. W., Boehm, K., Swaroop, M., et al. (1993). Widespread expression of the human and rat Huntington's disease gene in brain and nonneural tissues. *Nat. Genet.* 5, 259–265. doi: 10.1038/ng1193-259

Sulston, J. E., and Horvitz, H. R. (1977). Post-embryonic cell lineages of the nematode, *Caenorhabditis elegans*. *Dev. Biol.* 56, 110–156. doi: 10.1016/0012-1606(77)90158-0

Sumakovic, M., Hegermann, J., Luo, L., Husson, S. J., Schwarze, K., Olendrowitz, C., et al. (2009). UNC-108/RAB-2 and its effector RIC-19 are involved in dense core vesicle maturation in *Caenorhabditis elegans*. *J. Cell Biol.* 186, 897–914. doi: 10.1083/jcb.200902096

Tank, E. M., Rodgers, K. E., and Kenyon, C. (2011). Spontaneous age-related neurite branching in *Caenorhabditis elegans*. *J. Neurosci.* 31, 9279–9288. doi: 10.1523/JNEUROSCI.6606-10.2011

Terry, R. D., Gonatas, N. K., and Weiss, M. (1964). Ultrastructural studies in Alzheimer's presenile dementia. *Am. J. Pathol.* 44, 269–297.

The Association for Frontotemporal Degeneration. (2014). *The Association for Frontotemporal Degeneration [Online]*. Available at: http://www.theaftd.org (accessed March 18, 2014)

The Huntington's Disease Collaborative Research Group. (1993). A novel gene containing a trinucleotide repeat that is expanded and unstable on Huntington's disease chromosomes. *Cell* 72, 971–983. doi: 10.1016/0092-8674(93)90585-E

Therrien, M., Rouleau, G. A., Dion, P. A., and Parker, J. A. (2013). Deletion of C9ORF72 results in motor neuron degeneration and stress sensitivity in *C. elegans*. *PLoS ONE* 8:e83450. doi: 10.1371/journal.pone.0083450

Thinakaran, G., Borchelt, D. R., Lee, M. K., Slunt, H. H., Spitzer, L., Kim, G., et al. (1996). Endoproteolysis of presenilin 1 and accumulation of processed derivatives *in vivo*. *Neuron* 17, 181–190. doi: 10.1016/S0896-6273(00)80291-3

Thinakaran, G., Kitt, C. A., Roskams, A. J., Slunt, H. H., Masliah, E., Von Koch, C., et al. (1995). Distribution of an APP homolog, APLP2, in the mouse olfactory system: a potential role for APLP2 in axogenesis. *J. Neurosci.* 15, 6314–6326.

Tissenbaum, H. A., and Guarente, L. (2001). Increased dosage of a sir-2 gene extends lifespan in *Caenorhabditis elegans*. *Nature* 410, 227–230. doi: 10.1038/35065638

Tomioka, M., Adachi, T., Suzuki, H., Kunitomo, H., Schafer, W. R., and Iino, Y. (2006). The insulin/PI 3-kinase pathway regulates salt chemotaxis learning in *Caenorhabditis elegans*. *Neuron* 51, 613–625. doi: 10.1016/j.neuron.2006.07.024

Toth, M. L., Melentijevic, I., Shah, L., Bhatia, A., Lu, K., Talwar, A., et al. (2012). Neurite sprouting and synapse deterioration in the aging *Caenorhabditis elegans* nervous system. *J. Neurosci.* 32, 8778–8790. doi: 10.1523/JNEUROSCI.1494-11.2012

Tretiakoff, K. (1919). Contribution a l'Etude de L'Anatomie pathologique du Locus Niger de Soemmering avec quelques déductions relatives à la pathogénie des troubles du tonus musculaire et De La Maladie de Parkinson. University of Paris: Paris.

Treusch, S., Hamamichi, S., Goodman, J. L., Matlack, K. E., Chung, C. Y., Baru, V., et al. (2011). Functional links between Aβ toxicity, endocytic trafficking, and Alzheimer's disease risk factors in yeast. *Science* 334, 1241–1245. doi: 10.1126/science.1213210

Tsuda, H., Han, S. M., Yang, Y., Tong, C., Lin, Y. Q., Mohan, K., et al. (2008). The amyotrophic lateral sclerosis 8 protein VAPB is cleaved, secreted, and acts as a ligand for Eph receptors. *Cell* 133, 963–977. doi: 10.1016/j.cell.2008.04.039

Ulery, P. G., Beers, J., Mikhailenko, I., Tanzi, R. E., Rebeck, G. W., Hyman, B. T., et al. (2000). Modulation of beta-amyloid precursor protein processing by the low density lipoprotein receptor-related protein (LRP). Evidence that LRP contributes to the pathogenesis of Alzheimer's disease. *J. Biol. Chem.* 275, 7410–7415. doi: 10.1074/jbc.275.10.7410

Vaccaro, A., Patten, S. A., Ciura, S., Maios, C., Therrien, M., Drapeau, P., et al. (2012a). Methylene blue protects against TDP-43 and FUS neuronal toxicity in *C. elegans* and *D. rerio*. *PLoS ONE* 7:e42117. doi: 10.1371/journal.pone.0042117

Vaccaro, A., Tauffenberger, A., Ash, P. E., Carlomagno, Y., Petrucelli, L., and Parker, J. A. (2012b). TDP-1/TDP-43 regulates stress signaling and age-dependent proteotoxicity in *Caenorhabditis elegans*. *PLoS Genet.* 8:e1002806. doi: 10.1371/journal.pgen.1002806

Valentine, J. S., Doucette, P. A., and Zittin Potter, S. (2005). Copper-zinc superoxide dismutase and amyotrophic lateral sclerosis. *Annu. Rev. Biochem.* 74, 563–593. doi: 10.1146/annurev.biochem.72.121801.161647

Van Deerlin, V. M., Leverenz, J. B., Bekris, L. M., Bird, T. D., Yuan, W., Elman, L. B., et al. (2008). TARDBP mutations in amyotrophic lateral sclerosis with TDP-43 neuropathology: a genetic and histopathological analysis. *Lancet Neurol.* 7, 409–416. doi: 10.1016/S1474-4422(08)70071-1

van Dijk, J. G., Van Der Velde, E. A., Roos, R. A., and Bruyn, G. W. (1986). Juvenile Huntington disease. *Hum. Genet.* 73, 235–239. doi: 10.1007/BF00401235

van Ham, T. J., Thijssen, K. L., Breitling, R., Hofstra, R. M., Plasterk, R. H., and Nollen, E. A. (2008). *C. elegans* model identifies genetic modifiers of alpha-synuclein inclusion formation during aging. *PLoS Genet.* 4:e1000027. doi: 10.1371/journal.pgen.1000027

Vartiainen, S., Pehkonen, P., Lakso, M., Nass, R., and Wong, G. (2006). Identification of gene expression changes in transgenic *C. elegans* overexpressing human alpha-synuclein. *Neurobiol. Dis.* 22, 477–486. doi: 10.1016/j.nbd.2005.12.021

Vinceti, M., Maraldi, T., Bergomi, M., and Malagoli, C. (2009). Risk of chronic low-dose selenium overexposure in humans: insights from epidemiology and biochemistry. *Rev. Environ. Health* 24, 231–248. doi: 10.1515/REVEH.2009.24.3.231

von Koch, C. S., Zheng, H., Chen, H., Trumbauer, M., Thinakaran, G., Van Der Ploeg, L. H., et al. (1997). Generation of APLP2 KO mice and early postnatal lethality in APLP2/APP double KO mice. *Neurobiol. Aging* 18, 661–669. doi: 10.1016/S0197-4580(97)00151-6

Vonsattel, J. P., Myers, R. H., Stevens, T. J., Ferrante, R. J., Bird, E. D., and Richardson, E. P. (1985). Neuropathological classification of Huntington's disease. *J. Neuropathol. Exp. Neurol.* 44, 559–577. doi: 10.1097/00005072-198511000-00003

Vowels, J. J., and Thomas, J. H. (1992). Genetic analysis of chemosensory control of dauer formation in *Caenorhabditis elegans. Genetics* 130, 105–123.

Wang, J., Farr, G. W., Hall, D. H., Li, F., Furtak, K., Dreier, L., et al. (2009). An ALS-linked mutant SOD1 produces a locomotor defect associated with aggregation and synaptic dysfunction when expressed in neurons of *Caenorhabditis elegans. PLoS Genet.* 5:e1000350. doi: 10.1371/journal.pgen.1000350

Wang, P., Yang, G., Mosier, D. R., Chang, P., Zaidi, T., Gong, Y. D., et al. (2005). Defective neuromuscular synapses in mice lacking amyloid precursor protein (APP) and APP-Like protein 2. *J. Neurosci.* 25, 1219–1225. doi: 10.1523/JNEUROSCI.4660-04.2005

Wasco, W., Bupp, K., Magendantz, M., Gusella, J. F., Tanzi, R. E., and Solomon, F. (1992). Identification of a mouse brain cDNA that encodes a protein related to the Alzheimer disease-associated amyloid beta protein precursor. *Proc. Natl. Acad. Sci. U.S.A.* 89, 10758–10762. doi: 10.1073/pnas.89.22.10758

Wasco, W., Gurubhagavatula, S., Paradis, M. D., Romano, D. M., Sisodia, S. S., Hyman, B. T., et al. (1993). Isolation and characterization of APLP2 encoding a homologue of the Alzheimer's associated amyloid beta protein precursor. *Nat. Genet.* 5, 95–100. doi: 10.1038/ng0993-95

Weidemann, A., Eggert, S., Reinhard, F. B., Vogel, M., Paliga, K., Baier, G., et al. (2002). A novel epsilon-cleavage within the transmembrane domain of the Alzheimer amyloid precursor protein demonstrates homology with Notch processing. *Biochemistry* 41, 2825–2835. doi: 10.1021/bi015794o

Wen, J. Y., Kumar, N., Morrison, G., Rambaldini, G., Runciman, S., Rousseau, J., et al. (1997). Mutations that prevent associative learning in *C. elegans. Behav. Neurosci.* 111, 354–368. doi: 10.1037/0735-7044.111.2.354

Westlund, B., Parry, D., Clover, R., Basson, M., and Johnson, C. D. (1999). Reverse genetic analysis of *Caenorhabditis elegans* presenilins reveals redundant but unequal roles for sel-12 and hop-1 in Notch-pathway signaling. *Proc. Natl. Acad. Sci. U.S.A.* 96, 2497–2502. doi: 10.1073/pnas.96.5.2497

Weyer, S. W., Klevanski, M., Delekate, A., Voikar, V., Aydin, D., Hick, M., et al. (2011). APP and APLP2 are essential at PNS and CNS synapses for transmission, spatial learning and LTP. *EMBO J.* 30, 2266–2280. doi: 10.1038/emboj.2011.119

Wheeler, J. M., Guthrie, C. R., and Kraemer, B. C. (2010). The role of MSUT-2 in tau neurotoxicity: a target for neuroprotection in tauopathy? *Biochem. Soc. Trans.* 38, 973–976. doi: 10.1042/BST0380973

Wiese, M., Antebi, A., and Zheng, H. (2010). Intracellular trafficking and synaptic function of APL-1 in *Caenorhabditis elegans. PLoS ONE* 5:e12790. doi: 10.1371/journal.pone.0012790

Wiese, M., Antebi, A., and Zheng, H. (2012). Regulation of neuronal APL-1 expression by cholesterol starvation. *PLoS ONE* 7:e32038. doi: 10.1371/journal.pone.0032038

Willnow, T. E., Hilpert, J., Armstrong, S. A., Rohlmann, A., Hammer, R. E., Burns, D. K., et al. (1996). Defective forebrain development in mice lacking gp330/megalin. *Proc. Natl. Acad. Sci. U.S.A.* 93, 8460–8464. doi: 10.1073/pnas.93.16.8460

Willnow, T. E., Sheng, Z., Ishibashi, S., and Herz, J. (1994). Inhibition of hepatic chylomicron remnant uptake by gene transfer of a receptor antagonist. *Science* 264, 1471–1474. doi: 10.1126/science.7515194

Witan, H., Kern, A., Koziollek-Drechsler, I., Wade, R., Behl, C., and Clement, A. M. (2008). Heterodimer formation of wild-type and amyotrophic lateral sclerosis-causing mutant Cu/Zn-superoxide dismutase induces toxicity independent of protein aggregation. *Hum. Mol. Genet.* 17, 1373–1385. doi: 10.1093/hmg/ddn025

Wood-Kaczmar, A., Gandhi, S., and Wood, N. W. (2006). Understanding the molecular causes of Parkinson's disease. *Trends Mol. Med.* 12, 521–528. doi: 10.1016/j.molmed.2006.09.007

Wroe, R., Wai-Ling Butler, A., Andersen, P. M., Powell, J. F., and Al-Chalabi, A. (2008). ALSOD: the Amyotrophic Lateral Sclerosis Online Database. *Amyotroph. Lateral Scler.* 9, 249–250. doi: 10.1080/17482960802146106

Yao, C., Johnson, W. M., Gao, Y., Wang, W., Zhang, J., Deak, M., et al. (2013). Kinase inhibitors arrest neurodegeneration in cell and *C. elegans* models of LRRK2 toxicity. *Hum. Mol. Genet.* 22, 328–344. doi: 10.1093/hmg/dds431

Yochem, J., and Greenwald, I. (1993). A gene for a low density lipoprotein receptor-related protein in the nematode *Caenorhabditis elegans. Proc. Natl. Acad. Sci. U.S.A.* 90, 4572–4576. doi: 10.1073/pnas.90.10.4572

Yochem, J., Gu, T., and Han, M. (1998). A new marker for mosaic analysis in *Caenorhabditis elegans* indicates a fusion between hyp6 and hyp7, two major components of the hypodermis. *Genetics* 149, 1323–1334.

Yochem, J., Tuck, S., Greenwald, I., and Han, M. (1999). A gp330/megalin-related protein is required in the major epidermis of *Caenorhabditis elegans* for completion of molting. *Development* 126, 597–606.

Yokoseki, A., Shiga, A., Tan, C. F., Tagawa, A., Kaneko, H., Koyama, A., et al. (2008). TDP-43 mutation in familial amyotrophic lateral sclerosis. *Ann. Neurol.* 63, 538–542. doi: 10.1002/ana.21392

Yoo, B. C., Kim, S. H., Cairns, N., Fountoulakis, M., and Lubec, G. (2001). Deranged expression of molecular chaperones in brains of patients with Alzheimer's disease. *Biochem. Biophys. Res. Commun.* 280, 249–258. doi: 10.1006/bbrc.2000.4109

Yoon, I. S., Pietrzik, C. U., Kang, D. E., and Koo, E. H. (2005). Sequences from the low density lipoprotein receptor-related protein (LRP) cytoplasmic domain enhance amyloid beta protein production via the beta-secretase pathway without altering amyloid precursor protein/LRP nuclear signaling. *J. Biol. Chem.* 280, 20140–20147. doi: 10.1074/jbc.M413729200

Yu, G., Nishimura, M., Arawaka, S., Levitan, D., Zhang, L., Tandon, A., et al. (2000). Nicastrin modulates presenilin-mediated notch/glp-1 signal transduction and betaAPP processing. *Nature* 407, 48–54. doi: 10.1038/35024009

Zambrano, N., Bimonte, M., Arbucci, S., Gianni, D., Russo, T., and Bazzicalupo, P. (2002). feh-1 and apl-1, the *Caenorhabditis elegans* orthologues of mammalian Fe65 and beta-amyloid precursor protein genes, are involved in the same pathway that controls nematode pharyngeal pumping. *J. Cell Sci.* 115, 1411–1422.

Zambrano, N., Buxbaum, J. D., Minopoli, G., Fiore, F., De Candia, P., De Renzis, S., et al. (1997). Interaction of the phosphotyrosine interaction/phosphotyrosine binding-related domains of Fe65 with wild-type and mutant Alzheimer's beta-amyloid precursor proteins. *J. Biol. Chem.* 272, 6399–6405. doi: 10.1074/jbc.272.10.6399

Zarranz, J. J., Alegre, J., Gómez-Esteban, J. C., Lezcano, E., Ros, R., Ampuero, I., et al. (2004). The new mutation, E46K, of alpha-synuclein causes Parkinson and Lewy body dementia. *Ann. Neurol.* 55, 164–173. doi: 10.1002/ana.10795

Zhang, Y. W., Luo, W. J., Wang, H., Lin, P., Vetrivel, K. S., Liao, F., et al. (2005). Nicastrin is critical for stability and trafficking but not association of other presenilin/gamma-secretase components. *J. Biol. Chem.* 280, 17020–17026. doi: 10.1074/jbc.M409467200

Zheng, G., Marino', M., Zhao, J., and Mccluskey, R. T. (1998). Megalin (gp330): a putative endocytic receptor for thyroglobulin (Tg). *Endocrinology* 139, 1462–1465. doi: 10.1210/endo.139.3.5978

Zigman, W. B. (2013). Atypical aging in Down syndrome. *Dev. Disabil. Res. Rev.* 18, 51–67. doi: 10.1002/ddrr.1128

Zlokovic, B. V., Martel, C. L., Matsubara, E., Mccomb, J. G., Zheng, G., Mccluskey, R. T., et al. (1996). Glycoprotein 330/megalin: probable role in receptor-mediated transport of apolipoprotein J alone and in a complex with Alzheimer disease amyloid beta at the blood–brain and blood–cerebrospinal fluid barriers. *Proc. Natl. Acad. Sci. U.S.A.* 93, 4229–4234. doi: 10.1073/pnas.93.9.4229

20

Phospholipase A_2 – nexus of aging, oxidative stress, neuronal excitability, and functional decline of the aging nervous system? Insights from a snail model system of neuronal aging and age-associated memory impairment

Petra M. Hermann[1,2], Shawn N. Watson[1] and Willem C. Wildering[1,2,3] *

[1] Department of Biological Sciences, University of Calgary, Calgary, AB, Canada
[2] Department of Physiology and Pharmacology, University of Calgary, Calgary, AB, Canada
[3] Hotchkiss Brain Institute, University of Calgary, Calgary, AB, Canada

Edited by:
Shin Murakami, Touro University-California, USA

Reviewed by:
Deborah Baro, Georgia State University, USA
Srinivas Ayyadevara, Central Arkansas Veterans Healthcare System, USA

***Correspondence:**
Willem C. Wildering, Department of Biological Sciences, University of Calgary, 2500 University Drive NW, Calgary, AB T2N 1N4, Canada
e-mail: wilderin@ucalgary.ca

The aging brain undergoes a range of changes varying from subtle structural and physiological changes causing only minor functional decline under healthy normal aging conditions, to severe cognitive or neurological impairment associated with extensive loss of neurons and circuits due to age-associated neurodegenerative disease conditions. Understanding how biological aging processes affect the brain and how they contribute to the onset and progress of age-associated neurodegenerative diseases is a core research goal in contemporary neuroscience. This review focuses on the idea that changes in intrinsic neuronal electrical excitability associated with (per)oxidation of membrane lipids and activation of phospholipase A_2 (PLA_2) enzymes are an important mechanism of learning and memory failure under normal aging conditions. Specifically, in the context of this special issue on the biology of cognitive aging we portray the opportunities offered by the identifiable neurons and behaviorally characterized neural circuits of the freshwater snail *Lymnaea stagnalis* in neuronal aging research and recapitulate recent insights indicating a key role of lipid peroxidation-induced PLA_2 as instruments of aging, oxidative stress and inflammation in age-associated neuronal and memory impairment in this model system. The findings are discussed in view of accumulating evidence suggesting involvement of analogous mechanisms in the etiology of age-associated dysfunction and disease of the human and mammalian brain.

Keywords: aging, age-associated memory impairment (AMI), lipid peroxidation, phospholipases A2, neuronal excitability, neuronal plasticity, *Lymnaea stagnalis*

INTRODUCTION

Most organisms age, humans and the vast majority of other complex animals included. That is, the life functions required for their survival and reproduction weaken as they grow older due to natural processes that are still only partially understood and involve a complex combination of chemical, genetic, metabolic, molecular, physiological, ecological, and evolutionary features (see for instance Kirkwood and Austad, 2000; Ljubuncic and Reznick, 2009; Masoro and Austad, 2011).

Aging generally affects all aspects of an organism's biology including, in the case of humans and complex multicellular animals, the nervous system's ability to execute its control processes and support learning and memory functions. For example, declining learning and memory performance, weakening sensory, and motor functions, and slowing of reaction times are common symptoms of old age in humans and many vertebrate and invertebrate model systems (Burke and Barnes, 2006; Chawla and Barnes, 2007; Murakami, 2007; Partridge, 2008; Yeoman et al., 2012; Haddadi et al., 2014). Some of these changes, particularly in our own species, may involve pathological processes such as Alzheimer's and Parkinson's disease. However, even in the healthy aging brain where loss of neurons and circuits to cell death is generally not a significant factor, functional performance tends to decline with age (Peters et al., 1994; West et al., 1994; Rapp and Gallagher, 1996; Rasmussen et al., 1996; Gazzaley et al., 1997; Merrill et al., 2000, 2001; Keuker et al., 2003; Burke and Barnes, 2006). Why this happens, particularly what makes healthy aging neurons change the way in which they work and communicate with each other is the focus of this article. Specifically, we explore the idea that processes triggered by oxidative stress ensuing at the level of phospholipid bilayer membranes of cells and organelles play a central role in age-associated deterioration of the healthy aging nervous system (Note: while this review centers on non-pathological mechanisms of brain aging it should be kept in mind that many consider normal and pathological aging as two causally related extremes of a continuum in which it is not always clear where normal aging ends and pathological aging starts. See for instance Hung et al., 2010; Dai et al., 2014).

The idea that oxidative stress is a major factor in biological aging has a long history and extensive experimental support (Harman, 1956; Pérez et al., 2009; Hekimi et al., 2011; Speakman and Selman, 2011; Zimniak, 2011; Alcedo et al., 2013). Yet, despite its prominence in the conceptual framework of biological aging, understanding of how oxidative stress translates to functional decline of the aging nervous system remains incomplete. Here we examine how (per)oxidation of methylene-interrupted polyunsaturated fatty acids[1] (PUFAs) and subsequent activation of members of the phospholipase A_2 (PLA_2) family of fatty acylases may play a central role in declining excitability of aging neurons and age-associated memory impairment (AMI; see **Figure 1** for conceptual framework; see **Figure 2** for mechanisms and potential implications of PUFA peroxidation).

NEUROBIOLOGICAL CORRELATES OF NORMAL AGING

Considerable effort has been put into identifying neurobiological correlates of normal brain aging for several decades. The picture emerging from these studies is that structural and functional changes occurring in the normal aging brain are generally much more low-key and variable than those found in pathological aging brains. The list of physiological and biochemical symptoms of neuronal aging is extensive and includes evidence for oxidative stress, impaired energy and redox metabolism, Ca^{2+} signaling perturbation, accumulating damage to proteins, lipids, nucleic acids and organelles, declining dendritic complexity, alterations in synaptic density, distribution and function, changes in gene regulation, and molecular processes underlying remodeling of synapses (Barnes, 1994; Burke and Barnes, 2006; Mattson and Magnus, 2006; Esiri, 2007; Shankar, 2010; Toescu and Vreugdenhil, 2010; Yeoman et al., 2012).

While cell autonomous processes likely constitute an important facet of neuronal aging, evidence for significant cell non-autonomous (i.e., organismal) dimensions of neuronal aging is growing. For instance, it is evident that brain aging has vascular, immunological and endocrinological dimensions (Joseph et al., 2005; Aïd and Bosetti, 2011; Yirmiya and Goshen, 2011; Alcedo et al., 2013; Rincon and Wright, 2013; Sadagurski and White, 2013; Oakley and Tharakan, 2014; Tarumi and Zhang, 2014).

[1]Key concept 1 | Methylene-interrupted PUFAs. Poly-unsaturated fatty acids with one or more pairs of hydrogen unsaturated carbons in *cis*-arrangement separated by a hydrogen-saturated (bis-allylic) methylene bridge. Because the methylene moiety's bis-allylic C–H bonds are weaker than ordinary C–H bonds they are prone to free radical attack. The main PUFAs with more than one bis-allylic methylene site in the plasmamembranes of neurons are arachidonic acid (AA), docosahexanoic acid (DHA), and eicosapentaenoic acid (EPA).

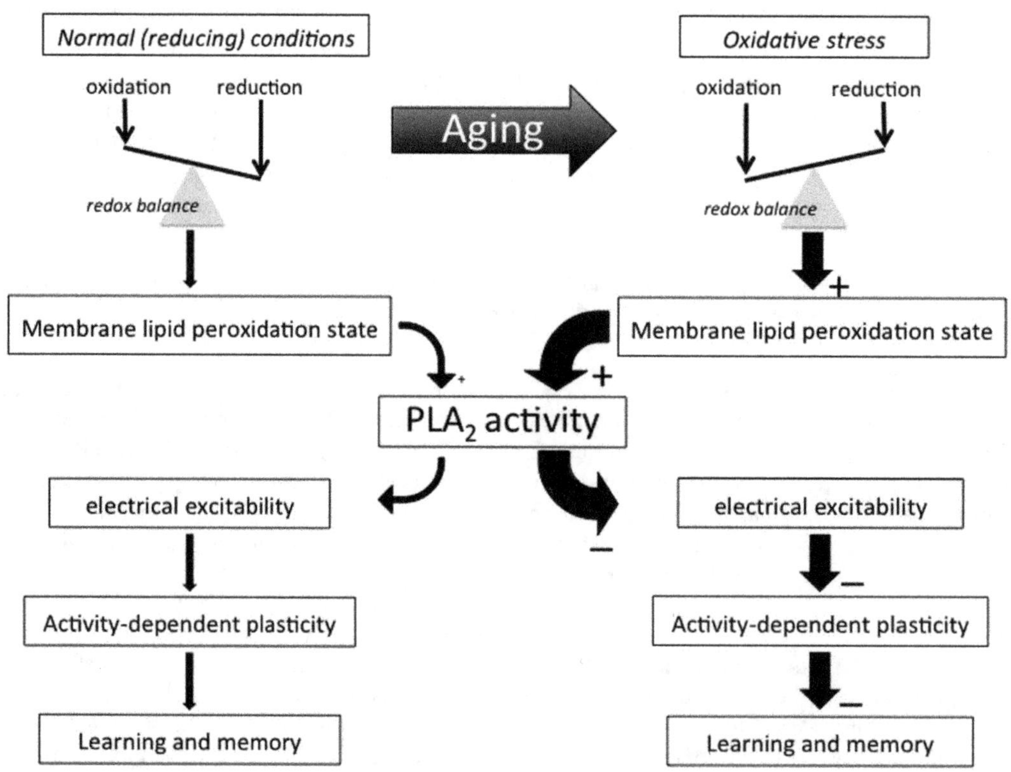

FIGURE 1 | Conceptual framework. This flow diagram outlines key concepts and hypotheses addressed in this essay and illustrate the way we propose they contribute to AMI. Many important biological processes involve redox reactions and many of life's macromolecules are sensitive to electrophilic attacks that may impair their ability to perform their normal functional or structural roles. Few of life's building blocks are as sensitive to oxidation as the poly-unsaturated fatty acids (PUFAs) making up much of cell and organelle membranes. Organisms generate electrophiles like reactive oxygen and nitrogen species as part of many essential live processes, including metabolism, host defense, and intercellular signaling processes. Active maintenance of an appropriate redox balance is therefore of the utmost importance for organismal function and survival. Biological aging tends to be associated with shifts in redox balance away from reducing towards oxidative conditions in many of an organism's molecular, cellular, and organismal systems and domains, including an advanced state of membrane PUFA peroxidation that recruits PLA_2 and induces a (PLA_2-dependent) decline in neuronal excitability and activity-dependent plasticity that manifests itself as AMI.

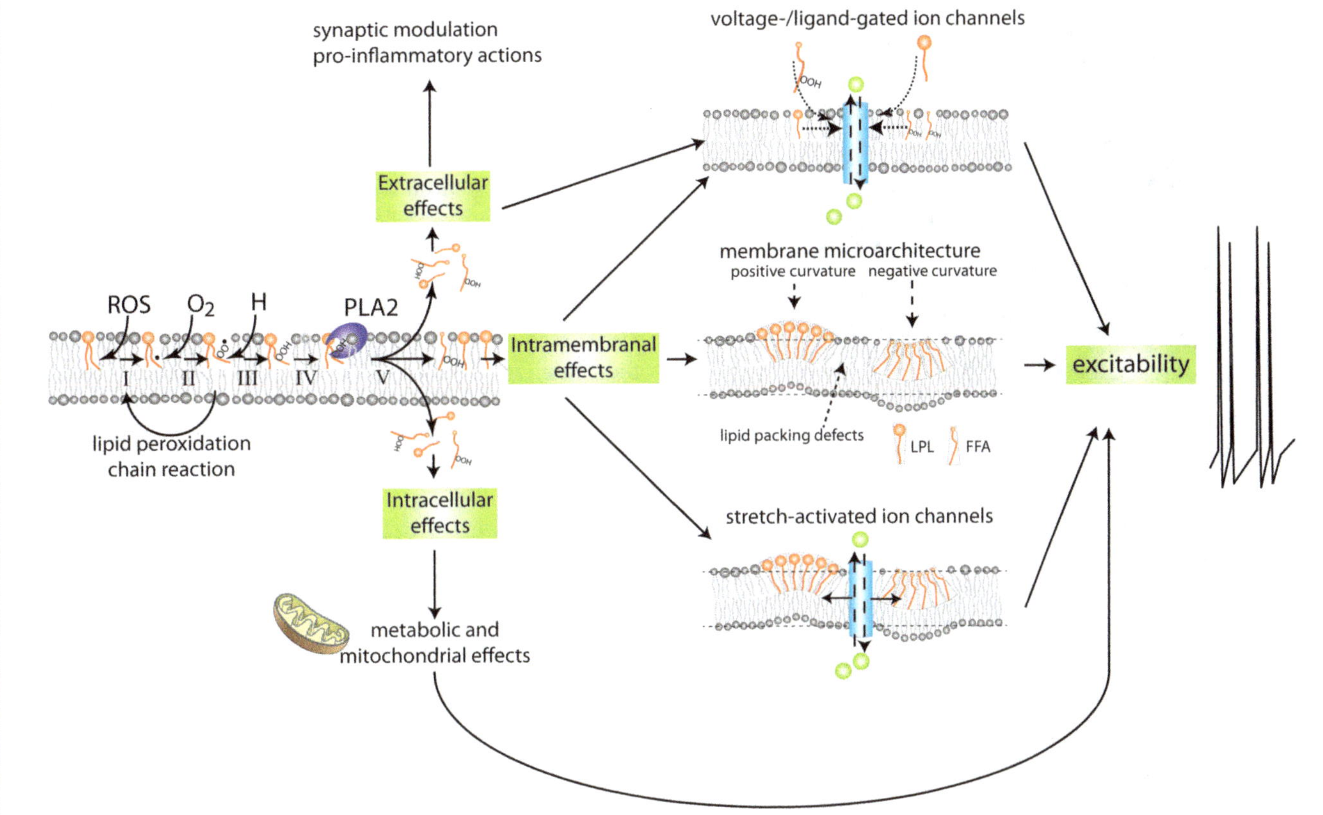

FIGURE 2 | Mechanism and possible implications of membrane lipid peroxidation and phospholipase A_2 activation. PUFAs are highly susceptible to (per)oxidation. Peroxidized PUFAs are prone to excision by members of the PLA_2 family of enzymes. The products of PLA_2's enzymatic activity, free fatty acids (FFAs) and lysophospholipids (LPLs), have a wide range of extracellular, intracellular, and intramembranal biological activities. This highly simplified diagram indicates a few of the mechanisms and targets with special relevance to the nervous system. FFAs and LPLs can themselves act as signaling molecules and modify gating behavior of various types of ion channels. In addition they can act as substrate for other lipid-based intra- and extracellular signaling cascades, including signaling systems regulating inflammation. Moreover, through their effect on membrane microarchitecture they may change functions of integral membrane proteins such as stretch-activated ion channels, alter lipid micro domain organization, disrupt organization of transmembrane signaling complexes, or alter other cellular processes such as membrane fission and fusion that are important in the regulation of intrinsic neuronal excitability, synaptic transmission, and molecular mechanisms underlying neuronal plasticity. See **Figure 6** for details on mechanisms involved in PUFA peroxidation.

One particularly intriguing organismal dimension to normal brain aging emerging in recent decades is the concept that the brain at least in part regulates its own destiny through insulin-like peptide signaling systems coupling nutrient availability and dietary conditions to the control of cell and organismal metabolism (e.g., Alcedo et al., 2013; Sadagurski and White, 2013). Furthermore, while there seems little doubt that many of the phenomena associated with neuronal aging are of a deteriorative nature, evidence for functional preservation and compensation has also been reported (see Barnes, 1994; Burke and Barnes, 2006 for review).

THE NEED FOR SIMPLIFICATION: *Lymnaea stagnalis* AS A MODEL FOR INTEGRATIVE MOLECULE-TO-BEHAVIOR INVESTIGATIONS OF NEURONAL AND BEHAVIORAL AGING

How all dietary, (bio)chemical, metabolic, molecular, cellular, physiological, system-, and organismal-level processes factor into biological aging of neurons and the nervous system and contribute to AMI remains one of the most important unsolved puzzles of neuroscience. Answering fundamental questions of this kind in a system as complex, dynamic, and inherently adaptive as the nervous system is not a trivial problem. With the goal of reducing the complexity of such undertaking, we adopted the pond snail *L. stagnalis* as our research platform (**Figure 3**). Since *Lymnaea* is not as widely known as other model systems in neuronal aging and AMI we will briefly summarize its most relevant features before continuing with the main focus of this review.

Lymnaea stagnalis is a freshwater pulmonate snail with a long and varied track record as a model system in a wide range of basic and applied biological research, including the study of behavioral, neural, and molecular aspects of associative learning and memory. It has a relatively simple central nervous system (CNS, **Figure 4**) of about 20,000–25,000 neurons organized in 11 ganglia. The CNS contains many individually identifiable neurons and well-mapped, behaviorally characterized neural circuits supporting direct behavior-to-molecule inferences about the foundations of neuronal function and dysfunction (see for instance Benjamin et al., 2000; Taylor and Lukowiak, 2000; Brembs, 2003; Benjamin

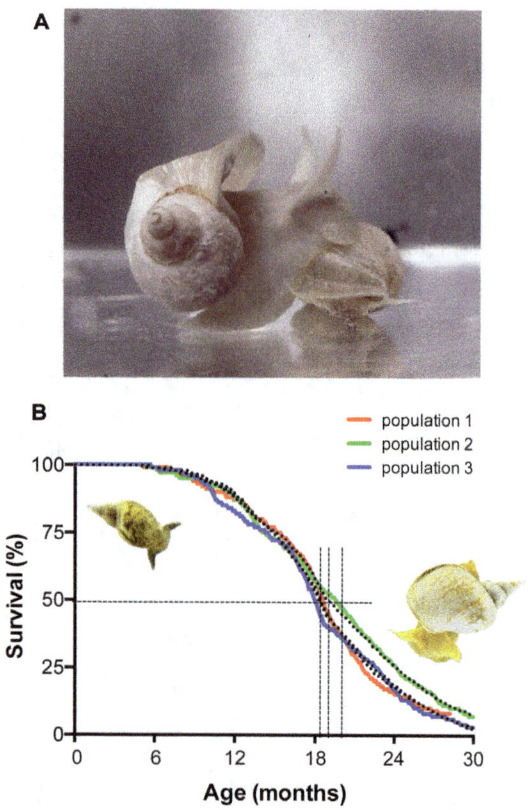

FIGURE 3 | *Lymnaea stagnalis*, the animal and its survival characteristics. (A) *L. stagnalis* is an obligate freshwater aquatic gastropod of the clade *Euthyneura*. The animals are bimodal breathers capable of absorbing oxygen through their skin and through ventilating a simple lung cavity to air. **(B)** Survival characteristics of populations of *Lymnaea* held in our aquatic facility. Shown are the census data for three different populations, representative for normal population survival in the facility (colored lines) fitted by a Weibull power law failure model (dotted lines). Under the conditions in our facility the median population age hovers around 1.5 years (vertical dotted lines median age ± 95% confidence interval) and individual maximum age routinely exceeds 2 years. Under standard culture conditions we maintain in our in house facility (i.e., *ad libitum* feeding of standard diet at 17–19°C water temperature under a 12:12 light:dark regimen) survival characteristics of healthy captive populations show very little variation and reach an average median age of 593 ± 13 days and average maximal age of 880 ± 10 days (arithmetic means ± SE of the mean, $n = 15$; for more details on aquaculture conditions see Watson et al., 2012a).

and Kemenes, 2010) including the biochemical, molecular, cell biological, and physiological foundations of neuronal aging and AMI.

Under laboratory conditions, *Lymnaea* can be effectively reared to ages and quantities required for aging research. Depending on variables like feeding regimen, animal density, day length and water temperature, the maximal age of the animals routinely exceeds 2.5 years with median ages of around 1.5 years under these conditions and age-dependent mortality follows Gompertz and Weibull survival characteristics indicative of aging (**Figure 3B**; see also Janse et al., 1988; Slob and Janse, 1988).

Lymnaea's application in aging studies dates back to the 1980s with the publication of several neurophysiological studies (Frolkis et al., 1984; Nagy et al., 1985; Janse et al., 1986), the first report of age effects on associative memory performance (Audesirk et al., 1982) and work on the general biology and population-level aspects of the species' aging process (Janse et al., 1988; Slob and Janse, 1988). Since then publications on various cell biological, endocrinological, neurophysiological, biophysical, behavioral, and reproductive aspects of aging in *Lymnaea* have appeared (Frolkis et al., 1989, 1991; Janse et al., 1989, 1999; Wildering et al., 1991; Klaassen et al., 1998; Janse and van der Roest, 2001; Arundell et al., 2006; Patel et al., 2006, 2010). Its use in research of the molecular and cellular foundations of AMI started in earnest with Hermann et al. (2007) followed by a series of other publications from our laboratory linking AMI and neuronal excitability changes to oxidative stress, inflammation, lipid peroxidation and declining glutathione (GSH) availability, and identifying PLA_2 as a central player in these phenomena (Watson et al., 2012a,b, 2013, 2014; Hermann et al., 2013; Beaulieu et al., 2014).

Lymnaea has quite a broad behavioral and sensory repertoire and can be taught to change many of its behaviors in response to a variety of chemical, mechanical, and even visual cues (Audesirk et al., 1982; Lukowiak et al., 1996; Sakakibara et al., 1998; Kawai et al., 2004; reviewed in Benjamin et al., 2000; Brembs, 2003; Lukowiak et al., 2006; Benjamin, 2012). Neurobiological substrates of several behavioral paradigms of associative learning and memory have been well characterized. In recent decades most research has focused on two training paradigms: classical conditioning of the animals' feeding behavior, a paradigm with critical involvement of a pair of interneurons called cerebral giant cells (CGCs), and operant conditioning of their aerial respiration, a paradigm with a multi-modal neuron called right pedal dorsal 1 (RPeD1) at its center (**Figures 4** and **5**; Spencer et al., 1999; Staras et al., 1999; for detailed review on the mechanisms and circuitry underlying these behaviors and learning paradigms see Benjamin et al., 2000; Brembs, 2003; Lukowiak et al., 2006; Benjamin, 2012). Using these two learning models, detailed insights in the molecular, cellular, neuronal network, and behavioral aspects of learning and memory have been obtained (Ribeiro et al., 2003, 2005; Kemenes et al., 2006a; Nikitin et al., 2006; Sadamoto et al., 2010; Wan et al., 2010; Dalesman and Lukowiak, 2012; Rosenegger and Lukowiak, 2013; reviewed in Benjamin et al., 2000 and Benjamin, 2012). Importantly, these studies show that, like other invertebrates, *Lymnaea* learning shares many key behavioral, molecular, and functional facets with learning in vertebrate model systems.

LIPID MEMBRANES AS A KEY THEATER OF AGING AND AGE-ASSOCIATED DECLINE OF THE NERVOUS SYSTEM

A large body of evidence indicates that oxidative stress is a prominent feature of both pathological and non-pathological forms of nervous system aging (Choi, 1995; Mattson and Magnus, 2006; Torres et al., 2011; Lopez et al., 2013; Orr et al., 2013; Haddadi et al., 2014). How oxidative stress contributes to age-associated disease processes of the brain and translates to functional decline of normal healthy aging neurons is not well understood. Here we explore the theory that processes associated with the high level of unsaturation of the lipid portion of neuronal membrane

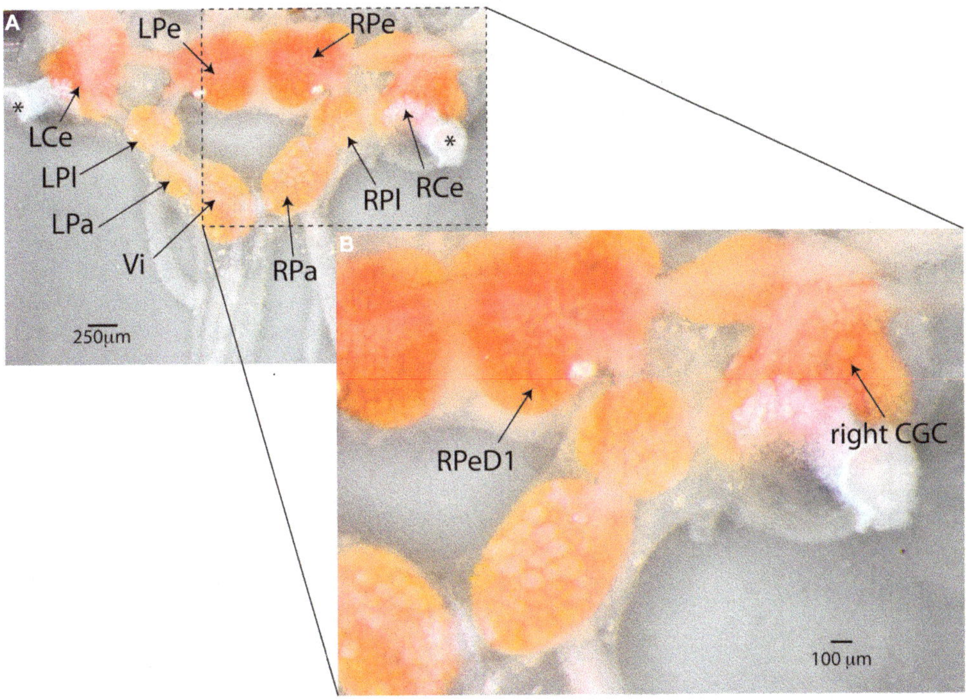

FIGURE 4 | *Lymnaea's* central nervous system and its identified neurons. (A) *Lymnaea's* central nervous system (CNS) is comprised of a circumesophagal ganglionic ring made up of nine ganglia plus two buccal ganglia that are not part of the inner ganglionic ring (LCe, left cerebral ganglion; RCe, right cerebral ganglion; LPe, left pedal ganglion; RPe, right pedal ganglion; LPl, left pleural ganglion; RPl, right pleural ganglion; LPa, left parietal ganglion; RPa, right parietal ganglion; Vi, visceral ganglion; the paired left and right buccal ganglia are not shown in this image. To expose location of neurons discussed in this paper, the cerebral commissure connecting LCe and RCe has been cut and LCe and RCe have been folded out laterally). Inside the ganglia somata of many neurons can be recognized. Many of these neurons are individually identifiable. **(B)** Enlargement of the boxed area in **(A)** showing the location of the two identified neurons that are the main focus of the paper. Right pedal dorsal 1 (RPeD1), located on dorsal surface of the RPe ganglion is a multi-modal neuron involved in the control of *Lymnaea's* aerial respiration and an important locus of operant-conditioning induced plasticity of the animals' respiratory behavior. The cerebral giant cell (GCG) indicated here is one of a bilaterally symmetrical pair of interneurons instrumental in the control of *Lymnaea's* feeding behavior. The CGCs are important loci of reward-conditioning of the animals feeding behavior. These composite images were generated from 15–20 images taken at different focal depths using DMap focus stacking algorithm in Zerene Stacker build T201404082055 (Zerene Systems, Richland, WA, USA).

constitute a key link between aging, oxidative stress, and the age-associated physiological and behavioral decline frequently observed in normal healthy aging animals and the etiology of age-associated disorders of the brain. Central to this idea are the inordinate sensitivity of methylene-interrupted PUFAs to electrophilic attacks and subsequent activation of PLA_2's, a family of enzymes involved in maintenance of membrane phospholipid integrity and membrane-associated lipid signaling processes (**Figure 2**).

Eukaryote cell and organelle membranes are functionally complex, dynamically regulated assemblies of mostly glycerophospholipids, fatty acids (FAs), sterols, proteins, glycoproteins, and glycolipids (Alberts et al., 2002). While most of life's structures are sensitive to oxidation, few are as susceptible to oxidative damage as phospholipid bilayer membranes (Zimniak, 2011). This elevated susceptibility to oxidation is due to a number of factors that conspire, as a manner of speaking, to create "perfect storm" conditions. First, under normal conditions solubility of molecular oxygen and many reactive oxygen and nitrogen species (RONS) in the lipid microenvironment of membranes is quite high (Subczynski and Wisniewska, 2000). Second, as mentioned, PUFAs are inordinately sensitive to attack by RONS and other electrophiles (Hulbert et al., 2007). Third, PUFAs that have undergone free radical attack are themselves reactive free radicals and are, because of the tightly packed molecular arrangement of phospholipids in bilayer membranes, capable of propagating potentially catastrophic lipid peroxidation cascades (Forlenza et al., 2007; Ballatori et al., 2009; Currais and Maher, 2013; Sultana et al., 2013). Neuronal membranes contain high levels of PUFAs such as arachidonic acids (AA), docosahexaenoic acids (DHA), and eicosapentaenoic acids (EPA), and are therefore particularly sensitive to (per)oxidation making lipid peroxidation potentially one of the major instruments of free radical-mediated injury and cell death in the nervous system.

Parenthetically, the idea that phospholipid membranes are one of the primary molecular theaters of aging and longevity has gained substantial traction in recent decades (for reviews see Pamplona, 2008; Zimniak, 2011). In fact, the observation that the level of lipid membrane unsaturation correlates inversely with longevity in mammals, birds, and even invertebrates led to formulation of the "Membrane hypothesis of aging" which essentially sees lipid

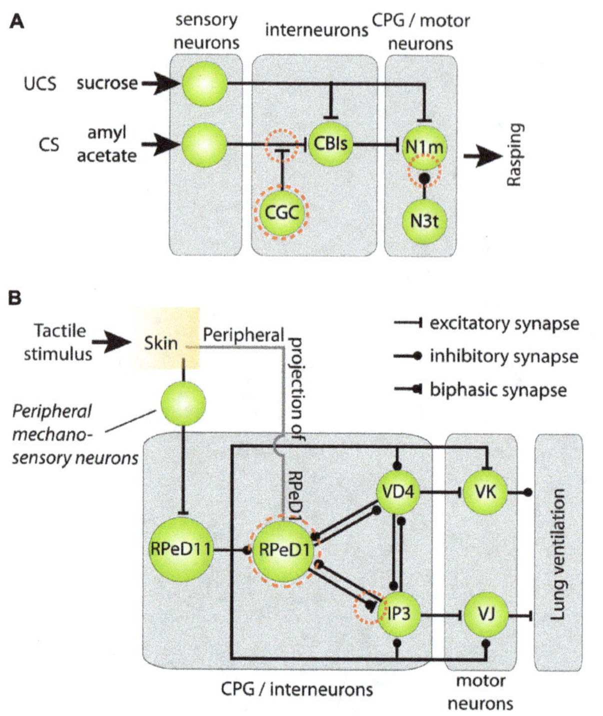

FIGURE 5 | Cellular models of classical reward and operant aversive conditioning in *Lymnaea*. (A) Parsimonious model of the neural mechanisms underlying classical chemical reward conditioning of *Lymnaea's* feeding behavior. Behavioral conditioning by peripheral application of sucrose as unconditioned stimulus (UCS) and amylacetate as conditioned stimulus (CS) induces a delayed persistent depolarization of the cerebral giant cells (CGC). This depolarization facilitates throughput of peripheral CS connections with cerebral-buccal interneurons (CBIs) thereby gating throughput of the CS to Neuron 1 medial (N1m) interneurons of the feeding circuit's central pattern generator (CPG) that play a pivotal role in the initiation of the three phase rasping cycle. At the same time, the spike frequency of the CPG interneuron N3t is reduced after behaviorally conditioning thereby releasing N1m from its inhibition. **(B)** Parsimonious model of the neural mechanisms underlying aversive operant conditioning of *Lymnaea's* aerial respiratory behavior. Aerial respiration involves opening and closing of an orifice giving access to the lung cavity (the pneumostome). The CPG driving the animals' aerial respiration behavior consists of three identified interneurons: right pedal dorsal 1 (RPeD1), visceral dorsal 4 (VD4) and (wide-acting) input 3 neuron (IP3). Spiking activity in RPeD1 initiates rhythmic pattern of spiking activity in VD4 and IP3 that in turn trigger electrical activity in, respectively, Visceral K (VK) pneumostome closer motor neurons and visceral J (VJ) pneumostome opener motor neurons. Aversive operant conditioning through tactile stimulation of the pneumostome area induces a hyperpolarization of RPeD1 and reduces the latter's ability to trigger rhythmic activity in IP3. Mechanosensory conditioning of the respiratory CPG's electrical activity through tactile stimulation of the pneumostome area involves both afferent projections of RPeD1 ("peripheral projections of RPeD1") and excitation of the 'whole-body withdrawal interneuron' RPeD11 by identified mechanosensory neurons. Dashed red circles in both circuit diagrams indicate neural loci of plasticity. Circuit diagrams shown were adapted from Benjamin et al. (2000), Taylor and Lukowiak (2000) and Benjamin and Kemenes (2010).

membranes as one of the weakest and therefore highest maintenance links in the biochemical armature of living organisms (Hulbert et al., 2007; Ungvari et al., 2011, 2013; Munro and Blier, 2012; Munro et al., 2013).

LIPID PEROXIDATION INDUCED PHOSPHOLIPASE A_2 ACTIVITY AND ITS CONSEQUENCES

One characteristic cellular response triggered by lipid peroxidation is activation of one or more PLA_2 family members that catalyze cleavage of FAs from the sn-2 position of glycero-phospholipids in plasma- and organelle membranes (Brown et al., 2003; Sun et al., 2004; Farooqui and Horrocks, 2006; Chen et al., 2008; Dennis et al., 2011). Although the precise underlying molecular mechanisms of lipid-peroxidation induced PLA_2 activation are still a matter of debate (see for instance Greenberg et al., 2008), it is generally thought to involve peroxidation induced changes in fatty acyl chain geometry (Niki, 1990; Salgo et al., 1992; Rashba-Step et al., 1997; Greenberg et al., 2008).

Activation of PLA_2 leads to the production of (peroxidized) free FAs (FFAs) and lysophospholipids (LPLs), both classes of molecules with potentially substantial biological activity (**Figure 6**; see below; Brown et al., 2003; Farooqui and Horrocks, 2006). For example, the molecular geometry of LPLs and FFAs is quite different from their mutual parent molecule (i.e., a phospholipid). They may therefore also cause changes in the micro-architecture and biophysical properties of phospholipid membranes and potentially affect membrane-associated signaling functions (**Figure 2**; Yu et al., 1992; Choi and Yu, 1995; Choe et al., 1995; Patel et al., 2001; reviewed in Piomelli et al., 2007). In addition, PLA_2 mediated FFA liberation is the starting point for the generation of an extensive array of lipid-based neuromodulators. That includes FFAs themselves (e.g., AA and DHA) and LPLs (e.g., lysolecithin) but also encompasses an extensive array of biologically active molecules such as eicosanoids, isoprostanes, and neuroprostanes generated by a variety of lipid metabolizing pathways. Many of these pathways act as direct effectors of signal transduction in the nervous system through either direct interaction with ion channels or binding to G-protein-coupled or nuclear receptors (reviewed in Piomelli et al., 2007; Sultana et al., 2013).

Poly-unsaturated fatty acid peroxidation generally also leads to the formation of electrophilic aldehydes such as acrolein, malondialdehyde (MDA), 4-hydroxy-2-nonenal (4-HNE; Pamplona, 2008, 2011). These highly reactive aldehydes can seriously compromise molecular integrity of cells and tissues through the formation of molecular adducts with phospholipids, proteins, and DNA. However, recent evidence suggests that these lipid-derived aldehydes may also induce adaptive responses driven to decrease oxidative damage and improve antioxidant defenses (see for instance Pizzimenti et al., 2013).

ANTIOXIDANT DEFENSES

Organisms are not defenseless against the actions of pro-oxidants. Rather, they posses a wide and varied array of enzymatic and non-enzymatic instruments to defend their structures and functions against oxidation that includes catalases, peroxidases, and dismutases, the GSH system and various other non-enzymatic anti-oxidants like vitamin C and vitamin E.

ENZYMATIC MECHANISMS

Because of its relatively low redox potential and high abundance, the tripeptide GSH is a versatile anti-oxidant involved as primary

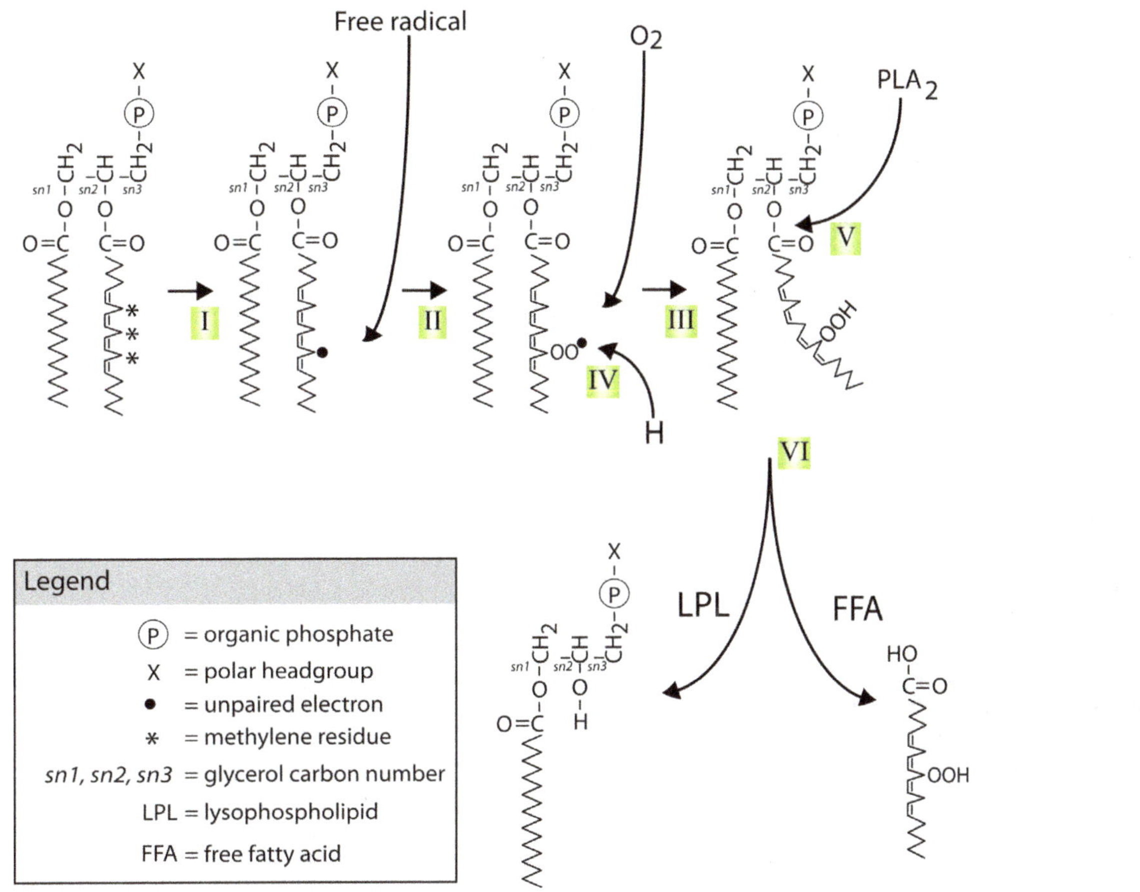

FIGURE 6 | Mechanisms of PUFAs peroxidation and hydrolysis. Neuronal glycerophospholipids contain high levels of methylene-separated PUFAs such as the 20:4 omega-6 fatty acid arachidonic acid (AA) shown attached at the second carbon of the phospholipid glycerol backbone (the sn-2 position) in the diagram. These PUFAs are very sensitive to free radical attack at their bis-allylic C-H bonds (indicated by *) and subsequent (per)oxidation. This process starts with (I) the formation of a C-centered radical (indicated by •) followed by (II) recombination with molecular oxygen that is normally present in abundance in lipid bilayers. The lipid peroxide radicals formed in step II can start a peroxidation chain reaction unless (IV) defused by reduction through for instance donation of a proton by vitamin E or neutralization by other chemical mechanisms. Peroxidation of these PUFAs (V) recruits members of the PLA_2 family of phospholipases. PLA_2 mediated hydrolysis of peroxidized PUFAs (VI) generates peroxidized FFAs and LPLs.

redox buffering of many intra- and extra-cellular compartments, including lipid membranes, and mitochondria (Mari et al., 2009; Ribas et al., 2014). In addition to its antioxidant actions, GSH also plays an important role in detoxification processes, including the detoxification of potentially harmful products of lipid peroxidation such as aforementioned aldehydes. This process is mediated by members of the glutathione-S-transferase (GST) family of enzymes (Zimniak, 2008; Ribas et al., 2014). GSH is one of the most abundant molecules in healthy cells and tissues. Its availability is a function of usage, *de novo* synthesis and redox regeneration. The rate-determining step in GSH synthesis is catalyzed by the enzyme γ-glutamylcysteine synthetase (GCL; Chen et al., 2005; Genovese et al., 2007). Perturbation of GCL activity has been shown to significantly reduce GSH availability. In the context of the current focus of lipid bilayer redox homeostasis as a instrument of neuronal aging it is thought provoking that several studies report age-related declines in in GSH levels and GCL activity in various cell types, including neurons (Toroser and Sohal, 2005, 2007; Zhu et al., 2006; Jacob et al., 2013; Watson et al., 2014). This suggests that anti-oxidant failure either with or without escalation of pro-oxidant activity may be a key facet of the progressive lipid peroxidation stress characteristic of aging.

NON-ENZYMATIC MECHANISMS

Non-enzymatic antioxidants such as Vitamins A, C, and E also play key roles in the defense against oxidative stress, including the maintenance of membrane redox homeostasis. Of these three vitamin families, Vitamin E is considered the major antioxidant present in membranes. Vitamin E is comprised of two families of closely related lipid-soluble compounds, the tocopherols, and tocotrienols. Alpha-tocopherol is the most abundant Vitamin E analog and according to recent insights has a preference for non-lipid raft PUFA-containing domains (Atkinson et al., 2010; Lemaire-Ewing et al., 2010). Alpha-tocopherol associates with membranes such that its active hydroxyl moiety is located at the lipid/water interface and not within the hydrocarbon matrix (Marquardt et al., 2013). As a consequence, α-tocopherol appears to exert its anti-oxidant activity at the surface of a membrane, possibly through the interception of diffusing ROS, or by means of terminating lipid radicals (Marquardt et al., 2013).

NON-TRADITIONAL, NON-ANTIOXIDANT ACTIONS OF α-TOCOPHEROLS

In addition, several studies provide an alternative, non-antioxidant, scenario for α-tocopherol's beneficial effects. That is, it is suggested that incorporation of α-tocopherols in membranes can structurally stabilize the membrane against lipid-peroxidation induced curvature stresses or normalize fatty acid signaling by acting as FFA trap through its ability to form hydrogen-bridges and engage in Vanderwaals interactions with FFAs (Atkinson et al., 2008; Lemaire-Ewing et al., 2010; Marquardt et al., 2013). Especially α-tocopherol's acyl tail has been shown to play a critical role in its membrane stabilizing effect (Kagan, 1989). Methylation of this hydroxyl group disrupts α-tocopherol's ability to engage in hydrogen-bridge formations. In this respect it is interesting to note that work from our lab shows that only non-methylated α-tocopherol is capable of reversing a decline in neuronal excitability due to age- or experimentally induced oxidative stress (Watson et al., 2012b).

LIPID PEROXIDATION AND (BRAIN) AGING

Considering that neuronal membranes tend to have a high PUFA content it is not surprising that lipid peroxidation and its byproducts are increasingly implicated in brain aging. For instance, accumulation of MDA, 4-HNE, acrolein is commonly reported in aged brains of vertebrate and invertebrate model systems (Terman and Brunk, 2006; Zhu et al., 2006; Watson et al., 2012b). Moreover, PLA_2s are also increasingly implicated in normal brain aging and the etiology of age-associated neurodegenerative disorders (Farooqui and Horrocks, 2006; Ong et al., 2010). How the products of PLA_2 activity exert their detrimental effects in the aging brain is, however, not always clear but may involve one or more of the scenarios outlined in the preceding sections.

INTRINSIC ELECTRICAL PROPERTIES AS A SUBSTRATE OF PLASTICITY

This review focuses on the role of intrinsic excitability of neurons in age-associated decline in behavioral plasticity. Decades of research on the cellular and molecular foundations of learning and memory have led to a "synapse-centric" view of learning and memory mechanisms that holds that memories are formed and stored through activity-dependent alterations of synaptic strength and neuronal circuit architecture (Bliss and Collingridge, 1993; Kandel, 2001). In this context non-synaptic mechanisms of plasticity, i.e., mechanisms involving changes in intrinsic electrical properties of neurons, have received much less attention. Yet, experimental evidence that changes in intrinsic neuronal electrical properties could be serving as part or whole of an engram beyond merely facilitating activity-dependent synaptic modulation goes back as far as the 1970s and the concept has gained substantial traction in recent years (reviewed in Benjamin et al., 2008; Mozzachiodi and Byrne, 2010; Sehgal et al., 2013; D'Angelo, 2014; for review of early work in this area see Byrne, 1987). For example, numerous studies have shown that eye blink trace conditioning in rodents induces an increase in intrinsic excitability of hippocampal CA1 and CA3 neurons through reduction of spike frequency adaptation caused by action potential afterhyperpolarizations (AHP) mediated by Ca^{2+}-dependent outward K^+ currents[2] (Coulter et al., 1989; Moyer et al., 1992, 2000; Disterhoft et al., 1996; Thompson et al., 1996; Oh et al., 2010; Sehgal et al., 2014; for review, see Christian and Thompson, 2003). There is also substantial evidence of non-synaptic forms of plasticity in invertebrates, particularly in gastropod mollusks. For instance, Alkon (1974, 1979) demonstrated that associative learning in the nudibranch snail *Hermissenda crasicornis* involved an increase in excitability of type B photo-receptor cell associated with a decrease in the types of voltage- and Ca^{2+}-sensitive K^+ currents mediating the AHP and spike frequency adaptation. In *Lymnaea*, long-term memory (LTM) for classical conditioning of feeding has been associated with a persistent Na^+-current dependent depolarization of the CGCs, two interneurons that act as gate-keepers to the feeding circuit and that play an essential role in chemosensory behavioral conditioning of the animals feeding behavior (Jones et al., 2003; Kemenes et al., 2006b; Nikitin et al., 2008, 2013). In the marine gastropod *Aplysia californica*, changes in intrinsic excitability of identified neurons in the central pattern-generating (CPG) network for feeding have been associated with the network's behavioral conditioning induced motor output (Sieling et al., 2014).

More examples of non-synaptic plasticity can be found in the literature (see reviews by Byrne, 1987; Benjamin et al., 2008; Mozzachiodi and Byrne, 2010; Sehgal et al., 2013; D'Angelo, 2014). For the purpose of the current review it is suffice to say that the idea of intrinsic excitability regulation as a non-synaptic instrument of plasticity is now on firmer ground than ever before. The balance of this paper focuses on the idea that the mechanisms controlling intrinsic neuronal excitability, particularly those underlying the control of repetitive action potential firing, are a key target of oxidative stress-associated aging processes and a root cause of functional decline of normal aging neurons and brains.

EVIDENCE FOR AGE-ASSOCIATED ALTERATIONS IN INTRINSIC ELECTRICAL PROPERTIES

Considering that neuronal electrical excitability is fundamental to brain function, substantial research on the neurobiological basis of behavioral aging has focused on the possibility that aging neurons undergo changes in intrinsic excitability. Neuronal excitability is

[2]Spike frequency adaptation, Action potential afterhyperpolarization (AHP), Ca^{2+}-activated K^+ currents – Spike frequency adaptation is a process by which the action potential firing rate of a neuron declines with time despite the maintenance of a constant excitatory stimulus. The action potential of most neurons is followed by an HP, a period of varying length of time during which the cells' membrane potential is lower than the resting potential preceding the action potential and during which the cell is less excitable than before. Various ionic mechanisms may contribute to the AHP including a class of outward K^+ currents activated either exclusively or in part by increase of intracellular free Ca^{2+} levels (i.e., Ca^{2+}-activated K^+ currents). The AHP as part of a negative feedback loop linking spiking frequency and opening of voltage-gated Ca^{2+} channels to activation of inhibitory Ca^{2+}-activated K^+ currents is a key component of spike frequency adaptation in most neurons (see Lewis et al., 1986; Sah, 1996; Sah and Davies, 2000 for more detail).

a complex function of a neuron's shape, the repertoire, distribution, and density of voltage- and ligand-gated ion channels in their plasma-membrane, the activity of ion pumps and various intra- and extracellular signaling systems and state variables, including intracellular Ca^{2+}-, metabolic-, and redox homeostasis (Bean, 2007; Beck and Yaari, 2008; Vacher et al., 2008; Nusser, 2012). There is evidence for age-associated changes in many of these parameters. It is beyond the scope of this paper to review this vast and diverse literature. For a more in-depth treatment of this subject the reader is referred to many excellent reviews available in this area (see Barnes, 1994; Burke and Barnes, 2006; Mattson and Magnus, 2006; Chawla and Barnes, 2007; Thibault et al., 2007; Mattson et al., 2008; Oh et al., 2010; Toescu and Vreugdenhil, 2010; Yeoman et al., 2012). Instead in the next paragraphs we briefly review key insights gained from vertebrate and invertebrate model systems suggesting that intensification of spike frequency adaptation mechanisms is an important facet of the normal neuronal aging process.

EVIDENCE FROM VERTEBRATE MODEL SYSTEMS

Most of the work on age-related intrinsic neuronal excitability changes in vertebrates has been done on the rodent hippocampus. On balance, the evidence from a large body of *in vitro* electrophysiological studies on different hippocampal regions of young and old mice, rats and rabbits suggest that most intrinsic neuronal electrical properties such as resting membrane potential, membrane time constant, input resistance, rheobase current, action potential threshold, and various aspects of action potential dynamics change very little across the lifespan (reviewed in Barnes, 1994; Burke and Barnes, 2006; Chawla and Barnes, 2007). However, "*a number of consistent changes do occur*" (Barnes, 1994). One of those changes involves alterations in voltage-gated Ca^{2+} currents, intracellular Ca^{2+}-homeostasis, Ca^{2+}-activated outward K^{+} currents and interactions between them enhancing the AHP and associated spike frequency adaptation of older neurons (Moyer et al., 1992; Tombaugh et al., 2005; reviewed in Oh et al., 2010). It should be noted, however, that even though the *in vitro* evidence for a role of these mechanisms in cognitive decline associated with normal brain aging is compelling, the idea is not undisputed (for review of this issue, see Burke and Barnes, 2006). Other studies report changes in voltage-activated Ca^{2+}- or Na^{+}-channel properties to age-associated decline in intrinsic excitability of various types of rodent neurons (Scott et al., 1988; Randall et al., 2012; Branch et al., 2014; for review see Annunziato et al., 2002; Foster, 2012).

EVIDENCE FROM INVERTEBRATE MODEL SYSTEMS

Several studies, particularly in gastropod mollusks, have looked into the question of intrinsic neuronal excitability changes in invertebrate neurons. For example, Frolkis et al. (1991, 1995) reported increased voltage-gated Ca^{2+} current densities and changes in other aspects of intrinsic electrical excitability in aged *Lymnaea* neurons. The same group reported changes in voltage-gated K^{+} currents amplitudes and inactivation kinetics in old *Lymnaea* neurons (Frolkis et al., 1989). Patel et al. (2006) reported a decline in intrinsic excitability associated with a decline in input resistance and an increase in AHP magnitude and duration in CGGs of older *Lymnaea* and Klaassen et al. (1998) observed a decline in excitability associated with a reduction in input resistance in aging RPeD1. We observed a decline in intrinsic excitability of CGCs in aged learning-impaired older animals and concluded that "*this decline in excitability is not due to changes in passive neurophysiological properties but rather involves alterations in active properties of the cells*" (Hermann et al., 2007). An age-associated decline in input resistance associated with lengthening membrane time constant was reported for at least three identified neurons in *Aplysia* (Rattan and Peretz, 1981).

Age-associated neurophysiological changes linked to behavioral impairment have been demonstrated in *Caenorhabditis elegans*, *Aplysia*, and *Lymnaea*. For instance, using a classical reward conditioning learning paradigm, we demonstrated in *Lymnaea* that a selective age-related impairment of appetitive LTM is associated with a decline in intrinsic excitability of the CGCs that is reflected in more pronounced spike frequency adaptation (**Figure 7**; Hermann et al., 2007). Along a similar vein, we also showed that age-related LTM impairment in aerial respiration operant-conditioning model is associated with enhanced spike frequency adaptation properties of RPeD1, an interneuron instrumental in the execution of this behavior and one of the cellular substrates of LTM in this learning paradigm (Watson et al., 2013). In addition, Janse et al. (1999) showed a correlation between reproductive senescence and reduced electrical excitability of the caudodorsal cells (CDCs), neuroendocrine cells producing *Lymnaea's* ovulation hormone and other neuropeptides involved in the regulation of reproductive behavior (Janse et al., 1999). In *Aplysia*, studies from the Peretz lab and a recent study by Kempsell and Fieber (2014) have linked age-associated behavioral and homeostatic deficiencies to declining neuronal excitability (Rattan and Peretz, 1981; Peretz, 1988; Skinner and Peretz, 1989). Interestingly, in the nematode *C. elegans* age-associated decline in chemotactic behavior is associated with a decline in sensory neuron excitability due to oxidation-induced enhancement of voltage-gated K^{+} currents (Cai and Sesti, 2009; Sesti et al., 2010).

HOW DOES OXIDATIVE STRESS CONTRIBUTE TO DECLINING EXCITABILITY OF AGING NEURONS?

How oxidative stress translates into functional decline and increased vulnerability to disease of the aging brain is only partly understood (Mattson and Magnus, 2006). First it should be noted that in the context of redox modulation of neuronal functions many pro-oxidants have both "good" and a "bad" aspects. For instance, under normal conditions pro-oxidants like RONS play important physiological roles in synaptic plasticity and memory formation (reviewed in Massaad and Klann, 2011; Milton and Sweeney, 2011). Yet, under conditions of oxidative stress the same mechanisms may affect neuronal plasticity and memory function in a negative manner (Hu et al., 2006; Negre-Salvayre et al., 2010; Massaad and Klann, 2011; Niki, 2012).

Second, many of the molecular instruments of neuronal excitability (i.e., membrane ion channels, receptors, vesicle fusion processes) are susceptible to oxidation or sensitive to alterations in cellular redox status (Annunziato et al., 2002; Dukoff et al.,

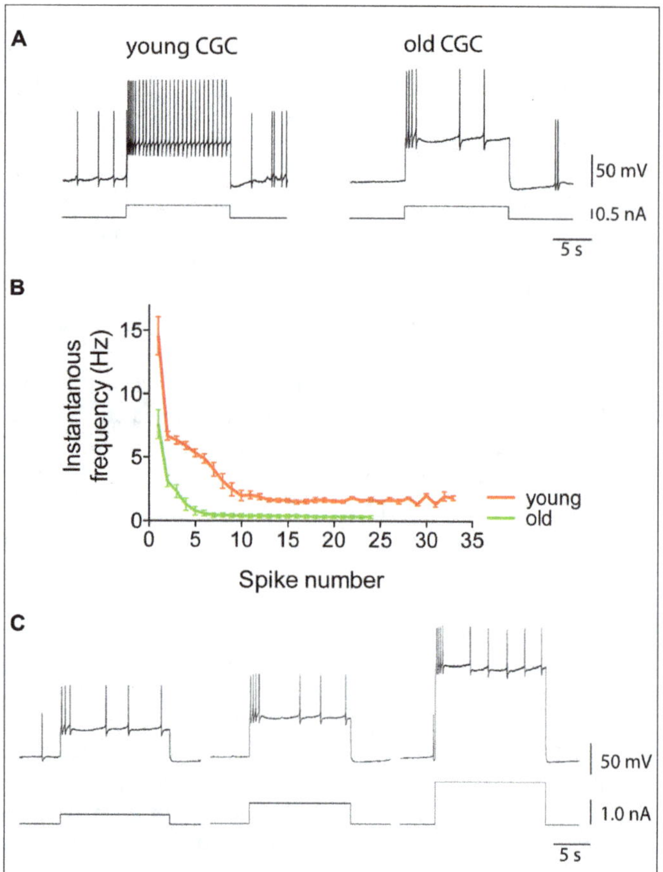

FIGURE 7 | Intrinsic electrical excitability of *Lymnaea* neurons declines with age. Using CGCs as example, this figure illustrates the characteristic age-associated enhancement of spike frequency adaptation that is also observed in other identified *Lymnaea* neurons, including RPeD1 (see for instance Watson et al., 2012b, 2013). **(A)** This figure shows examples of intracellular recordings of spiking activity evoked in young and old CGCs by injection of 0.5 nA depolarizing current. Identical current injection results in a non-accommodating response in young CGCs but a rapidly accommodating response in old CGCs. **(B)** Average instantaneous frequency response of young and old CGCs. Current injected in young CGCs evokes a high-frequency action potential burst followed by a steady non accommodating firing response. In contrast, current injected in old CGCs evokes a few action potentials and a rapidly accommodating response. **(C)** Example of reduced excitability in old CGCs. Increasing stimulus strength fails to evoke a high-frequency non-accommodating response in old CGCs. Adapted from Hermann et al. (2007) with permission from American Psychological Association (APA).

2014). For instance, a particularly salient example concerns the so-called A-current (I_A) family, a family of outward transient voltage-gated K^+ currents (i.e., they are self-inactivating) that plays important roles in the regulation of neuronal excitability (Adams and Galvan, 1986; Bean, 2007). It has long been known that I_A's inactivation properties are modulated by changes in intracellular redox conditions (Ruppersberg et al., 1991; Bähring et al., 2001). That is, under cytosolic reducing conditions the current displays its characteristic fast N-type inactivation behavior whereas under oxidizing conditions this inactivation process is slowed down. In a manner of speaking, this process turns I_A from a "temporary brake" into a "permanent brake" on a neuron's spiking ability. It has been suggested that these mechanisms may operate as a safety switch against metabolic overload by matching a neuron's energy demanding electrical activity to its metabolic capacity (Gulbis, 2002). The I_A family of ion channels is not the only type of ion channels susceptible to changes in cellular redox homeostasis. Many other types of ion channels playing significant roles in the control and execution of neuronal excitability, including voltage-gated Na^+ and Ca^{2+}, are subject to redox modulation (for review see Annunziato et al., 2002).

In addition, over the last number of decades it has become clear that many of the molecular correlates of neuronal excitability and processes are sensitive to the composition and micro-architecture of their membrane environment and/or are modulated by various membrane-derived lipid signaling moieties (for review see Piomelli et al., 2007; Dart, 2010; Rosenhouse-Dantsker et al., 2012). Maintaining lipid membrane homeostasis is therefore a crucial facet of the maintenance of functional integrity of neurons and the brain. Below we illustrate these ideas with some of the most salient examples.

MEMBRANE-ASSOCIATED CORRELATES OF NEURONAL EXCITABILITY CONTROL

There are numerous examples of lipid-mediated signaling in the nervous system. For instance, although there is still some debate whether its actions arise from direct or indirect interactions with ion channel proteins it is evident that AA, one of the most common PUFAs in the nervous system, can modulate a variety of ion channels, including voltage-gated Ca^{2+} channels, mechano-gated K^+ channels like TRAAK, TREK-1, and other members of the four-transmembrane/two-pore domain (4TM2P) family of background K^+ channels (Patel et al., 1998; Maingret et al., 1999; Roberts-Crowley et al., 2009). Alternatively, PUFAs like AA or EPA liberated from their plasma membrane environment can act as metabolic precursors for several signaling pathways active in the nervous system. This includes the eicosanoid pathway that generates a collection of signaling molecules (i.e., prostaglandins, prostacyclins, thromboxanes, lipoxins, and leukotrienes). Many eicosanoids regulate immune functions and inflammation but also double as neuromodulators (for review see Nigam and Schewe, 2000; Liang et al., 2007). Intriguingly, one of those eicosanoid neuromodulators, the 12-lipoxygenase (12-LOX) metabolite 12-HPETE has long been known as an activator of *Aplysia*'s S-type K^+-channels (Piomelli et al., 1987). These K^+ channels, later identified to belong to the TREK-1 family, are instrumental in non-synaptic forms of plasticity underlying behavioral modification of *Aplysia*'s gill withdrawal reflex (Hawkins, 1984) Similar PLA_2- and/or LOX-dependent arachidonic-acid modulated background K^+ channels have been described in *Lymnaea* (Kits et al., 1997; Lopes et al., 1998). Opening of these 4TM2P channels generates an outward current. It is, therefore, conceivable that elevated levels of PLA_2-activity associated with inflammation, oxidative stress, and aging induce a decline in neuronal excitability through activation of these 4TM2P background K^+ channels. An alternative route linking membrane oxidative stress to a decline in neuronal excitability involves aforementioned aldehyde byproducts of lipid peroxidation. As mentioned MDA, 4-HNE and acrolein can cause irreversible damage to many of the cells macromolecules through covalent conjugation (Farooqui and Horrocks, 2006) or engage in various signaling activities including pathways regulating mitochondrial function and other aspects of cell metabolism (Riahi et al., 2010; Ayala et al., 2014).

Yet another intriguing plausible explanation for the effects of lipid peroxidation on neuronal excitability involves structural rather than signaling arguments. Specifically, as noted before peroxidation very likely incites considerable changes in the molecular geometry of affected PUFAs that affect the way they "fit" in the membrane and may introduce considerable changes in the micro-architecture and biophysical properties of bilayer membranes including parameters such as membrane curvature, membrane viscosity, lipid composition, and distribution. These changes may have various implications for neuronal signaling functions, including the organization of transmembrane signaling complexes, vesicle fusion processes, receptor trafficking, and ion channel functions (Yu et al., 1992; Choi and Yu, 1995; Choe et al., 1995; Patel et al., 2001; reviewed in Piomelli et al., 2007). For example, membrane curvature stresses have been found an important factor in the regulation of neuronal electrical activity through the activation of stretch/mechano sensitive background K^+ channels known to contribute to the regulation of neuronal excitability (**Figure 2**; Patel et al., 2001). Also, the lipid architecture of presynaptic terminal membranes does play a vital role in synaptic Ca^{2+}-triggered exocytosis process raising the possibility that PUFA peroxidation interferes with synaptic functions (reviewed in Davletov and Montecucco, 2010).

Taken together, even though there are still a lot of loose ends in the conceptual framework we sketched here it seems evident that proper management of membrane redox status, lipid peroxidation and phospholipid lysis products generated by or with the aid of PLA_2 is likely critical for functional homeostasis of neurons and by extension the nervous system. Below we summarize and discuss evidence from recent work done in our laboratory trying to fit the pieces of this puzzle together.

PLA_2 – A LIPASE AT THE NEXUS OF AGING, OXIDATIVE STRESS, NEURONAL ELECTRICAL EXCITABILITY CONTROL AND FUNCTIONAL DECLINE OF THE AGING NERVOUS SYSTEM?

In the preceding paragraphs we explored the prospect for interplay between oxidative stress, lipid membrane factors, PLA_2, and changes in intrinsic neuronal excitability as a factor in functional decline of normal aging neurons. In this section we review the evidence that lipid peroxidation-induced PLA_2 activity lays at the root of inflammation-, age-, and oxidative stress-associated functional impairment of the nervous system in *Lymnaea* and put our findings in the context of a growing literature suggesting that we are dealing with an evolutionary widely conserved mechanism.

As described above, aging *Lymnaea* display associative LTM impairment in two functionally and anatomically distinct (i.e., appetitive and respiratory) learning paradigms (Hermann et al., 2007, 2013; Watson et al., 2012a, 2013, 2014; Beaulieu et al., 2014). In both instances, LTM failure was associated with reduced spontaneous action potential activity and enhanced spike frequency adaptation of the two key interneurons underlying both execution and plasticity of the respective behaviors (i.e., CGCs and RPeD1). Both behavioral and electrophysiological facets of age-associated respiratory and appetitive LTM impairment could be reproduced in young animals through treatment with 2,2′- azobis-2-methylpropanimidamide (AAPH), a water-soluble free radical generator commonly used to induce PUFA peroxidation, furthering the notion of plasmamembrane lipid peroxidation as a significant agent of neuronal and behavioral aging in *Lymnaea* (**Figure 8**). Evidence of increased FFA mobilization from brains and other tissues was found in both old and AAPH-treated young animals (Watson et al., 2013; Beaulieu et al., 2014). Moreover, treatment with the lipid-domain anti-oxidant α-tocopherol reversed decline in neuronal excitability in both experimental oxidative stressed and naturally aged neurons (Watson et al., 2012a,b). Remarkably, all these behavioral, electrophysiological, and biochemical symptoms of aging and experimental oxidative stress could be reversed by treatment with aristolochic acid, a broad spectrum PLA_2 inhibitor that inhibits both Ca^{2+}-dependent cPLA2 and Ca^{2+}-independent $iPLA_2$ (**Figure 8**; Vishwanath et al., 1988; Lopes et al., 1998; Carnevale and Cathcart, 2001).

No evidence was found of significant age-associated impairment or experimental oxidative stress-induced repression of transcription-independent short/intermediate term memory (S/ITM) in either of the two behavioral conditioning paradigms, suggesting that transcription-independent forms of memory appear impervious to aging or oxidative stress. As yet, we have no definitive answer to the question why LTM is selectively susceptible. However, preliminary evidence from our laboratory suggests that both aging and AAPH-induced oxidative stress in participation with PLA_2 alters aspects of mitochondrial functions that may affect their ability to contribute to intracellular Ca^{2+}-buffering. The molecular pathways underlying LTM formation in *Lymnaea* involve "traditional" conserved cAMP- and Ca^{2+}-sensitive CREB- and MAPK-dependent pathways (Ribeiro et al., 2003; Wagatsuma et al., 2006; Guo et al., 2010). It is therefore conceivable that dysregulation of intracellular Ca^{2+} homeostasis disrupts transcription-regulation pathways involved in LTM expression. Furthermore, the observation that PLA_2 inhibition rescues LTM is particularly intriguing in view of evidence implicating FFAs and PLA_2 in mitochondrial uncoupling in pancreatic β-cells (Ježek et al., 2010, 2014). Although speculative at this point in time, it is not unreasonable to postulate that a similar mechanism may underlie the PLA_2-associated LTM impairment in *Lymnaea*.

Intriguingly, selective appetitive LTM impairment could also be induced in young *Lymnaea* through systemic activation of their cellular immune system (Hermann et al., 2013). As before in naturally aged and experimentally oxidation-stressed young animals, inflammation-associated LTM impairment could be rescued by means of PLA_2 inhibition (Hermann et al., 2013). Together, our data indicate that the processes underlying *Lymnaea's*

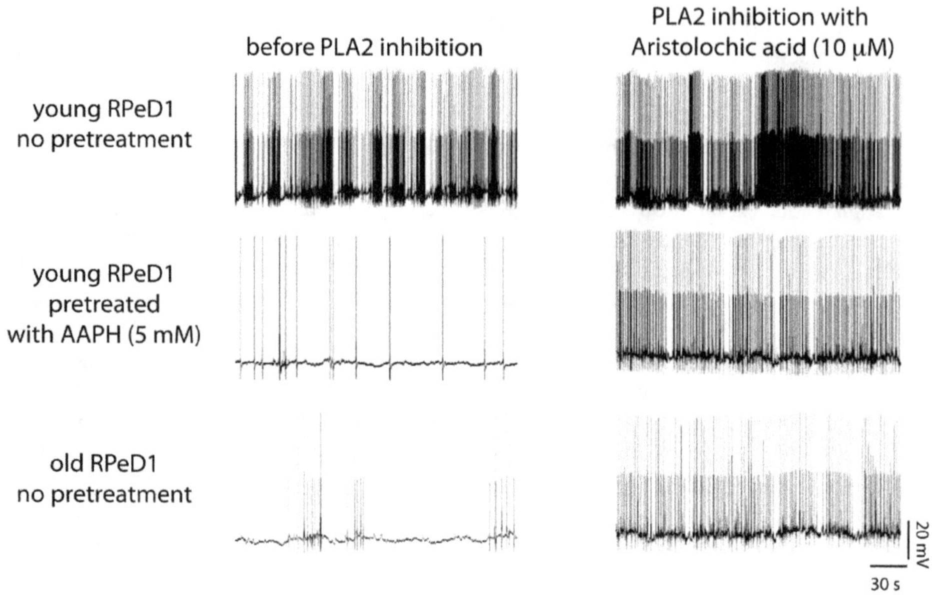

FIGURE 8 | Phospholipase A_2 (PLA_2) contributes to regulation of respiratory neural circuit activity in old and oxidative stressed young brains. Examples of action potential activity recorded from RPeD1 in isolated young central nervous systems (CNSs) pretreated for 30 min with either vehicle-only **(top row)** or the pro-oxidant 2,2-azobis (2-methylpropion-amidine) dihydrochloride (AAPH; **middle row**), and old CNSs maintained in vehicle-only **(bottom row)**, before **(left column)**, and after 30 min of treatment with the PLA_2 inhibitor aristolochic acid **(right column)**. Reprinted from Watson et al. (2013) with permission from Elsevier.

transcription-dependent forms of memory are particularly vulnerable to aging, oxidative stress, and inflammation and that PLA_2 plays a pivotal role in each of these models of associative LTM failure.

PLA_2's AS THERAPEUTIC TARGETS?

PLA_2's and deregulation of lipid metabolism are increasingly implicated in human age-, oxidative stress-, and inflammation-associated conditions including cardiovascular diseases and age-associated neurodegenerative diseases such as Alzheimer's disease (Sun et al., 2004; Farooqui and Horrocks, 2006; Adibhatla and Hatcher, 2008; Sanchez-Mejia et al., 2008; Chalimoniuk et al., 2009; Sanchez-Mejia and Mucke, 2010; Desbene et al., 2012; Gentile et al., 2012; Hui, 2012; reviewed in Sun et al., 2014). They are therefore, not surprisingly, increasingly targeted or considered as targets for therapeutic intervention (see for instance, Garcia-Garcia and Serruys, 2009; Quach et al., 2014). Particularly, it is intriguing that lipoprotein-associated phospholipase A_2 (Lp-PLA_2), also known as platelet-activating factor acetylhydrolase (PAF-AH) was identified as a potential factor in cerebrovascular oxidative stress and inflammation and risk factor for human dementia and subsequently drew considerable interest as a therapeutic target in Alzheimer's disease (Davidson et al., 2012; Acharya et al., 2013; Fitzpatrick et al., 2014). However, there are still a lot of unknowns surrounding the pathways, processes and conditions leading to PLA_2 activation in different cell types that should be resolved before effective and safe therapeutic targets and agents for the treatment and prevention of these increasingly germane age-associated public health concerns (Sun et al., 2014). For instance, whereas many studies implicate PLA_2 hyperactivity as a factor in the etiology of Alzheimer's disease (Sanchez-Mejia and Mucke, 2010; Gentile et al., 2012; Hui, 2012), other studies suggest that hypoactivity of intracellular PLA_2s ($cPLA_2$ and $iPLA_2$) are a contributing factor to memory impairment and Alzheimer's neuropathology (reviewed by Schaeffer et al., 2009).

RELEVANCE AND FUTURE DIRECTIONS

The evidence reviewed here infers close ties between inflammation, oxidative stress, lipid-peroxidation, PLA_2-activation, neuronal excitability, and AMI in *Lymnaea* and echo a rapidly growing evidence from basic, clinical, and epidemiological research that PLA2s, inflammation and oxidative stress are important factors in age-related cognitive decline and impairment in humans and other mammals (Sun et al., 2004, 2014; Phillis et al., 2006; Adibhatla and Hatcher, 2008; Lee et al., 2011). Considering this remarkable conservation we believe that *Lymnaea*'s extraordinary suitability for detailed, direct, and tightly integrated molecule-to-behavior dissection of the neurobiological substrates of AMI will in addition to furthering understanding of the biological foundations and parameters of aging potentially also generate valuable insights into mechanisms of and possible solutions for human AMI and other age-associated afflictions of our own nervous system. Before that goal can be achieved many questions need to be answered.

Among the unanswered questions requiring further attention is the identity of the ionic mechanisms through which the products of PLA_2-mediated fatty acyl hydrolysis exert their inhibitory influence on neuronal excitability. As outlined in the preceding pages, there are many possibilities to test ranging from FA dependent modulation of ion channels to alterations in autacoid modulation of synaptic functions and hypotheses encompassing elements of membrane architecture dependent regulation of neuronal electrical properties.

Another important puzzle to solve is what inhibition of PLA_2, one of the main tools of membrane homeostasis and repair, does to long-term cell/tissues homeostatic integrity. Considering the impact lipid peroxidation is expected to have on membrane structure and function, our finding that PLA_2 inhibition restored rather than aggravated neuro-physiological and behavioral correlates of aging, experimental oxidative stress, and inflammation is puzzling and urges further study.

Yet another intriguing perspective we are currently exploring is mitochondrial involvement in the lipid peroxidation- and PLA_2-dependent declining excitability and plasticity of aging *Lymnaea* neurons. Neurons critically depend on mitochondria to provide the energy to establish and maintain membrane excitability and engage in their quintessential and metabolically costly electrochemical signaling activities (Kann and Kovács, 2007; Mattson et al., 2008). Mitochondria are also a critical partner in intracellular free Ca^{2+} homeostasis and are one of the main sources of RONS and other pro-oxidants. There are many tight reciprocal links between neuronal electrical and mitochondrial activities and many neuronal excitability disorders appear to be associated with mitochondrial aberrancies (Kann and Kovács, 2007; Mattson et al., 2008; Surmeier et al., 2012). Moreover, there is also a substantial body of evidence indicating involvement of mitochondria-associated oxidative stress, lipid signaling, Ca^{2+} dysregulation in normal aging, and the pathogenesis of common age-associated neurological diseases including AD and PD in which lipid peroxidation and PLA_2 may be key partners (reviewed in Thibault et al., 2007; Mattson et al., 2008; Toescu and Vreugdenhil, 2010; Waldbaum and Patel, 2010). The *Lymnaea* model system we have developed provides an excellent platform to investigate these interactions between neuronal energy metabolism, electrical excitability, and plasticity in great detail.

The *Lymnaea* research platform we portrayed here will also be a great tool to investigate fundamental mechanisms of neuronal and behavioral aging and test other existing and emerging aging theories. For example, there is growing evidence that insulin and other insulin-like peptides (ILPs) modulate aspects of plasticity in the *Lymnaea* CNS and enhance learning abilities in older learning-impaired snails (Murakami et al., 2013; Pirger et al., 2014). These findings resonate very well with a rapidly expanding literature that ILPs and insulin resistance are a major endocrine factor in aging in general and aging of the nervous system in particular (Kim and Feldman, 2012; Alcedo et al., 2013). Moreover, because of its identified neurons the model system will allow us to explore many important fundamental scientific questions about aging neurons and brains like: do neurons age according to "plan" or do they fail at random? Are some neuronal physiological phenotypes more vulnerable to aging than others? Can we reverse the effects of aging without repercussion? What are the principles and mechanisms underlying robust and reliable complex brains? Are all changes observed in aging neurons mal-adaptive or are some perhaps compensatory and adaptive? Are neurons and brains life cycles subject to the same resource constraints and trade-offs as other types of cells and tissues in the animal body?

ACKNOWLEDGMENTS

This work was supported by a Discovery Grant from the National Science and Engineering Research Council (NSERC) of Canada to Willem C. Wildering.

REFERENCES

Acharya, N. K., Levin, E. C., Clifford, P. M., Han, M., Tourtellotte, R., Chamberlain, D., et al. (2013). Diabetes and hypercholesterolemia increase blood-brain barrier permeability and brain amyloid deposition: beneficial effects of the LpPLA2 inhibitor darapladib. *J. Alzheimers Dis.* 35, 179–198. doi: 10.3233/JAD-122254

Adams, P. R., and Galvan, M. (1986). Voltage-dependent currents of vertebrate neurons and their role in membrane excitability. *Adv. Neurol.* 44, 137–170.

Adibhatla, R. M., and Hatcher, J. F. (2008). Phospholipase A2, reactive oxygen species and lipid peroxidation in CNS pathologies. *BMB Rep.* 41, 560–567. doi: 10.5483/BMBRep.2008.41.8.560

Aïd, S., and Bosetti, F. (2011). Targeting cyclooxygenases-1 and -2 in neuroinflammation: therapeutic implications. *Biochimie* 93, 46–51. doi: 10.1016/j.biochi.2010.09.009

Alberts, B., Johnson, A., Lewis, J., Raff, M., Roberts, K., and Walter, P. (2002). *Molecular Biology of the Cell,* 4th Edn. New York: Garland Science.

Alcedo, J., Flatt, T., and Pasyukova, E. G. (2013). Neuronal inputs and outputs of aging and longevity. *Front. Genet.* 4:71. doi: 10.3389/fgene.2013.00071

Alkon, D. L. (1974). Associative training of Hermissenda. *J. Gen. Physiol.* 64, 70–84. doi: 10.1085/jgp.64.1.70

Alkon, D. L. (1979). Voltage-dependent calcium and potassium ion conductances: a contingency mechanism for an associative learning model. *Science* 205, 810–816. doi: 10.1126/science.223244

Annunziato, L., Pannaccione, A., Cataldi, M., Secondo, A., Castaldo, P., Di Renzo, G., et al. (2002). Modulation of ion channels by reactive oxygen and nitrogen species: a pathophysiological role in brain aging? *Neurobiol. Aging* 23, 819–834. doi: 10.1016/S0197-4580(02)00069-6

Arundell, M., Patel, B. A., Straub, V., Allen, M. C., Janse, C. K., O'Hare, D., et al. (2006). Effects of age on feeding behavior and chemosensory processing in the pond snail, *Lymnaea stagnalis. Neurobiol. Aging* 27, 1880–1891. doi: 10.1016/j.neurobiolaging.2005.09.040

Atkinson, J., Epand, R. F., and Epand, R. M. (2008). Tocopherols and tocotrienols in membranes: a critical review. *Free Rad. Biol. Med.* 44, 739–764. doi: 10.1016/j.freeradbiomed.2007.11.010

Atkinson, J., Harroun, T., Wassal, S. R., Stillwell, W., and Katsaras, J. (2010). The location and behavior of *alpha* -tocopherol in membranes. *Mol. Nutr. Food Res.* 54, 641–651. doi: 10.1002/mnfr.200900439

Audesirk, T. E., Alexander, J. E., Audesirk, G. J., and Moyer, C. M. (1982). Rapid, nonaversive conditioning in a freshwater gastropod. I. Effects of age and motivation. *Behav. Neural Biol.* 36, 379–390. doi: 10.1016/S0163-1047(82)90782-8

Ayala, A., Muñoz, M. F., and Argüelles, S. (2014). Lipid peroxidation: production, metabolism, and signaling mechanisms of malondialdehyde and 4-hydroxy-2-nonenal. *Oxid. Med. Cell. Longev.* 2014, 1–31. doi: 10.1155/2014/360438

Bähring, R., Milligan, C. J., Vardanyan, V., Engeland, B., Young, B. A., Dannenberg, J., et al. (2001). Coupling of voltage-dependent potassium channel inactivation and oxidoreductase active site of Kvbeta subunits. *J. Biol. Chem.* 276, 22923–22929. doi: 10.1074/jbc.M100483200

Ballatori, N., Krance, S. M., Notenboom, S., Shi, S., Tieu, K., and Hammond, C. L. (2009). Glutathione dysregulation and the etiology and progression of human diseases. *Biol. Chem.* 390, 191–214. doi: 10.1515/BC.2009.033

Barnes, C. A. (1994). Normal aging: regionally specific changes in hippocampal synaptic transmission. *Trends Neurosci.* 17, 13–18. doi: 10.1016/0166-2236(94)90029-9

Bean, B. P. (2007). The action potential in mammalian central neurons. *Nat. Rev. Neurosci.* 8, 451–465. doi: 10.1038/nrn2148

Beaulieu, E., Ioffe, J., Watson, S. N., Hermann, P. M., and Wildering, W. C. (2014). Oxidative-stress induced increase in circulating fatty acids does not contribute to phospholipase A2-dependent appetitive long-term memory failure in the pond snail *Lymnaea stagnalis. BMC Neurosci.* 15:56. doi: 10.1186/1471-2202-15-56

Beck, H., and Yaari, Y. (2008). Plasticity of intrinsic neuronal properties in CNS disorders. *Nat. Rev. Neurosci.* 9, 357–369. doi: 10.1038/nrn2371

Benjamin, P. R. (2012). Distributed network organization underlying feeding behavior in the mollusk *Lymnaea. Neural Syst. Circuits* 2:4. doi: 10.1186/2042-1001-2-4

Benjamin, P. R., and Kemenes, G. (2010). *Lymnaea* learning and memory. *Scholarpedia* 5, 4247. doi: 10.4249/scholarpedia.4247

Benjamin, P. R., Kemenes, G., and Kemenes, I. (2008). Non-synaptic neuronal mechanisms of learning and memory in gastropod molluscs. *Front. Biosci.* 13:4051–4057.

Benjamin, P. R., Staras, K., and Kemenes, G. (2000). A systems approach to the cellular analysis of associative learning in the pond snail *Lymnaea. Learn. Mem.* 7, 124–131. doi: 10.1101/lm.7.3.124

Bliss, T. V. P., and Collingridge, G. L. (1993). A synaptic model of memory: long-term potentiation in the hippocampus. *Nature* 361, 31–39. doi: 10.1038/361031a0

Branch, S. Y., Sharma, R., and Beckstead, M. J. (2014). Aging decreases L-type calcium channel currents and pacemaker firing fidelity in substantia nigra dopamine neurons. *J. Neurosci.* 34, 9310–9318. doi: 10.1523/JNEUROSCI.4228-13.2014

Brembs, B. (2003). Operant conditioning in invertebrates. *Curr. Opin. Neurobiol.* 13, 710–717. doi: 10.1016/j.conb.2003.10.002

Brown, W. J., Chambers, K., and Doody, A. (2003). Phospholipase A2 (PLA2) enzymes in membrane trafficking: mediators of membrane shape and function. *Traffic* 4, 214–221. doi: 10.1034/j.1600-0854.2003.00078.x

Burke, S. N., and Barnes, C. A. (2006). Neural plasticity in the ageing brain. *Nat. Rev. Neurosci.* 7, 30–40. doi: 10.1038/nrn1809

Byrne, J. H. (1987). Cellular analysis of associative learning. *Physiol. Rev.* 67, 329–439.

Cai, S.-Q., and Sesti, F. (2009). Oxidation of a potassium channel causes progressive sensory function loss during aging. *Nat. Neurosci.* 12, 611–617. doi: 10.1038/nn.2291

Carnevale, K. A., and Cathcart, M. K. (2001). Calcium-independent phospholipase A(2) is required for human monocyte chemotaxis to monocyte chemoattractant protein 1. *J. Immunol.* 167, 3414–3421. doi: 10.4049/jimmunol.167.6.3414

Chalimoniuk, M., Stolecka, A., Ziemińska, E., Stepień, A., Langfort, J., and Strosznajder, J. B. (2009). Involvement of multiple protein kinases in cPLA2 phosphorylation, arachidonic acid release, and cell death in in vivo and in vitro models of 1-methyl-4-phenylpyridinium-induced parkinsonism - the possible key role of PKG. *J. Neurochem.* 110, 307–317. doi: 10.1111/j.1471-4159.2009.06147.x

Chawla, M. K., and Barnes, C. A. (2007). Hippocampal granule cells in normal aging: insights from electrophysiological and functional imaging experiments. *Progr. Brain Res.* 163, 661–821. doi: 10.1016/S0079-6123(07)63036-2

Chen, C. T., Green, J. T., Orr, S. K., and Bazinet, R. P. (2008). Regulation of brain polyunsaturated fatty acid uptake and turnover. *Prostaglandins Leukot. Essent. Fatty Acids* 79, 85–91. doi: 10.1016/j.plefa.2008.09.003

Chen, J., Small-Howard, A., Yin, A., and Berry, M. J. (2005). The responses of Ht22 cells to oxidative stress induced by buthionine sulfoximine (BSO). *BMC Neurosci.* 6:10. doi: 10.1186/1471-2202-6-10

Choe, M., Jackson, C., and Yu, B. P. (1995). Lipid peroxidation contributes to age-related membrane rigidity. *Free Radic. Biol. Med.* 18, 977–984. doi: 10.1016/0891-5849(94)00217-8

Choi, B. H. (1995). Oxidative stress and Alzheimer's disease. *Neurobiol. Aging* 16, 675–678. doi: 10.1016/0197-4580(95)00065-M

Choi, J. H., and Yu, B. P. (1995). Brain synaptosomal aging: free radicals and membrane fluidity. *Free Radic. Biol. Med.* 18, 133–139. doi: 10.1016/0891-5849(94)00106-T

Christian, K. M., and Thompson, R. F. (2003). Neural substrates of eyeblink conditioning: acquisition and retention. *Learn. Mem.* 10, 427–455. doi: 10.1101/lm.59603

Coulter, D. A., Lo Turco, J. J., Kubota, M., Disterhoft, J. F., Moore, J. W., and Alkon, D. L. (1989). Classical conditioning reduces amplitude and duration of calcium-dependent afterhyperpolarization in rabbit hippocampal pyramidal cells. *J. Neurophysiol.* 61, 971–981.

Currais, A., and Maher, P. (2013). Functional consequences of age-dependent changes in glutathione status in the brain. *Antioxid. Redox Signal.* 19, 813–822. doi: 10.1089/ars.2012.4996

Dai, D.-F., Chiao, Y. A., Marcinek, D. J., Szeto, H. H., and Rabinovitch, P. S. (2014). Mitochondrial oxidative stress in aging and healthspan. *Longev. Healthspan* 3, 6. doi: 10.1186/2046-2395-3-6

Dalesman, S., and Lukowiak, K. (2012). How stress alters memory in 'smart' snails. *PLoS ONE* 7:e32334. doi: 10.1371/journal.pone.0032334

D'Angelo, E. (2014). *The Organization of Plasticity in the Cerebellar Cortex: From Synapses to Control*, Vol. 210 (Amsterdam: Elsevier), 31–58.

Dart, C. (2010). Lipid microdomains and the regulation of ion channel function. *J. Physiol.* 588, 3169–3178. doi: 10.1113/jphysiol.2010.191585

Davidson, J. E., Lockhart, A., Amos, L., Stirnadel-Farrant, H. A., Mooser, V., Sollberger, M., et al. (2012). Plasma lipoprotein-associated phospholipase A2 activity in Alzheimer's disease, amnestic mild cognitive impairment, and cognitively healthy elderly subjects: a cross-sectional study. *Alzheimers Res. Ther.* 4, 51. doi: 10.1186/alzrt154

Davletov, B., and Montecucco, C. (2010). Lipid function at synapses. *Curr. Opin. Neurobiol.* 20, 543–549. doi: 10.1016/j.conb.2010.06.008

Dennis, E. A., Cao, J., Hsu, Y. H., Magrioti, V., and Kokotos, G. (2011). Phospholipase A2 enzymes: physical structure. Biological function, disease implications, chemical inhibition, and therapeutic intervention. *Chem. Rev.* 111, 6130–6185. doi: 10.1021/cr200085w

Desbene, C., Malaplate-Armand, C., Youssef, I., Garcia, P., Stenger, C., Sauvée, M., et al. (2012). Critical role of cPLA2 in Abeta oligomer- induced neurodegeneration and memory deficit. *Neurobiol. Aging* 33, 1123.e17–1123.e29. doi: 10.1016/j.neurobiolaging.2011.11.008

Disterhoft, J. F., Thompson, L. T., Moyer, J. R., and Mogul, D. J. (1996). Calcium-dependent after hyperpolarization and learning in young and aging hippocampus. *Life Sci.* 59, 413–420. doi: 10.1016/0024-3205(96)00320-7

Dukoff, D. J., Hogg, D. W., Hawrsyh, P. J., and Buck, L. T. (2014). Scavenging ROS dramatically increases NMDA receptor whole cell currents in painted turtle cortical neurons. *J. Exp. Biol.* 217, 3346–3355. doi: 10.1242/jeb.105825

Esiri, M. M. (2007). Ageing and the brain. *J. Pathol.* 211, 181–187. doi: 10.1002/path.2089

Farooqui, A. A., and Horrocks, L. A. (2006). Phospholipase A2-generated lipid mediators in the brain: the good, the bad, and the ugly. *Neuroscientist* 12, 245–260. doi: 10.1177/1073858405285923

Fitzpatrick, A. L., Irizarry, M. C., Cushman, M., Jenny, N. S., Chi, G. C., and Koro, C. (2014). Lipoprotein-associated phospholipase A2 and risk of dementia in the Cardiovascular Health Study. *Atherosclerosis* 235, 384–391. doi: 10.1016/j.atherosclerosis.2014.04.032

Forlenza, O. V., Schaeffer, E. L., and Gattaz, W. F. (2007). The role of phospholipase A2 in neuronal homeostasis and memory formation: implications for the pathogenesis of Alzheimer's disease. *J. Neural Transm.* 114, 231–238. doi: 10.1007/s00702-006-0597-0

Foster, T. C. (2012). Dissecting the age-related decline on spatial learning and memory tasks in rodent models: N-methyl-D-aspartate receptors and voltage-dependent Ca2+ channels in senescent synaptic plasticity. *Prog. Neurobiol.* 96, 283–303. doi: 10.1016/j.pneurobio.2012.01.007

Frolkis, V. V., Kvitnitskaya-Ryzhova, T. Yu., and Martynenko, O. A. (1995). Aging of neurons in the mollusc *Lymnaea stagnalis* small parietal ganglion: a morpho-functional comparison in the same neuron. *Exp. Gerontol.* 30, 533–544. doi: 10.1016/0531-5565(95)00008-5

Frolkis, V. V., Martynenko, O. A., and Timchenko, A. N. (1989). Age-related changes in the function of somatic membrane potassium channels of neurons in the mollusc *Lymnaea stagnalis. Mech. Ageing Dev.* 47, 47–54. doi: 10.1016/0047-6374(89)90006-7

Frolkis, V. V., Martynenko, O. A., and Timchenko, A. N. (1991). Potential-dependent Ca channels of neurons in the mollusc *Lymnaea stagnalis* in aging: effect of norepinephrine. *Mech. Ageing Dev.* 58, 75–83. doi: 10.1016/0047-6374(91)90121-F

Frolkis, V. V., Stupina, A. S., Martinenko, O. A., Tòth, S., and Timchenko, A. I. (1984). Aging of neurons in the mollusc *Lymnaea stagnalis.* Structure, function and sensitivity to transmitters. *Mech. Ageing Dev.* 25, 91–102. doi: 10.1016/0047-6374(84)90132-5

Garcia-Garcia, H. M., and Serruys, P. W. (2009). Phospholipase A2 inhibitors. *Curr. Opin. Lipidol.* 20, 327–332. doi: 10.1097/MOL.0b013e32832dd4c7

Gazzaley, A. H., Thakker, M. M., Hof, P. R., and Morrison, J. H. (1997). Preserved number of entorhinal cortex layer II neurons in aged macaque monkeys. *Neurobiol. Aging* 18, 549–553. doi: 10.1016/S0197-4580(97)00112-7

Genovese, T., Mazzon, E., Esposito, E., Muia, C., Di Paola, R., Di Bella, P., et al. (2007). Role of endogenous glutathione in the secondary damage in experimental spinal cord injury in mice. *Neurosci. Lett.* 423, 41–46. doi: 10.1016/j.neulet.2007.05.058

Gentile, M. T., Reccia, M. G., Sorrentino, P. P., Vitale, E., Sorrentino, G., Puca, A. A., et al. (2012). Role of cytosolic calcium-dependent phospholipase A2 in Alzheimer's disease pathogenesis. *Mol. Neurobiol.* 45, 596–604. doi: 10.1007/s12035-012-8279-4

Greenberg, M. E., Li, X. M., Gugiu, B. G., Gu, X., Qin, J., Salomon, R. G., et al. (2008). The lipid whisker model of the structure of oxidized cell membranes. *J. Biol. Chem.* 283, 2385–2396. doi: 10.1074/jbc.M707348200

Gulbis, J. M. (2002). The beta subunit of Kv1 channels: voltage-gated enzyme or safety switch? *Novartis Found. Symp.* 245, 127–141. doi: 10.1002/0470868759.ch9

Guo, C. H., Senzel, A., Li, K., and Feng, Z. P. (2010). De novo protein synthesis of syntaxin-1 and dynamin-1 in long-term memory formation requires CREB1 gene transcription in *Lymnaea stagnalis*. *Behav. Genet.* 40, 680–693. doi: 10.1007/s10519-010-9374-9

Haddadi, M., Jahromi, S. R., Sagar, B. K., Patil, R. K., Shivanandappa, T., and Ramesh, S. R. (2014). Brain aging, memory impairment and oxidative stress: a study in *Drosophila melanogaster*. *Behav. Brain Res.* 259, 60–69. doi: 10.1016/j.bbr.2013.10.036

Harman, D. (1956). Aging: a theory based on free radical and radiation chemistry. *J. Gerontol.* 11, 298–300. doi: 10.1093/geronj/11.3.298

Hawkins, R. D. (1984). A cellular mechanism of classical conditioning in Aplysia. *J. Exp. Biol.* 112, 113–128.

Hekimi, S., Lapointe, J., and Wen, Y. (2011). Taking a "good" look at free radicals in the aging process. *Trends Cell Biol.* 21, 569–576. doi: 10.1016/j.tcb.2011.06.008

Hermann, P. M., Lee, A., Hulliger, S., Minvielle, M., Ma, B., and Wildering, W. C. (2007). Impairment of long-term associative memory in aging snails (*Lymnaea stagnalis*). *Behav. Neurosci.* 121, 1400–1414. doi: 10.1037/0735-7044.121.6.1400

Hermann, P. M., Park, D., Beaulieu, E., and Wildering, W. C. (2013). Evidence for inflammation-mediated memory dysfunction in gastropods: putative PLA2 and COX inhibitors abolish long-term memory failure induced by systemic immune challenges. *BMC Neurosci.* 14:83. doi: 10.1186/1471-2202-14-83

Hu, D., Serrano, F., Oury, T. D., and Klann, E. (2006). Aging-dependent alterations in synaptic plasticity and memory in mice that overexpress extracellular superoxide dismutase. *J. Neurosci.* 26, 3933–3941. doi: 10.1523/JNEUROSCI.5566-05.2006

Hui, D. Y. (2012). Phospholipase A(2) enzymes in metabolic and cardiovascular diseases. *Curr. Opin. Lipidol.* 23, 235–240.

Hulbert, A. J., Pamplona, R., Buffenstein, R., and Buttemer, W. A. (2007). Life and death: metabolic rate, membrane composition, and life span of animals. *Physiol. Rev.* 87, 1175–1213. doi: 10.1152/physrev.00047.2006

Hung, C.-W., Chen, Y.-C., Hsieh, W.-L., Chiou, S.-H., and Kao, C.-L. (2010). Ageing and neurodegenerative diseases. *Ageing Res. Rev.* 9(Suppl.)1, S36–S46. doi: 10.1016/j.arr.2010.08.006

Jacob, K. D., Hooten, N. N., Trzeciak, A. R., and Evans, M. K. (2013). Markers of oxidant stress that are clinically relevant in aging and age-related disease. *Mech. Ageing Dev.* 134, 139–157. doi: 10.1016/j.mad.2013.02.008

Janse, C., and van der Roest, M. (2001). cAMP and excitability in neuroendocrine cells during reproductive senescence. *Neurobiol. Aging* 22, 503–514. doi: 10.1016/S0197-4580(01)00211-1

Janse, C., van der Roest, M., and Slob, W. (1986). Age-related decrease in electrical coupling of two identified neurons in the mollusk *Lymnaea stagnalis*. *Brain Res.* 376, 208–212. doi: 10.1016/0006-8993(86)90920-0

Janse, C. K., Peretz, B., van der Roest, M., and Dubelaar, E. J. (1999). Excitability and branching of neuroendocrine cells during reproductive senescence. *Neurobiol. Aging* 20, 675–683. doi: 10.1016/S0197-4580(99)00021-4

Janse, C. K., Slob, W., Popelier, C. M., and Vogelaar, J. W. (1988). Survival characteristics of the mollusc *Lymnaea stagnalis* under constant culture conditions: effects of aging and disease. *Mech. Ageing Dev.* 42, 263–274. doi: 10.1016/0047-6374(88)90052-8

Janse, C. K., Wildering, W. C., and Popelier, C. M. (1989). Age-related changes in female reproductive activity and growth in the mollusc *Lymnaea stagnalis*. *J. Gerontol.* 44, B148–B155. doi: 10.1093/geronj/44.6.B148

Ježek, J., Jabùrek, M., Zelenka, J., and Ježek, P. (2010). Mitochondrial phospholipase A2 activated by reactive oxygen species in heart mitochondria induces mild uncoupling. *Physiol. Res.* 59, 737–747.

Ježek, P., Olejár, T., Smolková, K., Ježek, J., Dlasková, A., Plecitá-Hlavatá, L., et al. (2014). Antioxidant and regulatory role of mitochondrial uncoupling protein UCP2 in pancreatic beta-cells. *Physiol. Res.* 63(Suppl. 1), S73–S91.

Jones, N. G., Kemenes, I., Kemenes, G., and Benjamin, P. R. (2003). A persistent cellular change in a single modulatory neuron contributes to associative long-term memory. *Curr. Biol.* 13, 1064–1069. doi: 10.1016/S0960-9822(03)00380-4

Joseph, J. A., Shukitt-Hale, B., Casadesus, G., and Fisher, D. (2005). Oxidative stress and inflammation in brain aging: nutritional considerations. *Neurochem. Res.* 30, 927–935. doi: 10.1007/s11064-005-6967-4

Kagan, V. E. (1989). Tocopherol stabilizes membrane against phospholipase A, free fatty acids and lysophospholipids. *Ann. N. Y. Acad. Sci.* 570, 121–135. doi: 10.1111/j.1749-6632.1989.tb14913.x

Kandel, E. R. (2001). The molecular biology of memory storage: a dialogue between genes and synapses. *Science* 294, 1030–1038. doi: 10.1126/science.1067020

Kann, O., and Kovács, R. (2007). Mitochondria and neuronal activity. *Am. J. Physiol. Cell Physiol.* 292, C641–C657. doi: 10.1152/ajpcell.00222.2006

Kawai, R., Sunada, H., Horikoshi, T., and Sakakibara, M. (2004). Conditioned taste aversion with sucrose and tactile stimuli in the pond snail *Lymnaea stagnalis*. *Neurobiol. Learn. Mem.* 82, 164–168. doi: 10.1016/j.nlm.2004.06.003

Kemenes, G., Kemenes, I., Michel, M., Papp, A., and Müller, U. (2006a). Phase-dependent molecular requirements for memory reconsolidation: differential roles for protein synthesis and protein kinase A activity. *J. Neurosci.* 26, 6298–6302. doi: 10.1523/JNEUROSCI.0890-06.2006

Kemenes, I., Straub, V. A., Nikitin, E. S., Staras, K., O'Shea, M., Kemenes, G., et al. (2006b). Role of delayed nonsynaptic neuronal plasticity in long-term associative memory. *Curr. Biol.* 16, 1269–1279. doi: 10.1016/j.cub.2006.05.049

Kempsell, A. T., and Fieber, L. A. (2014). Behavioral aging is associated with reduced sensory neuron excitability in *Aplysia californica*. *Front. Aging Neurosci.* 6:84. doi: 10.3389/fnagi.2014.00084

Keuker, J. I., Luiten, P. G., and Fuchs, E. (2003). Preservation of hippocampal neuron numbers in aged rhesus monkeys. *Neurobiol. Aging* 24, 157–165. doi: 10.1016/S0197-4580(02)00062-3

Kim, B., and Feldman, E. L. (2012). Insulin resistance in the nervous system. *Trends Endocrinol. Metabol.* 23, 133–141. doi: 10.1016/j.tem.2011.12.004

Kirkwood, T. B. L., and Austad, S. N. (2000). Why do we age? *Nature*, 408, 233–238. doi: 10.1038/35041682

Kits, K. S., Lodder, J. C., and Veerman, M. J. (1997). Phe-Met-Arg-Phe-amide activates a novel voltage-dependent K+ current through a lipoxygenase pathway in molluscan neurones. *J. Gen. Physiol.* 110, 611–628. doi: 10.1085/jgp.110.5.611

Klaassen, L. J., Janse, C. K., and van der Roest, M. (1998). Multiple synaptic connections of a single neuron change differentially with age. *Neurobiol. Aging* 19, 341–349. doi: 10.1016/S0197-4580(98)00065-7

Lee, J., Kosaras, B., Del Signore, S. J., Cormier, K., McKee, A., Ratan, R. R., et al. (2011). Modulation of lipid peroxidation and mitochondrial function improves neuropathology in Huntington's disease mice. *Acta Neuropath.* 121, 487–498. doi: 10.1007/s00401-010-0788-5

Lemaire-Ewing, S., Desrumaux, C., Neel, D., and Laurent, L. (2010). Vitamin E transport, membrane incorporation and cell metabolism: is α-tocopherol in lipid rafts an oar in the lifeboat? *Mol. Nutr. Food Res.* 54, 631–640. doi: 10.1002/mnfr.200900445

Lewis, D. V., Huguenard, J. R., Anderson, W. W., and Wilson, W. A. (1986). Membrane currents underlying bursting pacemaker activity and spike frequency adaptation in invertebrates. *Adv. Neurol.* 44, 235–261.

Liang, X., Wu, L., Wang, Q., Hand, T., Bilak, M., McCullough, L., et al. (2007). Function of COX-2 and prostaglandins in neurological disease. *J. Mol. Neurosci.* 33, 94–99. doi: 10.1007/s12031-007-0058-8

Ljubuncic, P., and Reznick, A. Z. (2009). The evolutionary theories of aging revisited-a mini review. *Gerontology* 55, 205–216. doi: 10.1159/000200772

Lopes, C. M. B., Franks, N. P., and Lieb, W. R. (1998). Actions of general anaesthetics and arachidonic acid pathway inhibitors on K +currents activated by volatile anaesthetics and FMRFamide in molluscan neurones. *Br. J. Pharmacol.* 125, 309–318. doi: 10.1038/sj.bjp.0702069

Lopez, N., Tormo, C., De Blas, I., Llinares, I., and Alom, J. (2013). Oxidative stress in Alzheimer's disease and mild cognitive impairment with high sensitivity and specificity. *J. Alzheimers Dis.* 33, 823–829. doi: 10.3233/JAD-2012-121528

Lukowiak, K., Martens, K., Orr, M., Parvez, K., Rosenegger, D., and Sangha, S. (2006). Modulation of aerial respiratory behaviour in a pond snail. *Respir. Physiol. Neurobiol.* 154, 61–72. doi: 10.1016/j.resp.2006.02.009

Lukowiak, K., Ringseis, E., Spencer, G., Wildering, W. C., and Syed, N. I. (1996). Operant conditioning of aerial respiratory behaviour in *Lymnaea stagnalis*. *J. Exp. Biol.* 199, 683–691.

Maingret, F., Fosset, M., Lesage, F., Lazdunski, M., and Honoré, E. (1999). TRAAK is a mammalian neuronal mechano-gated K+ channel. *J. Biol. Chem.* 274, 1381–1387. doi: 10.1074/jbc.274.3.1381

Mari, M., Morales, A., Colell, A., Garcia-Ruiz, C., and Fernandez-Checa, J. C. (2009). Mitochondrial glutathione, a key survival antioxidant. *Antioxid. Redox Signal.* 11, 2685–2700. doi: 10.1089/ars.2009.2695

Marquardt, D., Williams, J. A., Kucerka, N., Atkinson, J., Wassal, S. R., Katsaras, J., et al. (2013). Tocopherol activity correlates with its location in a membrane: a new perspective on the antioxidant Vitamin E. *J. Am. Chem. Soc.* 135, 7523–7533. doi: 10.1021/ja312665r

Masoro E. J., and Austad, S. N. (2011). *Handbook of the Biology of Aging*. Amsterdam: Elsevier Academic Press.

Massaad, C. A., and Klann, E. (2011). Reactive oxygen species in the regulation of synaptic plasticity and memory. *Antioxid. Redox Signal.* 14, 2013–2053. doi: 10.1089/ars.2010.3208

Mattson, M. P., Gleichmann, M., and Cheng, A. (2008). Mitochondria in neuroplasticity and neurological disorders. *Neuron* 60, 748–766. doi: 10.1016/j.neuron.2008.10.010

Mattson, M. P., and Magnus, T. (2006). Ageing and neuronal vulnerability. *Nat. Rev. Neurosci.* 7, 278–294. doi: 10.1038/nrn1886

Merrill, D. A., Chiba, A. A., and Tuszynski, M. H. (2001). Conservation of neuronal number and size in the entorhinal cortex of behaviorally characterized aged rats. *J. Comp. Neurol.* 438, 445–456. doi: 10.1002/cne.1327

Merrill, D. A., Roberts, J. A., and Tuszynski, M. H. (2000). Conservation of neuron number and size in entorhinal cortex layers II, III, and V/VI of aged primates. *J. Comp. Neurol.* 422, 396–401. doi: 10.1002/1096-9861(20000703)422:3<396::AID-CNE6>3.0.CO;2-R

Milton, V. J., and Sweeney, S. T. (2011). Oxidative stress in synapse development and function. *Dev. Neurobiol.* 72, 100–110. doi: 10.1002/dneu.20957

Moyer, J. R., Power, J. M., Thompson, L. T., and Disterhoft, J. F. (2000). Increased excitability of aged rabbit CA1 neurons after trace eyeblink conditioning. *J. Neurosci.* 20, 5476–5482.

Moyer, J. R., Thompson, L. T., Black, J. P., and Disterhoft, J. F. (1992). Nimodipine increases excitability of rabbit CA1 pyramidal neurons in an age- and concentration-dependent manner. *J. Neurophysiol.* 68, 2100–2109.

Mozzachiodi, R., and Byrne, J. H. (2010). More than synaptic plasticity: role of nonsynaptic plasticity in learning and memory. *Trends Neurosci.* 33, 17–26. doi: 10.1016/j.tins.2009.10.001

Munro, D., and Blier, P. U. (2012). The extreme longevity of Arctica islandicais associated with increased peroxidation resistance in mitochondrial membranes. *Aging Cell* 11, 845–855. doi: 10.1111/j.1474-9726.2012.00847.x

Munro, D., Pichaud, N., Paquin, F., Kemeid, V., and Blier, P. U. (2013). Low hydrogen peroxide production in mitochondria of the long-lived Arctica islandica: underlying mechanisms for slow aging. *Aging Cell* 12, 584–592. doi: 10.1111/acel.12082

Murakami, S. (2007). Caenorhabditis elegans as a model system to study aging of learning and memory. *Mol. Neurobiol.* 35, 85–94. doi: 10.1007/BF02700625

Murakami, J., Okada, R., Sadamoto, H., Kobayashi, S., Mita, K., Sakamoto, Y., et al. (2013). Involvement of insulin-like peptide in long-term synaptic plasticity and long-term memory of the pond snail *Lymnaea stagnalis*. *J. Neurosci.* 33, 371–383. doi: 10.1523/JNEUROSCI.0679-12.2013

Nagy, I., Toth, S., and Lustyik, G. (1985). Verification of the membrane hypothesis of aging on the identified giant neurons of the snail *Lymnaea stagnalis* L. (Gastropoda, Pulmonata) by a combined application of intracellular electrophysiology and X-ray microanalysis. *Arch. Gerontol. Geriatr.* 4, 53–66. doi: 10.1016/0167-4943(85)90018-4

Negre-Salvayre, A., Auge, N., Ayala, V., Basaga, H., Boada, J., Brenke, R., et al. (2010). Pathological aspects of lipid peroxidation. *Free Radic. Res.* 44, 1125–1171. doi: 10.3109/10715762.2010.498478

Nigam, S., and Schewe, T. (2000). Phospholipase A(2)s and lipid peroxidation. *Biochim. Biophys. Acta* 1488, 167–181. doi: 10.1016/S1388-1981(00)00119-0

Niki, E. (1990). Free-radical initiators as source of water-soluble or lipid-soluble peroxyl radicals. *Methods Enzymol.* 186, 100–108. doi: 10.1016/0076-6879(90)86095-D

Niki, E. (2012). Do antioxidants impair signaling by reactive oxygen species and lipid peroxidation products. *FEBS Lett.* 586, 3767–3770. doi: 10.1016/j.febslet.2012.09.025

Nikitin, E. S., Balaban, P. M., and Kemenes, G. (2013). Nonsynaptic plasticity underlies a compartmentalized increase in synaptic efficacy after classical conditioning. *Curr. Biol.* 23, 614–619. doi: 10.1016/j.cub.2013.02.048

Nikitin, E. S., Kiss, T., Staras, K., O'Shea, M., Benjamin, P. R., and Kemenes, G. (2006). Persistent sodium current is a target for cAMP-induced neuronal plasticity in a state-setting modulatory interneuron. *J. Neurophysiol.* 95, 453–463. doi: 10.1152/jn.00785.2005

Nikitin, E. S., Vavoulis, D. V., Kemenes, I., Marra, V., Pirger, Z., Michel, M., et al. (2008). Persistent sodium current is a nonsynaptic substrate for long-term associative memory. *Curr. Biol.* 18, 1221–1226. doi: 10.1016/j.cub.2008.07.030

Nusser, Z. (2012). Differential subcellular distribution of ion channels and the diversity of neuronal function. *Curr. Opin. Neurobiol.* 22, 366–371. doi: 10.1016/j.conb.2011.10.006

Oakley, R., and Tharakan, B. (2014). Vascular hyperpermeability and aging. *Aging Dis.* 5, 114–125. doi: 10.14336/AD.2014.0500114

Oh, M. M., Oliveira, F. A., and Disterhoft, J. F. (2010). Learning and aging related changes in intrinsic neuronal excitability. *Front. Aging Neurosci.* 2:2. doi: 10.3389/neuro.24.002.2010

Ong, W. Y., Farooqui, T., and Farooqui A. A. (2010). Involvement of cytosolic phospholipase A2, calcium independent phospholipase A2 and plasmalogen selective phospholipase A2 in neurodegenerative and neuropsychiatric conditions. *Curr. Med. Chem.* 17, 2746–2763. doi: 10.2174/092986710791859289

Orr, W. C., Radyuk, S. N., and Sohal, R. S. (2013). Involvement of redox state in the aging of *Drosophila melanogaster*. *Antioxid. Redox Signal.* 19, 788–803. doi: 10.1089/ars.2012.5002

Pamplona, R. (2008). Membrane phospholipids, lipoxidative damage and molecular integrity: a causal role in aging and longevity. *Biochim. Biophys. Acta* 1777, 1249–1262. doi: 10.1016/j.bbabio.2008.07.003

Pamplona, R. (2011). Advanced lipoxidation end-products. *Chem. Biol. Interact* 192, 14–20. doi: 10.1016/j.cbi.2011.01.007

Partridge, L. (2008). Some highlights of research on aging with invertebrates. *Aging Cell* 7, 605–608. doi: 10.1111/j.1474-9726.2008.00415.x

Patel, A. J., Honoré, E., Maingret, F., Lesage, F., Fink, M., Duprat, F., et al. (1998). A mammalian two pore domain mechano-gated S-like K+ channel. *EMBO J.* 17, 4283–4290. doi: 10.1093/emboj/17.15.4283

Patel, A. J., Lazdunski, M., and Honoré, E. (2001). Lipid and mechano-gated 2P domain K(+) channels. *Curr. Opin. Cell Biol.* 13, 422–428. doi: 10.1016/S0955-0674(00)00231-3

Patel, B. A., Arundell, M., Allen, M. C., Gard, P., O'Hare, D., Parker, K., et al. (2006). Changes in the properties of the modulatory cerebral giant cells contribute to aging in the feeding system of *Lymnaea*. *Neurobiol. Aging* 27, 1892–1901. doi: 10.1016/j.neurobiolaging.2005.09.041

Patel, B. A., Arundell, M., Parker, K. H., Yeoman, M. S., and O'Hare, D. (2010). Microelectrode investigation of neuronal ageing from a single identified neurone. *Phys. Chem. Chem. Phys.* 12, 10065–10072. doi: 10.1039/c0cp00310g

Peretz, B. (1988). Long-term change of viability of neuron functioning and its possible behavioral consequences in the adult *Aplysia*. *J. Physiol.* 83, 217–223.

Pérez, V. I., Bokov, A., Remmen, H. V., Mele, J., Ran, Q., Ikeno, Y., et al. (2009). Is the oxidative stress theory of aging dead? *Biochim. Biophys. Acta* 1790, 1005–1014. doi: 10.1016/j.bbagen.2009.06.003

Peters, A., Leahu, D., Moss, M. B., and McNally, K. J. (1994). The effects of aging on area 46 of the frontal cortex of the rhesus monkey. *Cereb. Cortex* 4, 621–635. doi: 10.1093/cercor/4.6.621

Phillis, J. W., Horrocks, L. A., and Farooqui, A. A. (2006). Cyclooxygenases, lipoxygenases, and epoxygenases in CNS: Their role and involvement in neurological disorders. *Brain Res. Rev.* 52, 201–243. doi: 10.1016/j.brainresrev.2006.02.002

Piomelli, D., Astarita, G., and Rapaka, R. (2007). A neuroscientist's guide to lipidomics. *Nat. Rev. Neurosci.* 8, 743–754. doi: 10.1038/nrn2233

Piomelli, D., Volterra, A., Dale, N., Siegelbaum, S. A., Kandel, E. R., Schwartz, J. H., et al. (1987). Lipoxygenase metabolites of arachidonic acid as second messengers for presynaptic inhibition of *Aplysia* sensory cells. *Nature* 328, 38–43. doi: 10.1038/328038a0

Pirger, Z., Naskar, S., László, Z., Kemenes, G., Reglődi, D., and Kemenes, I. (2014). Reversal of age-related learning deficiency by the vertebrate PACAP and IGF-1 in a novel invertebrate model of aging: the pond snail (*Lymnaea stagnalis*). *J. Gerontol. A Biol. Sci. Med. Sci.* 69, 1331–1338. doi: 10.1093/gerona/glu068

Pizzimenti, S., Ciamporcero, E. S., Daga, M., Pettazzoni, P., Arcaro, A., Cetrangolo, G., et al. (2013). Interaction of aldehydes derived from lipid peroxidation and membrane proteins. *Front. Physiol.* 4:242. doi: 10.3389/fphys.2013.00242

Quach, N. D., Arnold, R. D., and Cummings, B. S. (2014). Secretory phospholipase A2 enzymes as pharmacological targets for treatment of disease. *Biochem. Pharmacol.* 90, 338–348. doi: 10.1016/j.bcp.2014.05.022

Randall, A. D., Booth, C., and Brown, J. T. (2012). Age-related changes to Na+ channel gating contribute to modified intrinsic neuronal excitability. *Neurobiol. Aging* 33, 2715–2720. doi: 10.1016/j.neurobiolaging.2011.12.030

Rapp, P. R., and Gallagher, M. (1996). Preserved neuron number in the hippocampus of aged rats with spatial learning deficits. *Proc. Natl. Acad. Sci. U.S.A.* 93, 9926–9930. doi: 10.1073/pnas.93.18.9926

Rashba-Step, J., Tatoyan, A., Duncan, R., Ann, D., Pushpa-Rehka, T. R., and Sevanian, A. (1997). Phospholipid peroxidation induces cytosolic phospholipase A2 activity: membrane effects versus enzyme phosphorylation. *Arch. Biochem. Biophys.* 343, 44–54. doi: 10.1006/abbi.1997.0134

Rasmussen, T., Schliemann, T., Sorensen, J. C., Zimmer, J., and West, M. J. (1996). Memory impaired aged rats: no loss of principal hippocampal and subicular neurons. *Neurobiol. Aging* 17, 143–147. doi: 10.1016/0197-4580(95)02032-2

Rattan, K. S., and Peretz, B. (1981). Age-dependent behavioral changes and physiological changes in identified neurons in *Aplysia* californica. *J. Neurobiol.* 12, 469–478. doi: 10.1002/neu.480120506

Riahi, Y., Cohen, G., Shamni, O., and Sasson, S. (2010). Signaling and cytotoxic functions of 4-hydroxyalkenals. *Am. J. Physiol. Endocrinol. Metab.* 299, E879–E886. doi: 10.1152/ajpendo.00508.2010

Ribas, V., Garcia-Ruiz, C., and Fernandez-Checa, J. C. (2014). Glutathione and mitochondria. *Front. Pharmacol.* 5:151. doi: 10.3389/fphar.2014.00151

Ribeiro, M. J., Schofield, M. G., Kemenes, I., O'Shea, M., Kemenes, G., and Benjamin, P. R. (2005). Activation of MAPK is necessary for long-term memory consolidation following food-reward conditioning. *Learn. Mem.* 12, 538–545. doi: 10.1101/lm.8305

Ribeiro, M. J., Serfozo, Z., Papp, A., Kemenes, I., O'Shea, M., Yin, J. C., et al. (2003). Cyclic AMP response element-binding (CREB)-like proteins in a molluscan brain: cellular localization and learning-induced phosphorylation. *Eur. J. Neurosci.* 18, 1223–1234. doi: 10.1046/j.1460-9568.2003.02856.x

Rincon, F., and Wright, C. B. (2013). Vascular cognitive impairment. *Curr. Opin. Neurol.* 26, 29–36. doi: 10.1097/WCO.0b013e32835c4f04

Roberts-Crowley, M. L., Mitra-Ganguli, T., Liu, L., and Rittenhouse, A. R. (2009). Regulation of voltage-gated Ca2+ channels by lipids. *Cell Calcium* 45, 589–601. doi: 10.1016/j.ceca.2009.03.015

Rosenegger, D., and Lukowiak, K. (2013). The participation of NMDA receptors, PKC, and MAPK in *Lymnaea* memory extinction. *Neurobiol. Learn. Mem.* 100, 64–69. doi: 10.1016/j.nlm.2012.12.008

Rosenhouse-Dantsker, A., Mehta, D., and Levitan, I. (2012). Regulation of ion channels by membrane lipids. *Compr. Physiol.* 2, 31–68. doi: 10.1002/cphy.c110001

Ruppersberg, J. P., Stacker, M., Pongs, O., Heinemann, S. H., Frank, R., and Koenen, M. (1991). Regulation of fast inactivation of cloned mammalian IK (A) channels by cysteine oxidation. *Nature* 352, 711–714. doi: 10.1038/352711a0

Sadagurski, M., and White, M. F. (2013). Integrating metabolism and longevity through insulin and IGF1 signaling. *Endocrinol. Metab. Clin. North Am.* 42, 127–148. doi: 10.1016/j.ecl.2012.11.008

Sadamoto, H., Kitahashi, T., Fujito, Y., and Ito, E. (2010). Learning-dependent gene expression of CREB1 isoforms in the molluscan brain. *Front. Behav. Neurosci.* 4:25. doi: 10.3389/fnbeh.2010.00025

Sah, P. (1996). Ca (2+)-activated K+ currents in neurones: types, physiological roles and modulation. *Trends Neurosci.* 19, 150–154. doi: 10.1016/S0166-2236(96)80026-9

Sah, P., and Davies, P. (2000). Calcium-activated potassium currents in mammalian neurons. *Clin. Exp. Pharm. Physiol.* 27, 657–663. doi: 10.1046/j.1440-1681.2000.03317.x

Sakakibara, M., Kawai, R., Kobayashi, S., and Horikoshi, T. (1998). Associative learning of visual and vestibular stimuli in *Lymnaea. Neurobiol. Learn. Mem.* 69, 1–12. doi: 10.1006/nlme.1997.3805

Salgo, M. G., Corongiu, F. P., and Sevanian, A. (1992). Peroxidation and phospholipase A2 hydrolytic susceptibility of liposomes consisting of mixed species of phosphatidylcholine and phosphatidylethanolamine. *Biochim. Biophys. Acta* 1127, 131–140. doi: 10.1016/0005-2760(92)90268-Z

Sanchez-Mejia, R. O., and Mucke, L. (2010). Phospholipase A2 and arachidonic acid in Alzheimer's disease. *Biochim. Biophys. Acta* 1801, 784–790. doi: 10.1016/j.bbalip.2010.05.013

Sanchez-Mejia, R. O., Newman, J. W., Toh, S., Yu, G. Q., Zhou, Y., Halabisky, B., et al. (2008). Phospholipase A2 reduction ameliorates cognitive deficits in a mouse model of Alzheimer's disease. *Nat. Neurosci.* 11, 1311–1318. doi: 10.1038/nn.2213

Schaeffer, E. L., Forlenza, O. V., and Gattaz, W. F. (2009). Phospholipase A2 activation as a therapeutic approach for cognitive enhancement in early-stage Alzheimer disease. *Psychopharmacol. (Berl).* 202, 37–51. doi: 10.1007/s00213-008-1351-0

Scott, B., Leu, J., and Cinader, B. (1988). Effects of aging on neuronal electrical membrane properties. *Mech. Ageing Dev.* 44, 203–214. doi: 10.1016/0047-6374(88)90022-X

Sehgal, M., Ehlers, V. L., and Moyer, J. R. (2014). Learning enhances intrinsic excitability in a subset of lateral amygdala neurons. *Learn. Mem.* 21, 161–170. doi: 10.1101/lm.032730.113

Sehgal, M., Song, C., Ehlers, V. L., and Moyer, J. R. (2013). Learning to learn - intrinsic plasticity as a metaplasticity mechanism for memory formation. *Neurobiol. Learn. Mem.* 105, 186–199. doi: 10.1016/j.nlm.2013.07.008

Sesti, F., Liu, S., and Cai, S. Q. (2010). Oxidation of potassium channels by ROS: a general mechanism of aging and neurodegeneration? *Trends Cell Biol.* 20, 45–51. doi: 10.1016/j.tcb.2009.09.008

Shankar, S. K. (2010). Biology of aging brain. *Indian J. Pathol. Microbiol.* 53, 595. doi: 10.4103/0377-4929.71995

Sieling, F., Bédécarrats, A., Simmers, J., Prinz, A. A., and Nargeot, R. (2014). Differential roles of nonsynaptic and synaptic plasticity in operant reward learning-induced compulsive behavior. *Curr. Biol.* 24, 941–950. doi: 10.1016/j.cub.2014.03.004

Skinner, T. L., and Peretz, B. (1989). Age sensitivity of osmoregulation and of its neural correlates in *Aplysia. Am. J. Physiol.* 256, R989–R996.

Slob, W., and Janse, C. K. (1988). A quantitative method to evaluate the quality of interrupted animal cultures in aging studies. *Mech. Ageing Dev.* 42, 275–290. doi: 10.1016/0047-6374(88)90053-X

Speakman, J. R., and Selman, C. (2011). The free-radical damage theory: accumulating evidence against a simple link of oxidative stress to ageing and lifespan. *BioEssays* 33, 255–259. doi: 10.1002/bies.201000132

Spencer, G. E., Syed, N. I., and Lukowiak, K. (1999). Neural changes after operant conditioning of the aerial respiratory behavior in *Lymnaea stagnalis. J. Neurosci.* 19, 1836–1843.

Staras, K., Kemenes, G., and Benjamin, P. R. (1999). Cellular traces of behavioral classical conditioning can be recorded at several specific sites in a simple nervous system. *J. Neurosci.* 19, 347–357.

Subczynski, W. K., and Wisniewska, A. (2000). Physical properties of lipid bilayer membranes: relevance to membrane biological functions. *Acta Biochim. Pol.* 47, 613–625.

Sultana, R., Perluigi, M., and Butterfield, D. A. (2013). Lipid peroxidation triggers neurodegeneration: a redox proteomics view into the Alzheimer disease brain. *Free Radic. Biol. Med.* 62, 157–169. doi: 10.1016/j.freeradbiomed.2012.09.027

Sun, G. Y., Chuang, D. Y., Zong, Y., Jiang, J., Lee, J. C.-M., Gu, Z., et al. (2014). Role of cytosolic phospholipase A2 in oxidative and inflammatory signaling pathways in different cell types in the central nervous system. *Mol. Neurobiol.* 50, 6–14. doi: 10.1007/s12035-014-8662-4

Sun, G. Y., Xu, J., Jensen, M. D., and Simonyi, A. (2004). Phospholipase A2 in the central nervous system: implications for neurodegenerative diseases. *J. Lipid Res.* 45, 205–213. doi: 10.1194/jlr.R300016-JLR200

Surmeier, D. J., Guzman, J. N., Sanchez, J., and Schumacker, P. T. (2012). Physiological phenotype and vulnerability in Parkinson's disease. *Cold Spring Harb. Perspect. Med.* 2, a009290. doi: 10.1101/cshperspect.a009290

Tarumi, T., and Zhang, R. (2014). Cerebral hemodynamics of the aging brain: risk of Alzheimer disease and benefit of aerobic exercise. *Front. Physiol.* 5:6. doi: 10.3389/fphys.2014.00006

Taylor B. E., and Lukowiak K. (2000). The respiratory central pattern generator of *Lymnaea*: a model, measured and malleable. *Respir. Physiol.* 122, 197–207. doi: 10.1016/S0034-5687(00)00159-6

Terman, A., and Brunk, U. T. (2006). Oxidative stress, accumulation of biological 'garbage', and aging. *Antiox. Redox Signal.* 8, 197–204. doi: 10.1089/ars.2006.8.197

Thibault, O., Gant, J. C., and Landfield, P. W. (2007). Expansion of the calcium hypothesis of brain aging and Alzheimer's disease: minding the store. *Aging Cell* 6, 307–317. doi: 10.1111/j.1474-9726.2007.00295.x

Thompson, L. T., Moyer, J. R., and Disterhoft, J. F. (1996). Transient changes in excitability of rabbit CA3 neurons with a time course appropriate to support memory consolidation. *J. Neurophysiol.* 76, 1836–1849.

Toescu, E. C., and Vreugdenhil, M. (2010). Calcium and normal brain ageing. *Cell Calcium* 47, 158–164. doi: 10.1016/j.ceca.2009.11.013

Tombaugh, G. C., Rowe, W. B., and Rose, G. M. (2005). The slow afterhyperpolarization in hippocampal CA1 neurons covaries with spatial learning ability in aged Fisher 344 rats. *J. Neurosci.* 25, 2609–2616. doi: 10.1523/JNEUROSCI.5023-04.2005

Toroser, D., and Sohal, R. S. (2005). Kinetic characteristics of native gamma-glutamylcysteine ligase in the aging housefly, *Musca domestica* L. *Biochem. Biophys. Res. Commun.* 326, 586–593. doi: 10.1016/j.bbrc.2004.11.066

Toroser, D., and Sohal, R. S. (2007). Age-associated perturbations in glutathione synthesis in mouse liver. *Biochem. J.* 405, 583–589. doi: 10.1042/BJ20061868

Torres, L. L., Quaglio, N. B., de Souza, G. T., Garcia, R. T., Dati, L. M., Moreira, W. L., et al. (2011). Peripheral oxidative stress biomarkers in mild cognitive impairment and Alzheimer's disease. *J. Alzheimers Dis.* 6, 59–68. doi: 10.3233/JAD-2011-110284

Ungvari, Z., Csiszar, A., Sosnowska, D., Philipp, E. E., Campbell, C. M., McQuary, P. R., et al. (2013). Testing predictions of the oxidative stress hypothesis of aging using a novel invertebrate model of longevity: the giant clam (*Tridacna derasa*). *J. Gerontol. A Biol. Sci. Med. Sci.* 68, 359–367. doi: 10.1093/gerona/gls159

Ungvari, Z., Ridgway, I., Philipp, E. E. R., Campbell, C. M., McQuary, P., Chow, T., et al. (2011). Extreme longevity is associated with increased resistance to oxidative stress in Arctica islandica, the longest-living non-colonial animal. *J. Gerontol. A Biol. Sci. Med. Sci.* 66, 741–750. doi: 10.1093/gerona/glr044

Vacher, H., Mohapatra, D. P., and Trimmer, J. S. (2008). Localization and targeting of voltage-dependent ion channels in mammalian central neurons. *Physiol. Rev.* 88, 1407–1447. doi: 10.1152/physrev.00002.2008

Vishwanath, B. S., Fawzy, A. A., and Franson, R. C. (1988). Edema-inducing activity of phospholipase A2 purified from human synovial fluid and inhibition by aristolochic acid. *Inflammation* 12, 549–561. doi: 10.1007/BF00914317

Wagatsuma, A., Azami, S., Sakura, M., Hatakeyama, D., Aonuma, H., and Ito, E. (2006). De Novo synthesis of CREB in a presynaptic neuron is required for synaptic enhancement involved in memory consolidation. *J. Neurosci. Res.* 84, 954–960. doi: 10.1002/jnr.21012

Waldbaum, S., and Patel, M. (2010). Mitochondrial dysfunction and oxidative stress: a contributing link to acquired epilepsy? *J. Bioenerg. Biomembr.* 42, 449–455. doi: 10.1007/s10863-010-9320-9

Wan, H., Mackay, B., Iqbal, H., Naskar, S., and Kemenes, G. (2010). Delayed intrinsic activation of an NMDA-independent CaM-kinase II in a critical time window is necessary for late consolidation of an associative memory. *J. Neurosci.* 30, 56–63. doi: 10.1523/JNEUROSCI.2577-09.2010

Watson, S. N., Lee, J. R., Risling, T. E., Hermann, P. M., and Wildering, W. C. (2014). Diminishing glutathione availability and age-associated decline in neuronal excitability. *Neurobiol. Aging* 35, 1074–1085. doi: 10.1016/j.neurobiolaging.2013.11.007

Watson, S. N., Risling, T. E., Hermann, P. M., and Wildering, W. C. (2012a). Failure of delayed nonsynaptic neuronal plasticity underlies age-associated long-term associative memory impairment. *BMC Neurosci.* 13:103. doi: 10.1186/1471-2202-13-103

Watson, S. N., Nelson, M. A., and Wildering, W. C. (2012b). Redox agents modulate neuronal activity and reproduce physiological aspects of neuronal aging. *Neurobiol. Aging* 33, 149–161. doi: 10.1016/j.neurobiolaging.2010.01.017

Watson, S. N., Wright, N., Hermann, P. M., and Wildering, W. C. (2013). Phospholipase A_2: the key to reversing long-term memory impairment in a gastropod model of aging. *Neurobiol. Aging* 34, 610–620. doi: 10.1016/j.neurobiolaging.2012.02.028

West, M. J., Coleman, P. D., Flood, D. G., and Troncoso, J. C. (1994). Differences in the pattern of hippocampal neuronal loss in normal ageing and Alzheimer's disease. *Lancet* 344, 769–772. doi: 10.1016/S0140-6736(94)92338-8

Wildering, W. C., van der Roest, M., de Vlieger, T. A., and Janse, C. K. (1991). Age-related changes in junctional and non-junctional conductances in two electrically coupled peptidergic neurons of the mollusc *Lymnaea stagnalis*. *Brain Res.* 547, 89–98. doi: 10.1016/0006-8993(91)90578-J

Yeoman, M. S., Scutt, G., and Faragher, R. (2012). Insights into CNS ageing from animal models of senescence. *Nat. Rev. Neurosci.* 13, 435–445. doi: 10.1038/nrn3230

Yirmiya, R., and Goshen, I. (2011). Immune modulation of learning, memory, neural plasticity and neurogenesis. *Brain Behav. Immun.* 25, 181–213. doi: 10.1016/j.bbi.2010.10.015

Yu, B. P., Suescun, E. A., and Yang, S. Y. (1992). Effect of age-related lipid peroxidation on membrane fluidity and phospholipase A2: modulation by dietary restriction. *Mech. Ageing Dev.* 65, 17–33. doi: 10.1016/0047-6374(92)90123-U

Zhu, Y., Carvey, P. M., and Ling, Z. (2006). Age-related changes in glutathione and glutathione-related enzymes in rat brain. *Brain Res.* 1090, 35–44. doi: 10.1016/j.brainres.2006.03.063

Zimniak, P. (2008). Detoxification reactions: relevance to aging. *Ageing Res. Rev.* 7, 281–300. doi: 10.1016/j.arr.2008.04.001

Zimniak, P. (2011). Relationship of electrophilic stress to aging. *Free Radic. Biol. Med.* 51, 1087–1105. doi: 10.1016/j.freeradbiomed.2011.05.039

Permissions

All chapters in this book were first published in FBBTINSDMPA & BCAMSTB, by Frontiers; hereby published with permission under the Creative Commons Attribution License or equivalent. Every chapter published in this book has been scrutinized by our experts. Their significance has been extensively debated. The topics covered herein carry significant findings which will fuel the growth of the discipline. They may even be implemented as practical applications or may be referred to as a beginning point for another development.

The contributors of this book come from diverse backgrounds, making this book a truly international effort. This book will bring forth new frontiers with its revolutionizing research information and detailed analysis of the nascent developments around the world.

We would like to thank all the contributing authors for lending their expertise to make the book truly unique. They have played a crucial role in the development of this book. Without their invaluable contributions this book wouldn't have been possible. They have made vital efforts to compile up to date information on the varied aspects of this subject to make this book a valuable addition to the collection of many professionals and students.

This book was conceptualized with the vision of imparting up-to-date information and advanced data in this field. To ensure the same, a matchless editorial board was set up. Every individual on the board went through rigorous rounds of assessment to prove their worth. After which they invested a large part of their time researching and compiling the most relevant data for our readers.

The editorial board has been involved in producing this book since its inception. They have spent rigorous hours researching and exploring the diverse topics which have resulted in the successful publishing of this book. They have passed on their knowledge of decades through this book. To expedite this challenging task, the publisher supported the team at every step. A small team of assistant editors was also appointed to further simplify the editing procedure and attain best results for the readers.

Apart from the editorial board, the designing team has also invested a significant amount of their time in understanding the subject and creating the most relevant covers. They scrutinized every image to scout for the most suitable representation of the subject and create an appropriate cover for the book.

The publishing team has been an ardent support to the editorial, designing and production team. Their endless efforts to recruit the best for this project, has resulted in the accomplishment of this book. They are a veteran in the field of academics and their pool of knowledge is as vast as their experience in printing. Their expertise and guidance has proved useful at every step. Their uncompromising quality standards have made this book an exceptional effort. Their encouragement from time to time has been an inspiration for everyone.

The publisher and the editorial board hope that this book will prove to be a valuable piece of knowledge for researchers, students, practitioners and scholars across the globe.

List of Contributors

Yenisel Cruz-Almeida
Pain Research and Intervention Center of Excellence, University of Florida, Gainesville, FL, USA

Mieniecia L. Black
Department of Aging and Geriatric Research, University of Florida, Gainesville, FL, USA

Evangelos A. Christou
Department of Applied Physiology and Kinesiology, University of Florida, Gainesville, FL, USA

David J. Clark
Department of Aging and Geriatric Research, University of Florida, Gainesville, FL, USA
Brain Rehabilitation Research Center, Malcom Randall VA Medical Center, Gainesville, FL, USA

Elisabetta Coppi, Elise Houdayer , Raffaella Chieffo, Francesca Spagnolo, Alberto Inuggi, Laura Straffi, Giancarlo Comi and Letizia Leocani
Neurological Department and Experimental Neurophysiology Unit, Institute of Experimental Neurology (INSPE), University Hospital-IRCCS San Raffaele, Milan, Italy

Marnie L. Vanden Noven, Hugo M. Pereira, Tejin Yoon, Alyssa A. Stevens, Kristy A. and Sandra K. Hunter
Exercise Science Program, Department of Physical Therapy, Marquette University, Milwaukee, WI, USA

Nielson
Department of Psychology, Marquette University, Milwaukee, WI, USA

David J. Clark and Sarah A. Ring
Brain Rehabilitation Research Center, Malcom Randall VA Medical Center, North Florida/South Georgia Veterans Health System, Gainesville, FL, USA
Department of Aging and Geriatric Research, University of Florida, Gainesville, FL, USA

Dorian K. Rose
Brain Rehabilitation Research Center, Malcom Randall VA Medical Center, North Florida/South Georgia Veterans Health System, Gainesville, FL, USA
Department of Physical Therapy, University of Florida, Gainesville, FL, USA

Eric C. Porges
Department of Aging and Geriatric Research, University of Florida, Gainesville, FL, USA

Marco Iosa, Augusto Fusco, Giovanni Morone and Stefano Paolucci
Clinical Laboratory of Experimental Neurorehabilitation, Fondazione Santa Lucia, Istituto di Ricovero e Cura a Carattere Scientifico (IRCCS), Rome, Italy

Rita Sleimen-Malkoun
CNRS, Institut des Sciences du Mouvement UMR 7287, Aix-Marseille Université, Marseille, France
Inserm, Institut de Neurosciences des Systèmes UMR_S 1106, Faculté de Médecine Timone, Aix-Marseille Université, Marseille, France

Jean-Jacques Temprado
CNRS, Institut des Sciences du Mouvement UMR 7287, Aix-Marseille Université, Marseille, France

S. Lee Hong
Ohio Musculoskeletal and Neurological Institute, Ohio University, Athens, OH, USA

Marika Berchicci
Department of Human Movement, Social and Health Sciences, University of Rome "Foro Italico", Rome, Italy

Giuliana Lucci
Neuropsychological Unit, IRCCS Santa Lucia Foundation, Rome, Italy

Rinaldo Livio Perri
Department of Human Movement, Social and Health Sciences, University of Rome "Foro Italico", Rome, Italy
Department of Psychology, University of Rome "La Sapienza", Rome, Italy

Donatella Spinelli and Francesco Di Russo
Department of Human Movement, Social and Health Sciences, University of Rome "Foro Italico", Rome, Italy
Neuropsychological Unit, IRCCS Santa Lucia Foundation, Rome, Italy

Marta Gonzalez-Freire, Stephanie A. Studenski and Luigi Ferrucci
Translational Gerontology Branch, National Institute on Aging, Intramural Research Program, National Institutes of Health, Baltimore, MD, USA
Longitudinal Studies Section, Baltimore Longitudinal Study of Aging, National Institute on Aging, National Institutes of Health, Baltimore, MD, USA

Rafael de Cabo
Translational Gerontology Branch, National Institute on Aging, Intramural Research Program, National Institutes of Health, Baltimore, MD, USA

Jolien Heetkamp
Department of Neuroscience, University Medical Center Groningen, University of Groningen, Groningen, Netherlands
Center for Human Movement Sciences, University Medical Center Groningen, University of Groningen, Groningen, Netherlands

Tibor Hortobágyi
Center for Human Movement Sciences, University Medical Center Groningen, University of Groningen, Groningen, Netherlands
Faculty of Health and Life Sciences, Northumbria University, Newcastle Upon Tyne, UK

Inge Zijdewind
Department of Neuroscience, University Medical Center Groningen, University of Groningen, Groningen, Netherlands

Wan X.Yao and Yufei Huang
Department of Kinesiology, Health, and Nutrition, College of Education and Human Development, USA
The University of Texas at San Antonio, San Antonio, TX, USA

Jinqi Li, Crystal G. Franklin and Jack L. Lancaster
Research Imaging Institute, The University of Texas Health Science Center at San Antonio, San Antonio, TX, USA

Zhiguo Jiang
Human Performance and Engineering Laboratory, Kessler Foundation Research Center, West Orange, NJ, USA
Department of Biomedical Engineering, New Jersey Institute of Technology, Newark, NJ, USA

Jia-Hong Gao
IDG/McGovern Institute for Brain Research, Peking University, Beijing, China

Guang H. Yue
Human Performance and Engineering Laboratory, Kessler Foundation Research Center, West Orange, NJ, USA

Christopher J. Hasson
Neuromotor Systems Laboratory, Department of Physical Therapy, Movement and Rehabilitation Sciences, Northeastern University, Boston, MA, USA

Dagmar Sternad
The Action Lab, Departments of Biology, Electrical and Computer Engineering, and Physics, Northeastern University, Boston, MA, USA

Morgan Newman, Esmaeil Ebrahimie and Michael Lardelli
School of Molecular and Biomedical Science, University of Adelaide, SA, Australia

Martine Therrien
Départment de Pathologie et Biologie Cellulaire, CRCHUM-Centre Hospitalier de l'Université de Montréal, Université de Montréal, Montréal, QC, Canada

J. Alex Parker
Départment de Pathologie et Biologie Cellulaire, Départment de Neurosciences, CRCHUM-Centre Hospitalier de l'Université de Montréal, Université de Montréal, Montréal, QC, Canada

Kevin Machino, Susan Wang, Hana Murakami and Shin Murakami
Department of Basic Sciences, College of Osteopathic Medicine, Touro University California, Vallejo, CA, USA

Christopher D. Link
Institute of Behavioral Genetics, University of Colorado, Boulder, Boulder, CO, USA

Scott J. Webster and Adam D. Bachstetter
Sanders-Brown Center on Aging, University of Kentucky, Lexington, KY, USA

Peter T. Nelson
Sanders-Brown Center on Aging, University of Kentucky, Lexington, KY, USA
Division of Neuropathology, Department of Pathology and Laboratory Medicine, University of Kentucky, Lexington, KY, USA

J. Alex Parker
Department of Neuroscience, CRCHUM, University of Montreal, Montreal, QC, Canada

Frederick A. Schmitt
Sanders-Brown Center on Aging, University of Kentucky, Lexington, KY, USA
Department of Neurology, University of Kentucky, Lexington, KY, USA

Linda J. Van Eldik
Sanders-Brown Center on Aging, University of Kentucky, Lexington, KY, USA
Department of Anatomy and Neurobiology, University of Kentucky, Lexington, KY, USA

Ilias Gkikas, Dionysia Petratou
Institute of Molecular Biology and Biotechnology, Foundation for Research and Technology-Hellas, Heraklion, Crete, Greece

NektariosTavernarakis
Institute of Molecular Biology and Biotechnology, Foundation for Research and Technology-Hellas, Heraklion, Crete, Greece
Department of Basic Sciences, Faculty of Medicine, University of Crete, Heraklion, Crete, Greece

Subhas Mukherjee, Mohammed A. Basar and Atanu Duttaroy
Department of Biology, Howard University, Washington, DC, USA

Claudette Davis
Department of Biology, Howard University, Washington, DC, USA
Biology Undergraduate Program, College of Science, George Mason University, Fairfax, VA, USA

Courtney Scerbak and Barbara E. Taylor
Institute of Arctic Biology, University of Alaska Fairbanks, Fairbanks, AK, USA
Department of Biology and Wildlife, University of Alaska Fairbanks, Fairbanks, AK, USA

Elena M. Vayndorf
Institute of Arctic Biology, University of Alaska Fairbanks, Fairbanks, AK, USA

Christian Neri
Laboratory of Neuronal Cell Biology and Pathology, Centre National de la Recherche Scientifique, UMR 8652, Paris, France
Sorbonnes Universités, UPMC Univ Paris 06, Paris, France

Monica Driscoll
Nelson Biological Laboratories, Department of Molecular Biology and Biochemistry, Rutgers, The State University of New Jersey, Piscataway, NJ, USA

Adanna G. Alexander and Chris Li
Department of Biology, City College of NewYork, NewYork, NY, USA
Department of Biology, The Graduate Center, City University of NewYork, NewYork, NY, USA

Vanessa Marfil
Department of Biology, City College of NewYork, NewYork, NY, USA

Petra M. Hermann
Department of Biological Sciences, University of Calgary, Calgary, AB, Canada
Department of Physiology and Pharmacology, University of Calgary, Calgary, AB, Canada

Shawn N. Watson
Department of Biological Sciences, University of Calgary, Calgary, AB, Canada

Willem C. Wildering
Department of Biological Sciences, University of Calgary, Calgary, AB, Canada
Department of Physiology and Pharmacology, University of Calgary, Calgary, AB, Canada
Hotchkiss Brain Institute, University of Calgary, Calgary, AB, Canada

Index

A

Agonist, 23, 26, 29, 108

Amyotrophic Lateral Sclerosis, 28, 81, 83, 86, 129, 137-141, 174, 178, 209, 211, 215-220

Anisotropy, 12, 15

Ankle Dorsiflexor Muscles, 16-17, 19-20, 24, 27

Augment Somatosensation, 5

B

Berg Balance Score, 1, 3-4

Bilateral Cortical Activation, 7, 13

Bilateral Motor Cortices, 12

C

Caenorhabditis Elegans, 120, 129-130, 138-142, 146-147, 171-172, 177-180, 186-187, 198-200, 202, 208-209, 213-220, 229, 236

Cardiorespiratory Fitness, 68, 74

Corpus Callosum, 8, 12-14, 37

Cortical Maps, 7-9, 11, 13

Cortical Representation, 7-8, 10, 13

D

Dim Task, 30-31, 33-35

Drosophila Spargel, 181, 183

E

Event-related Potential, 68

F

Fatiguing Contraction, 16-17, 19-21, 23-29, 87-88, 95

Frontotemporal Dementia, 129, 139, 141, 169, 206-207, 209, 213, 217-218

G

Gait Spatiotemporal Measurements, 30, 34

Gastrocnemius, 18-20, 23, 26, 108

H

Hand Motor Function, 8-9

Hand Motor Performance, 8-9, 11

High-cognitive Demand, 16-21, 23-27

Homoscedasticity, 2-3

Hyperphosphorylation, 132, 147, 200, 207, 213

I

Insulin Signaling, 171-172, 178-179, 181-187, 189-192, 194-198, 204, 206, 211, 217

Interhemispheric Interactions, 7-8, 12, 14, 99

Ipsilateral Silent Period, 7-10, 14, 98

Isometric Contractions, 16-17, 24, 27-29, 96-97, 99-100

M

Martin's Vigorimeter, 9

Mean Arterial Pressure, 20, 25

Mechanosensory Neurons, 130, 186-193, 195-197, 207, 212, 226

Mitochondrial Biogenesis, 78, 81, 181

Mobility Deficits, 30-31

Mobility Function, 1-5, 36, 82

Molting Defects, 203, 206

Monoaminergic Drive, 17, 26-27

Monofilament, 1-2, 4

Motoneurone Pool, 17, 25-26, 100

Motor Cortex Functioning, 8

Motor Overflow, 8, 14, 99

Motor Variability, 16, 66

Muscle Denervation, 76, 78, 83

Myocardial Oxygen Consumption, 25

N

Near Infrared Spectroscopy, 30

Neuromuscular Junction, 76-77, 79, 83-86, 137

Neuronal Insulin Signaling, 187

Nine Hole Peg Test, 7, 9, 13-14

O

Oogenesis, 181, 184-185

P

Peroxisome Proliferator Activated Receptor, 181

Physiological Aging, 7-8, 12-14, 173, 187

Physiological Arousal, 19, 38

Plantar Surface, 1-2, 4-5

Prefrontal Cortex, 29, 31, 37-38, 66, 68-69, 73-75, 102, 153-154, 168, 170, 175

Proteotoxicity, 134, 137, 140, 177, 186, 196, 198, 211, 213-214, 219

R

Rating Of Perceived Exertion, 20, 24
Resting Motor Threshold, 7-8, 89, 91

S

Sarcopenia, 40, 48-49, 52, 62, 76, 78, 80-86
Sensory Thresholds, 4
Simple Response Task, 68, 72
Skin Conductance, 30-31, 33-34
Somatosensation, 1, 3-5
Somatosensory Function, 1, 3, 5
Somatosensory Impairment, 1, 4
Somatosensory Information, 4-5
Somatosensory Screening, 2, 5
Spargel Expression, 183
Symptomatic Cardiovascular Disease, 2, 31
Synergist, 16, 26-27, 108

T

Tactile Perception, 1-4
Tibialis Anterior, 18, 20, 23, 26-27, 82, 99
Torque Fluctuations, 23-27
Transcallosal Inhibition, 7, 12
Transcranial Magnetic, 7-8, 14-15, 62, 72, 88-89, 100, 109
Transcranial MagneticStimulation, 7-8, 14-15, 72, 89, 100, 109
Transcriptional Coactivator, 181
Transmembrane Domain, 119, 201, 220

V

Vest Task, 30-31, 35
Vibrating Insoles, 1, 5